# Internal Medicine for Dental Treatments

Toshimi Chiba • Hiroyuki Yamada
Editors

# Internal Medicine for Dental Treatments

## Patients with Medical Diseases

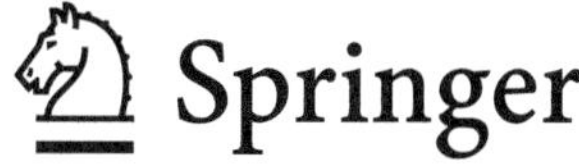

*Editors*
Toshimi Chiba
Division of Internal Medicine of Dentistry, Department of Oral Medicine
School of Dentistry, Iwate Medical University, Morioka
Iwate, Japan

Hiroyuki Yamada
Division of Oral and Maxillofacial Surgery, Department of Oral and Maxillofacial Reconstructive Surgery
School of Dentistry
Iwate Medical University, Morioka
Iwate, Japan

ISBN 978-981-99-3298-6 ISBN 978-981-99-3296-2 (eBook)
https://doi.org/10.1007/978-981-99-3296-2

Translation from the Japanese language edition: "Shika Ishi no tameno Naikagaku" by Toshimi Chiba and Hiroyuki Yamada, © Ishiyaku Pub,Inc. 2021. Published by Ishiyaku Pub,Inc.. All Rights Reserved.

This is a translated version of the book originally published in Japanese language. This has been facilitated using machine translation (by the service DeepL.com) followed by authors revising, editing and verifying the translated manuscript.



This Springer imprint is published by the registered company Springer Nature Singapore Pte Ltd.
The registered company address is: 152 Beach Road, #21-01/04 Gateway East, Singapore 189721, Singapore

Paper in this product is recyclable.

# Preface for the English Version

It is my great pleasure to publish *Internal Medicine for Dental Treatments: Patients with Medical Diseases* from Japan to the world. This is a very valuable book that describes diseases from the viewpoints of both physicians and dentists, and we believe that it will be shared by doctors from many countries.

While there are many books on internal medicine, not many have been written with a focus on dental problems. This book is a bidirectional book that is useful as a guide to deal with dental treatment problems that have emerged from the medical viewpoint. In Japan's super-aging society, the number of patients with various diseases is increasing even in dentistry, and knowledge of internal medicine is essential for dentists. However, there is a large gap between the knowledge of internal medicine learned in dental medical education and the individual events that require immediate judgment in the clinical dental practice. It is currently left to the dentist's own study to fill this gap. This book clearly describes the methods, rationale, and specific measures for approaching medical problems that arise during dental treatment, and is expected to become a must-have book for dentists to improve their skills and perform more patient-based dental care.

Currently, dentistry is mainly concerned with therapeutics, but we believe that diagnostics of lesions will become more useful in the future. In other words, in addition to early detection and early diagnosis of oral lesions, further minimally invasive treatment will be demanded by patients, and we believe there are already requests for such treatment. In order to respond to these demands, it will be even more desirable in the future to understand the pathophysiology of diseases and to proceed with dental treatment with knowledge of patients' comorbidities. This book adequately covers these demands of dental treatments. We are convinced that this book will be a textbook for dentists, dental students, and related professions, and we believe that it will also be useful for physicians. In keeping with its status as a specialized book, the descriptions are more in-depth and technical terms are used appropriately.

We hope you will read this book and make use of it in your daily practice and in the education of your students.

Morioka, Iwate, Japan — Toshimi Chiba
Morioka, Iwate, Japan — Hiroyuki Yamada

# Preface

This book is written by specialists in internal medicine, surgery, psychiatry, and obstetrics, and gynecology from all over Japan who are familiar with dental care, as well as dentists who are promoting cutting-edge dental care, and provides more practical contents for dental practice. The authors have been asked to write about typical diseases in each field that are often seen in actual practice, and to include recent topics that are suitable for medical doctors to read. Dentists, on the other hand, were asked to provide more detailed descriptions of items to be considered in actual clinical practice, including the dosages of drugs actually used in practice. We have also asked them to include as many clinical photographs as possible. The skin manifestations that correlate with visceral diseases are known as dermadrome. Similarly, findings on the oral mucosa are said to lead to the detection and diagnosis of systemic diseases, and recently the term "Oradrome" has been proposed, drawing further attention to the approach from oral symptoms to systemic diseases. This is the first book in Japan written by dentists and physicians on a single disease from this perspective. Another feature of this book is the inclusion of symptomatology. The background and mechanism of symptoms are essential for understanding the pathophysiology of the disease, so they are included in this book.

The aging of the population is the backdrop for the need for medical collaboration. In fact, it is my strong impression that the percentage of patients who have comorbidities and take multiple medications is increasing. It is common in daily medical practice to identify comorbidities and confirm pathophysiological conditions based on the medications taken. In such cases, it is necessary to check the patient's medication notebook, diabetes notebook, blood pressure notebook, warfarin notebook, osteoporosis-related medication record notebook, etc., and patients themselves have a wide range of information. Symptoms and conditions change on a daily basis, so it is always important to keep this information in mind. In addition, new drugs such as molecular-targeted drugs via various receptors have recently appeared on the market, not only for malignant diseases but also for lifestyle-related diseases, and it is necessary to keep up with medical information.

This book was written by doctors and dentists, so there is some overlap in content, but it is an important reminder of the importance of the subject matter. This book is highly recommended not only for dental students who aspire to become dentists, but also for dentists in clinical training, and dentists and dental hygienists who are active in the front line of dental care. It is also highly recommended for all doctors involved in dental care, as well as for all professionals working in medical facilities such as elderly care facilities. We are pleased to publish the first edition of this book, and we are confident that it will be of constant use to you. We hope that the contents of this book will be further developed and enhanced in the future.

Finally, I would like to express my sincere gratitude to the authors of this book.

Morioka, Iwate, Japan Toshimi Chiba

# Contents

# Part I

# Symptomatology

# 1 Respiratory/Infection Symptoms

Norihiko Funaguchi, Masahito Ogasawara, Takuji Kiryu, Takeshi Terashima, Yasuhiro Gon, Tetsuo Shimizu, and Hirofumi Sawai

## 1 Dyspnea

Norihiko Funaguchi

Dyspnea is a generalized subjective symptom of discomfort and effort during breathing. Dyspnea is a subjective sensation, and there are various expressions of dyspnea such as a feeling of insufficient air, a feeling of effort in respiratory movements, a feeling of tightness in the chest, and a feeling of suffocation. Dyspnea is not limited to respiratory diseases but also includes cardiac diseases, anemia, neurological diseases, metabolic diseases, and psychogenic diseases. Even healthy subjects complain of dyspnea during exercise. Not all respiratory failure patients with hypoxemia complain of dyspnea, and not all patients with dyspnea present with hypoxemia.

Dyspnea is a sensation, and the following sensory receptors are thought to be involved in the development of dyspnea. Central chemoreceptors in the medulla oblongata are stimulated mainly by an increase in $PaCO_2$ (partial pressure of carbon dioxide in arterial blood), and excitation of these receptors stimulates the respiratory center, resulting in increased respiration. Peripheral chemoreceptors are located in the carotid and aortic bodies and are strongly stimulated by a decrease in $PaO_2$ (partial pressure of oxygen in arterial blood). In addition, there are various receptors in the airways and lungs that affect respiration, many of which are innervated by the vagus nerve. When these receptors are stimulated, cough and bronchoconstriction occur, resulting in dyspnea. Mechanoreceptors in the chest wall, especially in respiratory muscles, are also associated with dyspnea. The presence of mechanoreceptors called muscle spindles, which are densely located in the intercostal muscles, is known among the respiratory muscles, and these receptors may be involved in the occurrence of dyspnea. And it is thought that stimuli from various sensory receptors are transmitted to the sensory cortex and are involved in the occurrence of dyspnea.

Dyspnea should be differentiated according to whether it is chronic or acute in nature, whether it occurs only on exertion or recurs paroxysmically at rest, and whether there are abnormal chest radiographs or not. Chronic obstructive pulmo-

N. Funaguchi · T. Kiryu (✉)
Department of Radiology, Asahi University Hospital, Gifu, Japan
e-mail: kiryu@hosp.asahi-u.ac.jp

M. Ogasawara
Division of Bioregulatory Pharmacology, Department of Pharmacology, Iwate Medical University, Yahaba, Iwate, Japan

T. Terashima
Department of Respiratory Medicine, Tokyo Dental College, Ichikawa General Hospital, Ichikawa, Chiba, Japan

Y. Gon · T. Shimizu
Division of Respiratory Medicine, Department of Internal Medicine, Nihon University School of Medicine, Itabashi-ku, Tokyo, Japan

H. Sawai
Kinki Health Care Center, Yodogawa-ku, Osaka, Japan


T. Chiba, H. Yamada (eds.), *Internal Medicine for Dental Treatments*,
https://doi.org/10.1007/978-981-99-3296-2_1

nary disease (COPD) is characterized by a gradual progression of dyspnea on exertion over a period of years. In bronchial asthma, dyspnea with paroxysmal cough and wheezing is common. In the case of heart failure, exertional dyspnea is seen with cardiac enlargement, but with worsening heart failure, dyspnea at rest and orthopnea may occur. Pulmonary thromboembolism and pneumothorax often present with sudden onset of dyspnea.

Dyspnea and shortness of breath may occur during strenuous exercise even in healthy individuals, but if shortness of breath occurs at rest or with minor exercise, the condition may be pathological. In order to determine whether dyspnea is pathological, it is necessary to evaluate the degree of dyspnea. The modified Medical Research Council (mMRC) scale (Table 1.1) [1] has been widely used as an objective measure of dyspnea. The modified Borg scale (Table 1.2) is a direct method for subjectively assessing the degree of dyspnea [2].

**Table 1.2** Modified Borg Scale. (Created based on [2])

| | |
|---|---|
| 0 | Nothing at all |
| 0.5 | Very, very weak |
| 1 | Very weak |
| 2 | Weak |
| 3 | – |
| 4 | Somewhat strong |
| 5 | Strong |
| 6 | – |
| 7 | Very strong |
| 8 | – |
| 9 | – |
| 10 | Very, very strong |

**Table 1.1** The modified Medical Research Council (mMRC) scale [1]

| Grade | Description of breathlessness |
|---|---|
| Grade 0 | I only get breathless with strenuous exercise |
| Grade 1 | I get short of breath when hurrying on level ground or walking up a slight hill |
| Grade 2 | On level ground, I walk slower than people of the same age because of breathlessness, or I have to stop for breath when walking at my own pace on the level |
| Grade 3 | I stop for breath after walking about 100 yards or after a few minutes on level ground |
| Grade 4 | I am too breathless to leave the house or I am breathless when dressing |

## 2 Shortness of Breath

Masahito Ogasawara

Shortness of breath is a feeling of difficulty in breathing, which may be a symptom of a serious illness, or it may be felt even in people without illness. Even healthy people may feel shortness of breath during mountain climbing or strenuous exercise. Shortness of breath is treated almost synonymously with dyspnea, a condition in which a person is unable to breathe properly. Shortness of breath is caused by the integration in the brain of sensory information from sensory receptors in the body (chemoreceptors, mechanical receptors in the lungs, pulmonary vascular receptors, and biochemical information from skeletal muscles) and the motor output system from the brain to the respiratory organs. When one of these pathways is disturbed, it is perceived as "shortness of breath." When any one of these pathways is impaired, we become aware of "shortness of breath." To be active without shortness of breath, the respiratory, circulatory, and myo-metabolic systems must work in good balance. When any one of these systems fails, shortness of breath is felt. The nervous system, the endocrine system, the blood (especially red blood cells), and the autonomic nervous system, including mental problems, are also involved in shortness of breath. When patients feel shortness of breath, they complain in various ways. Specifically, patients often complain of (1) a sense of chest or respiratory obstruction, (2) the need to exert effort to breathe, (3) the desire for oxygen or to breathe, (4) the inability to take large breaths, and (5) the rapid and ragged breathing. If the patient complains of shortness of breath or dyspnea, arterial blood gas measurement, chest X-ray, electrocardiography, and hematology should be performed immediately. The Hugh-Jones classification (Table 1.3) is frequently used to evaluate the degree of dyspnea, and is rated on a 5-point scale [3].

The etiology of shortness of breath and dyspnea can be divided into (1) pulmonary diseases (including pulmonary circulatory disturbances), (2) cardiac diseases, (3) upper respiratory diseases, (4) psychogenic diseases, (5) hematologic

**Table 1.3** Hugh-Jones classification. (Created based on [3])

| Grade | Description |
|---|---|
| I | Is the patient's breathing as good as that of other persons of the same age and build at work, when walking and climbing hills or stairs? |
| II | Is the patient able to walk with normal persons of the same age and build on the level but is unable to keep up on hills or stairs? |
| III | Is the patient unable to keep up with normal persons on the level but can walk about 1.6 km or more at one's own speed? |
| IV | Is the patient unable to walk more than 50 m on the level without a rest? |
| V | Is the patient feeling short of breath when talking or dressing and/or undressing or unable to leave one's house because of shortness of breath? |

diseases (anemia, leukemia, etc.), (6) metabolic diseases, (7) neuromuscular diseases, and (8) gas poisoning and oxygen deficiency.

However, the mode of onset and concomitant symptoms are particularly important in the differential diagnosis of shortness of breath and dyspnea. In the idiopathic and paroxysmal form, pulmonary embolism, spontaneous pneumothorax, bronchial asthma, aspiration of a foreign body into the upper airway, inhalation of poisonous gases, acute myocardial infarction, and hyperventilation syndrome are considered. Acute and progressive (onset within a few days) cases include acute pneumonia, pleurisy, acute heart failure, malignant tumor, diabetic ketoacidosis, metabolic acidosis due to acute renal failure, and acute exacerbation of chronic obstructive pulmonary disease. In the chronic course, chronic obstructive pulmonary disease, diffuse panbronchiolitis, bronchiectasis, interstitial pneumonia, and psychological factors are considered. Concomitant symptoms include (1) presence of fever, (2) edema, (3) blood sputum, (4) chest pain, (5) sputum, (6) wheezing, (7) dry cough, and (8) easy fatigability.

## 3 Wheezing/Stridor

Takuji Kiryu

Wheezing is a "noise" produced when the airways are narrowed. In general, "Stridor" means a low, relatively loud, mainly inspiratory sound that does not require a stethoscope. "Wheeze" refers to mainly expiratory, high-pitched, relatively quiet sounds that require a stethoscope.

The classification of wheezing is shown in the following (1–4). Each of these is briefly described below:

### 3.1 Wheezing from Narrowing of the Large Airway and Wheezing from Narrowing of the Small Airway

A large airway is an airway from the upper airway, including the nasal cavity, pharynx, and larynx, to the level of the trachea, and the "noise" emitted from this airway is almost synonymous with the "Stridor" described above. On the other hand, the small airway is the airway at the level of the lower respiratory tract, including the bronchi, bronchioles, and alveolar canal, and the "noise" emitted from this airway is almost synonymous with the "wheeze."

### 3.2 "Stridor" and "Wheeze"

Stridor, as described above, is a lower-pitched sound that does not require a stethoscope than wheeze during stenosis of "large airways"; wheeze is a relatively high-pitched sound that requires a stethoscope when a "narrow airway" is narrowed. The *Nanzando Medical Dictionary* states that "wheeze is specific to patients with bronchial asthma" [4].

### 3.3 Transient (Reversible) and Persistent (Irreversible) Wheezing

Transient (reversible) wheezing presents as a reversible, transient symptom when airway constriction is caused by sputum or other adherent materials. On the other hand, persistent (irreversible) wheezing is caused by "organic changes," such as inflammation or tumors, resulting in a narrowing of the airway, and presents with irreversible persistent symptoms.

### 3.4 Inspiratory and Expiratory Wheezing

Inspiratory wheezing is heard when breathing in, and expiratory wheezing is heard when breathing out. Generally, inspiratory wheezing is heard during narrowing of the central airway from the upper airway, such as the larynx and pharynx. Expiratory wheezing is often heard during narrowing of the peripheral airways, such as in bronchial asthma.

When "wheezing" is suspected in daily practice, it should be evaluated according to the following procedure. As mentioned above, "Stridor" often does not require a stethoscope, while "wheeze" often requires a stethoscope. Therefore, if you suspect "wheeze," use the stethoscope with attention to the inspiratory and expiratory state. If irreversible organic disease is suspected, imaging tests (plain radiograph, CT, MRI, etc.) should be performed, and if reversible functional disease is suspected, pulmonary function tests should be performed.

There are a variety of diseases that cause wheezing [5]. We divide them into two groups: diseases that cause "expiratory wheezing" and diseases that cause "inspiratory wheezing."

The following is a list of diseases that cause "inspiratory wheezing." These include glossoptosis, enlargement of tonsil, adenoiditis, laryngitis/epiglottitis, laryngeal trauma, vocal cord paralysis, laryngopharynx tumors, croup, foreign bodies, tracheal tuberculosis, rhinoscleroma, sarcoidosis, amyloidosis, recurrent polychondritis, tracheopathia osteoplastica, and tracheobronchomalacia.

The following is a list of diseases that cause "expiratory wheezing:"

bronchial asthma, chronic obstructive pulmonary disease, bronchitis and bronchiolitis, bronchiectasis, lung cancer, congestive heart failure, pneumoconiosis, eosinophilic granulomatosis with polyangiitis, etc.

## 4 Cough

Takeshi Terashima

### 4.1 Symptoms

Cough is the most common symptom of the respiratory system, and it is caused by a variety of diseases, including infectious diseases, allergies, and tumors. Just before coughing, the vocal cords are temporarily closed, and when the airway pressure rises to a certain degree, the vocal cords are opened at once, and the air is instantly expelled at high speed and with a strong force, accompanied by a coughing sound. Coughing is often initiated reflexively, but it can also be initiated voluntarily.

### 4.2 Pathogenesis and Developmental Mechanism

There are cough receptors in the airway that respond to mechanical or chemical stimuli. When cough receptors detect excessive stimuli, they excite the cough center in the medulla oblongata via the parasympathetic nervous system, resulting in a reflex cough. Irritant gases, sputum, and aspiration are the causes of irritation. When the airway epithelium is damaged by airway infection and the cough receptors are easily stimulated, or when the airway epithelium is hypersensitive in atopic cough, simple stimuli such as changes in temperature or humidity cause cough. The contraction of bronchial smooth muscle also stimulates the cough center. In bronchial asthma/cough variant asthma, airway hyperresponsiveness is increased, and changes in temperature and air pressure stimulate bronchial smooth muscle contraction, inducing cough.

### 4.3 Classification and Differential Diseases

Wet cough (cough with sputum) and dry cough (cough without sputum) are classified as acute

**Table 1.4** Causative diseases and conditions that cause cough

| | Acute cough | Subacute and chronic cough |
|---|---|---|
| Wet cough | Acute bronchitis | Chronic bronchitis |
| | Bacterial pneumonia | Chronic obstructive pulmonary disease (COPD) |
| | Pulmonary tuberculosis | Bronchiectasis |
| | Lung cancer | Postnasal drip |
| | | Pulmonary tuberculosis |
| | | Lung cancer |
| Dry cough | Common cold syndrome | Postinfectious cough |
| | Respiratory infection (virus, mycoplasma, chlamydia, pneumonia, etc.) | Pertussis |
| | Pneumothorax | Mycoplasma infection |
| | Pleurisy | Chlamydia pneumoniae infection |
| | Pulmonary thromboembolism | Bronchial asthma/ cough variant asthma |
| | Respiratory tract foreign body | Atopic cough |
| | Aspiration | Interstitial pneumonia |
| | | Gastroesophageal reflux disease |
| | | Drug-induced (angiotensin-converting enzyme (ACE) inhibitor) |

and chronic according to their duration. In wet cough, cough plays an important role in the removal of secretions from the airways. According to the duration, there are three types of cough: acute cough that is mild within 3 weeks, subacute cough that lasts 3–8 weeks, and chronic cough that lasts more than 8 weeks. The causative diseases are listed in Table 1.4.

### 4.4 Clinical Examination and Diagnosis

In addition to the presence, character, and duration of sputum, the cause of the cough should be investigated based on physical examination, imaging examination, and respiratory function test, referring to information such as the trigger of the cough, presence of infectious symptoms, medical history, medication history, and smoking history.

### 4.5 Treatment

Fundamental treatment of the causative disease is the first priority. In asthma/cough variant asthma, inhaled steroids and other agents should be used to reduce airway hyperresponsiveness, and long-acting beta-2 stimulants should be used to achieve adequate bronchodilation. In chronic obstructive pulmonary disease (COPD), smoking cessation is the first priority. In bacterial infections, appropriate antimicrobial therapy is expected to decrease the volume of sputum and reduce airway irritation. Histamine $H_1$ receptor antagonists are effective in atopic cough. Cough has the role of removing foreign substances and sputum, and it is not advisable to stop coughing unnecessarily with antitussive agents. On the other hand, coughing itself can stimulate the airways and cause further coughing, and severe coughing can cause physical exhaustion and muscle pain.

### 4.6 Cough Reflex and Aspiration

If the cough reflex is impaired, even if saliva, sputum, etc. enter the respiratory tract from the oral cavity, there is a risk of pneumonia due to the inability of the cough to evacuate the airway after aspiration.

## 5 Sputum

Yasuhiro Gon, Tetsuo Shimizu

### 5.1 What Is Sputum?

Sputum is a condition in which the secretions produced by the mucous membrane of the lower respiratory tract (the pathway from the trachea to the bronchi, bronchioles, and alveoli) pathologically increase and are expectorated outside the body. Airway secretions are secreted by bronchial glands, goblet cells, Clara cells, type II alveolar epithelium, and other airway constituent cells. Physiologically, it protects the respiratory tract mucosa by removing fine particles (pollen, dust, etc.) in the air, along with ciliary movement of the respiratory tract.

Physiologically, it protects the respiratory tract mucosa by removing fine particles (pollen, dust, etc.) in the air, along with ciliary movement of the respiratory tract. Inflammation of the lower respiratory tract increases the production of airway secretions, and sputum is usually expectorated with cough. Sputum contains a glycoprotein called mucin, and the viscosity of sputum is affected by the composition of mucin. The color and viscosity of sputum change depending on the cause of increased production of airway secretions.

## 5.2 Causes of Sputum

Inflammation of the lower respiratory tract accounts for the majority of sputum production, although inflammation, tumor, and pulmonary congestion are common causes. Inflammation is divided into infectious and noninfectious diseases, and infectious diseases include cold syndrome, acute bronchitis, pneumonia, pulmonary tuberculosis, and pulmonary mycosis, in which microorganisms such as bacteria, viruses, tubercle bacilli, and fungi infect the lower respiratory tract, causing inflammation and sputum production. The most common noninfectious diseases are bronchial asthma, chronic obstructive pulmonary disease (COPD), and bronchiectasis. Bronchial asthma tends to cause cough, sputum, and wheezing due to allergic chronic airway inflammation, while COPD causes cough, sputum, and shortness of breath due to chronic airway inflammation caused by inhalation of toxic substances such as tobacco smoke. In COPD, chronic airway inflammation due to inhalation of toxic substances such as tobacco smoke causes cough, sputum, and shortness of breath. In bronchiectasis, part of the bronchi is dilated, and the dilated bronchi are chronically infected with microorganisms such as bacteria, and cough, sputum, and bloody sputum are likely to be observed. In bronchiectasis, part of the bronchi is dilated, and the dilated bronchi are chronically infected with microorganisms such as bacteria, and cough, sputum, and bloody sputum are likely to be observed.

## 5.3 Points of Examination

The main point of examining a patient complaining of sputum is to first check whether the expectoration of sputum is accompanied by cough. If it is not accompanied by cough, it is often oral secretions such as saliva. Next, check the color of the sputum (Table 1.5, Fig. 1.1). Yellow or green purulent sputum is a finding suggestive of bacterial infection of the lower respiratory tract, and acute bronchitis or bacterial pneumonia should be suspected. The color of sputum from infections other than bacterial infections and noninfectious diseases is often clear to white. Bloody sputum is a condition in which blood is mixed with sputum, and if it is accompanied by bloody sputum, there is a possibility of pulmonary tuberculosis, bronchiectasis, or lung tumor. In addition, the presence of symptoms associated with sputum (fever, wheezing, shortness of breath) should be checked, and the cause of sputum should be diagnosed by chest X-ray and sputum examination.

## 5.4 Sputum Examination

Sputum examination includes bacterial examination test and cytodiagnosis and is useful for

**Table 1.5** Sputum color and diseases

| Sputum color | Disease |
|---|---|
| Purulent (yellow, green) | Bacterial infection (acute bronchitis, pneumonia) |
| White, clear | Chronic obstructive pulmonary disease, bronchial asthma, and viral infection |
| Bloody sputum | Pulmonary tuberculosis, bronchiectasis, and lung tumor |

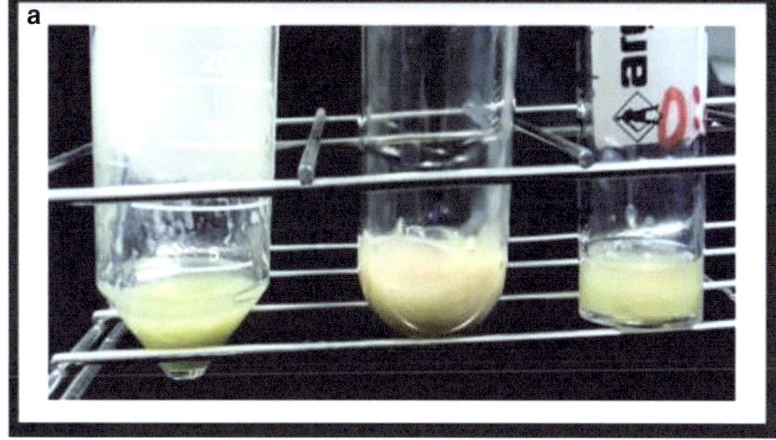

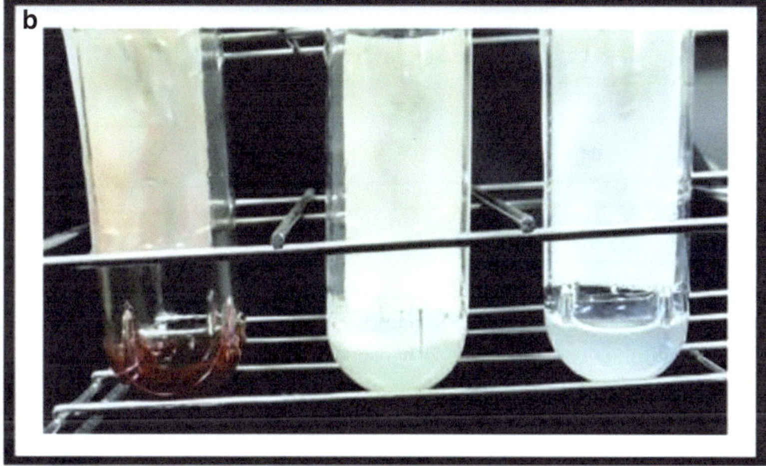

**Fig. 1.1** Color of sputum. (**a**) Purulent. (**b**) Bloody sputum, white, clear. (Photo provided by Dr. Hiroyuki Nishiyama, Department of Clinical Laboratory, Nihon University Itabashi Hospital)

diagnosis and differentiation of infectious diseases and lung tumors. Bacteriological tests include standard bacteriological tests to detect standard bacteria such as *Streptococcus pneumoniae* and mycobacterium test to detect *Mycobacterium tuberculosis* and *nontuberculous mycobacteria*. Bacteriological tests not only identify the causative microorganism but also examine the effect of antimicrobial agents on the causative microorganism by drug susceptibility test. Cytodiagnosis is useful in the diagnosis of pulmonary malignant tumor by examining the presence of malignant cells in sputum. For bacteriological examination, it is important to collect good-quality sputum containing a large amount of lower respiratory tract secretions with little saliva. In the Geckler classification (Table 1.6), the number of squamous cells and neutrophils in sputum is measured microscopically, and specimens with less squamous cells and more neutrophils are suitable for bacteriological examination.

**Table 1.6** Geckler classification

| | Squamous epithelial cells | Neutrophils | |
|---|---|---|---|
| Geckler | Number of cells/field of view (100 times) | Number of cells/field of view (100 times) | Quality |
| 1 | >25 | <10 | No good |
| 2 | >25 | 10–25 | No good |
| 3 | >25 | >25 | No good |
| 4 | 10–25 | >25 | Good |
| 5 | <10 | >25 | Good |

## 6 Fever

Hirofumi Sawai

### 6.1 Body Temperature

Body temperature is measured in the axilla, oral cavity, and rectum and is 0.3–0.5 °C higher in the oral cavity and 0.6–1.0 °C higher in the rectum than in the axilla. The axillary temperature in normal subjects is usually 36.0–37.0 °C, with a diurnal variation that is lower in the early morning and 0.5–1.0 °C higher in the afternoon and evening. A body temperature of 37.5 °C or higher is called fever, 38.0 °C or higher is called high fever, and 37.0–37.5 °C is called slight fever.

### 6.2 Causes of Fever

Infectious diseases (e.g., bacteria, viruses, mycoplasma, chlamydia, fungi, tuberculosis) are the most common causes of fever, but it is caused by malignant tumors (e.g., cancer, leukemia, malignant lymphoma), collagen diseases (e.g., systemic lupus erythematosus), inflammatory bowel diseases (e.g., ulcerative colitis, Crohn's disease), central nervous system diseases (e.g., brain stem hemorrhage), hyperthyroidism, heat attack, anemia, pregnancy, drug fever (fever due to adverse effects of drugs), etc.

### 6.3 Symptoms of Fever

Heart sensation, general malaise, headache, anorexia, drowsiness, sweating, myalgia, arthralgia, etc. are observed, and high fever causes chills, shivering, convulsions, delirium, etc.

### 6.4 Types of Fever

1. Continued Fever (Fig. 1.2)
   A sustained high fever with a diurnal variation of less than 1 °C. It is seen in lobar pneumonia, miliary tuberculosis, typhoid fever, etc.
2. Remittent F(Fig. 1.3)
   A persistent fever with a diurnal variation of more than 1 °C. It is seen in many infectious diseases, malignant tumors, etc.
3. Intermittent Fever (Fig. 1.4)
   It is a condition in which the diurnal variation is more than 1 °C and the temperature

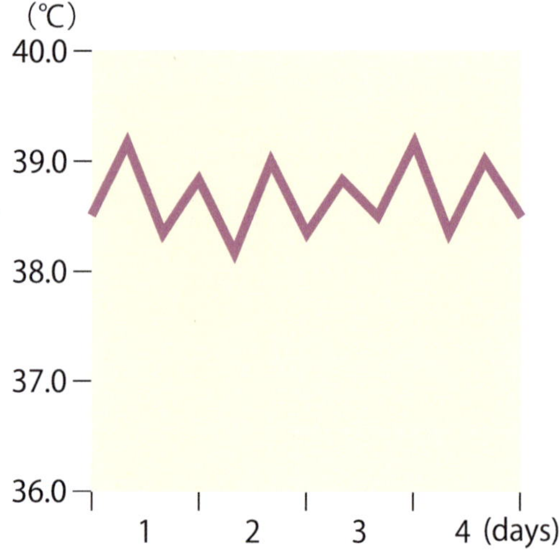


**Fig. 1.2** Continued fever

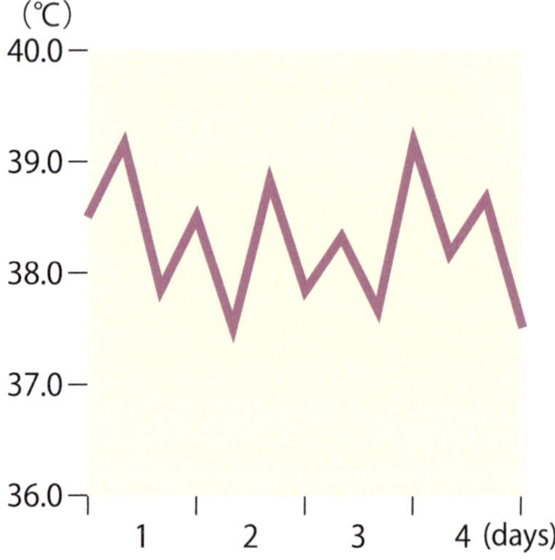


**Fig. 1.3** Remittent fever

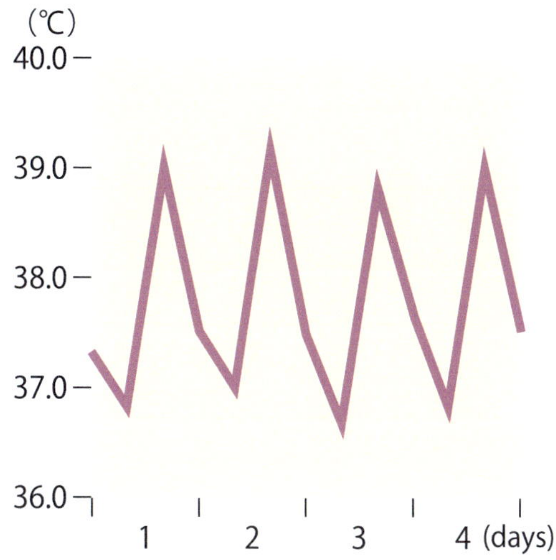


**Fig. 1.4** Intermittent fever

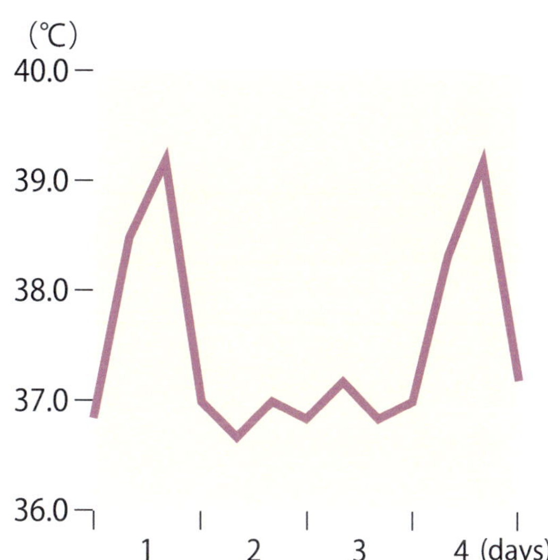


**Fig. 1.5** Periodic fever

drops lower than 37 °C. It is seen in infectious diseases, drug fever, etc.

4. Periodic Fever (Fig. 1.5)

   In vivax malaria or malarial malaria, fever recurs periodically (every 3 or 4 days).

5. Pel-Ebstein Fever

   In Hodgkin's disease, several days of fever follow an afebrile period of several days and return to the afebrile period.

## 6.5 Fever of Unknown Origin (FUO)

When fever persists for more than 3 weeks and its cause cannot be identified after 3 days of hospitalization or more than three outpatient examinations, it is called (classical) fever of unknown origin (FUO). The major causes of FUO are infectious diseases (tuberculosis, infective endocarditis, intra-abdominal abscess, etc.), malignant tumors, and collagen diseases.

## References

1. Launois C, et al. Correlation of respiratory symptoms and spirometric lung patterns in a rural community setting, Sindh, Pakistan:a cross sectional survey. BMC Pulm Med. 2012;12:61.
2. Borg G. Psychophysical bases of perceived exertion. Med Sci Sports Exerc. 1982;14(5):377–8.
3. Hugh Jones P, et al. A simple standard exercise test and its use for measuring exertion dyspnoea. Br Med J. 1952;1:65–71.
4. Nanzando's medical dictionary. 19th ed. Tokyo: Nanzan-do; 2007 (in Japanese).
5. Divakaran S, et al. Clinical problem-solving: all that wheezes…. N Engl J Med. 2017;377:477–84.

# 2 Cardiovascular Symptoms

Masashi Watanabe, Hiroshige Ohashi, Tomonori Segawa, Masahito Ogasawara, Akihiko Hasegawa, and Shin Inoue

## 1 Shock [1, 2]

Masashi Watanabe

Shock is a condition in which circulatory disturbance leads to systemic tissue perfusion impairment and tissue dysfunction. If it persists, tissue perfusion impairment leads to irreversible cellular and organ damage and multiple organ failure, which is life-threatening. The main symptom is hypotension, which is caused by a decrease in cardiac output or a decrease in peripheral vascular resistance or both.

In the treatment of shock, it is important to recognize and intervene early, when the metabolic mechanisms are working effectively (pre-shock).

The pathophysiology is classified into four categories according to the cause: (1) hypovolemic shock, (2) cardiogenic shock, (3) obstructive shock, and (4) distributive shock.

### 1.1 Diagnosis

As mentioned above, shock is a condition in which circulatory disturbances lead to systemic tissue perfusion disturbances and organ damage due to impaired tissue oxygen metabolism. A fall in blood pressure (systolic blood pressure below 90 mmHg) is one criterion, but a fall in blood pressure is not synonymous with shock. Vital signs (state of consciousness, blood pressure, pulse rate, respiratory rate, temperature) and clinical findings such as urine output, skin pallor, cold sweat, and peripheral circulation should be combined to make a comprehensive judgment. If it takes more than 2 s for the capillaries to refill after the nail bed is compressed and the pressure is released, this suggests a peripheral circulatory disturbance.

The original version of the chapter has been revised. A correction to this chapter can be found at https://doi.org/10.1007/978-981-99-3296-2_21

M. Watanabe
Department of Medicine, School of Life Dentistry at Tokyo, The Nippon Dental University, Chiyoda-ku, Tokyo, Japan

H. Ohashi
Asahi University Hospital, Gifu, Japan

T. Segawa
Department of Cardiology, Asahi University Hospital, Gifu, Japan

M. Ogasawara (✉)
Division of Bioregulatory Pharmacology, Department of Pharmacology, Iwate Medical University, Yahaba, Iwate, Japan

A. Hasegawa
Division of Internal Medicine, Department of Comprehensive Medical Sciences, Meikai University School of Dentistry, Sakado, Saitama, Japan

S. Inoue
Department of Internal Medicine, Showa University Dental Hospital, Ota-ku, Tokyo, Japan



T. Chiba, H. Yamada (eds.), *Internal Medicine for Dental Treatments*,
https://doi.org/10.1007/978-981-99-3296-2_2

### 1.2 Assessment of Causative Disease

1. Hypovolemic Shock.

   It is caused by loss of circulating blood or plasma volume due to trauma, rupture of an aortic aneurysm, gastrointestinal bleeding, severe pancreatitis, intestinal obstruction, severe diarrhea or vomiting, or burns, resulting in a decrease in cardiac output. It is associated with peripheral vasoconstriction due to reactive sympathetic tone.
2. Cardiogenic Shock.

   It is associated with acute myocardial infarction, myocarditis, mitral insufficiency due to papillary muscle rupture, ventricular septal perforation, cardiac rupture, dilated cardiomyopathy, reduced cardiac output due to arrhythmia, and peripheral vasoconstriction due to reactive sympathetic tone.
3. Obstructive Shock.

   It is caused by pulmonary embolism, cardiac tamponade, tension pneumothorax, and supine hypotensive syndrome caused by compression of the inferior vena cava by the pregnant uterus. Treatment of the causative obstruction is necessary.
4. Distributive Shock.

   It is caused by a decrease in body vascular resistance, an increase in vascular permeability, and a decrease in stroke volume due to a decrease in preload caused by venous dilation without any of the above abnormalities. Causes include anaphylaxis, septicemia, and neurogenesis.

### 1.3 Severity and Prognosis

The severity of the disease is assessed by APACHE II score, SOFA score, and blood lactate level.

### 1.4 Treatment

Treatment and diagnosis should be performed simultaneously, since the shock condition needs to be improved and the cause should be investigated. The main treatment for shock is respiratory and circulatory control. The main treatment for shock is respiratory and circulatory control: A, airway; B, breathing; C, disability; and D, consciousness assessment immediately and treatment initiated. Patients who present with shock need to be promptly evaluated for ABCD, and physical examination and treatment perform simultaneously. Vital signs should be assessed repeatedly and evaluate changes over time to determine response to therapy. Prioritize tests that can be performed at the bedside (emergency room or ward), such as blood tests, electrocardiography, ultrasound, and portable radiography. If a CT scan or MRI scan is performed in a patient who is not yet out of shock, it should be performed in an environment where the patient's condition can be adequately monitored and immediate action can be taken if symptoms worsen. After the patient is resuscitated and has recovered from the shock, additional imaging tests need to be performed to make a final diagnosis. Serum lactate is useful in assessing the severity of the disease.

## 2 Edema [3–5]

Hiroshige Ohhashi

### 2.1 The Pathophysiology of Edema

Edema is a generalized or localized accumulation of excess fluid in the tissues between blood vessels and cells. When edema occurs, the eyelids and lower limbs swell, and in severe cases, pleural effusion and ascites appear; digital impression is observed when the swollen area is compressed. When the edema is localized, it is called localized edema, and when it is seen in the whole body, it is called generalized edema.

About 60% of the human body is water, and about 40% is intracellular water (intracellular fluid), and the remaining 20% is extracellular. Of the extracellular fluid, about 5% is blood flowing in blood vessels, and the remaining 15% is interstitial fluid between blood vessels and cells. Edema appears when interstitial fluid increases disproportionately. Hydrostatic pressure and colloid osmotic

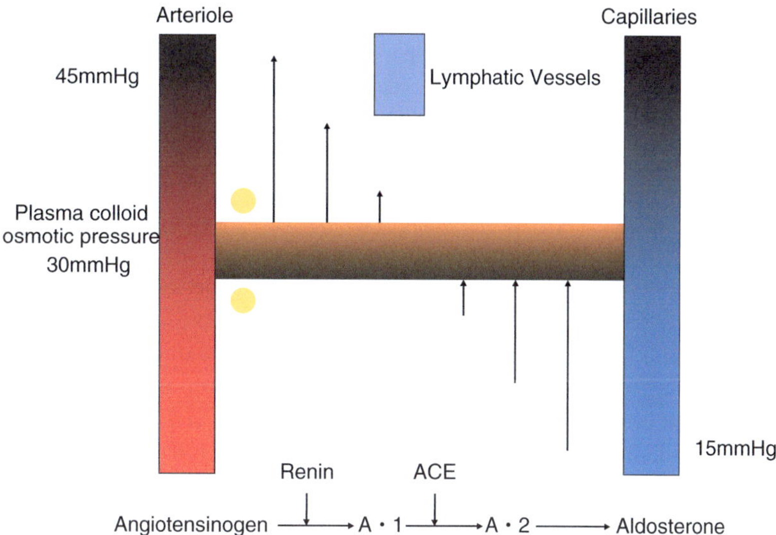


**Fig. 2.1** Edema occurs due to decreased colloid osmotic pressure caused by low albumin levels, increased venous pressure, and increased permeability of capillaries

pressure inside and outside the capillary wall play a major role in the movement of water.

In summary, a decrease in plasma colloid osmotic pressure, an increase in venous pressure, an increase in capillary permeability, and an obstruction of the lymphatic system are the causes of edema development (Fig. 2.1)

## 2.2 Differentiation of Edema

Edema can be classified as generalized or localized. Most generalized edema is caused by cardiac disease, renal disease, liver disease, or nutritional disorders, and it is necessary to differentiate between them by paying attention to the characteristic findings of each disease. Localized edema is usually caused by thrombophlebitis or chronic lymphangitis and is due to obstruction of veins or lymphatic vessels.

Generalized edema is observed in the following pathophysiology and differs from localized edema in its onset mechanisms.

1. Nephrotic Syndrome.

   In nephrotic syndrome, hypoproteinemia and hypoalbuminemia are the main causes of edema. When a large amount of protein (>3.5 g/day) leaks into the urine, hypoalbuminemia (<3.0 g/dL) occurs, leading to hyperlipidemia and edema. Hypoalbuminemia decreases the colloid osmotic pressure in the blood, and edema develops due to the transfer of water to the tissues. In addition, a decrease in effective arterial blood volume leads to a decrease in cardiac output and an increase in renal reabsorption of water and sodium, resulting in edema (under filling edema).

   In some cases of nephrotic syndrome, the effective arterial blood flow is not decreased, and in these cases, water and sodium retention in the distal renal tubules is increased (over filling edema).

2. Renal Failure.

   In the oliguric phase of acute renal failure, a rapid decrease in glomerular filtration rate (GFR) leads to water and sodium retention and the appearance of edema.

   In chronic renal failure, glomerular sodium filtration is reduced due to a decrease in GFR, but the sodium balance per unit nephron is maintained. However, edema is caused by excessive sodium and water intake in this condition.

3. Heart Failure.

   In heart failure, blood flow to the kidneys is decreased, the renin-angiotensin system is increased, reabsorption of sodium and water in the tubules is increased, and edema appears. In addition, venous pressure increases in the periphery, causing water to move into the interstitium, which may contribute to the development of edema. In heart failure, sympathetic nervous system activity is often increased, which may contribute to the development of edema via the renin-angiotensin system.

The presence of findings indicative of cardiac disease, such as cardiomegaly, together with findings such as dyspnea, pulmonary rales, venous distension, and hepatomegaly, indicates that the edema is due to heart failure.

4. Hepatic Edema: A Nutritionally Impaired Edema.

   In liver cirrhosis and nutritional disorders, albumin synthesis, which maintains plasma colloid osmotic pressure, is decreased, causing water to move into the interstitium and edema to occur. On the other hand, because the effective circulating blood volume is decreased, the renin-angiotensin system is increased, sodium accumulates, and edema is enhanced. In liver cirrhosis, a large amount of ascites causes an increase in abdominal pressure and a delay in venous return from the lower limbs, which contributes to enhanced edema of the lower limbs.
5. Endocrine Edema.

   Hypothyroidism, also called myxedema, is characterized by edema of the face and lower legs without surface imprint (non-pitting edema).
6. Idiopathic Edema.

   Idiopathic edema refers to cases in which there is no causative disease for edema and the cause is unknown. The diagnosis is made by exclusion, but most patients are female in their 20 s–50 s and are characterized by intermittent edema. It is characterized by a large difference in body weight between morning and evening because water excretion changes with body position. When the difference in body weight between morning and evening is more than 1.4 kg, it is defined as idiopathic edema.
7. Drug-Induced Edema.

   Edema can also be induced by drugs. Shosaikoto containing glycyrrhiza, stronger neo-minophagen C, and estrogen agonist have aldosterone-like effects and can cause sodium retention.Ca antagonists may induce edema by increasing local vascular permeability.

# 3 Cyanosis

Tomonori Segawa

## 3.1 Disease Overview

Cyanosis is a condition in which the skin and mucous membranes, such as the lips, oral mucosa, fingertips, nail beds, and earlobes, show a dark purple color. The concentration of reduced hemoglobin in the blood of capillaries is 2.0–2.5 g/dL under normal conditions, but cyanosis appears when the concentration of reduced hemoglobin in the blood of these subcutaneous capillaries is 5 g/dL or higher and in arterial blood 3 g/dL or higher. It can be caused by abnormal hemoglobinemia, such as methemoglobinemia, which is seen when methemoglobin levels are 0.5 g/dL or higher. However, it should be noted that cyanosis is not always a symptom of hypoxemia, as it may not be present in carbon monoxide poisoning or anemia.

## 3.2 Pathology and Physiology

In normal subjects, arterial blood oxygen saturation is 100%, venous blood oxygen saturation is 70%, and intrapapillary blood oxygen saturation is 85%. If the hemoglobin concentration is 12.5 g/dL, the capillary-reduced hemoglobin concentration is 1.875 g/dL, and cyanosis occurs when capillary oxygen saturation falls below 60%. In the case of central cyanosis with decreased arterial oxygen saturation, when arterial oxygen saturation is less than 75%, blood oxygen saturation in capillaries is less than 60%, and cyanosis appears. In peripheral cyanosis, in which arterial oxygen saturation is not decreased, vascular resistance in the capillaries is increased, blood flow in the capillaries is highly decreased, oxygen saturation decreases due to increased oxygen release, and reduced hemoglobin concentration increases.

## 3.3 Classification

It is classified into central and peripheral based on the mechanism of onset.

1. Central cyanosis: It is thought to appear in the whole body due to a decrease in oxygen saturation of arterial blood. Causes include respiratory failure and right-left shunts. In respiratory failure, cyanosis is caused by inadequate oxygenation of pulmonary arterial blood due to hypoventilation, ventilation perfusion ratio inequality, and diffusion impairment. Causes include pulmonary diseases (acute respiratory distress syndrome, chronic obstructive pulmonary disease, emphysema, etc.) and heart failure with pulmonary edema. Congenital heart diseases with a right-left shunt include tetralogy of Fallot, complete transposition of great vessels, total anomalous pulmonary venous return, and Eisenmenger's syndrome.
2. Peripheral cyanosis: It is caused by severe hypotension and peripheral circulatory failure. The former includes shock, low cardiac output syndrome, and severe heart failure without pulmonary edema. The latter are caused by vascular spasm (Raynaud's phenomenon, cold exposure), arterial occlusive disease (thromboembolism, arteriosclerosis obliterans), and venous occlusive disease (thromboembolism, thrombophlebitis).

### 3.4 Differential Diagnosis

Central cyanosis is present in both the skin and mucous membranes. However, in patients with patent ductus arteriosus, cyanosis is seen only in the lower extremities, and dissociative cyanosis is not seen in the upper extremities. In central cyanosis, the partial pressure of oxygen in the arterial blood and oxygen saturation are both decreased, and 100% oxygen inhalation improves cyanosis in pulmonary disease and ventilation disorders, but not in cyanotic congenital heart disease. If the cause of cyanosis due to cardiac or pulmonary disease is not clear, the presence of abnormal hemoglobin such as methemoglobinemia should be suspected.

Peripheral cyanosis is found mainly in the superficial layers of the skin, such as the fingertips and auricles, but not in the mucous membranes, such as the oral mucosa and ocular conjunctiva. Arterial oxygen partial pressure and oxygen saturation are normal, but venous oxygen saturation is highly depressed, making it relatively easy to distinguish from central cyanosis. Peripheral cyanosis does not improve with 100% oxygen inhalation and is strongly influenced by environmental temperature, so it is generally improved by keeping the patient warm. Peripheral cyanosis is usually present in cardiogenic shock, but mixed findings may occur in patients with pulmonary edema.

## 4 Palpitation

Masahito Ogasawara

The heart repeats contraction and dilation, which are transmitted as pulse waves from the heart to the periphery, and the electrical excitation and beating of the heart occur regularly in a fixed rhythm. Everyone has experienced a strong and rapid heartbeat immediately after running at full speed or strenuous exercise or a pounding heartbeat when under stress or anxiety, such as when speaking in public. These are "normal palpitations" when the heart is working normally. However, when the heartbeat or pulse is disturbed, it is recognized as an unpleasant symptom and is called "pathological palpitation." Individuals differ in whether they feel palpitations or not. A thorough history of the circumstances and triggers of palpitations, their onset, termination, duration, and frequency of occurrence is necessary. If possible, the patient should be interviewed in detail about the characteristics of palpitations, not just "palpitations." Subjective symptoms (chest pain, chest tightness, disturbance of consciousness, shortness of breath, dyspnea, etc.) and objective symptoms (anemia, goiter, protruding eyes, edema, hand tremor, etc.) associated with palpitations should be noted.

The causes of pathological palpitations can be divided into (1) cardiac causes and (2) noncardiac causes. Electrocardiography is indispensable in determining the cause of palpitations. A heart rate of 100 beats per minute or more is called tachycardia, and a heart rate of less than 60 beats per minute is called bradycardia.

The pulse can be examined by the patient himself, and it is important to note the pulse rate and the rhythm of the pulse. Three fingers are placed together parallel to the radial artery, and when equal force is applied, each finger touches the pulse on its belly, and the beats per minute are counted. Abnormalities of the pulse include tachycardia, bradycardia, and arrhythmia.

Tachycardia is mainly caused by (1) an increased demand for oxygen in systemic tissues and (2) a decrease in cardiac output. In the former case, tachycardia is often caused by, other than cardiac disease anemia, fever, infection, hypoglycemia, hyperthyroidism, pheochromocytoma, drug-induced (use of beta-receptor-acting drugs in chronic obstructive pulmonary disease and bronchial asthma), and taste (tobacco and alcohol). In the latter case, a decrease in single cardiac output is compensated for by increasing the number of heartbeats. Atrial fibrillation and atrial flutter are caused by heart rhythm. Cardiovascular disorders can also cause tachyarrhythmias due to damage to cardiomyocytes caused by pressure or volume loading. Other disorders include valvular disease (aortic stenosis, aortic regurgitation, mitral stenosis, mitral regurgitation, etc.), left-right shunt disease (atrial septal defect, ventricular septal defect), hypertensive heart disease, and cardiomyopathy.

In athletes, the resting heart rate may be less than 40 beats per minute, and bradycardia is not always a pathological condition. When symptoms such as fainting, hypotension, and heart failure are induced, it is considered pathological bradycardia, and treatment is necessary. In addition to sick sinus syndrome and atrioventricular block, which are caused by the heart itself, drug-induced (digitalis, beta-blockers, acetylcholinesterase inhibitors such as donepezil hydrochloride used in the treatment of dementia), hyperkalemia, hypothyroidism, hypoadrenalism, vagal tone, and hypothermia associated with systemic diseases have been listed. Palpitations caused by irregular pulse are often due to cardiac diseases, such as extrasystoles (atrial extrasystoles, ventricular extrasystoles) and tachycardiac atrial fibrillation. In addition to cardiac and systemic diseases, there are also arrhythmias caused by psychogenic factors (panic disorder, anxiety neurosis, hyperventilation syndrome).

## 5 Chest Pain

Masahito Ogasawara

Chest pain and chest symptoms are one of the most frequent complaints. There is a wide variety of conditions, some of which are life-threatening and urgent and should be treated with caution. When a patient complains of chest pain, the following points should be considered. (1) whether it is a first occurrence or recurrent, (2) presence or absence of triggers, (3) character, (4) location, radiating pain, (5) time of onset of chest pain, (6) duration, (7) pattern of onset (suddenness), (8) accompanying symptoms, and (9) presence or absence of risk factors.

Chest pain can be caused by a variety of diseases, including chest wall, respiratory, circulatory, mediastinal, and extrathoracic (especially gastrointestinal) tissues, depending on the source.

In chest pain originating from the chest wall, tender points are observed, and the character of the pain may change with pressure, suggesting intercostal neuralgia, myalgia, herpes zoster, trauma to the chest wall, fracture, or bone metastasis of malignancy. Especially in chest pain caused by the musculoskeletal system of the chest wall, the intensity of pain changes with body movement and position. It is not uncommon for patients to complain that the pain becomes stronger when they take a deep breath. In herpes zoster, a bullous eruption along the intercostal nerves may be accompanied by pain and a sense of itching.

Chest pain originating from the respiratory organs may be caused by diseases that affect the pleura, such as pleurisy, pneumothorax, and malignant tumors of the pleura, since there are no pain nerves in the lung parenchyma. However, pleural infiltration of lung cancer and pneumonia may also be recognized as chest pain when inflammation reaches the pleura or when the pulmonary vasculature is suddenly pulled.

Chest pain of cardiovascular origin includes diseases of life-threatening importance. Chest pain in ischemic heart disease (angina pectoris, myocardial infarction) covers a relatively large area of the anterior chest and is unlikely to be indicated by an index finger. Chest pain in angina pectoris and myocardial infarction is relatively widespread. In effort angina, there are many triggers for chest pain, including exercise, heavy lifting, cold exposure, and psychological stress. The duration of pain is in "minutes" and is remitted with rest or sublingual nitroglycerin. If chest pain recurs repeatedly or lasts more than 30 min, myocardial infarction is considered a possibility. In acute myocardial infarction, it is not uncommon for patients to complain of referred pain such as toothache, epigastric pain, and radiating pain to the left arm. In addition, patients with poorly controlled diabetes mellitus often have autonomic neuropathy and do not complain of chest pain. It is important not to exclude the possibility of myocardial infarction because of the absence of chest pain.

Aortic dissection is the most important aortic disease. In this disease, chest pain is sudden and sharp, with a "tearing" sensation. As the disease progresses, the extent of the pain shifts or increases. Other conditions include aortic valve stenosis, mitral valve prolapse, and epicarditis. In these diseases, a heart murmur can often be heard by auscultation, but chest pain is not often the main symptom.

Gastroesophageal reflux disease (GERD) is a common cause of chest pain in the digestive system. The main symptom of gastroesophageal reflux disease is "heartburn," which often begins within 30 min after eating. However, many patients do not complain of typical heartburn symptoms and present with a variety of symptoms, including chest pain, chest discomfort, and reflux of food.

Among these, acute myocardial infarction, acute aortic dissection, pulmonary artery thromboembolism, and tension pneumothorax are the most urgent. Chest pain, dyspnea, and gastrointestinal symptoms often accompany these diseases, and it is important to refer them to a specialist as soon as possible.

## 6 Tachycardia, Bradycardia

Akihiko Hasegawa

### 6.1 Pulse

The pulse rate (heart rate) is considered to be 60–90 beats per minute in healthy individuals.

Tachycardia is defined as a pulse rate of 100 beats per minute or more.

Bradycardia is defined as a pulse rate of less than 60 beats per minute (some consider it less than 50) (Table 2.1).

The pulse is measured by placing the index, middle, and ring fingers on the radial artery and

**Table 2.1** Main causes of tachycardia and bradycardia

| Tachycardia (≥100 beats/min) | Bradycardia (<60 beats/min) |
|---|---|
| Tachyarrhythmia: | Bradyarrhythmia: |
| Sinus tachycardia, paroxysmal supraventricular tachycardia (PSVT), (tachycardiac) atrial fibrillation, atrial flutter, and ventricular tachycardia | Sinus bradycardia, sick sinus syndrome, atrioventricular block, and (bradycardiac) atrial fibrillation |
| Physical exercise | Aging |
| Excitement | Intense physical excercise habit |
| Mental stress | Vasovagal reflex |
| Strong pain stimulation | Neurogenic shock |
| Heart failure | Hypothyroidism |
| Respiratory disease | Medications (β-blockers, antiarrhythmic drugs, diltiazem, verapamil, digitalis) |
| Anemia | |
| Hypoglycemia | |
| Fever | |
| Dehydration | |
| Hyperventilation syndrome | |
| Shock (except neurogenic shock) | |
| Hyperthyroidism | |
| Pheochromocytoma | |
| Panic disorder | |
| Medications (dopamine, adrenaline, isoproterenol, nifedipine, antipsychotic drugs) | |

palpating the radial artery. If the pulse is regular, the number of 15-s periods is multiplied by four; if the pulse is irregular, the number of 1-min periods is counted. In some cases, the pulse rate and heart rate do not match (pulse rate ≤ heart rate). This is because the pulse wave may not be transmitted to the radial artery even if there is a heartbeat and is often seen in arrhythmias such as atrial fibrillation and extrasystoles.

Pulse rate (heart rate) fluctuates according to the balance between sympathetic and parasympathetic nerves, which are autonomic nerves.

In both tachycardia and bradycardia, palpitations (the subjective symptoms of the heartbeat itself, which is usually unnoticeable, and of irregularity in the heartbeat) are often noticed.

## 6.2 Tachycardia

Sinus tachycardia, paroxysmal supraventricular tachycardia, (tachycardiac) atrial fibrillation, atrial flutter, and ventricular tachycardia are the most common arrhythmias that produce tachycardia.

Physical exercise, excitement, mental stress, and strong pain stimuli increase sympathetic nerve activity, resulting in an increase in heart rate and tachycardia.

In heart failure, respiratory disease, anemia, hypoglycemia, fever, and dehydration, physiological compensatory mechanisms lead to increased heart rate and tachycardia.

In hyperventilation syndrome, tachycardia occurs due to increased sympathetic activity.

In shock (hypovolemic shock, cardiogenic shock, obstructive shock, distributive shock (septic shock, anaphylactic shock)), a blood pressure decrease activates the sympathetic nervous system, resulting in tachycardia.

Tachycardia is caused by excessive secretion of thyroid hormones in hyperthyroidism and catecholamines in pheochromocytoma.

Anxiety disorders, especially panic disorder, cause sudden onset of severe anxiety and overactivity of the sympathetic nervous system, resulting in tachycardia, chest discomfort, and sweating.

Dihydropyridine Ca antagonists (especially nifedipine), which are commonly used as antihypertensive agents, may cause reflex tachycardia due to a blood pressure decrease caused by vasodilation.

## 6.3 Bradycardia

Sinus bradycardia, sick sinus syndrome, atrioventricular block (especially complete atrioventricular block), and (bradycardiac) atrial fibrillation are the most common arrhythmias that produce bradycardia.

The pulse rate decreases with age. This is thought to be due to a decrease in the heart rate response to catecholamines and a decrease in coronary artery blood flow that occurs with aging.

People with intense physical exercise habits, especially long-distance runners, often have bradycardia at rest. This is the result of the body's adaptation to be able to run long distances faster with less pulse and blood volume.

The vasovagal reflex is caused by a decrease, in sympathetic tone due to pain, anxiety, or fear, and by an increase in parasympathetic tone, resulting in hypotension, bradycardia, and syncope.

Neurogenic shock is one of distributive shock in which autonomic nervous system dysfunction due to spinal cord injury results in bradycardia and hypotension.

In hypothyroidism, bradycardia occurs due to decreased thyroid hormone action.

Beta-blockers suppress sympathetic nerves, and non-dihydropyridine Ca antagonists (diltiazem, verapamil) suppress atrioventricular (AV) **node** conduction by inhibiting Ca current-dependent conduction, which may result in a decrease in heart rate and bradycardia. Digitalis suppresses AV node conduction by increasing vagal (parasympathetic) nerve activity, resulting in a decrease in heart rate. Severe bradycardia may occur in digitalis intoxication.

# 7 Hypertension and Hypotension

Shin Inoue

## 7.1 Blood Pressure Variation

Blood pressure fluctuates constantly, mainly under the influence of sympathetic and parasympathetic nervous activity. Normally, blood pressure begins to fall after going to bed, reaches its lowest point around 3–4 am, and then gradually rises, increasing sharply on awakening and following daytime activity. This is called diurnal blood pressure variation. In daily life, blood pressure constantly fluctuates due to physical activities such as work, rest, defecation, urination, conversation, and walking, and emotions such as anger and anxiety also affect it. With age, blood pressure rises due to increased sympathetic nerve activity during early morning awakening, resulting in early morning hypertension, which is called morning surge and is a risk factor for arteriosclerosis. In addition to the autonomic nervous activity described above, circulating plasma volume, electrolytes, and the dynamics of various hormones affect blood pressure fluctuations. The factors responsible for the rise and fall in blood pressure will be outlined.

1. Increase in Blood Pressure.

   In general, there are no subjective symptoms when blood pressure is elevated. However, with increased sympathetic nerve activity, patients may complain of headache, stiffness in the shoulders, nervousness, and flushing. Furthermore, mucosal bleeding such as nasal bleeding may occur when blood pressure rises. When abnormalities in blood pressure are observed, multiple measurements should be taken, and if necessary, the difference between the right and left sides and between the upper and lower limbs should be checked. It is also important to check the heart rate and the presence of arrhythmia.

   In the elderly, blood pressure tends to rise upon awakening, and early morning hypertension is more likely to occur in the winter than in the summer. In addition, elderly patients tend to have a greater physical burden when they visit the hospital, and their blood pressure and heart rate tend to increase during the visit. It is necessary to measure blood pressure after taking a break in the waiting room. According to the "Guidelines for the Management of Hypertension 2019," hypertension is defined as a systolic blood pressure of 130 mmHg or higher or a diastolic blood pressure of 80 mmHg or higher measured several times, but please refer to another section for details [6].

   When blood pressure is elevated in an outpatient dental clinic, it is important to conduct a thorough interview. In addition to the patient's medical history, the presence of daily blood pressure measurements and their values, as well as the history and results of physical examinations, will be helpful for future treatment. Even if the patient is being treated for hypertension, if the blood pressure is high at the time of visit, the prescription and the blood pressure at the outpatient clinic should be examined. Furthermore, it is necessary to confirm that the patient is taking the medication as directed.

   White coat hypertension with normal home blood pressure generally does not require medical treatment, but when the blood pressure is markedly elevated at the time of visit, dental phobia and psychiatric disorders such as social anxiety disorder may be suggested in some cases. If the blood pressure is markedly elevated, dental treatment is difficult, and anxiolytics and beta-blockers are administered beforehand. If control is not good, concomitant use of antidepressants such as selective serotonin reuptake inhibitors (SSRIs) or treatment under sedation by a dental anesthesiologist should be considered.

   When chest pain, back pain, headache, or paralysis is observed along with elevated blood pressure, urgent treatment is necessary because of the possibility of dissecting aneurysm of the aorta or cerebral hemorrhage. In addition, hypertension in patients younger than 35 years of age should be differentiated from secondary hypertension such as endocrine disorders such as primary aldosteronism, Cushing's disease, hyperthyroidism, or renal vascular hypertension.

2. Decrease in Blood Pressure.

   Hypotension is broadly classified into orthostatic hypotension, acute hypotension, and chronic hypotension. Acute hypotension includes various types of shock. Chronic hypotension is classified into asymptomatic constitutional hypotension, essential hypotension of unknown cause and symptomatic, and symptomatic hypotension clearly caused by other diseases. The criteria for hypotension are often defined as 90/50 mmHg or less, but no clear criteria have been established for the indication of treatment. The following subjective symptoms, physical findings, and the presence or absence of shock are important.

   Dizziness or light-headedness when standing up are subjective symptoms of decreased blood pressure. Patients may also complain of decreased alertness and drowsiness and may say that they have anemia, which should be described as cerebral anemia. Younger patients complain of tachycardia, palpitations, and cold sweats due to sympathetic reflexes when blood pressure falls rapidly. If the blood pressure falls further, syncopal attack may occur. For shock and fainting, please refer to another section. In the elderly, transient cerebral ischemia may lead to impaired consciousness, dysarthria, hemiplegia, and impaired vision.

   Autonomic nerve function plays a role in lowering blood pressure, and parasympathetic (vagal) nerve activity is important. In children and adolescents, orthostatic disorder (OD), in which blood flow to the body and brain is decreased during waking, has received attention as a cause of school absenteeism [7]. When moving from the supine to the standing position, approximately 500–700 mL of blood descends from the upper body to the lower body; two autonomic mechanisms including baroreceptors are involved in the blood pressure regulation and cerebral blood flow maintenance. One is venous baroreceptors in the atria and vena cava, which monitor changes in blood volume based on the degree of stretch, and carotid sinus baroreceptors, which monitor changes in blood volume based on the degree of stretch. The other is the arterial baroreceptor in the carotid sinus and aorta, which senses changes in arterial pressure and transmits them to the vasomotor center. The cardiac vasomotor center in the medulla oblongata synthesizes these informations and transmits commands to the centrifugal vagus and sympathetic nerves. As a result, cardiac output may be temporarily lowered by about 20% during orthostasis compared with lying down, but blood pressure is maintained at a constant level by constricting the venous vessels mainly in the lower body. In the case of orthostatic dysregulation, it is assumed that the venous blood vessels in the lower body do not constrict during waking, suggesting a malfunction of this regulatory mechanism.

   The vasovagal reflex is thought to account for most of the hypotension that occurs during dental treatment, but pain and intraoral stabbing against a background of anxiety and stress stimulate the cardiovascular motor center in the medulla oblongata via the vagal afferent branch, resulting in a decrease in heart rate and blood pressure due to vasodilation. For more information about this, please refer to the guidelines of the Japanese Dental Society of Anesthesiology [8]. In general, patients recover within a few minutes without any sequelae, but in repeated cases, psychiatric disorders or autonomic abnormalities should be considered. If anxiety is strong, dental phobia should be considered and anxiolytic agents and beta-blockers should be administered, but combined use of antidepressants such as SSRIs may be effective. Adequate sedation and systemic management with the cooperation of a dental anesthesiologist is also recommended.

In the elderly, orthostatic hypotension is more likely to occur after a meal because of increased vagal activity and concentration of blood in the gastrointestinal tract. The presence or absence of antihypertensive medication, its type and dosage, and the concomitant use of calcium channel blockers and grapefruit juice should be noted. In the summer, dehydration and heat stroke may affect the patient, but elderly patients are more likely to fall and suffer fractures as their blood pressure decreases.

In addition, myocardial infarction and drug anaphylaxis tend to have a poor prognosis. It is important to note risk factors such as allergies, obesity, and diabetes. NSAIDs (nonsteroidal anti-inflammatory drugs) tend to cause painless gastric ulcers, and hypotension due to gastrointestinal bleeding should be noted. Shy-Drager syndrome, amyloid neuropathy, and Addison's disease are other conditions that can cause chronic, intractable hypotensive attacks and should be differentiated.

## References


1. Sugimoto T, et al., editors. Internal medicine. 9th ed. Tokyo: Asakura Shoten; 2008. p. 413–5. (in Japanese).
2. Nishida J, et al., editors. Internal medicine for the odontology. Revised 4 ed. Tokyo: Nankaido; 2018. p. 44–5. (in Japanese).
3. Uchiyama S, Tomino K, Imai Y, editors. Nephrology for specialists. 2nd ed. Tokyo: Igaku Shoin; 2009. p. 77–83. (in Japanese).
4. Fukagawa M, Yasuda T, editors. Manual of kidney diseases for residents. 3rd ed. Tokyo: Igaku Shoin; 2017. p. 33–6. (in Japanese).
5. Fukai T, Kurokawa K, supervisors. Harrison's principles of internal medicine. 5th ed. Tokyo: Medical Science International; 2015. (in Japanese).
6. The Japanese Society of Hypertension, Committee for the Preparation of Hypertension. Guidelines for the Management of Hypertension 2019. Tokyo: Life Science Publishing; 2019. (in Japanese).
7. Tanaka H. Instantaneous orthostatic hypotension, postural tachycardia syndrome and neurally mediated syncope in children. Pediatr Cardiol Card Surg. 2001;17(1):8–19.
8. The Japanese Dental Society of Anesthesiology. Guidelines for treatment of vasovagal reflex during dental treatment. The Japanese Dental Society of Anesthesiology; 2018 (in Japanese). http://kokuhoken.net/jdsa/publication/file/guideline/guideline_vasovagalreflex.pdf.

# 3 Digestive Symptoms

Shogo Ohkoshi, Jiro Nishida, Takahiko Kudo, Tatsushi Omatsu, Shinya Maejima, and Yukihide Nishimura

## 1 Weight Loss/Weight Increase

Shogo Ohkoshi

Body mass index (BMI) is calculated by dividing body weight (kg) by the square of height (m), and the range of 18.5–25 is considered normal. BMI of 22 is considered to be the weight least susceptible to disease, and the square of height (m) multiplied by 22 is the standard weight. However, because body weight depends on the skeletal system of the individual, the degree of weight loss or gain is important and often associated with diseases.

Weight loss occurs when metabolic catabolism (wasting) continues to exceed food and water intake. Weight loss may be defined as a loss of 5% or more of body weight within 6 months without excessive exercise or dieting, but any subjective symptoms, regardless of duration or severity, should be treated with caution because they may indicate a hidden disease. Age is also an important factor when considering the cause of weight loss. Gastrointestinal symptoms such as decreased appetite, dysphagia sensation, and diarrhea, metabolic and endocrine symptoms such as thirst and sweating, and psychiatric symptoms such as insomnia and anxiety should be noted. Diseases that cause weight loss include the following.

### 1.1 Malignant Tumor

The most common cancers that cause weight loss are those of the digestive system, such as pancreatic cancer and advanced gastric cancer. Esophageal cancer causes symptoms of dysphagia, and colorectal cancer causes symptoms of intestinal obstruction such as abdominal pain, diarrhea, anemia, and constipation. In general, patients who experience weight loss can be considered to be in an advanced stage.

S. Ohkoshi (✉)
School of Life Dentistry at Niigata, The Nippon Dental University, Niigata, Japan
e-mail: okoshi@ngt.ndu.ac.jp

J. Nishida
Department of Gastroenterology, Tokyo Dental College, Ichikawa General Hospital, Ichikawa, Chiba, Japan

T. Kudo
Department of Gastroenterology, Health Sciences University of Hokkaido, Sapporo, Hokkaido, Japan

T. Omatsu
Molecular Gastroenterology and Hepatology, Graduate School of Medical Science, Kyoto Prefectural University of Medicine, Kyoto, Japan

S. Maejima
Matsumoto Dental University, Shiojiri, Nagano, Japan

Y. Nishimura
Department of Rehabilitation Medicine, Iwate Medical University School of Medicine, Yahaba, Iwate, Japan



T. Chiba, H. Yamada (eds.), *Internal Medicine for Dental Treatments*,
https://doi.org/10.1007/978-981-99-3296-2_3

### 1.2 Endocrine and Hematologic Diseases and Chronic Infectious Diseases

When diabetes mellitus progresses and hyperglycemia persists, body catabolism increases, resulting in weight loss. Patients often complain of dry mouth due to hyperglycemia. Diabetes mellitus is also a common complication of pancreatic cancer. Hyperthyroidism is also a typical disease causing weight loss. It is common in young women and is accompanied by characteristic symptoms such as swelling of the thyroid gland, protrusion of the eyes, and sweating. Blood diseases such as malignant lymphoma, chronic diseases such as tuberculosis, and hypoadrenalism also cause weight loss.

### 1.3 Mental Illness

Depression is one of the most frequent and common disorders that cause weight loss. It is caused by a decrease in appetite food intake. The presence or absence of symptoms such as insomnia is helpful in diagnosis. Anorexia nervosa occurs in young women. It is associated with an extreme aversion to weight gain and repeated vomiting. In alcoholics, weight loss is caused by constant drinking and reduced nutritional intake. It is important to interview the patient's life history as well as drug addiction.

### 1.4 Chronic Diarrhea

When diarrhea continues, mainly due to gastrointestinal diseases, weight loss occurs due to malabsorption. Intestinal diseases such as Crohn's disease, ulcerative colitis, and infectious enteritis are considered. Since the pancreas is an organ that secretes digestive enzymes, chronic pancreatitis also causes weight loss due to diarrhea.

### 1.5 Diseases of the Elderly

In general, weight loss occurs gradually with age. However, weight loss becomes more pronounced with the onset of other diseases. In dementia, physical activity gradually declines, and the amount of food eaten also decreases, resulting in weight loss. Recently, "frailty" has been attracting attention. It mainly refers to cases in which weight loss, muscle weakness, and walking speed decrease with aging. In addition, "sarcopenia" refers to a decrease in muscle mass. It is important as a precursor to the transition to "bedridden" in the elderly.

The accumulation of visceral fat causes the metabolic syndrome. This induces hypertension, diabetes mellitus, and hyperlipidemia, leading to the progression of arteriosclerosis and ultimately to diseases such as myocardial infarction, cerebral infarction, and chronic kidney disease. On the other hand, when weight gain occurs in patients with chronic heart failure, renal failure, or ascites due to liver cirrhosis, it indicates excessive accumulation of water in the body, and diuretics are necessary.

## 2 Jaundice

Jiro Nishida

Jaundice is a yellowish pigmentation of the skin and mucous membranes seen when serum bilirubin levels are elevated. The standard levels of total serum bilirubin range from 0.2 to 1.0 mg/dL, but when the levels are elevated approximately 2 mg/dL, a yellowish pigmentation can be confirmed on the examination of the bulbar conjunctiva. When the levels exceed approximately 4 mg/dL, jaundice can be diagnosed by physical examination of the skin (Fig. 3.1).

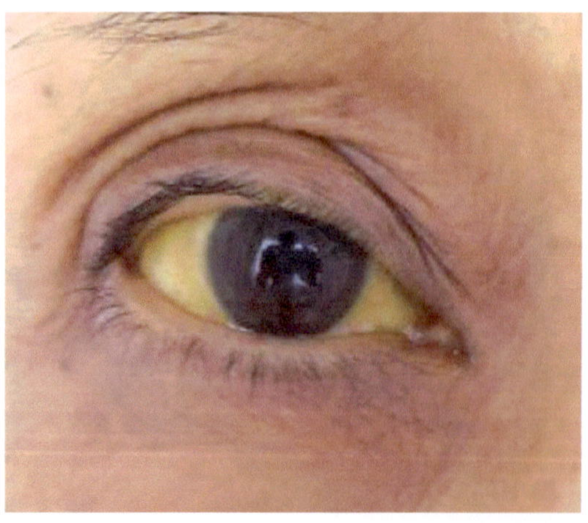

**Fig. 3.1** Jaundice observed in the bulbar conjunctiva

Carotenosis is an orange discoloration of the palms and soles caused by the excessive consumption of carotene-rich foods such as oranges and pumpkins and can be distinguished from jaundice because of the absent of the bulbar conjunctival pigmentation.

Bilirubin is produced by the release of hemoglobin from senescent red blood cells. Before conjugation to glucuronic acid in hepatocytes, bilirubin is called indirect bilirubin and is non-soluble. After glucuronic acid conjugation, it is called direct bilirubin, which is water-soluble and excreted into bile, and intestinal bacteria convert the bilirubin to urobilinogen, which is excreted in stool and urine. Some of urobilinogen is reabsorbed from the intestine and transported into the liver (enterohepatic circulation). Jaundice is caused by increased

serum bilirubin levels due to various pathophysiological disorders.

The classification of jaundice is as follows.

### 2.1 Indirect Type Predominant Hyperbilirubinemia

In hemolytic anemia, erythrocyte destruction is increased, and the production of indirect bilirubin is excessive and cannot be fully conjugated by hepatocytes. In addition to a decrease in hemoglobin concentration and increased indirect bilirubin, there is an increased reticulocyte count, decreased serum haptoglobin, and an increased urinary and fecal urobilin. In liver failure due to end-stage cirrhosis or fulminant hepatitis, indirect type hyperbilirubinemia may be observed because of decreased hepatocyte conjugation capacity.

### 2.2 Hepatocellular Jaundice

This is typically seen in acute hepatitis A and B, but it is also seen in various hepatic disorders such as alcoholic, drug-induced, and autoimmune hepatitis. With hepatocyte degeneration and necrosis, transaminases (AST (aspartate transaminase) and ALT (alanine transaminase)) increase rapidly, and hyperbilirubinemia appears due to impaired transport and conjugation of bilirubin in the liver. Jaundice observed in end-stage cirrhosis and fulminant hepatitis is also classified as hepatocellular in its pathogenesis.

### 2.3 Intrahepatic Bile Stasis

This is a jaundice caused by impaired bile excretion in the capillary bile ducts between the hepatocytes, without any obvious mechanical obstruction of the biliary system. The most common causes of intrahepatic cholestasis are drug-induced acute cases and, in chronic cases, primary biliary cholangitis (PBC) and primary sclerosing cholangitis (PSC).

### 2.4 Obstructive Jaundice

This is caused by mechanical obstruction of the biliary system and presents with direct type hyperbilirubinemia. The obstruction may be caused by biliary stones (e.g., common bile duct stones), biliary infections (e.g., cholangitis), or malignant tumors (e.g., cholangiocarcinoma or pancreatic head cancer). The diagnosis can be made by confirming the dilatation of the bile ducts in and outside the liver by imaging studies.

### 2.5 Constitutional Jaundice

Inborn errors of bilirubin metabolism in the liver include Crigler-Najjar syndrome and Gilbert's syndrome, which are characterized by indirect bilirubin predominance, and Dubin-Johnson syndrome and Rotor syndrome, which are characterized by direct bilirubin predominance. Gilbert's syndrome occurs in 3–7% of the Japanese population and is frequently encountered in daily practice.

## 3 Nausea and Vomiting [1, 2]

Takahiko Kudo

### 3.1 Definitions

Nausea is an urgent, unpleasant feeling of wanting to vomit up the contents of the stomach. Vomiting is a vigorous expulsion of gastric contents, which may or may not be accompanied by nausea.

## 3.2 Pathophysiology

Vomiting is thought to be mediated by the vomiting center located in the dorsal nucleus of the vagus in the medulla oblongata. There are two main stimulation pathways to the vomiting center, and vomiting is thought to be induced by central and peripheral stimulation.

1. Central Stimulation

   It is caused by direct stimulation of the vomiting center by mechanical stimuli such as increased cerebral pressure and stroke, chemical stimuli such as anticancer drugs, and sensory stimuli such as mental stress and foul odor.
2. Peripheral Stimulation

   Vomiting occurs when the vomiting center is stimulated by gastrointestinal stimuli such as dyspepsia, toxins, drugs, and inflammation or by vagal stimuli from the vestibular nerve of the inner ear and cerebellum caused by motion sickness and dizziness.

## 3.3 Causal Disease

Nausea and vomiting are caused by a variety of diseases, which can be divided into central and peripheral disorders (Table 3.1).

## 3.4 How to Proceed with the Diagnosis

Because of the wide variety of diseases that cause nausea and vomiting, as shown in Table 3.1, it is often difficult to make a diagnosis immediately. When a patient with vomiting is seen, it is very important to determine the urgency and severity of the disease by accurately ascertaining vital signs (state of con-

**Table 3.1** Diseases that cause nausea and vomiting

| Central irritant disorder | |
|---|---|
| Increased intracranial pressure | Brain hypertension, hemorrhage with increased cerebral pressure, subarachnoid hemorrhage, brain tumor, and meningitis |
| Cerebral circulatory disorder | Shock, hypoxic encephalopathy, cerebral infarction, and encephalitis |
| Upper central stimulation | Anorexia nervosa, epilepsy, depression, aversion, fear, stress, and visual/olfactory/gustatory stimulation |
| Addiction | Morphine, digitalis, antibacterials, anticancer drugs, antihypertensive drugs, aminophylline, colchicine, alcohol, etc. |
| Systemic disease | Diabetic ketoacidosis, uremia, and adrenal insufficiency |
| Others | Morning sickness and pregnancy toxemia |
| | |
| Peripheral irritation disorder | |
| Digestive disorder | |
| • Malignant tumor | Gastric cancer, colorectal cancer, esophageal cancer, liver cancer, pancreatic cancer, and small intestinal cancer |
| • Esophageal | Mallory-Weiss syndrome, gastroesophageal reflux disease (GERD), and esophageal hiatal hernia |
| • Gastrointestinal diseases | Acute gastritis, peptic ulcer, acute enteritis, acute appendicitis, food poisoning, parasite, peritonitis, intestinal obstruction, and pyloric stenosis |
| • Biliary and pancreatic diseases | Cholelithiasis, acute cholecystitis, acute cholangitis, and acute pancreatitis |
| • Liver diseases | Cirrhosis and acute hepatitis |
| Cardiovascular diseases | Congestive heart failure, angina pectoris, and acute myocardial infarction |
| Urological diseases | Ureteral calculus, renal calculus, pyelonephritis |
| Otolaryngological diseases | Otitis media, Meniere's disease, motion sickness, direct pharyngeal irritation |
| Eye disease | Glaucoma |
| Gynecological diseases | Uterine adnexitis, menstrual molimen, and climacteric disturbance |

**Table 3.2** Symptoms associated with vomiting and diseases that should be differentiated from the medical history

| | |
|---|---|
| Sudden severe headache and disturbance of consciousness | Subarachnoid hemorrhage |
| Abdominal pain, pediatric, and mucous feces | Intussusception |
| Chest pain, shortness of breath, and cold sweat | Myocardial infarction |
| Female, nausea during fasting, and the symptom improves after eating | Morning sickness |
| Fever and pericardial umbilical pain | Appendicitis |
| Binge eating and persistent orbital pain | Acute pancreatitis |
| Persistent upper abdominal pain, abdominal pain after meals, and history of gallstones | Attack of biliary colic |
| Fever, headache, and disturbance of consciousness | Meningitis |
| Abdominal pain, deep tachypnea, and disorientation | Diabetic ketoacidosis |
| Abdominal pain, constipation, and full stomach | Intestinal obstruction |
| Anorexia, constipation, thirst, and polyuria | Hypercalcemia |
| Bacterial gastroenteritis due to ingestion of raw foods and the presence of others with the same symptoms | Bacterial gastroenteritis |
| Fever and psychiatric symptoms | Encephalitis |
| NSAIDs oral | Gastric ulcer |
| Cirrhosis of the liver, abdominal pain, and fever | Idiopathic bacterial peritonitis |

sciousness, temperature, blood pressure, pulse rate, respiratory rate, presence of shock, and temperature of the extremities). In some cases, it is possible to narrow down the differential from the accompanying symptoms and medical history (Table 3.2).

## 3.5 Important Points of Physical Examination

Vital signs (state of consciousness, temperature, blood pressure, pulse rate, respiratory rate, presence of shock, and temperature of extremities), muscle weakness, body size (lean or obese), jaundice and rash, and the presence of seizures and involuntary movements are most important. Although the physical examination in the dental office is limited, the following points should be considered when performing the physical examination, keeping in mind systemic diseases that may cause nausea and vomiting (Table 3.3).

**Table 3.3** Points to consider when performing a physical examination

| | |
|---|---|
| Conjunctiva | Anemia and jaundice |
| Head | Bruise and presence of trauma |
| Eye | Difference of ocular pupil and presence of nystagmus |
| Exhaled | Ammonia odor, acetone odor, and fecal odor |
| Cervical | Cervical rigidity, thyroid gland, and presence of enlarged lymph nodes |
| Chest | Cardiopulmonary disease |
| Abdominal | Muscular defenses, presence of ascites, hepatomegaly, abdominal masses, and tarry stool |
| Back | Percussive pain |

When vomiting occurs, it is important to observe the vomitus for the presence of indigestible materials, blood, and bile. If vomiting occurs suddenly during dental treatment, be careful to avoid aspiration. If the situation is judged to be urgent, it is important to arrange for emergency transportation to a higher-order medical institution immediately.

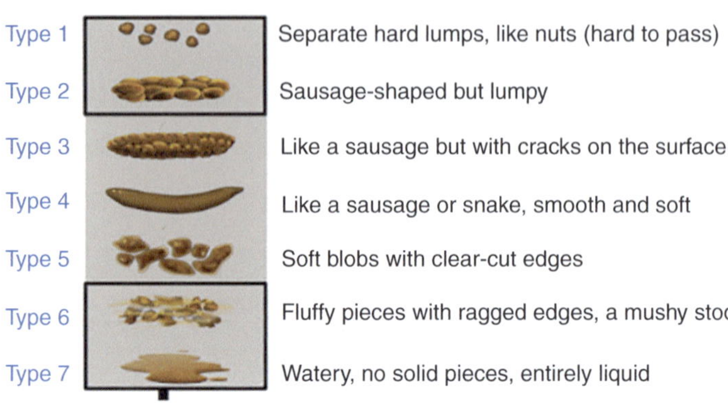


**Fig. 3.2** The Bristol Stool Form Scale [3]. *Type 1*: Separate hard lumps like nuts (hard to pass). *Type 2*: Sausage-shaped but lumpy. *Type 3*: Like a sausage but with cracks on the surface. *Type 4*: Like a sausage or snake, smooth and soft. *Type 5*: Soft blobs with clear-cut edges. *Type 6*: Fluffy pieces with ragged edges, a mushy stool. *Type 7*: Watery, no solid pieces, and entirely liquid

# 4 Diarrhea

Tatsushi Omatsu

## 4.1 Overview

Diarrhea is defined as frequent discharge of muddy to liquid stools with high water content and a stool weight exceeding 200 g/day. The composition of stool is 60–70% water, 15–20% mucosal cells detached from the intestinal tract, 10–15% intestinal bacteria and their carcasses, and 5–10% indigestible food residues, with very little food debris and mostly water. When the water content in stool is 70–80%, it is soft stool; when 80–90%, it is muddy stool; and when more than 90%, it is watery stool. The shape of stool is generally expressed by the Bristol Stool Form Scale, and diarrhea is classified into type 6 and type 7 (Fig. 3.2) [3–5].

## 4.2 Disease [6–8]

About 9 L of water enters the gastrointestinal tract daily, of which 2 L is from oral intake such as meals and drinking water, and 7 L is from secretions such as saliva, gastric juice, bile, pancreatic juice, and intestinal juice. Ninety-nine percent of this water is absorbed in the small intestine (approximately 7.5 L) and large intestine (approximately 1.5 L). Therefore, even a small decrease in water absorption in the intestine or a small increase in secretions is sufficient to cause diarrhea. Four mechanisms of diarrhea are described below.

1. Osmotic Diarrhea

   It is caused by water-soluble solutes, which are not easily absorbed by the intestinal tract, remaining in the intestine and causing water retention. Such solutes include magnesium salts and polyethylene glycol, which are used as laxatives for constipation. High-fructose corn syrup is used as a sweetener in place of sugar, but it is not readily absorbed, and osmotic diarrhea occurs when a large amount is ingested. Lactulose, which is used as a laxative, has a similar mechanism.
2. Secretory Diarrhea

   Diarrhea occurs when the secretion of water and electrolytes into the intestinal tract exceeds absorption. Infection is the most common cause of secretory diarrhea, and the secretion is increased by enterotoxin secreted by bacteria. Unabsorbed dietary fat and bile acids stimulate secretion in the colon and cause diarrhea. Excessive production of hormones that stimulate intestinal secretion, such as VIP (vasoactive intestinal peptide) and gastrin, from endocrine tumors also causes diarrhea.

**Table 3.4** Main conditions and diseases causing diarrhea

| | |
|---|---|
| Acute diarrhea | |
| Infectious | Viral infections: norovirus, rotavirus |
| | Bacterial infection: *Campylobacter*, *Salmonella*, *Vibrio parahaemolyticus*, *Pathogenic escherichia coli*, and *Pseudomembranous enteritis* |
| Toxic | Food poisoning (toxin-producing bacteria): *Staphylococcus aureus* and *Bacillus cereus* |
| | Heavy metals: arsenic and mercury |
| Drug-induced | Massive laxative ingestion, anticancer drugs, and antimicrobial drugs |
| Allergic | Eosinophilic gastroenteritis and food allergy |
| Others | Binge eating, ingestion of indigestible food, ischemic colitis, and psychogenic |
| Chronic diarrhea | |
| Infectious | Viral infections: Cytomegalovirus |
| | Bacterial infection: Intestinal tuberculosis |
| | Parasites: Entamoeba histolytica and Giardia lamblia |
| Functional | Irritable bowel syndrome |
| Inflammatory bowel disease | Ulcerative colitis and Crohn's disease |
| Drug-induced | Collagenous colitis (mainly caused by proton pump inhibitors and NSAIDs) |
| Malabsorption | Celiac disease, chronic pancreatitis, and lactose intolerance |
| After surgical | Resection or bypass of the stomach or intestines |
| Endocrine tumors | VIPoma, Gastrinoma, and carcinoid |
| Systemic disease | Hyperthyroidism and diabetes mellitus |

3. Mucosal-Damaging Diarrhea

   Inflammatory bowel diseases, such as ulcerative colitis and Crohn's disease, and various bacterial enteritis cause damage to the intestinal mucosa, resulting in increased permeability and the discharge of large amounts of leachate into the intestinal lumen, as well as impaired absorption, resulting in diarrhea.
4. Diarrhea Due to Decreased Transit Time and Surface Area

   When the gastrointestinal tract is short and has a small surface area, such as post gastric or intestinal resection, or when intestinal motility is increased due to irritable bowel syndrome or hyperthyroidism, water absorption is insufficient, resulting in diarrhea.

Clinically, diarrhea is classified into two groups: acute diarrhea, which occurs rapidly and usually resolves in a few days to a week, and chronic diarrhea, which lasts more than 3–4 weeks (Table 3.4). In terms of frequency, acute diarrhea is often caused by infectious enteritis caused by viruses or bacteria, and chronic diarrhea is often caused by irritable bowel syndrome.

## 4.3 Diagnosis and Treatment

The interview should be included detailed information about the stool, such as duration, frequency, and characteristics (presence of blood, pus, or mucus); dietary information for the days prior to the onset; information about outbreaks, such as epidemics at home or at work; physical symptoms, such as nausea, vomiting, abdominal pain, fever, and changes in weight and appetite; medication, overseas travel, and history of abdominal surgery. During the medical examination, the presence of high fever, bloody stools, and dehydration should always be checked as symptoms suggestive of more serious conditions. For dehydration, check for thirst, decreased urine output, decreased blood pressure, tachycardia, and decreased skin turgor (when it takes more than 2 s for the skin to return to its original flat state after being picked up and released). If there is blood in the stool, consultation with a specialist should be considered.

### 4.4 Treatment

The basic treatment of diarrhea is to prevent or correct dehydration by replacing fluids and electrolytes. If oral intake is possible, oral rehydration solution containing electrolytes and carbohydrates should be recommended. Patients with diarrhea occasionally refrain from taking fluids because they feel that taking fluids will increase the frequency of toilet, therefore the risk of dehydration should be explained and patients should be advised to drink small amounts of fluids frequently. If oral intake is difficult due to frequent vomiting, fluid infusion should be administered. Most cases of infectious diarrhea resolve with correction of dehydration alone, and therefore, easy administration of antibiotics should be avoided. If specific infectious enterocolitis that requires antimicrobial therapy is suspected, consultation with a specialist should be considered. As for antidiarrheals, diarrhea is a defensive response to expel enterotoxins and pathogens from the intestinal tract, and therefore, easy use of antidiarrheals should be avoided.

## 5 Anorexia and Nausea [9, 10]

Shinya Maejima

### 5.1 Conditions in Which the Symptoms Appear

Anorexia is a decrease or loss of appetite.

The appetite center is located in the hypothalamus, which balances and regulates feeding through two mechanisms: facilitation and inhibition. The hypothalamus receives signals from the periphery, and instinctive appetite is generated. It is then transmitted to higher centers in the cerebral cortex, where it is recognized and integrated into feeding behavior. For example, elevated blood glucose, as a humoral signal in the circulating blood, suppresses the facilitatory mechanism in the hypothalamus and stimulates the inhibitory mechanism, which is related to the cessation of feeding behavior. In addition, gastric wall stretch is transmitted from vagal afferents to the medulla oblongata as a neural signal, which is then transmitted to the hypothalamus as a signal in the central nervous system, stimulating inhibitory mechanisms. Because of the complexity of the factors involved, the etiology of anorexia varies widely (Table 3.5).

**Table 3.5** Diseases that cause anorexia

| |
|---|
| A. Internal disease |
| 1. Digestive disorders |
| (a) Oral diseases such as oral hypofunction |
| (b) Esophageal disease |
| (c) Gastric and duodenal diseases |
| (d) Small intestinal and colorectal disease |
| (e) Liver and biliary tract diseases |
| (f) Pancreatic disease |
| (g) Peritoneal disease |
| 2. Diseases other than digestive organs |
| (a) Cerebral nerve disease |
| (b) Metabolic and endocrine disorders |
| (c) Respiratory disease |
| (d) Cardiovascular disease |
| (e) Renal disease |
| (f) Blood disorders |
| (g) Infectious disease |
| B. Mental illness |
| (a) Organic mental disorder (dementia) |
| (b) Anorexia nervosa |
| (c) Mood disorder (depression) |
| (d) Schizophrenia |
| (e) Neurotic disorders and stress-related disorders |
| C. Drugs and addiction |
| (a) Drugs such as anticancer drugs, industrial drugs, alcohol, etc. |
| D. Pregnancy |
| (a) Hyperemesis gravidarum |

Anorexia is a common feature and nonspecific symptom of a variety of organic diseases. It is often associated with psychological factors or problems in daily life, or it may be the result of a serious underlying disease such as cancer.

Nausea is a subjective symptom of feeling as if one is about to vomit and is accompanied by a feeling of discomfort in the pharynx, anterior chest, and upper abdomen. It may also be accompanied by pallor, cold sweats, increased salivation, and other autonomic nervous system changes. Nausea is a common precursor to vomiting that is a reflex discharge of gastric contents.

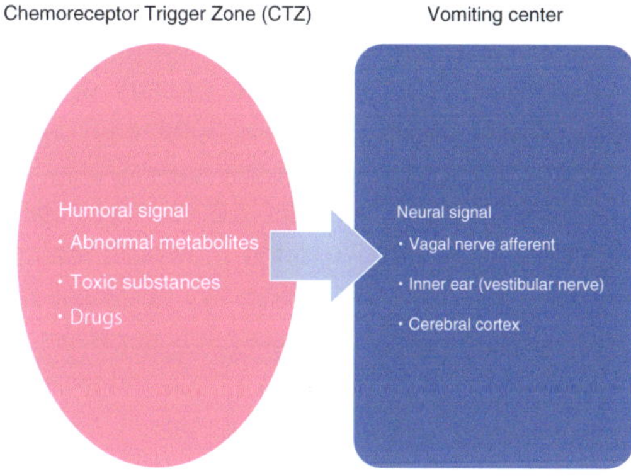


**Fig. 3.3** Stimulus transmission of nausea

The vomiting center in the medulla oblongata is involved, and the pathway of transmission differs depending on the etiology of the nausea. Abnormalities in the stomach, intestinal tract, and other internal organs are transmitted to the vomiting center via the vagus nerve. Abnormalities of the vestibular organs in the inner ear also stimulate the vomiting center via the vestibular nerve. As a humoral signal, the chemoreceptor trigger zone (CTZ) in the caudal margin of the fourth ventricle detects toxic substances in the blood or spinal fluid and stimulates the vomiting center (Fig. 3.3).

The fact that the CTZ is an anatomical region that is not protected by the blood-brain barrier makes it suitable as a defense mechanism against toxic substances.

## 5.2 Differentiated Diseases

Persistent nausea often leads to anorexia. The first step is to thoroughly differentiate between medical and psychiatric disorders. If medical disease is suspected, gastroenterological disease should be diagnosed next. Drugs, poisoning, and, in women of appropriate age, pregnancy should also be considered (Fig. 3.4).

**Fig. 3.4** Etiology of anorexia and nausea

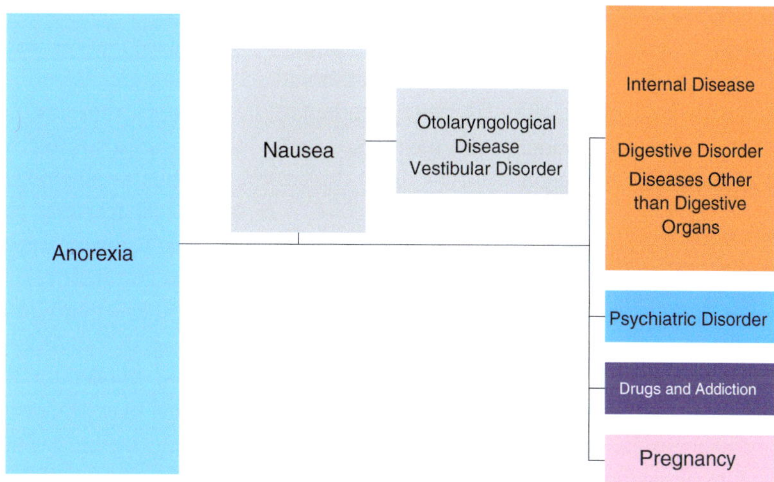

## 6 Dysphagia [11, 12]

Yukihide Nishimura

Swallowing refers to the process of recognizing food, taking it into the mouth, chewing it, sending it to the pharynx, and passing it through the esophagus. In general, the swallowing process is divided into three phases, oral, pharyngeal, and esophageal phases, but it is also often referred to as a five-phase process that includes a preceding phase during which food is recognized and a preparation phase during which food is chewed to form a food mass (Fig. 3.5).

### 6.1 Causes of Dysphagia

It is classified into two categories: organic causes such as postoperative pharyngeal cancer of the oral cavity, pharynx, larynx, and esophagus, and functional causes such as cerebrovascular disorders and degenerative diseases such as Parkinson's disease. As the population ages, the effects of aging should also be considered. Aging increases the threshold of saltiness and bitterness in the sense of taste. The atrophy of salivary glands and the decrease in the number of remaining teeth make it difficult to form food masses by mastication. In addition, the onset of the swallowing reflex is delayed and the speed of the swallowing reflex movement decreases. In addition, immobility, lack of use, and unnecessary fasting should be taken into consideration, as well as incompatibility of tracheal cannulae and dentures, which can also cause dysphagia.

### 6.2 Symptoms of Dysphagia

The most common causes of dysphagia are swallowing, coughing, hoarseness, dehydration, low nutrition, xerostomia, oral contamination, fever, and pneumonia. Repeated saliva swallowing tests and water swallowing tests are simple and useful screening tests for dysphagia. The swallowing process itself can be visualized and evaluated by swallowing contrast examination. Swallowing endoscopy is simple and can be performed at the bedside, and it can evaluate the movement of the vocal cords, pyriform sinus, and the presence of residual material in the epiglottic vallecula. However, it has several disadvantages, including the inability to see the moment of swallowing and the fact that small aspirations may be missed.

### 6.3 Rehabilitation Treatment of Feeding and Swallowing Disorders

Unnecessary fasting management can lead to oral contamination and a decrease in swallowing function. Adequate oral care should be actively provided to prevent aspiration pneumonia and to facilitate early oral intake.

Swallowing training can be broadly divided into indirect training without food and direct training with food.

Indirect training includes ice massage, aperture training, shakia training, blowing training, and tube swallowing training. As treatment for the preparatory and oral phases, it is necessary to strengthen the muscles of the tongue and perioral muscles and to improve the range of motion. Chewing gum is also effective. As treatment for the pharyngeal phase, efforts should be made to strengthen the neck muscles and improve the range of motion. It is also important to induce pharyngeal reflexes and to strengthen the closure of the nasopharynx and pharynx. Swallowing and coughing are also effective. Strengthening of the respiratory muscles, cough training, and vocal training are also effective. Direct training includes conscious swallowing, breath-holding swallowing, neck rotation, and bite volume control. Feeding using positions with neck flexion and rotation and multiple swallowing are also effective. Other environmental adjustments include adjusting the environment, posture, and eating patterns, thickening liquids, adjusting medications that may decrease swallowing function, and adapting dentures. Gastrostomy should be considered when tube feeding needs to be continued for more than 1 month. Patients with a gastrostomy are often able to take food orally over time, so it is advisable to reevaluate swallowing function at appropriate times.

Pre-oral (anticipatory) phase:

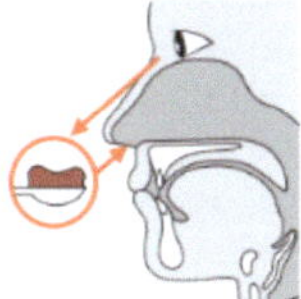

The period of recognition of food. It leads to appetite, saliva secretion, and movement of the digestive tract.

Oral preparation phase:

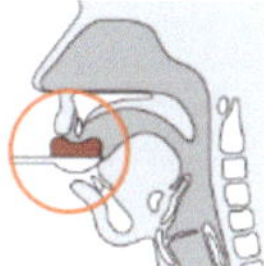

The period when food is chewed and mixed with saliva to form a food mass.

Oral phase:

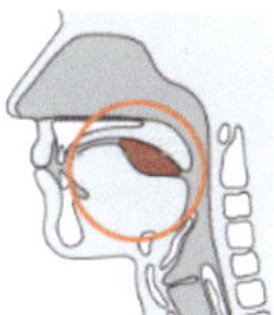

This is the period when food masses formed in the oral cavity are delivered to the pharynx by tongue movement. It is important that the tongue is firmly attached to the anterior part of the palate to deliver the food mass.

Pharyngeal phase:

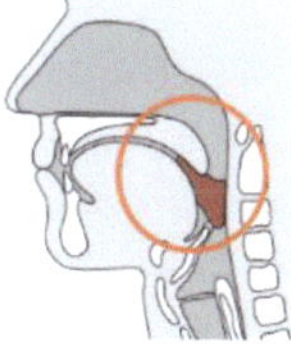

The swallowing reflex is the time when the food mass is delivered from the pharynx to the esophagus. It is usually complete in about 0.5 seconds.

Esophageal phase:

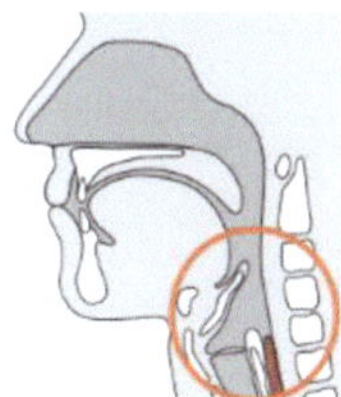

The period during which the food mass passes through the esophageal inlet and is transported to the stomach. The upper esophageal sphincter prevents reflux into the pharynx, and the lower esophageal sphincter prevents gastroesophageal reflux.

**Fig. 3.5** Five stages of feeding and swallowing

Patients with dysphagia are at increased risk for dehydration and undernutrition. Dehydration and malnutrition can further exacerbate dysphagia and interfere with rehabilitation therapy. It is important to understand the importance of nutritional management.

## References


1. Asaka M, Kanno K, Chiba T, editors. Gastroenterology. Tokyo: Nishimura Shoten; 2013. p. 146–50. (in Japanese)
2. Yazaki Y, supervised. New clinical internal medicine. 10th ed. Tokyo: Igaku Shoin; 2020. p. 41–3. (in Japanese).
3. The Japanese Society of Gastroenterology. Evidence-based clinical practice guidelines for irritable bowel syndrome 2020. 2nd ed. Tokyo: Nankodo; 2020. (in Japanese).
4. O'Donnell LJD, et al. Detection of pseudodiarrhoea by simple clinical assessment of intestinal transit rate. Br Med J. 1990;300(6722):439–40.
5. Longstreth GF, et al. Functional bowel disorders. Gastroenterology. 2006;130(5):1480–91.
6. Japanese Society of Laboratory Medicine. Guidelines for clinical laboratory medicine JSLM 2018 - laboratory approaches/symptoms/diseases. Tokyo: Japanese Society for Clinical Laboratory Medicine; 2021. p. 179–81. (in Japanese).
7. Makuuchi M, et al., editors. Guidelines for the treatment of digestive diseases today. 3rd ed. Tokyo: Igaku Shoin; 2010. p. 20–2. (in Japanese).
8. MSD manual professional version professional/gastrointestinal disorders/symptoms of gastrointestinal disorders/diarrhea. https://www.msdmanuals.com/ja-jp/.
9. Imura H, et al. Integrated handbook of internal medicine, vol. 3. Tokyo: Nakayama Shoten; 1996. p. 8–16, 306–10. (in Japanese).
10. Hesketh PJ. Chemotherapy-induced nausea and vomiting. N Engl J Med. 2008;358:2482–94.
11. Supervised by the Japan Society for Rehabilitation Medicine. Core textbook of rehabilitation medicine and medical care. Tokyo: Igaku Shoin; 2022. (in Japanese).
12. Yonemoto K. Contemporally textbook of rehabilitation medicine. 3rd ed. Tokyo, Ishiyaku Publishers, Inc. (in Japanese).

# 4 Neurological and Psychosomal Symptoms

Hiroaki Ooboshi, Kotaro Otsuka, Kenzo Koizumi, Masayo Fukuhara, Hideo Niwa, Kazuhiro Muramatsu, and Toshimi Chiba

## 1 Headache

Hiroaki Ooboshi

Headache is one of the most common neurological symptoms experienced by most people. Headache can also be caused by ingestion of cold confectionery such as shaved ice, and most headaches are functional in nature without any lesions. However, headache can be caused by a wide variety of causes, and attention should be paid to serious organic diseases, such as subarachnoid hemorrhage, that require urgent transport to a specialist. Many headaches are associated with the dental field and chronic headache has a significant impact on quality of life, so it is important to identify the cause of the headache and provide adequate treatment.

In the brain parenchyma, there are no nociceptors (pain receptors). In the cranium, pain is felt by stimulation of the meninges and vascular walls on the surface of the brain and by stimulation of cranial nerves related to pain perception (trigeminal nerve, glossopharyngeal nerve, and vagus nerve). Outside the cranium, nociceptive sensory nerves distributed in the periosteum, fascia, and scalp that cover the cranium, may detect the nociceptive stimuli sensory as headache.

To understand the pathogenesis of headache, it is helpful to refer to the international classification used by the Japanese Headache Society [1] (Table 4.1). Primary headaches without lesions (functional headaches), such as migraine, often recur and are referred to as chronic headaches. Secondary headache (symptomatic headache) associated with intracranial or related organ lesions, such as cerebrovascular disease, brain tumors, and meningitis, should be discriminated. Other types of headache include painful cerebral neuropathy. Headaches directly related to the dental field are

H. Ooboshi
Department of Internal Medicine, Fukuoka Dental College, Fukuoka, Japan

K. Otsuka (✉)
Department of Neuropsychiatry, Iwate Medical University School of Medicine, Yahaba, Iwate, Japan
e-mail: kotaro29@df6.so-net.ne.jp

K. Koizumi
Department of Neurology, Tokyo Dental College, Ichikawa General Hospital, Ichikawa, Chiba, Japan

M. Fukuhara
Division of General Internal Medicine, Kyushu Dental University Faculty of Dentistry, Kitakyushu, Fukuoka, Japan

H. Niwa
Department of Neurology and Head and Neck Surgery, Nihon University School of Dentistry at Matsudo, Matsudo, Chiba, Japan

K. Muramatsu
Yokohama Tsurumi Rehabilitation Hospital, Yokohama, Kanagawa, Japan

T. Chiba
Division of Internal Medicine of Dentistry, Department of Oral Medicine, Iwate Medical University, Morioka, Iwate, Japan
e-mail: toschiba@iwate-med.ac.jp


T. Chiba, H. Yamada (eds.), *Internal Medicine for Dental Treatments*,
https://doi.org/10.1007/978-981-99-3296-2_4

**Table 4.1** Classification of headache [1]

| **Part 1: The primary headaches** |
|---|
| 1. Migraine |
| 2. Tension-type headache |
| 3. Trigeminal autonomic cephalalgias |
| 4. Other primary headache disorders |
| **Part 2: The secondary headaches** |
| 5. Headache attributed to trauma or injury to the head and/or neck |
| 6. Headache attributed to cranial and/or cervical vascular disorder |
| 7. Headache attributed to nonvascular intracranial disorder |
| 8. Headache attributed to a substance or its withdrawal |
| 9. Headache attributed to infection |
| 10. Headache attributed to disorder of homeostasis |
| 11. Headache or facial pain attributed to disorders of the cranium, neck, eyes, ears, nose, sinuses, teeth, mouth, or other facial or cervical structures |
| 12. Headache attributed to psychiatric disorder |
| **Part 3: Painful cranial neuropathies and other facial pain and other headaches** |
| 13. Painful lesions of the cranial nerves and other facial pains |
| 14. Other headache disorders |

included in "headache or facial pain due to disorders of the skull, neck, eyes, nose, sinuses, teeth, mouth, or other facial and neck tissues" in the secondary headache category. The following is an overview of the most common headaches, featuring points of the differential diagnosis.

## 1.1 Migraine

Migraine is a representative type of chronic headache and its incidence is relatively high. Classic migraine is characterized by pulsating headache following the aura, such as scintillating scotoma (a darkening of the center of a flickering light) or paresthesia. However, migraine without aura is more common. It is often associated with nausea and is more likely to occur in young women and those with a family history of migraine. The diagnostic criteria in Table 4.2 are used. The mechanism of migraine is still unknown, but it has been proposed that it may be due to constriction or dilation of blood vessels in the head or abnormal neural activity in the brain. Triptans (serotonin receptor agonists) are often effective in cases of

**Table 4.2** Diagnostic criteria of migraine [1]

| A. At least five fulfilling B–D |
|---|
| B. Headache attacks lasting 4–72 h |
| C. Headache has at least two of the following four characteristics: |
| 1. Unilateral location |
| 2. Pulsating (throbbing) quality |
| 3. Moderate or severe pain intensity (which interferes with daily life) |
| 4. Aggravation by or causing avoidance of routine physical activity (e.g., walking or climbing stairs) |
| D. During headache at least one of the following: |
| 1. Nausea and/or vomiting |
| 2. Photophobia and phonophobia |
| E. Secondary headache can be ruled out. |
| In the case of "migraine with aura," migraine can be diagnosed if there are two or more scintillating scotoma |

moderate or severe attacks that do not improve with conventional analgesics. Prophylactic treatment (calcium channel blockers, beta-blockers, antiepileptic drugs, and antidepressants) is recommended for patients who have more than two attacks per month.

## 1.2 Tension-Type Headache

It is the most common chronic headache among primary headaches. It is caused by tension in the neck and shoulders and often presents as a persistent, nonpulsatile, dull pain centered in the occipital to posterior cervical region but may be described as a tightening of the entire head. It is rarely associated with nausea and is not accompanied by aura. Continued muscle tension causes an inflammatory response associated with circulatory insufficiency and the production of pain-inducing substances such as prostaglandins. In recent years, it is often caused by long staring at a monitor in the same posture during office work or continuing unnatural postures during sleep, etc. Mental stress is an important cause as well. According to the frequency, headaches are classified as (1) rare recurrent tension-type headache (less than 1 day/month), (2) frequent recurrent tension-type headache (1–14 days/month), or (3) chronic tension-type headache (more than 15 days/month).

Non-pharmacological treatments, such as headache exercises, are recommended to relieve muscle tension. As for drug therapy, analgesics such as NSAIDs (nonsteroidal anti-inflammatory drugs) are usually effective and useful in the treatment of recurrent tension-type headache attacks. However, excessive use of these drugs may lead to drug abuse headache and gastrointestinal problems. Non-pharmacological treatment and prophylactic agents such as antidepressants are recommended, especially in chronic headache.

### 1.3 Cluster Headache

Trigeminal and autonomic headaches are characterized by unilateral headache and ipsilateral head parasympathetic autonomic symptoms, and cluster headache is a typical example. Cluster headache is characterized by pulsating pain in the back of the eye or around the eye, which appears several times a day. The pain is intense and stabbing and is accompanied by conjunctival hyperemia on the same side as the pain, tears, nasal obstruction, anterior forehead and facial sweating, contracted pupils, and drooping eyelids. It is most common in men in their 20s–40s and some are associated with family history. Once the attack occurs, it lasts several weeks to several months. Most recur after a remission period of months to years.

### 1.4 Headache Due to Cerebrovascular Disorder

Subarachnoid hemorrhage is the most common cerebrovascular disorder that causes headache. Rupture of an aneurysm in the subarachnoid space causes bleeding in the subarachnoid space, which stimulates nociceptors in the meninges, resulting in headache. The headache is described as a severe headache with an inexperienced pain like being hit by a hammer. If the amount of hemorrhage is large, the patient will be, from the beginning, in a state of impaired consciousness or cardiopulmonary arrest due to increased cerebral pressure, but if the amount of hemorrhage is small, the patient will present with only headache. However, rebleeding from a cerebral aneurysm often occurs within 24 h, and if this occurs, the condition is severe, so prompt transport to a neurosurgical specialist is necessary if headache from subarachnoid hemorrhage is suspected [2].

In the case of cerebral hemorrhage, headache is also caused by stretching and traction of the brain surface tissue as the hematoma increases. In the case of cerebral hemorrhage, headache is rarely the main symptom because it is accompanied by neurological symptoms and disturbance of consciousness.

Arterial dissection can occur inside or outside the cranium. In Japan, vertebral arteries are the common site of arterial and that causes ischemia in the posterior inferior cerebellar artery territory occurring at a young age (dorsolateral infarction of the medulla oblongata, Wallenberg's syndrome). The vertebral artery ascends through the transverse process foramen of the cervical vertebrae and is easily dissected by hyperextension of the neck. Although symptoms of cerebral infarction or subarachnoid hemorrhage may occur from the onset, occipital and posterior neck pain is often present, making it an important disorder in the differential diagnosis of headache.

### 1.5 Headache Due to Infection

The headache is caused by infectious inflammation of the meninges. In the case of meningitis, nuchal rigidity is a symptom of meningeal irritation, but it is often not apparent in the early stages of infection. Photophobia, the feeling of being dazzled by light, is another characteristic symptom of meningeal irritation. Since meningitis is an infectious disease, fever is an important diagnostic point. In the case of encephalitis, in which the inflammation is mainly in the brain parenchyma, headache is not as prominent as in meningitis, and neurological symptoms and disturbance of consciousness are the main symptoms.

## 2 Sleep Disorder

Kotaro Otsuka

### 2.1 About Sleep

Sleep is composed of REM (rapid eye movement) and non-REM cycles, and the quality of sleep varies with age. REM sleep is accompanied by rapid eye movement, brain activity, and dreaming. In non-REM sleep, δ-wave is related to slow wave sleep (SWS) and is most dominant in stege IV, sleep is deep, eye movement is not accompanied in deep sleep, and memory is reinforced. After sleep onset, shallow non-REM sleep becomes deep non-REM sleep, and REM sleep appears about 90 min after sleep onset. After that, non-REM sleep and REM sleep appear alternately, repeating four to five times in a 90-min cycle.

For example, non-REM sleep is reduced and REM sleep is increased in the elderly. Insomnia in the elderly is related to various factors such as body temperature rhythm, melatonin secretion, autonomic nervous system activity, and mental health. In addition, it is not uncommon for people to be active until late at night due to changes in their living environment. In the treatment of dental patients, it is not uncommon for them to complain of insomnia, to take sleeping pills, and to experience delirium. In this article, an overview of sleep disorders and their relationship to dental treatment are described.

## 2.2 Sleep Disorders

The International Classification of Sleep Disorders, third edition (ICSD-3), classifies sleep-wake disorders into the following groups: insomnia disorders, sleep-related breathing disorders, central disorders of hypersomnolence, circadian rhythm sleep-wake disorders, sleep-related movement disorders, parasomnias, and other sleep disorders [1].

### 2.2.1 Insomnia (Insomnia Disorder)

In this article, we mainly focus on insomnia (insomnia disorder) as a sleep disorder. Insomnia disorder is defined as the appearance of insomnia symptoms, social dysfunction during the daytime, and QOL (quality of life) impairment. The insomnia symptoms include difficulty falling asleep, midway awakening, early morning awakening, and disturbance of sound sleep. In insomnia, drowsiness, general malaise, hypomotility, and gastrointestinal symptoms may occur, and hypertension and hyperglycemia may occur when sleep duration is shortened. Recently, polysomnography has been used for differential diagnosis, and insomnia disorders are associated with shortened total sleep time, decreased slow wave sleep, and low sleep efficiency.

It has been reported that ICU patients have fragmented sleep, with an increased proportion of shallow sleep and loss of REM and deep sleep [3], and that acute symptoms and hospitalization can cause sleep deprivation due to various factors such as environment, respirator, anxiety, pain, and medication, resulting in short-term delirium, respiratory failure, cardiovascular instability, and immunosuppression. In the long term, mental health problems such as depression and anxiety, sleep disorders, and increased mortality have been reported [4].

In addition to medication, non-pharmacological treatments should be considered. For example, it is important to identify lifestyle and physical conditions that may be contributing to insomnia. A wide variety of factors are associated with sleep, including stress, intake of stimulants such as caffeine and nicotine, effects of aging, alcohol consumption, changes in lifestyle, lack of exercise, effects of physical illness, effects of medications, and effects of mental disorders. It is important to address these factors and provide guidance on sleep hygiene. Other approaches such as cognitive behavioral therapy may also be considered. In addition, medication such as sleeping pills should be administered with attention to the development of physical dependence such as tolerance and withdrawal symptoms.

## 2.3 Considerations for the Use of Sleeping Pills

1. Tolerance: Tolerance to benzodiazepines is caused by a decrease in $GABA_A$ receptors in short-term use and by a decrease in the interaction between GABA binding sites and benzodiazepine binding sites in long-term use [5]. Consideration should be given to changing to a drug with a longer duration of action, a nonbenzodiazepine, an orexin receptor antagonist, or a melatonin receptor agonist.

2. Carryover effect: The effects of sleeping pills persist after the next morning, resulting in symptoms such as daytime drowsiness, lightheadedness, weakness/headache, and general malaise. As a countermeasure, it is advisable to administer a sleeping pill with a shorter duration of action, change the sleeping pill, or reduce the dose [6] or change to a drug with less muscle relaxant effect.
3. Adverse effects of alcohol: Alcohol intake causes an increase in midstream awakenings, a decrease in deep sleep, and an increase in shallow sleep.
4. Cross-tolerance: The development of tolerance to similar drugs by the formation of drug resistance is called cross-tolerance, and there is a possibility that cross-tolerance to benzodiazepines may emerge.

## 3 Syncope

Kenzo Koizumi

Syncope is defined as "a transient loss of consciousness resulting from a transient generalized decrease in cerebral blood flow (global cerebral ischemia) characterized by a sudden, brief, and spontaneous complete recovery of consciousness" [7]. Decreased blood pressure (hypotension) and generalized cerebral hypoperfusion are the main pathogeneses. When arterial blood pressure decreases, the baroreceptor reflex system maintains arterial pressure by the action of the sympathetic nervous system, but syncope occurs when this compensatory mechanism does not work effectively. When cerebral blood flow is suddenly interrupted, complete loss of consciousness occurs within 6–8 s, and loss of consciousness also occurs when systolic blood pressure falls below 50 and 60 mmHg in the upright position [8].

**Table 4.3** Classification of syncope

| Classification of syncope |
|---|
| **Reflex (neuromodulatory) syncope** |
| **Vasovagal** |
| Orthostatic load |
| Emotional (fear, pain, use of instruments in dental procedures, hematophobia) |
| **Situational** |
| Urination |
| Stimulation of the digestive tract (swallowing, defecation) |
| Coughing, sneezing |
| Post-exercise |
| Others (laughing, brass band) |
| **Carotid sinus syndrome** |
| Atypical (atypical symptoms without precursors or obvious triggers) |
| **Syncope due to orthostatic hypotension** |
| **Drug-induced** |
| Vasodilators, diuretics, phenothiazines, and antidepressants |
| **Decreased circulating blood volume** |
| Hemorrhage, diarrhea, vomiting, etc. |
| **Primary dysautonomia** |
| Pure autonomic failure, multiple system atrophy, Parkinson's disease, and Lewy body dementia |
| **Secondary dysautonomia** |
| Diabetes mellitus and amyloidosis |
| Spinal cord injury |
| Autonomic neuropathy |
| Paraneoplastic autonomic neuropathy and renal failure |
| **Cardiac syncope** |
| **Arrhythmia** |
| Bradycardiac: Sinus failure, bradycardia-tachycardia syndrome, and atrioventricular block |
| Tachycardiac: Supraventricular and ventricular (WPW syndrome, Brugada syndrome, long QT syndrome) |
| **Organic heart disease** |
| Aortic stenosis, acute myocardial infarction/ischemia, and hypertrophic cardiomyopathy |
| Cardiac tumor (Benign tumors include myxomas and papillary fibroelastomas, etc., malignant tumors include sarcomas and mesotheliomas, etc., and metastatic malignancies.) |
| Pericardial disease/tamponade, congenital coronary artery anomalies, and prosthetic valve dysfunction |
| **Cardiopulmonary and macrovascular** |
| Pulmonary embolism, acute aortic dissection, and pulmonary hypertension |

### 3.1 Classification (Table 4.3)

#### 3.1.1 Reflex Syncope

Vasovagal syncope is the most common type of syncope encountered in daily practice, and a characteristic history is helpful. It tends to occur during prolonged standing (crowded train, morning assembly) and is associated with prodromal symptoms (darkening of the eyes, hyperhidrosis, nausea, abdominal discomfort, visual and auditory disturbances). It is triggered by sleep deprivation, general malaise, alcohol consumption, high temperature, pain, and mental stress. Situational syncope is induced by certain circumstances, and micturition syncope is more likely to occur in middle-aged and older men after drinking. Carotid sinus syndrome is caused by rotation of the head and compression of the neck.

#### 3.1.2 Syncope Due to Orthostatic Hypotension

Orthostatic hypotension is diagnosed when the systolic blood pressure drops by 20 mmHg or more within 3 min after standing up from the supine position. A decrease in circulating blood volume (hemorrhage or dehydration) or an abnormality in any part of the baroreceptor reflex system can cause a severe drop in blood pressure during orthostasis. In particular, the elderly have a low baroreceptor reflex function, and a history of lifestyle-related diseases (cardiovascular disease, diabetes mellitus) or the effects of medications for these diseases tend to cause hypotension. Degenerative diseases of the central nervous system may be associated with autonomic neuropathy, and syncope may be the trigger for diagnosis.

#### 3.1.3 Cardiac Syncope

Cardiac syncope is associated with a higher risk of mortality and sudden death than noncardiac syncope. Attention should be paid to the presence of syncope that occurs during exercise or in the supine position, syncope preceded by chest pain or palpitations, a family history of sudden death, and a history of cardiac disease. Arrhythmias cause a decrease in cardiac output, and acute coronary syndromes (myocardial infarction, angina pectoris) cause syncope due to myocardial pump failure or arrhythmia. It has been reported that about 20% of patients with painless acute coronary syndromes present to the clinic complaining of syncope or presyncope [9].

### 3.2 Diseases That Can Easily Be Mistaken for Syncope: Epilepsy

Epileptic seizures result from excessive discharge of cerebral neurons and are essentially different from the pathogenesis of syncope but are often difficult to differentiate. Symptoms that are highly specific to epilepsy include tongue bite, head rotation, urinary incontinence, preictal haze, preictal hallucinations, and myalgia [10]. Although convulsive-like symptoms may also occur in syncope (convulsive syncope), they can be distinguished from epilepsy by the fact that syncope precedes convulsions, are of short duration (several seconds to tens of seconds), and are not followed by dizziness.

## 4 Disturbance of Consciousness

Masayo Fukuhara

### 4.1 Level of Consciousness

In order to provide safe dental care, we should always pay attention to vital signs. The evaluation of consciousness is especially important. Consciousness has two components: level of consciousness (arousal) and recognition function. When both of them are normal, it is called clear consciousness, and when one or both of them are disturbed, it is called disturbance of consciousness.

The absence of any disturbance of consciousness is called clear consciousness, depending on the severity of the level of consciousness, from somnolence (awakening by light stimuli but falling into a sleepy state when the stimuli are removed) to coma (complete lack of response to painful stimuli).

The Japan Coma Scale (JCS) is a scale of consciousness level used in Japan (Table 4.4) [11]. The JCS is also called the 3–3–9 degree scale because of the way it is classified, and the higher the number, the more severe the consciousness disorder. A normal person is described as "0." At first glance, it may seem difficult, but in reality, it is better to think about how to deal with a person who seems to have a consciousness disorder. If a person is lying in front of you, the first thing you would do is to call out to him or her. If the person has opened his or her eyes before you call out to him or her, ask a question or speak lightly to him or her. If the person does not open his or her eyes, we will call out loudly or shake the person. If the person still does not respond, we will give a painful stimulus.

**Table 4.4** Japan Coma Scale (JCS) (modified with permission from [11])

| | |
|---|---|
| I. The patient is awake without any stimulation (expressed in one digit) | |
| 1 | Almost fully conscious |
| 2 | Unable to recognize time, place, or person |
| 3 | Unable to recall name or date of birth |
| II. The patient can be aroused (then reverts to previous state after cessation of stimulation) (expressed in two digits) | |
| 10 | Easily by being spoken to (or is responsive with purposeful movements, phrases, or word) |
| 20 | With loud voice or shaken of shoulders (or is almost always responsive to very simple words like yes or no or to movements) |
| 30 | Only by repeated mechanical stimuli |
| III. The patients cannot be aroused with any applied mechanical stimuli (expressed in three digits) | |
| 100 | Responds with movements to avoid the stimulus |
| 200 | Responds with slight movements including decerebrate and decorticate posture |
| 300 | Does not respond at all except for change of respiratory rate and rhythm |

In addition, additional information such as R (restlessness), I (incontinence of urine and feces), A (loss of spontaneity), etc. is added and indicated as JCS 1-R, 200-I, etc.

Let us understand the word "disorientation." Disorientation is the ability to correctly recognize one's situation, such as date, time, season, place, and person. In order to check one's awareness of time and place, you can ask questions such as "What year and month is today?"

A special disorder of consciousness is delirium. Delirium is a reversible disorder of consciousness in which the disturbance of the level of consciousness itself is mild but is accompanied by difficulty concentrating attention, cognitive decline, sleep disturbance (insomnia), excitement (restlessness), and hallucinations (especially visual hallucinations). Simply put, it is an agitated disturbance of consciousness. The onset is acute or subacute, the symptoms are variable, and they tend to increase at night. It can be caused by brain disease, systemic disease, or drugs, especially those that affect the central nervous system. One of the triggering factors is surgery, and it often occurs after surgery. Particular attention should be paid in the elderly.

**Table 4.5** AIUEO-TIPS

| | | |
|---|---|---|
| A | Alcoholism and acidosis | Acute alcoholism and metabolic acidosis |
| I | Insurin | Hypoglycemia and diabetic ketoacidosis |
| U | Uremia | Uremia |
| E | Endocrine, encephalopathy | Endocrine disease and hepatic encephalopathy |
| O | Oxygen and opiate | Hypoxemia and narcotic drug |
| T | Trauma, temperature, and tumor | Traumatic injury, abnormality of body temperature, and brain tumor |
| I | Infection | Infectious disease (meningitis, encephalitis) |
| P | Psychiatric, porphyria, and pharmacology | Psychiatric disease, porphyria, and drug-induced |
| S | Syncope, stroke/SAH, seizure, and shock | Syncope, cerebral stroke/subarachnoid hemorrhage, seizure, and shock |

Table 4.5 shows AIUEO-TIPS for major diseases that should be differentiated in disorders of consciousness. Originally, AEIOU-TIPS was used in overseas countries as a way to remember the differential disorders of consciousness in emergency. The term "tips" means "knack." There are various kinds of diseases including those for neurological diseases, diseases that cause hypoxia (cardiac diseases, respiratory diseases, asphyxia), shock, hepatic failure, renal failure, and metabolic (blood glucose and electrolyte abnormalities) and infectious diseases.

When a patient suddenly becomes unconscious during dental treatment, a differential diagnosis should be made based on other vital signs (pulse, blood pressure, respiration, temperature), other symptoms (presence of hemiplegia, neurological signs such as convulsions), transcutaneous arterial oxygen saturation ($SpO_2$), and medical history. If hemiplegia or pupillary abnormalities are present, stroke (cerebrovascular disease) should be considered first. If accompanied by convulsive seizures, epilepsy should be considered. If the patient is being treated with antidiabetic drugs (oral hypoglycemic agents, insulin), consider the possibility of hypoglycemia. If a drop in blood pressure accompanies impaired consciousness, consider the cause of shock. Transient loss of consciousness due to vasovagal reflex (transient bradycardia and decrease in blood pressure due to pain stimulation against a background of anxiety and tension) that occurs during dental treatment is frequent but transient, and if it persists, other diseases should be considered. Asphyxia causing hypoxia, cardiac disease, and respiratory disease should also be considered. Although rare, anaphylactic shock and poisoning caused by anesthetics and other drugs should be considered.

### 4.2 Delirium

Delirium is particularly common in the elderly, in patients with dementia, and in patients with severe physical complications. The risk factors for delirium are known to be dementia, mild cognitive impairment, history of delirium, impairment of life function, visual impairment, hearing impairment, severe physical illness, depression, transient cerebral ischemia or stroke, alcohol dependence, and the elderly [12]. According to the diagnostic criteria of the American Psychiatric Association [13], delirium (1) impairs attention and consciousness, (2) tends to occur over a short period of time and fluctuates in severity over the course of a day, (3) is associated with disorientation and other cognitive deficits, (4) does not occur in neurocognitive disorders or coma, (5) is not associated with other existing, established, or ongoing neurocognitive disorders and does not occur in the context of a marked decrease in arousal level as in coma, and (6) is caused by physical illness or substance intoxication.

The triggering factors are as follows [14]:

1. Environmental factors: hospitalization, brightness, noise, and ICU admission
2. Physical factors: pain, dehydration, low nutrition, immobilization by intravenous infusion, and drains or restraints
3. Sensory factors: loss of vision and hearing
4. Psychological factors: psychological stress
5. Anxiety, depression, and sleep-related factors: insomnia, disturbance of day-night rhythm, and sleep-related disorders

Therefore, preventive interventions include the following [15, 16]:

1. Cognitive function and disorientation: provide adequate lighting, clocks, and calendars, and facilitate visitation.
2. Dehydration and constipation: Recommendations for moderate drinking and appropriate fluid replacement.
3. Hypoxia: Management of oxygen saturation.
4. Limitation of movement: Recommendations for walking and rehabilitation.
5. Infection: Treatment of infection and removal of unnecessary catheter.
6. Multidrug combination therapy: Multidrug combination therapy.
7. Pain: Do not overlook pain when communication is limited.
8. Low nutrition: Guidance on nutritional support. Dentures: Appropriate adjustment.
9. Sensory impairment: Provide assistance to ensure that vision and hearing function properly.
10. Sleep disorders: Minimize nighttime treatment and maintain quietness.

The administration of psychotropic drugs is also considered as a symptomatic pharmacotherapy.

## 5 Convulsion

Masayo Fukuhara

A convulsion is a seizure in which a muscle contracts involuntarily, that is, independently of the person's will. It may occur in the whole body or in some muscles.

In most cases, short convulsive attacks lasting a few seconds to a few minutes occur. Along with convulsions, abnormal body sensation, unresponsiveness (behavioral arrest), and disturbance of consciousness may be observed. Vomiting and urinary and fecal incontinence may also occur with loss of consciousness. Headache, general malaise, clouding of consciousness, and weakness of the extremities may also occur after the seizure.

**Table 4.6** Causes of convulsions (diseases and conditions)

| | |
|---|---|
| 1. Central nervous system disease | Epilepsy, cerebrovascular disease (stroke)/encephalitis, meningoencephalitis/trauma/brain tumor |
| 2. Other than central disease | Metabolic abnormalities: Electrolyte abnormalities (Na, Ca) and blood glucose abnormalities (hyperglycemia, hypoglycemia)<br>Hypoxia<br>Hepatic failure: Hepatic encephalopathy<br>Renal failure: Uremia<br>Drug addiction<br>Febrile convulsion |

There are various causes of convulsions. Table 4.6 shows the diseases and conditions that can cause convulsions. The order is not necessarily the most common, but they are the ones that need to be differentiated.

Repeated convulsions caused by repetitive hyperexcitability of cortical neurons (epileptic firing) are included in epilepsy. For more information on epilepsy, please refer to "Epilepsy" in Chap. 16.

Convulsions may occur as an acute symptom of stroke (cerebrovascular disease), and examination of hemiplegia and other neurological symptoms is necessary. Regarding blood glucose abnormalities, both hyperglycemia and hypoglycemia can cause convulsions. If the patient has underlying diabetes mellitus, it is important to check the blood glucose control status. In addition, hypoglycemia may occur in patients who are taking diabetes medication (oral diabetes medication, insulin). Furthermore, when diabetes mellitus is complicated by infection, blood glucose may rise suddenly and hyperglycemia may occur. Hypoxia can cause convulsions, and it is necessary to differentiate between the diseases that cause them.

The following is an explanation of febrile convulsions. Febrile convulsions are the most common cause of childhood convulsions. Its characteristics are shown in Table 4.7. A tonic-clonic seizure is a seizure in which the whole body becomes stiff, the hands and feet stick out strongly, and there is a repetition of a tonic phase with fine convulsions and a clonic phase with rhythmic movements.

**Table 4.7** Concept and characteristics of febrile convulsions (especially simple febrile convulsions)

| | |
|---|---|
| Concept | Convulsive seizures occurring in infancy associated with fever (usually >38 °C)<br>A clear cause of seizure, such as central nervous system infection or metabolic disease, should be excluded |
| Susceptible age | 6 months to 6 years |
| Duration | Mostly 20 min or less |
| Seizure | Symmetric tonic-clonic seizure |
| Associated with fever | Often at the onset of fever |
| Frequency | Majority is less than four times a year |
| EEG | Normal |
| Prognosis | Simple type has a good prognosis |

In addition, it should be remembered that anaphylactic shock and poisoning caused by anesthetics and other drugs occur rarely.

In case of convulsions, it is important to check the vital signs and to secure the airway. Consider the cause of the convulsions and respond accordingly. If convulsions persist for a long time or occur many times in a short time, it is called "status epilepticus," which is prone to hypoxic conditions and requires immediate treatment.

Physiological abnormalities of muscle tone, such as cramp in the leg or temporary twitching of the eyelids, are also called "cramps," but these do not require treatment in most cases.

## 6 Dizziness: Vertigo

Hideo Niwa

There is a wide range of vertigo symptoms. Some of the terms to describe vertigo represent dizziness, presyncope, disequilibrium, and light headedness. The diagnosis of vertigo can be difficult because patients may not be able to accurately describe their vertigo symptoms. However, a detailed interview is important because vertigo can be diagnosed to some extent by interviewing the patient. In this section, we describe vertigo diseases that dentists should pay attention to.

## 6.1 Benign Paroxysmal Positional Vertigo

Benign paroxysmal positional vertigo (BPPV) is the most frequent form of peripheral vertigo and is more common in patients over 50 years of age [17]. It is believed that floating otoliths in the semicircular canal cause vertigo symptoms. Vertigo occurs with head movement (turning over, sitting upright). The onset is sudden and the duration of vertigo is usually less than 1 min. The Dix-Hallpike maneuver shows characteristic downwardly and torsionally beating nystagmus, and the direction of nystagmus observed in the supine position is opposite to that observed on sitting upright. There are no cochlear symptoms (hearing loss, tinnitus) associated with vertigo, although nausea and vomiting may occur. Treatment is mainly medication, but in the case of otoliths suspended from the semicircular canal, the Epley method is used to return the otolith to its original location. If nausea and vomiting are severe, anti-dizziness drugs and antiemetics should be used. The patient may recover autonomously and wait-and-see approach may be taken.

## 6.2 Vestibular Neuritis

Vestibular neuritis is a disorder of peripheral vertigo in which vertigo symptoms occur suddenly, most commonly in patients in their 30s–50s, with no difference in gender. It is thought to be caused by a viral infection of the vestibular nerve and has been reported to occur after upper respiratory tract infections [18]. The onset of rotatory vertigo accompanied by sudden severe nausea and vomiting may last for several days. It is a disorder of the vestibular system without cochlear symptoms. Vertigo gradually resolves from a few days to a few weeks, but a feeling of light headedness may persist for several months. In most cases, the lateral semicircular canal is affected, and rotatory nystagmus toward the healthy side and a tendency to fall to the affected side are observed. The Dix-Hallpike maneuver does not show any characteristic nystagmus. Drug therapy consists of anti-dizziness drugs and antiemetics. Antianxiety drugs may also be used.

## 6.3 Meniere's Disease

Meniere's disease is characterized by repeated symptoms of vertigo, hearing loss, and tinnitus. Meniere's disease occurs in a wide range of age groups, from 20 to 60 years old, and tends to be more common in women. Meniere's disease is mainly thought to be endolymphatic hydrops, which a clear fluid can be found to increase in the membranous labyrinth of the inner ear. Treatments focused on sedation of vertigo and improvement of hearing loss in the paroxysmal phase. Osmotic diuretics, antivertigo drugs, and anxiolytic drugs are used, and surgical treatment such as injection of gentamicin into the middle ear or endolymphatic sac decompression may be performed in patients who do not respond to pharmacotherapy. During the interictal period, patients should improve their lifestyle to prevent the onset of seizures. In Europe and the United States, patients are advised to limit salt, water, caffeine, and alcohol intake [19].

## 6.4 Central Vertigo

About a quarter of patients with cerebellar or brainstem abnormalities complain of vertigo symptoms [20]. Central vertigo includes cerebral hemorrhage, cerebral infarction, and vestibular system tumors, and dizziness and gait ataxia appear more frequently than vertigo. Vertical nystagmus appears in central vertigo, and downbeat nystagmus is associated with cerebellar and brainstem disorders, while upbeat nystagmus is associated with medullary lesions. However, it should be noted that brainstem infarction in the vertebrobasilar artery region and vestibular nerve system tumors may cause nystagmus as well as peripheral vertigo. Central tumors include auditory nerve tumors, which are schwannomas derived from the vestibular nerve. The tumor progresses slowly, and symptoms such as tinnitus, hearing loss, and facial nerve palsy appear as the tumor grows. Surgical treatment should be taken into consideration and when the tumor is small, stereotactic radiotherapy (gamma knife) is used.

### 6.5 Cardiovascular System-Related Dizziness

Although cardiovascular system-related dizziness is infrequent, when floating sensation persists for several months, or intermittent or short dizziness symptoms appear during physical movement, abnormal blood pressure, orthostatic hypotension, bradyarrhythmia, and cerebrovascular disease should be considered, and cardiovascular system examination is necessary [21].

Eventually if a patient complains of dizziness or vertigo, it is important to consult a specialist (otolaryngology or neurology) to improve the patient's QOL.

## 7 Higher Brain Dysfunction [22, 23]

Kazuhiro Muramatsu

The human brain has three main functions: (1) motor functions to move limbs and face, (2) perceptual functions to sense sounds, smells, and touch; and (3) higher brain functions to control memory, cognition, emotion, and language. In other words, damage to function (3) results in higher brain dysfunction.

The brain is responsible for higher functions, with the cerebrum and thalamus playing a particularly important role. Brain damage can be partial (localized) or generalized (diffuse) and occur in various regions. Depending on the location, extent, and severity of the damage, higher brain dysfunction has qualitatively and quantitatively different aspects, including language, action, recognition, and memory.

In the examination of higher brain functions, patients are asked to perform various tasks, but none of the tasks can be performed using only one psychological process. If an MRI or CT scan has already been taken, it is practical to use the images to predict possible symptoms and to focus on them during the examination. If the patient's level of consciousness or attention is impaired, he or she may not be able to follow many of the instructions given in the examination of higher brain dysfunction, and the correct evaluation may not be possible.

### 7.1 Aphasia

Aphasia is a loss of language ability due to brain damage. The aspects of language that are impaired in aphasia can be roughly divided into four categories: speech, comprehension, calling, and recitation.

The center of brain regions related to language is thought to be located mainly around the Sylvian fissure in the left cerebral hemisphere (peri-Sylvian fissure language area). In the majority of right-handed people, and in more than 70% of left-handed people, the language area is located in the left hemisphere. The posterior part of the inferior frontal gyrus is called Broca's area, and the posterior part of the superior temporal gyrus is called Wernicke's area. Broca's aphasia is characterized by slurred speech (nonfluent), word distortion (dysarthria), mild comprehension impairment, and poor recitation. Wernicke's aphasia is smooth (fluent) speech, no dysarthria, severe comprehension impairment, and poor recitation (Fig. 4.1).

The terms alexia and agraphia are used to refer to conditions in which the ability to read and write is an acquired impairment as a result of brain injury.

### 7.2 Apraxia

There are three main types of apraxia: ideomotor apraxia, ideational apraxia, and limb kinetic apraxia.

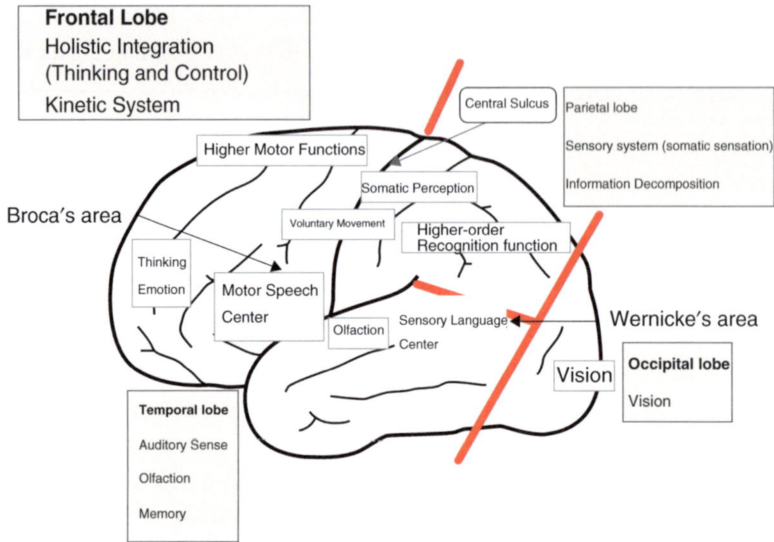


**Fig. 4.1** Language area

**Table 4.8** Tests of ideational apraxia

| |
|---|
| 1. Wave goodbye |
| 2. Come on in |
| 3. Do the soldier's salute |
| 4. Imitate brushing your teeth as if you were holding a toothbrush |
| 5. Imitate combing your hair as if you were holding a comb |
| 6. Imitate locking the door |
| 7. Imitate hitting a nail as if you were holding a hammer |
| First of all, it is carried out by verbal command, and when it is not done well, the examiner shows the act and makes it imitate |

### 7.2.1 Ideomotor Apraxia

It is an impairment of the ability to perform a learned intentional action. It occurs in right-handed people with left hemispheric damage and affects the left and right upper limbs. The actions are impaired (Table 4.8).

In the case of ideational apraxia, the patient is unable to perform the serial manipulation of multiple objects in daily life. For example, a candle, a candleholder, and a match are prepared, and a person is instructed, "Please light the candle using these items."

### 7.2.2 Limb Kinetic Apraxia

It is a condition in which the performance of actions, mainly with the hands and fingers, is incomplete, coarse, or interrupted. Patients have difficulties in using chopsticks or fastening buttons.

### 7.2.3 Oral-Facial Apraxia

Intentional execution of movements using the muscles of the lower face, tongue, larynx, and pharynx is impaired. In severe cases, patients are unable to open their mouths when asked to do so but can open their mouth in natural situations such as eating or in reflexes such as yawning. This symptom is caused by damage to the left hemisphere.

### 7.2.4 Dressing Apraxia

It is a symptom of an inability to put on individual clothes or to put them on in the wrong way. It occurs in right hemisphere injuries.

## 7.3 Agnosia

We know what an object is when we see it, and we know who a person is when we see their face. We can also hear sounds and spoken words and understand their source and meaning. These easily and immediately recognizable abilities can be impaired despite the fact that we can see and hear.

### 7.3.1 Visual Agnosia

It is a cognitive impairment of visually presented objects, and recognition through other senses (e.g., touch) is well maintained. Although the visual acuity and field of vision are sufficient to recognize the object, the patient is unable to recognize the object. It is caused by damage to the bilateral occipital lobes.

#### 7.3.2 Prosopagnosia

You see a familiar face, and you do not know who it is. On the other hand, you can recognize someone by listening to his or her voice. Not only can they not say the name of a person they knew before their illness, but they also cannot tell what kind of person the person is, such as their occupation.

#### 7.3.3 Cortical Deafness

It is a condition of deafness caused mainly by lesions of the bilateral temporal lobes. The patient is said to be deaf and unresponsive to loud sounds, whether pure tones, speech sounds, or environmental sounds.

#### 7.3.4 Tactile Agnosia

Inability to recognize objects by touch, despite the absence of somatosensory disturbance. It appears on the hand contralateral to the cerebral hemispheric lesion (mainly in the parietal lobe).

### 7.4 Memory Disorder

The inability to remember new things and the difficulty in recalling old experiences and knowledge are disorders of declarative memory. The term "declaration" refers to the ability to consciously express memory information regardless of its verbal nature. Procedural memory is a memory that can be preserved in clinical amnesic patients, and it can be preserved in movements, actions, and behaviors.

## 8 General Malaise

Toshimi Chiba

### 8.1 Concept

General malaise is a subjective symptom of feeling tired or languid. It is synonymous with easy fatigability and fatigue. Even healthy people feel general malaise due to physical or mental overwork, stress, lack of sleep, etc., and it is called physiological overwork. However, pathological malaise is considered when the patient does not recover even after rest or when the workload is not so heavy as to make the patient feel tired.

### 8.2 Pathophysiology

Physical fatigue is caused by hypotension, chronic inflammation, hormone secretion abnormalities, low nutrition, electrolyte abnormalities, and drugs, while mental fatigue is caused by depression and neurosis.

### 8.3 Differentiated Diseases

1. Psychoneurotic diseases: neurosis, psychosomatic disorders, depression, and schizophrenia are considered as mental fatigue.
2. Infectious diseases: General malaise is often observed in patients with slight fever due to infectious diseases. In elderly patients, only malaise may be present without noticing slight fever. In addition, anorexia may lead to low nutrition. Bacterial infections such as endocarditis, tuberculosis, and abscesses, fungal infections, parasitic infections, and viral infections such as AIDS are common causes.
3. Chronic inflammatory diseases: General malaise may be observed in sarcoidosis and collagen diseases.
4. Neuromuscular diseases: General malaise may be observed in myasthenia gravis, multiple sclerosis, etc.
5. Endocrine and metabolic diseases: Endocrine diseases include Addison's disease, hypothyroidism, and anterior hypopituitarism, which cause hypotension. Diabetes mellitus is a representative metabolic disease, and vitamin $B_1$ deficiency also causes malaise mainly in the lower limbs.
6. Drugs: Alcohol, narcotics, organic solvents, heavy metals, and pesticides may cause general malaise.
7. Water-electrolyte imbalance: Hyponatremia associated with vomiting and diarrhea, and other symptoms such as hypopotassemia, hyperpotassemia, hypocalcemia, hypercalce-

mia, hypophosphatemia, and hypermagnesemia may cause general malaise.

8. Chronic diseases of each organ
   (a) Hematologic diseases: Persistent malaise may be observed in iron-deficiency anemia. Pallor of the skin and mucous membranes may occur.
   (b) Respiratory disease: Respiratory tract infection may cause general malaise with cough and sputum.
   (c) Cardiac disease: Heart failure, valvular heart disease, arrhythmia, etc. may cause general malaise, accompanied by heart murmur and hypertension.
   (d) Gastrointestinal diseases: Anemia due to peptic ulcer or chronic gastritis may cause general malaise.
   (e) Liver disease: General malaise and jaundice may be observed due to liver dysfunction.
   (f) Renal disease: Edema and hypoproteinemia may be accompanied by general malaise.
9. Malignancy: General malaise due to latent malignancy may occur.

## 8.4 Diagnosis and Examination

On physical examination, fever is suspicious for infection, yellowing of the ocular conjunctiva for liver disease, edema for renal disease, eyelid conjunctiva for anemia, and protruding eyeballs and the presence of a neck mass for thyroid disease.

In screening tests, positive urine protein indicates renal disease, and positive urine sugar indicates diabetes mellitus. In blood tests, decreased hemoglobin (Hb) concentration is considered to be anemia; abnormal of white blood counts (WBC) or leukocyte fraction indicates leukemia. In blood biochemistry tests, elevated CRP is suspected to be infectious disease, and elevated AST (aspartate transaminase) and ALT (alanine transaminase) indicate liver disease. BUN (blood urea nitrogen) and creatinine (Cr) are useful in screening for renal disease, serum Na, K, and Cl for electrolyte abnormalities and T3, T4, and TSH for thyroid disease. Chest radiography should be performed when cardiac or pulmonary disease is suspected, and electrocardiogram should be performed when cardiac disease is suspected.

## References

1. Headache Classification Committee of the International Headache Society (IHS). The International Classification of Headache Disorders, 3rd edition. Cephalalgia. 2018;38(1):1–211.
2. The Japan Stroke Society Committee on Guidelines for the Management of Stroke, editor. Japanese guidelines for the management of stroke 2015. Tokyo: Kyowa Kikaku; 2015. p. 186–90. (in Japanese).
3. Elliott R, et al. Characterisation of sleep in intensive care using 24-hour polysomnography: an observational study. Crit Care. 2013;17(2):r46.
4. Knauert MP, et al. Sleep and sleep disordered breathing in hospitalized patients. Semin Respir Crit Care Med. 2014;35(5):582–92.
5. Mishima K, editor. Clinical guideline for proper usage and tapering of hypnotics. Tokyo: Jihou; 2014. (in Japanese).
6. Uchiyama M, editor. Guideline for response and treatment of sleep disorders. 3rd ed. Tokyo: Jihou; 2019. (in Japanese).
7. The Japanese Circulation Society. Guidelines for diagnosis and treatment of cardiovascular diseases (2011 Joint Study Group Report). Guidelines for diagnosis and management of syncope (2012 revised edition). (in Japanese). https://www.j-circ.or.jp/cms/wp-content/uploads/2020/02/JCS2012_inoue_h.pdf.
8. Wieling W, et al. Symptoms and signs of syncope: a review of the link between physiology and clinical clues. Brain. 2009;132(Pt 10):2630–42.
9. Brieger D, et al. Acute coronary syndromes without chest pain, an underdiagnosed and undertreated high-risk group: insights from the Global Registry of Acute Coronary Events. Chest. 2004;126(2):461–9.
10. Sheldon R, et al. Historical criteria that distinguish syncope from seizures. J Am Coll Cardiol. 2002;40(1):142–8.
11. Shigemori M, et al. Guidelines for the management of severe head injury, 2nd edition. Neurol Med Chir (Tokyo). 2012;52:1–30.
12. Inouye SK, et al. Delirium in elderly people. Lancet. 2014;383(9920):911–22.
13. Supervisory translation Saburo Takahashi et al. DSM-5 diagnostic and statistical manual of mental disorders. Tokyo: Igaku Shoin; 2014. p. 588. (in Japanese).
14. Japanese Society of General Hospital Psychiatry, Delirium Guideline Revision Group, editor. Clinical guideline for delirium treatment guideline for delirium, 2nd ed. Tokyo: Seiwa Shoten; 2015. p. 33–34. (in Japanese).

15. Kawai E, et al. Delirium in the elderly and dementia patients: a multidisciplinary team aims to improve the prognosis without missing the signs—Delirium in the elderly and dementia patients. (in Japanese).
16. NICE guidelines [CG103] Delirium: prevention, diagnosis and management; 2010.
17. Muncie HL, Sirmans SM, James E. Dizziness. Approach to evaluation and management. Am Fam Physician. 2017;95(3):154–62.
18. Schessel DA, Minor LB, Nedzelski J. Meniere's disease and other peripheral vestibular disorders. In: Gaertner RS, Murphy MB, editors. Cummings otolaryngology head and neck surgery. 4th ed. Philadelphia: Mosby; 2004. p. 3231–2.
19. Harcourt J, Barraclough K, Bronstein AM. Meniere's disease. BMJ. 2014;349:24–7.
20. Neuhauser HK. Epidemiology of vertigo. Curr Opin Neurol. 2007;20(1):40–6.
21. Longo D, et al. Harrison's principles of internet medicine. 18th ed. McGraw-Hill Professional; 2011. p. 178–81.
22. Ishiai J. Higher brain dysfunction studies. 3rd ed. Tokyo: Ishiyaku Shuppan; 2022. (in Japanese).
23. Hirayama K. Understanding and examination of higher brain dysfunction. Tokyo: Chugai Igaku Sha; 2017. (in Japanese).

# Endocrine/Renal/Blood/Other Symptoms

5

Yoshiharu Yajima, Keiko Naruse, Kimihiro Matsumoto, Masahiro Ieko, Toshimi Chiba, Yoshihiro Matsukawa, Natsumi Ikumi, and Ryoichi Tanaka

## 1 Dehydration

Yoshiharu Yajima

### 1.1 Introduction

Dehydration is caused by the loss of body fluid either external environment or internal biophysiological factors. Because the amount of body fluid volume depends on the balance between extracellular water and serum sodium concentration, dehydration is classified according to serum sodium concentration. Severe dehydration can lead to life-threatening conditions. Moreover, inappropriate treatment can elicit serious complications.

### 1.2 Symptoms

Typical symptoms appeared in dehydration status, such as dry mouth, weakness, lightheadedness, indifference, anorexia, nausea and vomiting, headache, dizziness, hypotension, convulsion (seizure), somnolence, coma, etc.

### 1.3 Physical Findings to Be Confirmed

Basic vital signs informations such as body temperature, blood pressure, pulse rate, frequency of respiration, and level of consciousness would be confirmed as soon as possible. Also skin condi-

Y. Yajima
Division of Internal Medicine, The Nippon Dental University School of Life Dentistry at Tokyo, Chiyoda-ku, Tokyo, Japan

K. Naruse
Department of Internal Medicine, School of Dentistry, Aichi Gakuin University, Nagoya, Aichi, Japan

K. Matsumoto
Department of Internal Medicine, Tokyo Dental College, Ichikawa General Hospital, Ichikawa, Chiba, Japan

M. Ieko
Department of Nursing, Faculty of Health and Medical Sciences, Sapporo University of Health Sciences, Sapporo, Hokkaido, Japan

T. Chiba (✉)
Division of Internal Medicine of Dentistry, Department of Oral Medicine, Iwate Medical University, Morioka, Iwate, Japan
e-mail: toschiba@iwate-med.ac.jp

Y. Matsukawa
Department of Internal Medicine, Tsurumi University Dental Hospital, Yokohama, Kanagawa, Japan

N. Ikumi
Nihon University School of Medicine, Itabashi-ku, Tokyo, Japan

R. Tanaka
Division of Dental Radiology, Department of Reconstructive Oral and Maxillofacial Surgery, Iwate Medical University School of Dentistry, Yahaba, Iwate, Japan



T. Chiba, H. Yamada (eds.), *Internal Medicine for Dental Treatments*,
https://doi.org/10.1007/978-981-99-3296-2_5

tion or turgor and local moisture level in the tongue, oral mucosa, and axilla, and enophthalmos can reflect the severity of dehydration.

## 1.4 Causes

### 1.4.1 Poor Intake of Water and Salt

Oral diseases, anorexia and malnutrition due to gastrointestinal diseases, intake difficulties due to living and working environment, cranial nerve diseases with oral intake difficulties, some eating disorders, and malabsorption due to gastrointestinal edema caused by hypoproteinemia.

### 1.4.2 Loss of Water and Salt

1. Loss from urine: osmotic diuresis due to disease, salt-losing nephropathy, and diuretic use
2. Loss from the gastrointestinal tract: Leakage into the interstitium due to vomiting, diarrhea, intestinal obstruction, or peritonitis
3. Loss from the skin: Leakage into the interstitium due to sweating by exercise, work, high temperature environment, or burns

## 1.5 Disease Classification

### 1.5.1 Hypertonic Dehydration

A state in which the serum Na concentration is high. Both extracellular and intracellular fluid are decreased. Water is lost, and intracellular dehydration increases, resulting in a strong complaint of thirst. It is seen in children and elderly patients with high fever.

### 1.5.2 Isotonic Dehydration

A state in which the serum sodium concentration is maintained. Extracellular fluid is decreased, but intracellular fluid is maintained. It is seen in large amounts of diarrhea, vomiting, and burns.

### 1.5.3 Hypotonic Dehydration

A state in which the serum sodium concentration is low. The extracellular fluid is decreased, but the intracellular fluid is maintained. Peripheral circulatory insufficiency is likely to occur because salts are lost in larger amounts. Although infrequent, it is seen in adrenal insufficiency, salt-losing nephropathy, and inappropriate correction of dehydration.

## 1.6 Dehydration in Children

In childhood, the balance of the body is maintained with a high level of extracellular fluid, but the kidney concentrating ability is immature and the body is small, so there is little extracellular fluid in reserve. Therefore, the loss of water and salt can easily lead to dehydration. When dehydration is evident, it is important to consider the possibility that the patient may already be severely dehydrated. In addition, the patient may not be able to report his or her symptoms appropriately; sufficient consideration is required.

## 1.7 Dehydration in Elderly

Elderly patients are often receiving medications for underlying diseases. For example, concomitant use of diuretics, laxatives, and some diabetic agents may predispose them to dehydration due to polyuria and diarrhea. The elderly have a relatively low extracellular fluid volume and, as in children, can easily become dehydrated due to changes in physical condition. Dehydration and heat stroke can easily occur in elderly patients with reduced ability to adapt to the environment, especially if they have poor appetite and difficulty in fluid and salt intake.

## 1.8 Heat Attach and Dehydration

Heat attach is a general term for conditions caused by impaired body adaptation to hot environments; dehydration in hot environments is particularly referred to as heat attach. High temperature, high humidity, strong solar and radiant heat, and light or no wind under high temperature conditions all interfere with the body's ability to dissipate heat. Heat attach develops when the balance between heat production and dissipation in the body is disturbed due to these environmental factors, and the body temperature rises significantly. The heat release response to adapt to the environment is controlled by the sweating response and skin blood flow response, which are controlled by the heat regulatory center; it depends on the individual's ability to regulate body temperature, the presence or absence of underlying illness, and even the physical condition. Therefore, even healthy subjects are at risk of severe hypertonic or hypotonic dehydration when heat dissipation is not appropriate due to poor physical condition in a hot environment. According to a survey of heat attach in Japan, electrolyte abnormalities were observed in about 6% of emergency cases [1]. Hypertonic dehydration and hypotonic dehydration are also observed in a low frequency, so it is important to take appropriate treatments at an early stage. In particular, events related to dental care, such as sleep deprivation induced by dental pain, decreased fluid intake due to oral diseases, and malnutrition, can be assumed. In order to provide safe treatment, it is important to consider environmental factors, the physical condition of each patient, and the ability to regulate body temperature and to provide appropriate guidance to prevent dehydration before and after treatment.

## 2 Hypoglycemia

Keiko Naruse

### 2.1 Conditions in Which the Symptom Appears

Hypoglycemia is defined as autonomic and central nervous system symptoms associated with low blood glucose levels. Clinical symptoms usually occur when the blood glucose level falls below 60 mg/dL, but the level of blood glucose that leads to the appearance of symptoms may vary depending on the underlying disease or condition of the patient.

Glucose is the most important substance in energy production, which is taken up by cells to produce ATP through the glycolytic system and TCA (tricarboxylic acid) cycle. In particular, the brain depends on glucose for most of the energy production under physiological conditions, and a decrease in blood glucose is a crisis on the basis of life support. Insulin is the only hormone that lowers blood glucose in the human body. On the other hand, there are several hormones that increase blood glucose (counter regulatory hormones) such as glucagon, catecholamine, glucocorticoids, and growth hormone. In healthy subjects, insulin secretion is first suppressed in response to a decrease in blood glucose, followed by an increase in secretion of counter regulatory hormones, which increases blood glucose by increasing glycogenolysis and gluconeogenesis in the liver (Fig. 5.1). Under normal conditions, hypoglycemia is usually avoided by this function.

Diabetes patients taking insulin or oral hypoglycemic agents may experience hypoglycemia due to failure of this regulation. In addition to insulin, sulfonylureas (SU) and fast-acting insulin secretagogues (glinides) are diabetic drugs that are likely to cause hypoglycemia.

### 2.2 Symptoms

Autonomic nerve symptoms usually appear as subjective symptoms when the blood glucose level is below 60 mg/dL, but the blood glucose threshold at which subjective symptoms appear varies from patient to patient. Catecholamine secretion by hypoglycemic stimuli induces tremor, tachycardia (palpitations), and anxiety, while acetylcholine secretion from sympathetic preganglionic neurons induces hunger and sweating (cold sweats). In spite of the secretion of counter regulatory hormones, if blood glucose decreases further, glucose deficiency in neurons causes a variety of central nervous system symptoms, such as malaise, drowsiness, dizziness, diplopia, headache, cognitive decline, and abnormal behavior, eventually leading to life-threatening conditions such as convulsions (seizures) and coma (Fig. 5.1). In diabetic patients with severe autonomic neuropathy, or when blood glucose levels fall slowly, central nervous system symptoms may appear without autonomic symptoms.

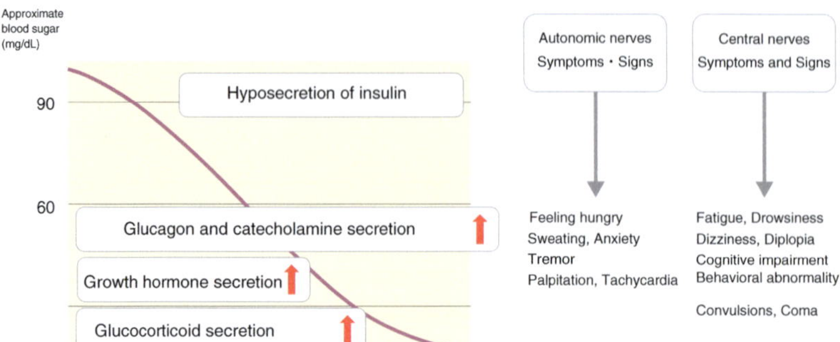


**Fig. 5.1** Hormone secretion, symptoms, and signs during hypoglycemia

### 2.3 Differential Diagnosis

The most common cause of hypoglycemia is drug-induced hypoglycemia in diabetic patients, and the use of antidiabetic agents should be confirmed. If drug-induced hypoglycemia is ruled out, differential diagnosis is proceeded by simultaneous measurement of serum insulin and C-peptide during hypoglycemia.

#### 2.3.1 Drug-Induced Hypoglycemia During Treatment of Diabetes Mellitus

Hypoglycemia is more likely to occur in diabetic patients undergoing treatment with insulin or insulin secretagogues (sulfonylurea and glinide) when the amount of food intake is reduced or when excessive exercise is involved. In particular, elderly diabetic patients with impaired renal function, decreased metabolism, and/or excretion of drugs should be carefully monitored for hypoglycemia.

#### 2.3.2 Insulinoma

It is a type of pancreatic endocrine tumor in which pancreatic beta cells are tumorized. Insulinoma autonomously oversecretes insulin, resulting in hypoglycemia. Some tumors are associated with multiple endocrine neoplasia type 1. Although most of the tumors are benign, less than 10% of them are malignant.

#### 2.3.3 Insulin Autoimmune Syndrome and Insulin Receptor Dysregulation

Insulin autoimmune syndrome is a condition in which insulin autoantibodies are produced in the absence of prior insulin therapy. Hypoglycemia is likely to occur when insulin and autoantibodies dissociate. In type B insulin resistance syndrome, autoantibodies against the insulin receptor are produced in an acquired state.

#### 2.3.4 Hypoglycemia Associated with Endocrine Disorders

In adrenocortical insufficiency and anterior hypopituitarism (ACTH deficiency), hypoglycemia may result from reduced hepatic gluconeogenesis due to inadequate cortisol secretion.

#### 2.3.5 Postgastrectomy Syndrome

After gastrectomy (especially when the pylorus is removed), food reaches the small intestine quickly and causes a rapid increase in blood glucose, resulting in a time lag between the insulin secretory response and hypoglycemia 2–3 h after eating (late dumping syndrome).

## 3 Anemia

Kimihiro Matsumoto

The supply of oxygen to systemic tissues in response to their oxygen demand is achieved by the transport of mature erythrocytes produced by the hematopoietic system to each organ and tissue and by the dissociation of oxygen at peripheral hypoxic sites due to the unique properties of hemoglobin. Anemia as a symptom is defined as a decrease in the number of red blood cells or hemoglobin concentration that can cause tissue hypoxia, in contrast to the commonly used "anemia" such as dizziness, lightheadedness, and transient loss of consciousness. A hemoglobin concentration of less than 13.0 g/dL in adult males, less than 12.0 g/dL in adult females and children, and less than 11.0 g/dL in the elderly and pregnant women, according to the World Health Organization (WHO) criteria, is widely used.

## 3.1 Conditions in Which the Symptom Appears

### 3.1.1 Iron Deficiency Anemia: IDA

About one-third of women of reproductive age have ferritin deficiency due to menstruation, while gastric ulcer, hemorrhoids, and malignant tumors of the gastrointestinal tract such as gastric and colorectal cancer are the main causes of IDA. Chronic hemorrhage causes iron loss, resulting in low iron stores and low ferritin levels in the body. The mean corpuscular volume (MCV) of red blood cells is low.

### 3.1.2 Anemia of Chronic Disease: ACD

It refers to microcytic anemia caused by impaired iron utilization associated with chronic inflammation such as rheumatoid arthritis, tuberculosis, and bedsore infection, for which iron therapy is ineffective. Recently, the hepcidin-mediated pathogenesis of this disease has been clarified.

### 3.1.3 Hereditary Anemia

Hemolysis due to hereditary quantitative and/or qualitative hemoglobin abnormalities, which leads to microcytic anemia.

### 3.1.4 Megaloblastic Anemia

It is caused by atrophic gastritis, loss of vitamin $B_{12}$ after several years of gastrectomy, or folate deficiency due to vegetarianism, ileocecal lesions, or folate metabolism antagonists such as methotrexate. It is often complicated by pancytopenia and/or neuropathy.

### 3.1.5 Hemolytic Anemia

This anemia is caused by severe valvular heart disease, march, or DIC (disseminated intravascular coagulation) and TTP (thrombotic thrombocytopenic purpura) which is from intravascular mechanical hemolysis when passing through narrower intravalvular spaces or microvascular thrombi. In addition, autoimmune hemolytic anemia (AIHA) due to production of red cell autoantibodies or extravascular hemolysis due to allogeneic antibody reaction after blood transfusion (in the spleen) is also prevalent. It is increased indirect bilirubin, LDH (lactate dehydrogenase), and reticulocytes. In intravascular hemolysis, free hemoglobin causes hypertension, renal dysfunction, and a marked decrease in haptoglobin.

### 3.1.6 Renal Anemia

Erythropoietin, an erythropoietic hormone secreted by the kidneys, is markedly reduced in patients with chronic renal failure. Erythropoiesis-stimulating agents (ESAs) are effective.

### 3.1.7 Aplastic Anemia: AA

It is caused by autoimmune hematopoietic stem cell damage caused by T cells. In addition to immunosuppressive therapy (IST), the efficacy of thrombopoietin (TPO) derivatives has recently been demonstrated.

### 3.1.8 Myelodysplastic Syndrome (MDS)

It was refractory to iron and was called refractory anemia. Recently, epigenomic mutations in hematopoietic stem cells have been identified. In addition, blood transfusion therapy is indicated for low-risk type, which defines without increased blasts. Concomitant use of blood transfusion therapy and azacitidine, a hypomethylating agent (HMA), or bone marrow transplantation are indicated for the high-risk form, which progresses to leukemia (acute myelogenous leukemia) in a relatively short time.

### 3.1.9 Hematopoietic Tumor

Hematopoietic failure is caused by loss of normal hematopoiesis due to leukemia and myeloma, which are tumors that have infiltrated the bone marrow. A decrease in platelets and leukocytes, which have a short half-life, is followed by a delayed decrease in erythrocytes, which have a long half-life.

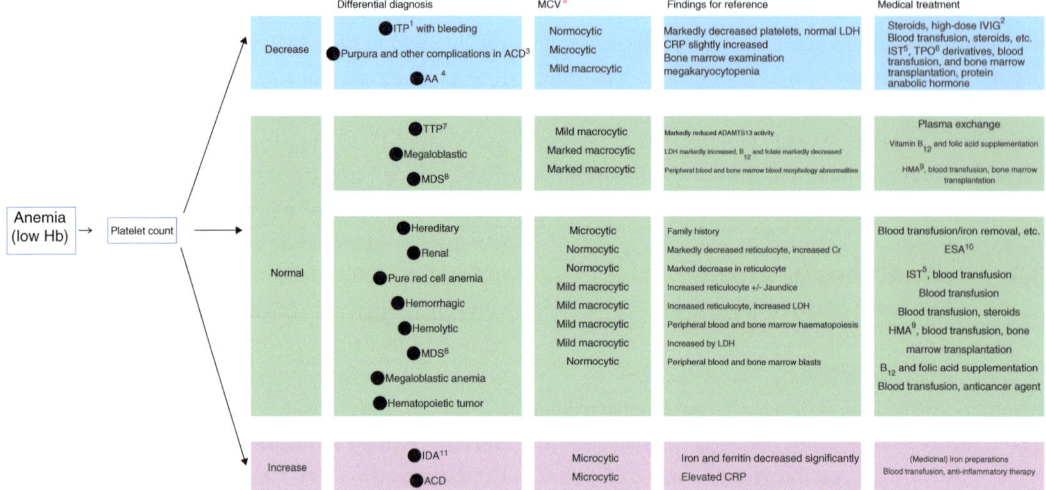


1 immune thrombocytopenic purpura: ITP, 2 intravenous immunoglobulin replacement: IVIG, 3 anemia of chronic disease: ACD, 4 aplastic anemia: AA, 5 immunosuppressive therapy: IST, 6 thrombopoietin: TPO, 7 thrombotic thrombocytopenic purpura: TTP, 8 myelodysplastic syndrome: MDS, 9 hypomethylating agents: HMA, 10 erythropoiesis stimulating agents: ESA, 11 iron deficiency anemia: IDA

*MCV: Mean red blood cell volume (fl)
Microcytic: 80 or less, Normocytic: 81-99, Macrocytic: 100 or more

**Fig. 5.2** Differentiation and treatment of anemia

### 3.2 Differential Diagnosis (Fig. 5.2)

In order to differentiate the above anemia conditions, among the erythrocyte indices calculated by the combination of erythrocyte count, hemoglobin, and hematocrit, MCV indicating the size of erythrocytes and reticulocyte count, an indicator of hematopoiesis WBC (white blood cells), PLT (platelet count), LDH, CRP (C-reactive protein), renal function, bilirubin levels, etc. are used for differentiation. Various confirmatory tests are performed to confirm the diagnosis, and specific treatment is given.

## 4 Bleeding Tendency

Masahiro Ieko

### 4.1 Conditions in Which the Symptom Appears

Hemorrhagic tendency is a general term for subcutaneous hemorrhage or organ hemorrhage without a clear trigger such as trauma or a situation in which normal hemostasis is not achieved [2]. Bleeding symptoms include (1) subcutaneous hemorrhage such as petechial hemorrhage, (2) mucosal hemorrhage such as nasal hemorrhage, (3) organ and intra-articular hemorrhage, and (4) hematoma formation and hemostasis difficulties [2]. The pathogenesis of bleeding tendency can often be inferred from clinical symptoms, and even small bleeding spots should not be overlooked.

The mechanism of bleeding tendency is recognized when some or more of the normal hemostatic mechanisms are disturbed. These include (1) abnormalities in platelets (number or function), (2) abnormalities in coagulation factors, (3) abnormalities in the vessel wall or capillaries, and (4) abnormalities in the fibrinolytic system [2]. The patient's medical history should also be noted. Hepatic disorders may lead to thrombocytopenia and decreased coagulation factors, and cerebrovascular disorders may be due to antiplatelet medication. Major hemorrhagic disorders are listed in Table 5.1 [2].

**Table 5.1** Symptoms of bleeding tendency and representative diseases

| |
|---|
| **Thrombocytopenia: petechial hemorrhage and subcutaneous and mucosal hemorrhage are the main symptoms** |
| Idiopathic thrombocytopenic purpura (ITP) |
| Thrombotic thrombocytopenic purpura (TTP) |
| Other thrombocytopenia (pancytopenia, leukemia) |
| **Abnormal platelet function: subcutaneous and mucosal bleeding are the main symptoms** |
| Glanzmann's thrombasthenia |
| Bernard-Soulier syndrome |
| Other platelet dysfunctions (platelet release disorder, essential thrombocythemia) |
| **Blood coagulation disorders: visceral bleeding and hematoma formation are the main symptoms (subcutaneous and mucosal bleeding and difficulty in stopping bleeding are the main symptoms in von Willebrand disease)** |
| Hemophilia |
| von Willebrand disease |
| Other coagulation factor abnormalities (hepatic disorder, afibrinogenemia, factor XIII deficiency) |
| **Vascular wall and capillary abnormalities: subcutaneous bleeding is the main symptom** |
| Hereditary hemorrhagic telangiectasia (Osler disease) |
| IgA vasculitis (Henoch-Schönlein purpura) |
| Other vascular wall and capillary abnormalities (purpura simplex, senile purpura, scurvy, Cushing's syndrome) |
| **Abnormalities of the fibrinolytic system: various bleeding symptoms** |
| $\alpha_2$-Plasmin inhibitor deficiency |
| Disseminated intravascular coagulation (DIC) |

## 4.2 Hemorrhagic Diseases Differentiated by Symptoms

### 4.2.1 Hemorrhagic Tendency, Mainly Subcutaneous and Mucosal Bleeding

Purpura is a general term for subcutaneous and submucosal hemorrhage, which is divided into (1) petechiae (1–5 mm in diameter), (2) ecchymosis (within 1 cm in diameter), and (3) suggillation (relatively large subcutaneous hemorrhage) according to size [3]. It is important to differentiate subcutaneous hemorrhage from erythema and telangiectasia. If the reddish purple color does not disappear when a transparent glass plate is pressed, it is considered to be subcutaneous hemorrhage [2], whereas if it disappears, it is considered to be erythema, telangiectasia, and pigmentation.

Purpura is often due to platelet abnormalities or abnormalities of the vascular wall or capillaries, and idiopathic thrombocytopenic purpura (ITP), von Willebrand disease, or thrombasthenia should be considered. If there are abnormalities in the number of red or white blood cells, aplastic anemia should be suspected, and if there are abnormalities in the morphology of white blood cells or enlarged lymph nodes, acute leukemia should be suspected. If there is renal dysfunction, abdominal pain, or arthralgia, consider IgA vasculitis (Henoch-Schönlein purpura), and if there is joint swelling or joint changes, consider thrombocytopenia associated with autoimmune disease. If telangiectasias are present, consider hepatic disorders such as cirrhosis and Osler disease. Thrombotic thrombocytopenic purpura (TTP) associated with renal or psychiatric disorders is not associated with severe hemorrhage symptoms. Although extremely rare, autoimmune hemorrhagic disease caused by autoantibodies against coagulation factors, such as acquired hemophilia A caused by coagulation factor VIII autoantibodies, should also be considered.

Senile purpura is characterized by well-defined planar subcutaneous hemorrhagic spots on the extensor side of the forearms and the dorsal surfaces of the hands, and simple purpura, which is more common in young women, is characterized by round, pale purpura, but no strong bleeding tendency.

### 4.2.2 Hemorrhagic Tendency Mainly Due to Organ Bleeding and Difficulty in Stopping Bleeding

Organ hemorrhage includes (1) intracranial hemorrhage (cerebral hemorrhage, epidural hematoma, etc.), (2) gastrointestinal hemorrhage (gastric hemorrhage, intestinal hemorrhage, etc.), (3) urinary hemorrhage (renal hemorrhage, bladder hemorrhage, etc.), (4) respiratory hemorrhage (pharyngeal hemorrhage, bronchial hemorrhage, etc.), and (5) others (intra-articular hemorrhage, ocular hemorrhage, etc.). In case of organ bleeding or hematoma formation, abnormalities in coagulation factors should be considered first, followed by abnormalities in fibrinolytic activity ($\alpha_2$-plasmin inhibitor (PI) deficiency or disseminated intravascular coagulation (DIC).

Hemophilia (congenital coagulation factor VIII or IX deficiency) is often associated with intramuscular or intra-articular bleeding. Congenital coagulation factor XIII deficiency is considered for bleeding tendency from the neonatal period to early infancy, and hemophilia is considered after infancy. Alpha$_2$-PI deficiency is associated with posterior bleeding (rebleeding from the hemostatic site). Difficulty in hemostasis during surgery can be caused by any bleeding mechanism, and von Willebrand disease is the most frequent cause of hemostasis during tooth extraction. Gastrointestinal hemorrhage and postoperative hematoma are also observed in liver diseases due to thrombocytopenia and decreased coagulation factors. Organ hemorrhage, hematoma formation, and purpura associated with solid cancer and sepsis are considered to be DIC.

## 5 Rash/Eruption [4–6]

Yoshihiro Matsukawa, Natsumi Ikumi

We can visually obtain medical information (visual examination) at a first visit of patients.

In other words, valuable information can be obtained from the skin at the beginning of medical examination, and this alone could establish a differential diagnosis.

A rash is a change on the skin, and an appropriate evaluation with palpation and visual examination is fundamental in dermatologic treatment.

Rashes are classified according to the mechanism of occurrence into (1) primary eruptions (eruptions on the healthy skin) (Fig. 5.3a) and (2) secondary eruptions (eruptions sequel to other eruptions). In addition, there is (3) a rash associated with specific skin lesions, and these three types cover almost all rashes (Fig. 5.3b, c).

Table 5.2 shows the classification of rashes and brief explanations.

Apart from these rashes, a rash associated with a specific disease is called a specific rash

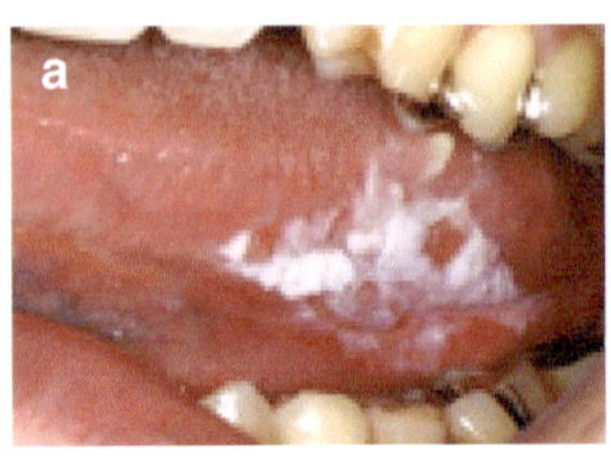


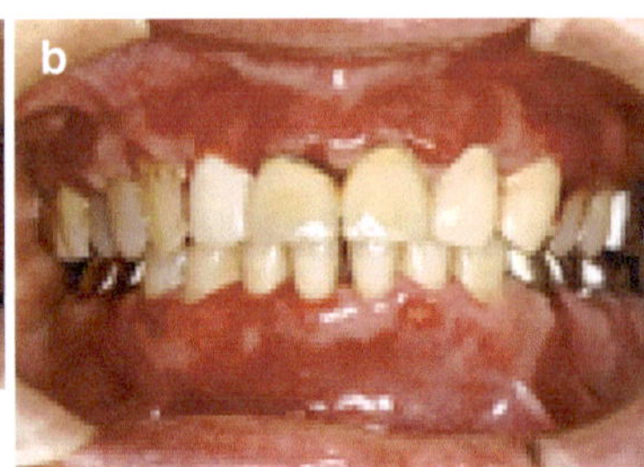


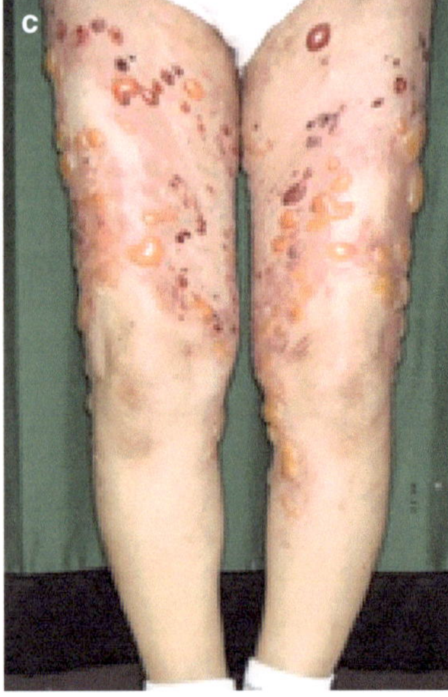


**Fig. 5.3** Diseases recognized in dental disease. (**a**) Oral leukoplakia (primary eruption). (**b**) Pemphigoid (specific skin rash). (**c**) Bullous pemphigoid (primary eruption + specific skin rash)

**Table 5.2** Classification of rash

| 1. Primary eruption (Notes 1 and 2) | 2. Secondary eruption (Note 3) | 3. Specific rash |
|---|---|---|
| **Macule** | Excoriation | Erythroderma[j] |
| Erythema | Erosion[g] | Melanosis |
| Purpura[a] | Ulcer[h] | Livedo[k] |
| Pigmented macule[b] | Scar | Poikiloderma |
| Leukoderma | Fissure | Lichen[l] |
| Telangiectasia | | Lichenification |
| Papule[c] | Callus[i] | Papilloma |
| Nodule[d] | Atrophy | Condyloma |
| Tumor[e] | Scale | Plaque[m] |
| Bulla vesicle | Crust | Acne[n] |
| Pustule | Abscess | Comedo[n] |
| Cyst | (Note 3) The first five rashes show skin defects | Sycosis[n] |
| Wheal[f] | | Herpes |
| (Note 1) A rash that does not rise from the skin is called a macule, whereas other primary eruptions do rise from the skin.<br>(Note 2) Erythema fades with pressure, but purpura does not fade because it is hemorrhage. Erythema and purpura can be distinguished by glass compression (glass compression method). | | Pemphigus[o]<br>Impetigo<br>Pityriasis<br>Xerosis<br>Ichthyosis<br>Sclerosis<br>Aphtha[p]<br>Leukoplakia |

Explanation of [a–p] in the table

[a] Caused by hemorrhage

[b] Melanin, hemosiderin, etc.

[c] Less than 10 mm in diameter

[d] 10–30 mm in diameter

[e] More than 30 mm in diameter

[f] Disappearance within 24 h

[g] Defects involving the basal layer of the epidermis

[h] Defects involving the dermis and subcutaneous tissue

[i] Localized proliferation and thickening of the epidermal keratin (corn)

[j] More than 80% of the body is erythematous and desquamated (exfoliative dermatitis)

[k] Livedo reticularis

[l] Clustered papules that persist and do not change into other eruptions

[m] Raised lesions 20–30 mm in diameter (e.g., xerosis)

[n] Lesions of hair follicles

[o] Autoimmune disease presenting as bullae

[p] Erosion/ulcer with round halation

and is important in the diagnosis of infectious diseases and rheumatic diseases (Table 5.3).

To understand rash is useful not only in the diagnosis of skin lesions but also in the comprehensive treatment of systemic diseases.

**Table 5.3** Examples of specific rashes

| | |
|---|---|
| Koplik spot | → Measles or rubella |
| Rosacea (Rose rash) | → Syphilis |
| Heliotrope rash | → Dermatomyositis |
| Malar rash (butterfly rash) | → Systemic lupus erythematosus: SLE |
| Discoid rash | → SLE |
| Salmon-colored rash | → Adult-onset still disease: AOS |
| Erythema annulare | → Sjögren's syndrome, Lyme disease, rheumatic fever, etc. |

# 6 Inspection/Palpation/Percussion/Auscultation

Toshimi Chiba

## 6.1 How to Proceed with the Examination

As soon as the patient enters the examination room, pay attention to the patient's gait, facial expression, and movements, and begin the examination. The same attention should be paid to facial features, facial expressions, and conversation when obtaining information about the patient's medical history during the medical interview.

1. Physical examination: To confirm vital signs, respiratory rate, blood pressure, pulse rate, and body temperature should be checked. It is important to check the head and neck, chest, abdomen, extremities, and neurological findings to ascertain the general condition of the patient and to detect negative findings (no abnormal findings) as well as positive findings.
2. Present status: These are the objective findings and physical findings obtained from inspection, palpation, percussion, auscultation, and neurological examination. The medical record should be accurate, detailed, and to the point. It should be written in such a way that the patient's condition can be ascertained by reviewing the medical record.
3. Inspection: A method of medical examination in which findings are obtained by observing

the external appearance of the patient. Compare the left and right to observe the movements of the trunk and limbs and skin abnormalities. The extent and size of abnormal findings should be noted.

4. Palpation: A method of medical examination by touching parts of the body with the hands and fingers. It is mainly useful for the examination of the abdomen, and in the head and neck region, it is also useful for determining the character of masses such as enlarged lymph nodes and thyroid glands.
5. Percussion: The size and position of internal organs and the presence or absence of pathological conditions are determined from the character of the sound produced by tapping the body surface with the fingers and the echoes transmitted to the fingers. Tympanic sound is a high-pitched, reverberant sound and is found in pneumothorax with a large air content and emphysema. It is also useful for percussion of the stomach bubble and dilated intestine due to intestinal obstruction.
6. Auscultation: It is useful for diagnosis of lesions in especially lungs, heart, abdominal organs, and blood vessels; there are two types of stethoscopes: the membrane type for listening to high tone sounds and the bell type for listening to low tone sounds.

   Based on the information obtained during the above physical examination, reconfirm the problems and points to be noted. List the differential diagnosis by considering expected diagnosis.

## 6.2 Head and Neck Examination

### 6.2.1 Skin and Nail Examination

The skin is the largest organ in the body and can often be examined by visual inspection of the exposed skin. Changes in the skin and nails reflect the status of the disease, with cyanosis suggestive of cardiac or pulmonary disease, jaundice suggestive of liver disease, and hyperpigmentation suggestive of hormonal secretion abnormalities such as Addison's disease or hemochromatosis due to hemosiderin deposition. The dorsum of the hands is a predominant region of basal cell carcinoma and keratosis, as well as findings in the ala of the nose, orbital region, and auricle. Malignant melanoma often presents with dark black pigmentation with induration. Petechiae or ecchymosis suggests hematologic disease or cachexia.

In addition, edema is seen systemically in cardiac disease, renal disease, liver cirrhosis, malnutrition, severe anemia, and endocrine disease, and angioneurotic edema (Quincke's edema) may appear transiently on the face and extremities due to increased vascular permeability. Turgor reduction is observed in dehydration. The rash may be a skin symptom of a systemic disease; butterfly rash is an erythematous rash that appears as a butterfly spreading its wings over the nose and cheeks, which systemic lupus erythematosus or dermatomyositis is observed. Erythema nodosum is found mainly on the lower legs and forearms and is associated with hemolytic streptococcal infection, Behcet's disease, ulcerative colitis, and Crohn's disease. Heliotrope erythema is a characteristic of dermatomyositis with purplish-red erythema and swelling of the upper eyelids. Palmar erythema is a reddish lesion on the thenar eminence, the hypothenar eminence, and the proximal of the fingers and is seen in chronic liver dysfunction such as cirrhosis. Other characteristic eruptions include Raynaud's phenomenon, which causes inadequate peripheral blood circulation in the extremities when exposed to cold, and spider angioma of the face and anterior chest seen in liver cirrhosis.

Changes in fingernails are often seen due to chronic diseases, such as cardiopulmonary disease in the case of clubbed finger, liver cirrhosis in the case of white changes, and linear nail hemorrhage in the case of infective endocarditis.

### 6.2.2 Head Examination

1. Inspection: The size, symmetry, and presence of skin lesions should be observed. Hair removal varies widely among individuals; pay attention to localized or age-inappropriate hair removal.
2. Palpation: Check for tenderness of the scalp.

### 6.2.3 Facial Examination

After observing the entire face, the eyes, nose, ears, and mouth should be examined in this order. Inspection of the face is the mainstay of the examination. The morphology and asymmetry of the face suggest various syndromes and pathological abnormalities. The facial expressions include anguish-like face, febrile face, abnegation-like face, masked face, Hippocratic face, moon face, myxedema-like face, and acromegaly face. Cushing's syndrome of moon face and hemiplegia of the face in Bell's palsy are observed, and in acromegaly, the forehead, especially the brow arch, cheekbones, and mandible are prominent, and the skin is dry and rough.

### 6.2.4 Eye Examination

The eyes can be an indicator of systemic disease and should be examined carefully. If the patients wear glasses, remove them before examining the head and neck. Bilateral ocular proptosis is seen in hyperthyroidism, and unilateral ocular proptosis is seen in orbital inflammation, tumors, cyst, and vascular lesions and often in paranasal inflammation. Ptosis is caused by partial myopathy or oculomotor paralysis. Palpebral xanthoma is associated with dyslipidemia, yellow coloring of the bulbar conjunctiva suggests liver disease, and redness suggests allergy or dry eye. The palpebral conjunctiva becomes pale and less red in anemia, and hyperemia of the palpebral conjunctiva and bulbar conjunctiva is seen in inflammation.

### 6.2.5 Ear Examination

The position, size, and shape of the auricle should be examined. The auricular and surrounding skin should be examined for the presence of pigmentation and precancerous lesions. In patients with gout, gouty nodes are suspected to be associated with atherosclerosis of the ear lobe crease.

### 6.2.6 Nasal Examination

The shape of the nose and the skin should be observed. In patients with liver cirrhosis and heavy drinkers of alcohol, dilatation of small veins at the nasal apex is observed.

### 6.2.7 Examination of the Lips

Examine the shape and coloration. The cleft lip should be examined for congenital diseases, and swelling and thickening should be seen in acromegaly, nephrotic syndrome, etc. Pallor should be seen in anemia, and dark red should be seen in polycythemia, and check for cyanosis of the lip.

### 6.2.8 Neck Examination

1. Inspection: Examine the neck for swelling and asymmetry. The trachea and thyroid cartilage should be positioned in the midline. If there is goiter, the neck appears swollen. The sternoclcidomastoid muscle should be checked for left-right difference, contour, redness, and swelling.
2. Palpation: The lymph nodes, thyroid gland, and salivary glands should be palpated. The position of the thyroid cartilage, cricoid cartilage, and sternocleidomastoid muscle should also be confirmed. It is common to palpate with the second to fourth finger pulp, and the findings are evaluated by checking the site, number, size, shape, hardness, surface irregularity, and presence or absence of tenderness, mobility, pulsation, and conglomerate.

   Palpation of the bilateral thyroid glands is useful in detecting enlarged thyroid glands, nodules, and infection. In addition, lymphadenopathy is also useful for diagnosing malignant tumors; the left supraclavicular lymph node, called the Virchow's node, is swollen due to metastasis of abdominal malignant

tumor, often metastasis of gastric cancer. Supraclavicular nodes may become swollen due to metastasis of malignant tumors from the breast, lung, etc. Malignant lymphoma, lymphocytic leukemia, lymph node tuberculosis, and infectious mononucleosis caused by Epstein-Barr virus (EBV) may also cause lymphadenopathy of the neck.
3. Auscultation: If there is swelling of thyroid, check for a vascular murmur.

## 7 Interpretation of Chest Radiograph

Ryoichi Tanaka

### 7.1 Introduction

The chest radiograph is a basic examination with a lot of information. Therefore, obtaining an accurate finding is difficult without a thorough knowledge of the composition of the chest radiograph. In this article, we describe the basics of reading plain chest radiographs and their use.

### 7.2 Basics of Plain Chest Radiographs

"Plain" is the basic imaging method without contrast media such as barium (conventionally used to confirm atrial dilatation and to identify esophageal hiatal hernia).

The first thing to do when interpreting an image is to be aware of its orientation and position. There are three basic orientations such as "frontal," "lateral," or "oblique." Also there are three basic positions such as "upright," "sitting," or "lying." In "lying" position, "supine," "prone," and "lateral decubitus" are included. It is important to properly select the orientation of the image according to the patient's condition and the purpose of the examination. Also, the appearance of the images will differ depending on the orientation, so careful interpretation is required.

The significance of each orientation is as follows:

1. Standing position: The basic body position. Gravity is applied toward the feet.

   Because pulmonary blood flow increases on the bottom side of the lung, the pulmonary vascular shadow is narrower in the upper lung fields and thicker in the lower lung fields. When stomach bubble is seen, the lower part of the bubble is often composed of gastric juice, which is characterized by the formation of a horizontal plane. In the sitting or supine position, elevation of the diaphragm, changes in the distribution of pulmonary vascular shadows (the difference between the upper and lower lung fields disappears), and changes in cardiac shadows (enlargement due to elevation of the diaphragm and dorsal deviation by gravity) are seen.
2. Frontal: The basic direction. Normally, the film and detector are placed just in front of the chest wall, and the X-ray enters from the dorsal (posterior) side and exits from the ventral (anterior) side. This is the posterior-anterior view (PA view). To determine the correct frontal view, the vertebral bodies should be located between the sternoclavicular joints on both sides, and the sternoclavicular joints should be located in the fourth posterior intercostal space. If the sternoclavicular joints are misaligned, mediastinal shadows and lung field density may be modified. Recently because computed tomography (CT) has replaced the role of lateral and oblique chest radiographs, the lateral and oblique chest radiographs are less frequently performed. The lateral decubitus position is useful in the diagnosis of pleural effusion, but it has also been largely replaced by CT.
3. Deep inspiratory position: This is the basic respiratory position for imaging. However, a stable maximum inspiratory position may not be obtained in the elderly, children, or patients with disabilities. Inadequate inspiration can cause elevation of the diaphragm, increased

lung field density, enlarged cardiac shadow, and enhanced pulmonary vascular shadow. Therefore, it is important to know the degree of insufflation. In the deep inspiratory position, the right diaphragm is usually located in the sixth or seventh anterior intercostal space, and the left diaphragm is located 1–1.5 intercostal spaces below it.

## 7.3 Basics of Image Reading

It is important to confirm that the images are taken in the correct position and orientation. When reading images, it is advisable to determine the order of observation to avoid oversight. In general, the images should be read from the outside to the inside. It is advisable to compare the densities of the lung fields at the same height on both sides to avoid the effects of gravity.

The key points are the cardiothoracic ratio, the pulmonary blood flow distribution, and the presence of enlarged mediastinal shadow.

Although pneumonia is often seen as a common disease, in the supine position, pleural effusions may be mistaken for pneumonia because of increased radiopacity of lung field due to overlapping. In pneumonia, the contrast of the pulmonary blood vessels is lost, and the contrast of the bronchi appears as a translucent tract because of the accumulation of exudate in the alveoli around the blood vessels (Fig. 5.4). Aspiration pneumonia occurs more frequently on the dorsal side of the lower lobe of the right lung, because the right main bronchial bifurcation is shallower and aspirated contents tend to move to the "right," "lower," and "dorsal" side due to the effect of gravity in the upright or supine position. In aspiration pneumonia, a high opacity is often seen close to the right heart border. However, because the lesion located dorsal, normal lung tissue is present near the right heart border, and the right heart (right atrium) border remains clear. The depth of the lesion can be inferred from the frontal view alone (Fig. 5.5).

For the dentists, it is necessary to note the following: aspiration and accidental ingestion of foreign bodies, subcutaneous emphysema mainly in the neck caused by air tools, anaphylaxis caused by dental anesthetics, and pulmonary edema secondary to anaphylaxis. In general, foreign bodies can be identified by plain radiographs because many of them are high absorbers of X-rays, but it should be noted that some materials may be difficult to identify by X-rays (Fig. 5.6).

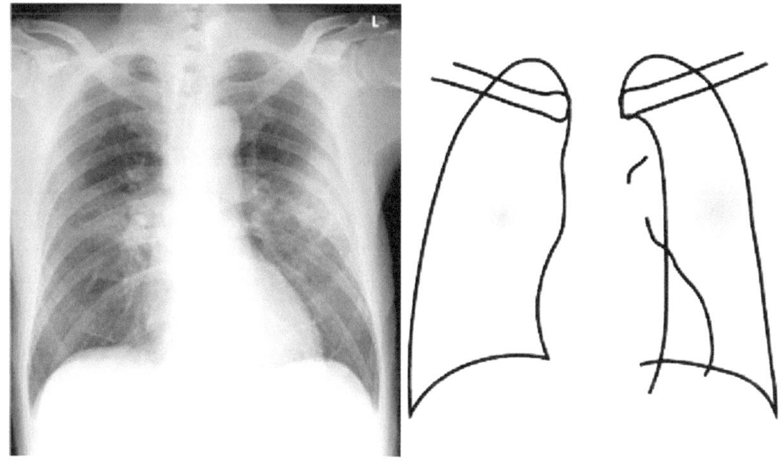


**Fig. 5.4** Bacterial pneumonia. The bilateral middle lung fields show an increase in density (infiltrative shadow) with indistinct margins. In the same area, the border of the pulmonary vascular shadow is unclear, indicating intrapulmonary involvement

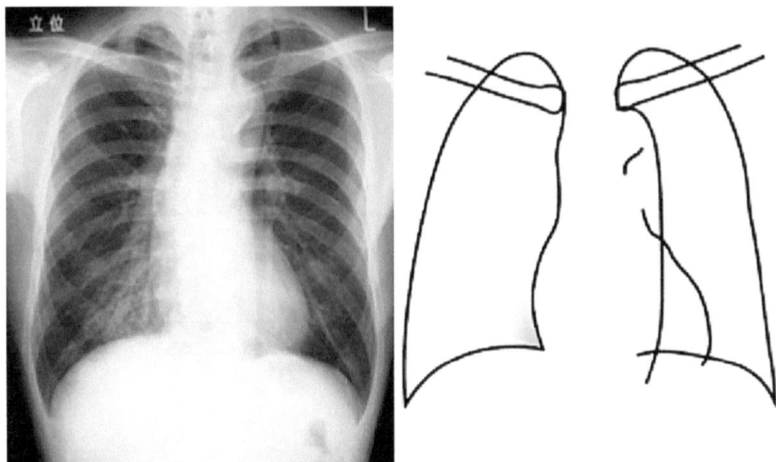


**Fig. 5.5** Aspiration pneumonia. An infiltrative shadow with air bronchogram is seen on the dorsal aspect of the right lower lobe. The bronchial translucency is an indication of an intrapulmonary lesion, as is the blurring of pulmonary vascular margins. In this case, the right atrium was clearly contoured, indicating that the lesion was not adjacent to the right atrium and was therefore located dorsally. Based on this information, the aspiration pneumonia is strongly suspected

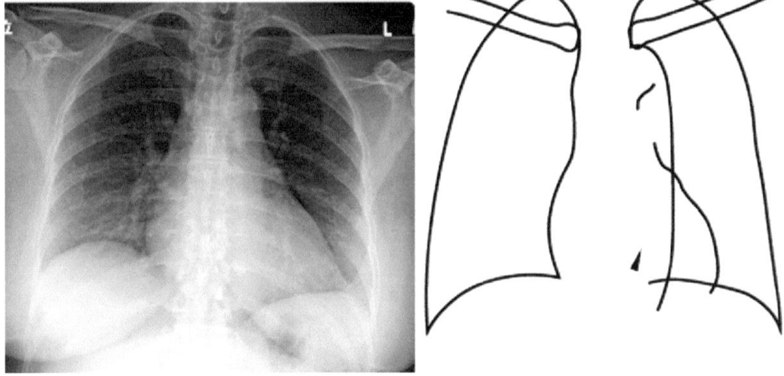


**Fig. 5.6** Foreign body in esophagus (accidental ingestion of foreign body). This is a case of accidental ingestion of a healing abutment. A dense foreign body was found in the lower esophagus. Since there is no lung structure in this part, it can be judged as accidental ingestion rather than aspiration

In addition, acute pulmonary edema associated with acute respiratory distress syndrome (ARDS), a condition related to anaphylaxis, should be noted. A bilateral infiltrating shadow at the lung hilum is a typical finding, and butterfly pulmonary opacities or a batwing sign can be seen (Fig. 5.7). If a patient complains of respiratory symptoms after dental treatment, it is important to keep this syndrome in mind and not to overlook the imaging findings.

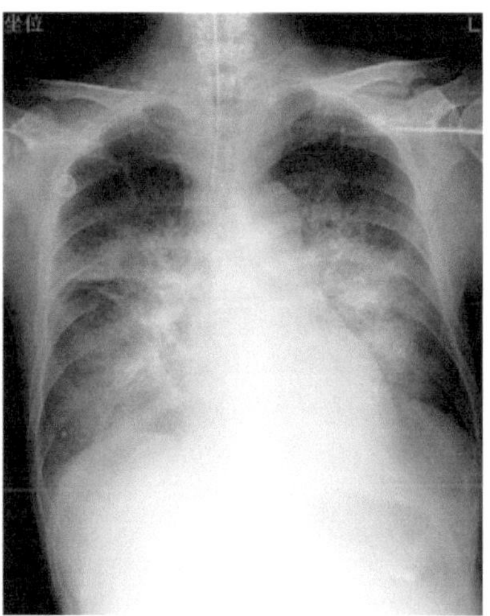

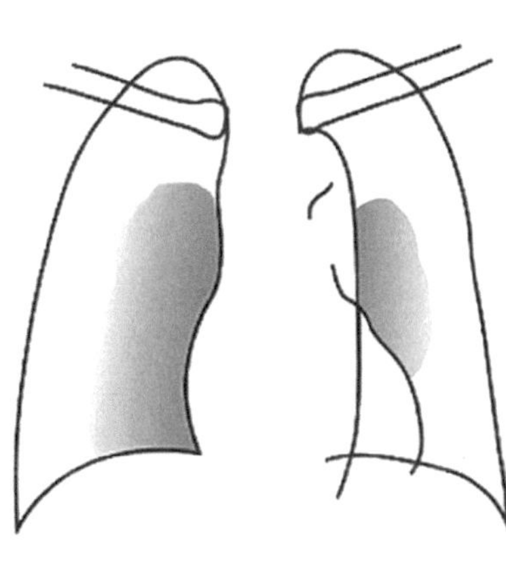

**Fig. 5.7** Acute pulmonary edema. A typical butterfly pulmonary opacities is that an infiltrative shadow that extends around the bilateral hilum is shown. Acute pulmonary edema can be caused by a variety of factors, but when it is caused by anaphylaxis, it is more likely to have an acute outcome and requires an emergency response. In the dental field, dental anesthesia is a potential cause of pulmonary edema, and acute pulmonary edema should be considered when patients complain of dyspnea

## References


1. Kanda J, et al. Relationship between blood sodium concentration and severity of heat stroke and muscle symptoms in heat stroke. KANTO J Jpn Assoc Acute Med. 2010;31:132–3. (in Japanese).
2. Ieko M. Clinical aspects of thrombohaemostasis—for residents I. 2. Differential diagnosis of bleeding tendency. Jpn J Thromb Hemost. 2007;18(6):555–8. (in Japanese).
3. Tomiyama Y. Clinical aspects of thrombohaemostasis—for residents I. 3. Classification and causes of purpura. Jpn J Thromb Hemost. 2007;18(6):559–62. (in Japanese).
4. Nakagawa Y. Atlas of oral mucosal diseases. (Kouku Nenmaku Shikkan Atlas). 2nd ed. Tokyo: Quintessence Publishing; 2018. (in Japanese).
5. Tomita Y, supervisor. Standard textbook of dermatology (Hyoujun Hifuka-gaku). 10th ed. Tokyo: Igaku Shoin; 2017. p. 42–51, 158–185. (in Japanese).
6. Klippel JH, Stone JH, Crofford LJ, White P, editors. Primer on the rheumatic diseases. Germany: Springer; 2008.

# Part II

# Diseases

# 6 Respiratory Diseases

Norihiko Funaguchi, Noritaka Ohga, Yoshimasa Kitagawa, Takuji Kiryu, Tadahide Noguchi, Yoshiyuki Mori, Takeshi Terashima, Hitoshi Miyashita, Tetsu Takahashi, Yasuhiro Gon, Tetsuo Shimizu, Yu Ohashi, Keisuke Hosokawa, Shigeru Sakurai, Kazuro Satoh, Toshimi Chiba, and Atsushi Ogawa

N. Funaguchi · T. Kiryu
Department of Radiology, Asahi University Hospital, Gifu, Japan

N. Ohga · Y. Kitagawa
Hokkaido University Faculty of Dental Medicine, Sapporo, Hokkaido, Japan

T. Noguchi
Department of Dentistry, Oral and Maxillofacial Surgery, School of Medicine, Jichi Medical University, Shimotsuke, Tochigi, Japan

Y. Mori
Department of Dentistry, Oral and Maxillofacial Surgery, Saitama Medical Center, Jichi Medical University, Saitama, Japan

T. Terashima (✉)
Department of Respiratory Medicine, Tokyo Dental College, Ichikawa General Hospital, Ichikawa, Chiba, Japan
e-mail: terasima@tdc.ac.jp

H. Miyashita
Department of Dentistry and Oral Surgery, Tohoku Medical and Pharmaceutical University Hospital, Sendai, Miyagi, Japan

T. Takahashi
Southern Tohoku Fukushima Hospital, Fukushima, Japan

Y. Gon · T. Shimizu
Division of Respiratory Medicine, Department of Internal Medicine, Nihon University School of Medicine, Itabashi-ku, Tokyo, Japan

Y. Ohashi
Division of Oral and Maxillofacial Surgery, Department of Oral and Maxillofacial Reconstructive Surgery, School of Dentistry, Iwate Medical University, Yahaba, Iwate, Japan

K. Hosokawa · S. Sakurai
Division of Behavioral Sleep Medicine and Sleep Disorders Center, Iwate Medical University, Morioka, Iwate, Japan

K. Satoh
Division of Internal Medicine of Dentistry, Department of Oral Medicine, Iwate Medical University, Morioka, Iwate, Japan

Division of Orthodontics, Department of Developmental Oral Health Science, School of Dentistry, Iwate Medical University, Morioka, Iwate, Japan

T. Chiba
Division of Internal Medicine of Dentistry, Department of Oral Medicine, Iwate Medical University, Morioka, Iwate, Japan

A. Ogawa
Division of Oral and Maxillofacial Surgery, Department of Oral and Maxillofacial Reconstructive Surgery, School of Dentistry, Iwate Medical University, Morioka, Iwate, Japan


T. Chiba, H. Yamada (eds.), *Internal Medicine for Dental Treatments*,
https://doi.org/10.1007/978-981-99-3296-2_6

## Acronyms

| | |
|---|---|
| AIDS | Acquired immunodeficiency syndrome |
| CAP | Community-acquired pneumonia |
| CRP | C-reactive protein |
| HAP | Hospital-acquired pneumonia |
| HIV | Human immunodeficiency virus |
| NHCAP | Nursing and healthcare-associated pneumonia |

# 1 Pneumonia [1]

Norihiko Funaguchi

## 1.1 Concept

Pneumonia is an acute inflammation of the lung parenchyma (alveolus) caused by infection with a variety of pathogenic microorganisms. Bacterial pneumonia is the most frequent.

## 1.2 Epidemiology

Since 2011, pneumonia has been the third leading cause of death in Japan, but since pneumonia and aspiration pneumonia have been classified separately since 2017, pneumonia has been ranked fifth and aspiration pneumonia sixth in 2019 statistics. More than 95% of pneumonia deaths were among people aged 65 years or older.

## 1.3 Cause and Classification

There are three types of pneumonia: community-acquired pneumonia (CAP), which occurs in people with no or minimal underlying disease; hospital-acquired pneumonia (HAP), which occurs in patients hospitalized for any disease (after 48 h of hospitalization); and healthcare-associated pneumonia (NHCAP), which occurs mainly in elderly people receiving medical care or nursing care. *Streptococcus pneumoniae*, *Haemophilus influenzae*, *Moraxella catarrhalis*, and *Legionella* are the causative organisms of bacterial pneumonia in CAP. The most important causative organisms of atypical pneumonia in CAP are *Mycoplasma pneumoniae* and *Chlamydophila pneumonia* (chlamydia). It is important to differentiate between bacterial pneumonia and atypical pneumonia, since the effective antimicrobial agents are different for each pneumonia (Fig. 6.1). The frequency of *Staphylococcus aureus* and *Pseudomonas aeruginosa*, including MRSA, is higher in HAP.

**Fig. 6.1** Differentiation between bacterial pneumonia and atypical pneumonia

1. under 60 years of age
2. no or mild underlying disease
3. have a persistent cough
4. lack of findings on chest auscultation
5. no sputum or no causative organism proved by rapid diagnostic method
6. white blood cell count of less than 10,000 μL

| Differential criteria | Suspected atypical pneumonia | Suspected bacterial pneumonia |
|---|---|---|
| Out of 5 items from 1 to 5 | 3 or more items | Less than 2 items |
| Out of 6 items from 1 to 6 | 4 or more items | Less than 3 items |

In NHCAP, aspiration pneumonia is more frequent, and oral *Streptococcus* and anaerobic bacteria should be considered. For *Legionella*, it is important to ask about the history of travel to hot springs and use of circulatory bathtubs. If there is a history of long-term use of steroids or immunosuppressive drugs, it is necessary to differentiate between fungus, *Mycobacterium tuberculosis*, and cytomegalovirus as opportunistic infections.

## 1.4 Symptoms

Symptoms such as fever, cough, sputum, chest pain, and dyspnea are often observed. Bacterial pneumonia is often accompanied by purulent sputum. Mycoplasma pneumonia is characterized by a persistent dry cough without sputum. In addition, malaise, anorexia, and disturbance of consciousness may be observed.

## 1.5 Clinical Examination

The number of leukocytes in the peripheral blood is increased in pneumonia caused by general bacteria, but in atypical pneumonia such as mycoplasma pneumonia, the number of leukocytes is often not increased. Sputum Gram's stain and culture and blood culture should be performed before starting treatment with antimicrobial agents. The urine antigen test for *Streptococcus pneumoniae* and *Legionella pneumophila* and the mycoplasma antigen test using pharyngeal swabs are useful for rapid diagnosis.

Chest roentgenogram shows infiltrative shadows, slit-glass shadows, and other shadows. Chest CT findings are broadly divided into alveolar pneumonia (lobar pneumonia) and bronchopneumonia. In the former, non-distracting infiltrative shadows and slit-glass shadows with bronchial translucency are seen (Fig. 6.2a), and *Streptococcus pneumoniae* and *Legionella pneumophila* are the most common causative organisms that induce severe pneumonia. In the latter case, infiltrative shadows with regional distribution, lobular central granular shadows, branched shadows, and bronchial wall thickening are seen (Fig. 6.2b), and most bacterial pneumonias including atypical pathogens such as *Mycoplasma* and *Haemophilus influenzae* show this pattern.

## 1.6 Treatment

It is evaluated that the presence of sepsis and severity of CAP determines the method of treatment (Fig. 6.3); the NHCAP and HAP determine the risk of aspiration pneumonia and whether the patient is terminal stage of disease or senility and further evaluate the presence of sepsis and severity of pneumonia and the risk of bacterial resistance.

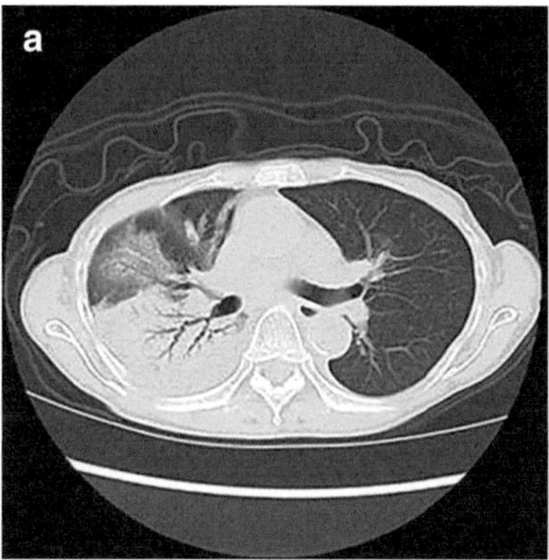


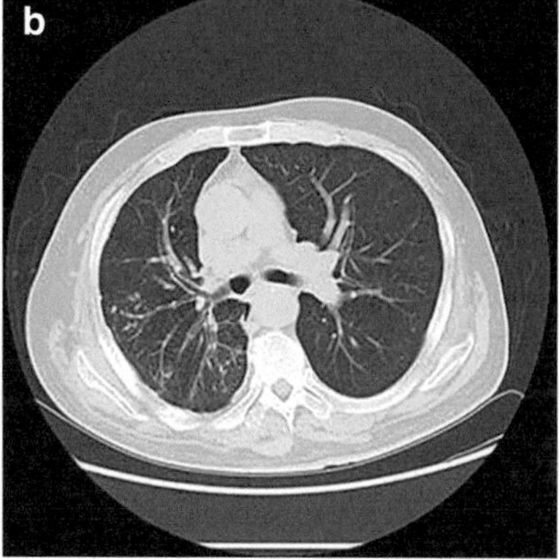


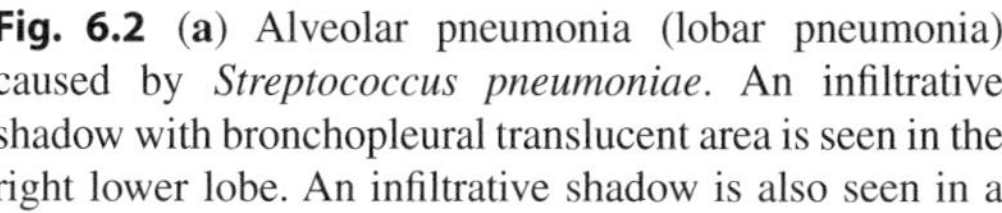

**Fig. 6.2** (**a**) Alveolar pneumonia (lobar pneumonia) caused by *Streptococcus pneumoniae*. An infiltrative shadow with bronchopleural translucent area is seen in the right lower lobe. An infiltrative shadow is also seen in a part of the right upper lobe. (**b**) Bronchopneumonia caused by *Haemophilus influenzae*. Regional granular shadow in the right upper lobe, light infiltrative shadow, and bronchial wall thickening are seen

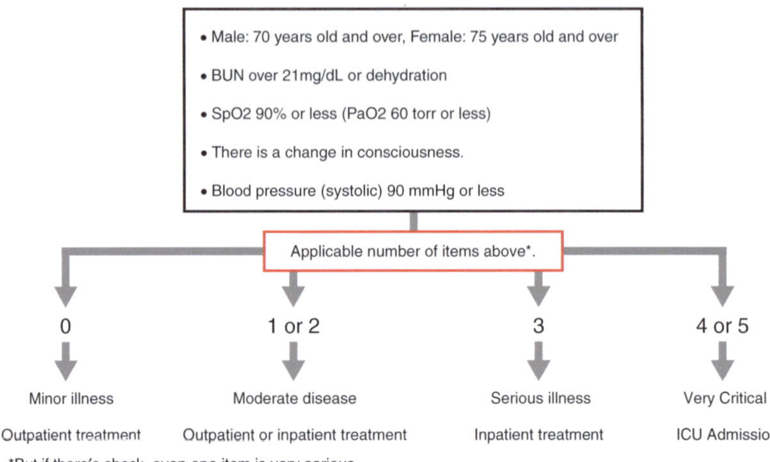


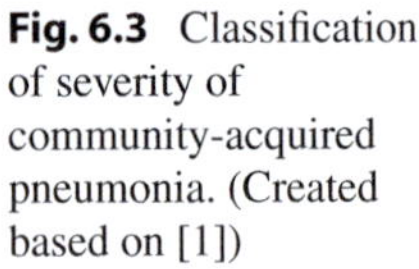
**Fig. 6.3** Classification of severity of community-acquired pneumonia. (Created based on [1])

Empiric therapy is used to identify the causative organism based on the patient's age, underlying medical condition, symptoms, and laboratory findings and to select an antimicrobial agent. It is important to administer sufficient doses of antimicrobial agents at an early stage. When the causative organism and drug susceptibility are determined by sputum culture, targeted therapy is used to select a more appropriate antimicrobial agent. For bacterial pneumonia, $\beta$-lactams such as penicillins and cephems are effective. For atypical pneumonia and *Legionella pneumophila*, $\beta$-lactams are not effective, and macrolides, quinolones, and tetracyclines are effective.

## 1.7 Aspiration Pneumonia

### 1.7.1 Concept

Aspiration pneumonia is a general term for pneumonia caused by aspiration of oral and pharyngeal contents such as saliva containing bacteria, food, and vomit containing gastric juice into the respiratory tract. Aspiration pneumonia accounts for more than 70% of pneumonia in the elderly.

### 1.7.2 Causes and Classification

Aspiration is caused by a decrease in the swallowing and coughing reflexes due to aging or disease. There are two types of aspiration: overt aspiration (aspiration of food or vomit) and silent aspiration (aspiration of small amounts of saliva during sleep or when unconscious). Many elderly patients with recurrent pneumonia are suspected of having aspiration pneumonia caused by silent aspiration.

Risk factors for aspiration pneumonia include cerebrovascular disease, neuromuscular disease that may cause dysphagia, consciousness disorder, severe dementia, gastroesophageal reflux, and multiple antipsychotic medications.

### 1.7.3 Clinical Examination

Hypoxemia, increased peripheral blood leukocyte count, and elevated C-reactive protein are observed. Chest CT shows a predominantly dorsal inferior lung field with ground glass appearance or infiltrative shadows.

### 1.7.4 Treatment

In the acute phase of severe aspiration pneumonia, patients are often forced to stop eating and drinking, and fluid replacement and tube feeding are performed. When the patient's condition improves with treatment, swallowing function is assessed and oral intake is considered. Evaluation of swallowing function includes repeated saliva swallowing tests, revised water swallowing tests, swallowing contrast examination, and swallowing endoscopy. Bacteria that cause aspiration pneumonia include anaerobes such as *Peptostreptococcus*, *Prevotella*, and *Fusobacterium*, as well as *Staphylococcus aureus* and Gram-negative enteric bacteria.

Antibacterial agents such as penicillins containing $\beta$-lactamase inhibitors, carbapenems, and clindamycin are used for treatment.

To prevent aspiration, oral care and swallowing rehabilitation should be performed. It is important to maintain a mildly elevated head position after eating and at bedtime. To raise the level of consciousness, sedative drugs and sleep-promoting drugs should be reduced or discontinued. ACE (angiotensin-converting enzyme) inhibitors and cilostazol should be considered to improve swallowing function. Patients with severe dysphagia or repeated aspirations may require a gastrostomy; however, gastrostomy alone does not prevent silent aspiration, and aspiration pneumonia cannot be completely prevented, so it is important to take measures to prevent aspiration.

## 1.8 Pneumonia as an Opportunistic Infection

### 1.8.1 Pneumocystis Pneumonia

1. Etiology: The pathogen is *Pneumocystis jirovecii*, a fungus, and it is an opportunistic infection that occurs mainly when cellular immunity is markedly impaired.

   It is one of the most common AIDS-related opportunistic infections, and HIV-positive individuals are at increased risk if their peripheral blood CD4 lymphocyte count is less than 200/μL. In non-HIV-positive individuals, risk factors include long-term use of steroids and immunosuppressive drugs, use of biological agents such as anti-TNF-alpha antibodies, and various immunocompromised states such as after bone marrow or organ transplantation.
2. Symptoms: Dry cough, fever, progressive dyspnea, and general malaise.
3. Laboratory tests: Elevated LDH and CRP, hypoxemia, and elevated β-D-glucan and KL-6.

   Chest X-rays show bilateral diffuse ground glass appearances. In chest CT, bilateral diffuse ground glass appearances with shading are typical. A normal area just below the pleura is seen as a characteristic image.

   The diagnosis is made by direct detection of the organism in sputum examination or bronchial lavage fluid by bacterioscopy with Giemsa or Grocott staining or by detection by PCR.
4. Treatment: Sulfamethoxazole and trimethoprim combination is the first choice, and pentamidine and atovaquone are the other therapeutic agents.

## 1.9 Notes from Dentistry Perspective

Yoshimasa Kitagawa, Noritaka Ohga

### 1.9.1 Oral Diseases and Prevention of Pneumonia and Aspiration Pneumonia

#### Etiology and Pathophysiology

When dysphagia occurs, nutritional disorder due to impaired food intake and pneumonia due to aspiration (inflow of food into the respiratory tract) become problems. The swallowing and coughing reflexes of healthy elderly people are similar to those of young people in their 20s, but the swallowing and coughing reflexes of elderly people with aspiration pneumonia are clearly blunted.

The causes of aspiration pneumonia due to dysphagia are as follows: cerebral vascular disease causing bulbar paralysis or pseudobulbar paralysis, postoperative oral cancer (with reconstructive surgery using a pedicled or free flap at the resection site), heavy drinking of alcohol, admission to a nursing home (bedridden state), total parenteral nutrition due to inability of oral ingestion, abnormal occlusion due to denture incompatibility, oral dryness, and poor oral hygiene.

Silent aspiration of saliva or regurgitated gastric contents into the respiratory tract while the patient is asleep is one of the most common causes of aspiration pneumonia. It is said that most pneumonia in the elderly is caused by aspiration due to the decline in swallowing function caused by aging, and it is an urgent need for measures of this problem in this super-aged society.

### Clinical Symptoms

Bacterial aspiration pneumonia generally develops over a period of days or weeks rather than hours. After a few days, the patient becomes sick and often presents with a fever of 37.5 °C or higher, malaise, and sputum production. Blood tests often show abnormally high levels of C-reactive protein (CRP) and peripheral blood leukocyte counts of 9,000/μL or higher, even though there are no obvious infection focuses in the oral cavity. Some patients also show weight loss and anemia, reflecting a more chronic course. Sputum often does not have a stench if the course of the disease is at least 1 week or less. Gram's stain of the sputum shows polymorphic leukocytes and multiple bacterial species. Sputum is often unsuitable as a specimen for anaerobic culture, because it cannot be avoided to be contaminated by oral indigenous bacteria.

### Diagnostic Imaging

On chest X-ray, consolidation is seen in the inferior lung segment due to the effect of gravity. Consolidation may be seen in the basal segment of the inferior lobe if the patient aspirates in the upright position and in the posterior segment of the superior lobe (usually right side) or the segment of inferior lobe if the patient aspirates supine position. The diagnosis of alveolar infiltrates on CT imaging is also very important (Fig. 6.4). In this case, the patient should be treated in collaboration with a respiratory physician. Aspiration pneumonia may be complicated by necrotizing pneumonia and pyothorax.

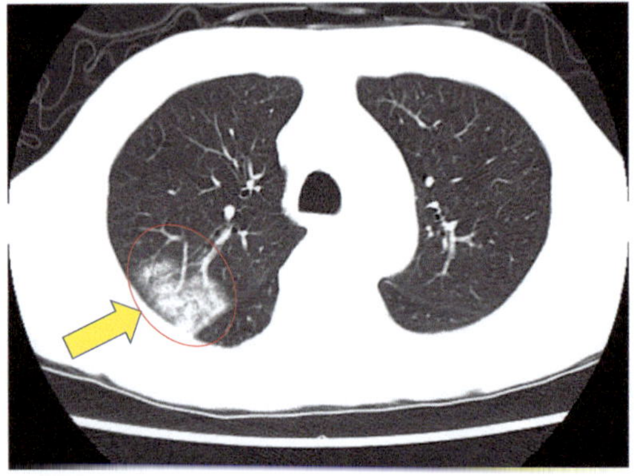

**Fig. 6.4** CT image of aspiration pneumonia

### Prevention of Aspiration Pneumonia and Oral Care

The importance of oral care in the prevention of aspiration pneumonia has been recognized in clinical practice over the past 20 years and is becoming common knowledge among healthcare staffs. To prevent aspiration pneumonia, it is important to reduce the number of oral bacteria by continuous oral care. Detailed oral care procedures are the subject of a separate article, but the basic principle is the mechanical cleaning of the teeth and oral soft tissues with toothbrushes, sponge brushes, and interdental brushes, combined with chemical cleaning methods such as gargling agents to ensure the prevention of oral infections.

Here, we would like to introduce a study conducted by Yoneyama et al. in Japan that pioneered the evidence for the prevention of aspiration pneumonia by oral care. In this study, the effects of oral care on the prevention of pneumonia were investigated over a 2-year period in 11 facilities throughout Japan. Three-hundred sixty-six residents of the facilities were randomly divided into two groups: an oral care group and a non-oral care group. Of the 366 residents, 184 received professional oral care over a 2-year period as the oral care group, whereas 182 did not receive any additional professional oral care. Of the 182 patients in the non-oral care group, 34 (19%) developed new pneumonia, compared with 21 (11%) in the oral care group. Furthermore, 30 patients (16%) in the non-oral care group died of pneumonia, compared with 14 patients (7%) in the oral care group (Fig. 6.5). This study of oral care for the prevention of aspiration pneumonia

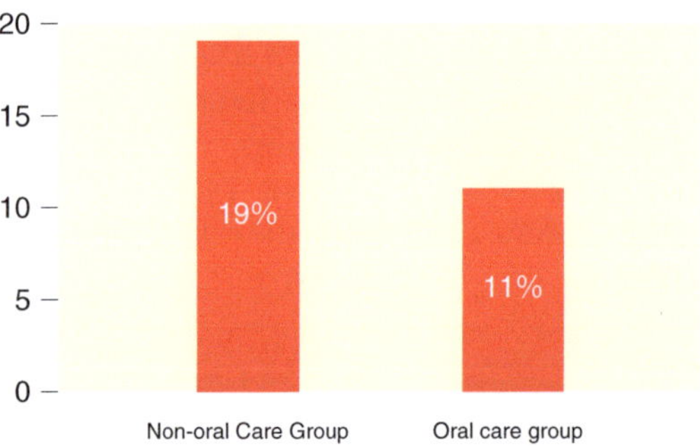


**Fig. 6.5** Comparison of the incidence of pneumonia between the non-oral care group and the oral care group

in elderly people requiring nursing care was published in the Lancet [2] and has received high praise both in Japan and overseas.

Thus, comprehensive oral care, including self-care performed daily by the patient and professional care performed by dentists, dental hygienists, and other specialists, is recognized as one of the top priorities in the prevention of aspiration pneumonia in the multidisciplinary cooperation among dentists, dental hygienists, physicians, nurses, speech therapists, physical therapists, and dietitians.

## 2 Chronic Obstructive Pulmonary Disease (COPD)

Takuji Kiryu

### 2.1 Concept

Chronic obstructive pulmonary disease (COPD) is a pulmonary disease caused by prolonged inhalation of tobacco smoke and other toxic substances. Respiratory function tests (Fig. 6.6) show airflow obstruction. Airflow obstruction is caused by a combination of peripheral airway lesions and emphysematous lesions in various proportions. Clinically, it presents with slowly progressive dyspnea on exertion and chronic cough and sputum, but these symptoms may be absent. The Japanese Respiratory Society Committee for the Preparation of the Fifth Edition of the COPD Guidelines define it as [3].

### 2.2 Epidemiology

COPD is mostly caused by smoking, and the prevalence of COPD in Japan is 8.6%, and the estimated number of patients is more than five million, but the number of people actually receiving medical care is several hundred thousand. According to the 2015 WHO report, COPD is the fourth leading cause of death. In Japan, it has been the tenth leading cause of death since 2014.

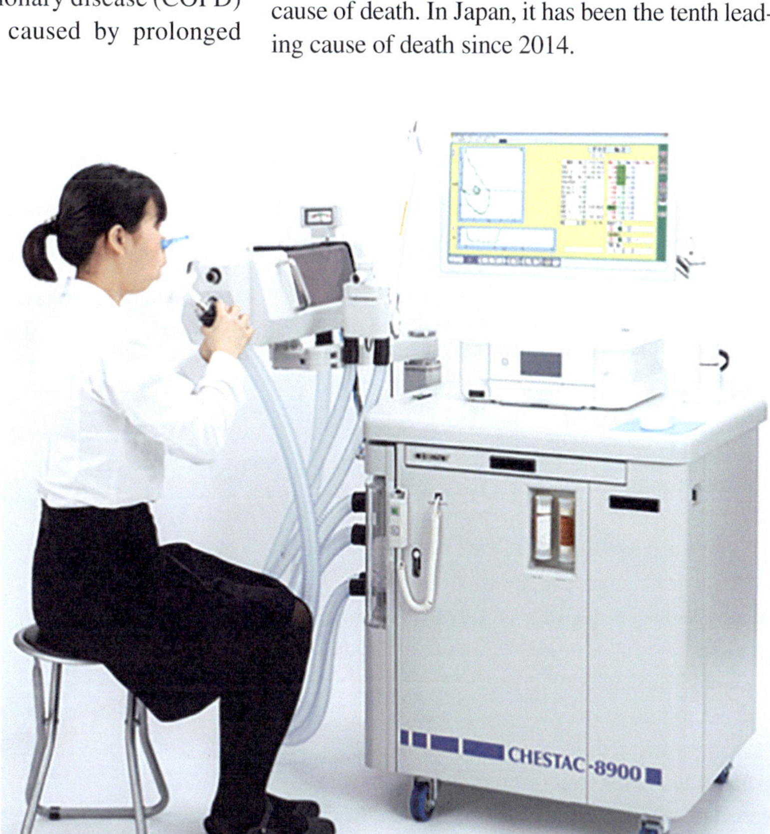


**Fig. 6.6** Respiratory function test. (Courtesy of CHEST M.I., INC.)

## 2.3 Pathogenesis

Risk factors for COPD include exogenous factors such as tobacco smoke, air pollution, respiratory infections, and occupational factors and endogenous factors such as genetic predisposition. Cigarette smoking is the most important risk factor for COPD. About 90% of COPD patients have a history of smoking, and mortality from COPD is about ten times higher in smokers than in nonsmokers.

Except for $\alpha_1$-antitrypsin deficiency, no endogenous factor has been identified as the responsible gene for COPD. In addition to the normal $\alpha_1$-antitrypsin gene (M-type), there are dysfunctional $\alpha_1$-antitrypsin genes (S-type and Z-type). In patients homozygous for ZZ or heterozygous for SZ, which are more common in Europeans and Americans, the level of $\alpha_1$-antitrypsin in the blood is severely reduced and emphysema develops. In Japanese, however, $\alpha_1$-antitrypsin deficiency is very rare.

## 2.4 Diagnosis

The diagnostic criteria for COPD are the following three items:

1. The presence of exposure factors such as a history of long-term smoking.
2. Respiratory function test after bronchodilator inhalation: the ratio of forced expiratory volume in 1 s to forced vital capacity less than 70%.
3. Exclude other diseases that may cause airflow obstruction.

There are two types of COPD: emphysematous COPD and non-emphysematous COPD. In emphysematous COPD, emphysematous lesions predominate and emphysematous shadows are seen predominantly on plain chest X-ray (Fig. 6.7) and computed tomography of the chest (chest CT) (Fig. 6.8), whereas in non-emphysematous COPD, peripheral airway lesions predominate and emphysematous shadows are absent or mild on the above imaging findings.

The staging of COPD is classified into stage I (mild), stage II (moderate), stage III (severe), and stage IV (very severe) according to the degree of decline in the ratio of forced expiratory volume in 1 s to forced vital capacity (FEV1/FVC%).

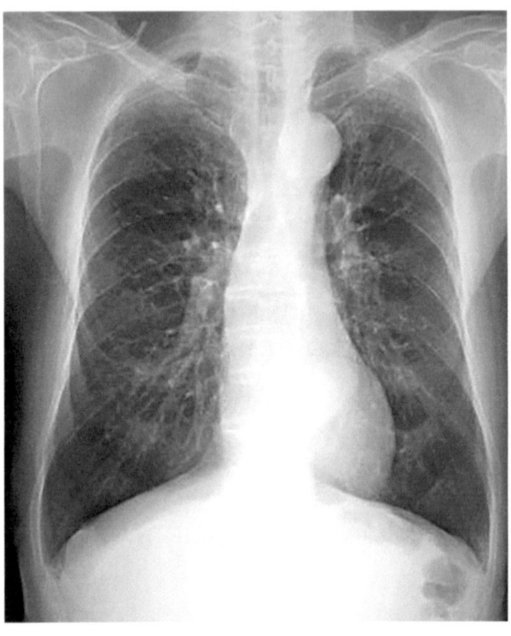

**Fig. 6.7** Chest X-ray. An 81-year-old man. Heavy smoker. Chronic obstructive pulmonary disease/stage III (severe). Increased pulmonary field permeability, diaphragmatic flatness, and drop heart are observed

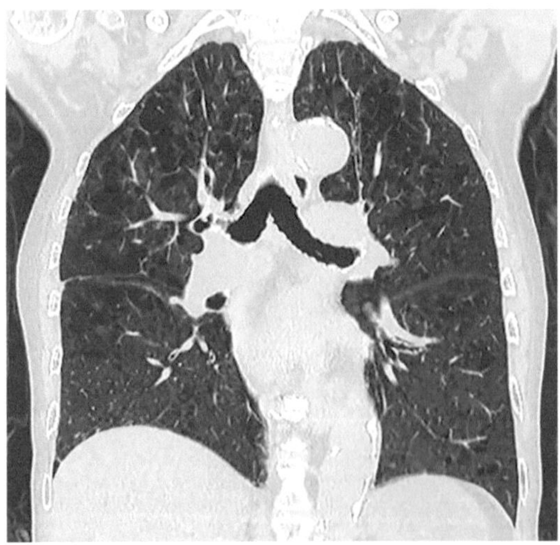

**Fig. 6.8** Chest CT. Seventy three years old. Female. Heavy smoker. Nodular hypoabsorbed areas are scattered or fused together

## 2.5 Clinical Findings

Clinical findings in COPD include shortness of breath, chronic cough, sputum, wheezing, weight loss, and anorexia. Physical examinations include prolonged expiration, pursed mouth breathing, barrel-shaped rib cage, hypertrophy of the sternocleidomastoid muscle, cyanosis, clubbed fingers, and diminished breath sounds on auscultation. A plain chest X-ray (Fig. 6.7) shows increased lung field lucency and a flattened diaphragm, and a chest CT (Fig. 6.8) shows emphysematous changes and airway wall thickening. Respiratory function tests show obstructive ventilatory impairment.

## 2.6 Treatment

The goal of COPD management is to improve the current situation and reduce future risk. Specifically, the severity of COPD should be assessed, smoking cessation should be strictly adhered to, and drug therapy should be combined with nondrug therapies such as respiratory rehabilitation and oxygen therapy.

The mainstay of pharmacotherapy is bronchodilators. There are three classes of bronchodilators: anticholinergics, $\beta_2$-stimulants, and methylxanthines. When the effect of a single agent is insufficient, multiple agents should be used in combination. Inhalants are recommended because of the balance of action and side effects.

## 2.7 Notes from Dentistry Perspective

Tadahide Noguchi, Yoshiyuki Mori

### 2.7.1 The Relationship Between Smoking and the Oral Cavity

#### Effect on Periodontal Disease

The risk factors for periodontal disease are bacterial, environmental, and host factors. Smoking is the greatest environmental risk factor, and smokers have a higher incidence of periodontal disease than nonsmokers, and periodontal disease progresses more rapidly over time. The major effects of nicotine are vasoconstriction and damage to fibroblasts. The vasoconstrictor effect of nicotine causes a decrease in blood flow in the gingival subepithelial vascular network and oxygen desaturation and increases the number and chemotaxis of neutrophils but decreases phagocytosis and collagen production, which exacerbates periodontal disease and reduces the ability to repair periodontal tissues. In addition, it suppresses the antigen-presenting function of macrophages and thus has a suppressive effect on immune function. These effects have been shown in many epidemiological studies [4, 5].

#### Effects on the Oral Mucosa

Direct effects on the oral mucosa also play a major role in the development and progression of mucosal diseases and oral cancer. In the case of oral mucosal diseases, there are reports of increased gingival melanin pigmentation caused by nicotine and increased mucosal keratosis and leukoplakia caused by tobacco chemicals, smoke, and thermal stimulation. Nicotinic keratosis occurs frequently in cigarette and pipe tobacco users and is characterized by extensive white patches on the mucous membrane of the palate with a relatively uniform color tone and petechial erythema coincident with the opening of the minor salivary glands [6] (Fig. 6.9).

Smoking is the greatest risk factor for oral cancer, and it has been shown that initiators and promoters of carcinogenesis are present among the approximately 4,000 chemicals in tobacco smoke.

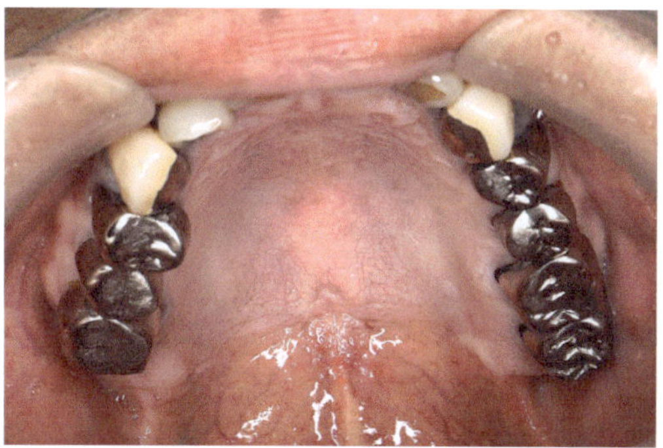

**Fig. 6.9** Nicotinic keratosis. Widespread white patches on the mucous membrane of the palate with petechial erythema coincident with the opening of the minor salivary glands

**New Types of Cigarettes (Noncombustible/ Heated Cigarettes, Electronic Cigarettes)**

Noncombustible/heated cigarettes and electronic cigarettes are new tobacco products, which are inhaled by heating leaf tobacco to produce a nicotine-containing aerosol (noncombustible/ heated cigarettes) or by heating liquid (with or without nicotine) to produce an aerosol (e-cigarettes). However, heated cigarettes, like conventional cigarettes, are addictive due to nicotine and contain toxic substances including carcinogens. In addition, it has been pointed out that the mechanism of generating aerosol by heating decomposes liquid components other than nicotine to generate a complex mixture, which can change into carcinogenic substances [7].

We believe that it will take a considerable amount of time to obtain chemical evidence for the effects of new tobacco products on the oral mucosa.

### 2.7.2 Dental Treatment of Patients with COPD

**Pretreatment Evaluation**

Contact the patient's physician and provide information in advance about the patient's activities of daily living and the degree of dyspnea according to the Hugh-Jones classification (Table 6.1) [8]. Evaluate for the presence of fever, cough, or worsening of the underlying disease, such as respiratory distress.

**Table 6.1** Fletcher, Hugh-Jones classification [8]

| |
|---|
| I. The patient is able to perform most of the same exertions as a normal person of the same age and can walk and climb stairs as well as a normal person |
| II. The patient is able to perform most of the same exertions as a normal person of the same age but cannot climb hills or stairs as well as a normal person |
| III. Cannot walk as well as an able-bodied person even on level ground but can walk more than 1 mile (1.6 km) at his own pace |
| IV. You cannot walk 50 yards (46 m) without resting |
| V. The patient is aware of breathlessness in conversation and in dressing and undressing. Cannot go out due to shortness of breath |

**Preparation**

Transcutaneous arterial blood oxygen saturation ($SpO_2$) is measured using a pulse oximeter.

The patient puts on the device during treatment and compares the status before, during, and after treatment. If there is an obvious decrease in $SpO_2$ from the normal value before treatment, we suspect that the patient's condition is worsening and consult with the attending physician or a specialist to determine whether to continue treatment. In addition, prepare for oxygen administration in case of hypoxemia, and prepare a suction catheter for sputum aspiration. In addition, because of the possibility of oxygen administration, pay attention to the location of combustible materials such as gas burners and alcohol torches.

**Treatment Position**

Deal with the patient in a sitting position. Raise the chair to a comfortable position. In the supine position, the pressure of the abdominal organs interferes with the movement of the diaphragm.

**Treatment Time**

The treatment time should be short, and care should be taken to avoid aspiration during treatment.

**Management by Intravenous Sedation**

It is recommended that intravenous sedation be performed in contact with the patient's physician.

Consideration of the above positions and caution against hypoxemia. Administer oxygen at low flow rates. Prolonged administration of high oxygen concentrations may suppress hypoxic ventilatory stimulation and exacerbate alveolar hypoventilation, resulting in $CO_2$ narcosis.

## 3 Bronchial Asthma

Takeshi Terashima

### 3.1 Concept

Bronchial asthma is a chronic inflammatory disease of the airways, characterized by spontaneous or remission with treatment of symptoms such as wheezing and dyspnea.

### 3.2 Pathophysiology

Airway inflammation involves eosinophils, lymphocytes (mainly Th2 lymphocytes), infiltrating cells (mainly mast cells), airway epithelium, nerves, airway smooth muscle, and secretory glands. Mast cells stimulated by antigens release chemical transmitters such as leukotrienes and histamine, which cause airway edema and bronchial smooth muscle contraction. Eosinophils release granule proteins and detach the airway epithelium, exposing sensory nerve endings and causing increased airway hypersensitivity (narrowing of the airway lumen at the slightest stimulus). When chronic inflammation persists, the airway lumen is narrowed by various stimuli, causing symptoms of airflow limitation.

### 3.3 Epidemiology

The prevalence of bronchial asthma is on the increase, especially in children. The prevalence of asthma in adults in Japan is about 5%.

### 3.4 Categories

There are various clinical phenotypes of bronchial asthma, especially severe bronchial asthma, and the conventionally used phenotypes include atopic asthma, which is an allergic disease, asthma in the elderly, and aspirin-induced asthma. Type II inflammation centered on Th2 lymphocytes is involved in atopic asthma, whereas elderly asthma and obese asthma are more common in nonatopic asthma, and mechanisms other than type II inflammation are thought to be involved.

### 3.5 Symptoms

Symptoms include wheeze, cough, dyspnea, chest tightness, and sputum production. Symptoms appear paroxysmal and recurrent and resolve spontaneously or with treatment. Symptoms tend to appear at night and in the early morning.

### 3.6 Mechanism of Pathogenesis

Genetic predisposition as individual risk factors, childhood viral infection, exposure to allergens such as mites and fungi, air pollution, and smoking as environmental factors have been estimated for the development of bronchial asthma. On the other hand, factors that cause exacerbation of symptoms and acute attacks in patients who have already developed bronchial asthma include exposure to allergens, air pollution, respiratory infection, changes in weather (temperature, humidity, air pressure), food, alcohol, exercise, and irritants (smoke, odor).

### 3.7 Clinical Examination and Diagnosis

Symptoms are important for diagnosis. Repeated episodes of paroxysmal dyspnea, wheezing, and cough, as well as spontaneous or remission of symptoms with treatment, support the diagnosis. The characteristic whistle-like sound wheeze is useful on auscultation during exacerbations, but it is not always heard during non-exacerbations. The presence of obstructive ventilatory impairment (forced expiratory volume in 1 s/forced vital capacity <70%) on spirometry is also helpful. The reversibility of airflow limitation is important, and inhalation of a $\beta_2$-stimulant is considered reversible if the forced expiratory volume in 1 s increases by more than 12% and more than 200 mL. An increase in expiratory nitric oxide concentration and eosinophil count in sputum and peripheral blood also suggests the presence of airway inflammation and bronchial asthma. In the atopic form, serum IgE is high, antigen-specific IgE is positive, and the inhalation test using antigen is positive. Imaging tests, such as chest X-ray and CT, are useful not for diagnosing bronchial asthma but for differentiating other diseases with similar symptoms, such as COPD (chronic obstructive pulmonary disease), heart failure, pneumonia, and lung cancer.

## 3.8 Severity

The severity of the chronic phase is classified according to the frequency and intensity of asthma exacerbations, impact on daily life, and nocturnal symptoms. The severity of exacerbations is assessed by the ability to talk and walk, the ability to lie down, the state of consciousness, and the degree of hypoxemia estimated from transcutaneous arterial blood oxygen saturation ($SpO_2$) [9].

## 3.9 Treatment

There are two types of treatment: one for long-term management in the chronic phase and the other for exacerbations. In the long-term management, it is important to avoid or eliminate risk factors that cause exacerbations and to maintain sufficient bronchodilation by reducing airway inflammation with drug therapy. The goal is to keep respiratory function as normal as possible and to be able to lead a normal life without restrictions. Inhalants with few side effects and localized airway effects are the mainstay of pharmacotherapy.

### 3.9.1 Chronic Phase

Inhaled corticosteroids with anti-inflammatory properties are used as first-line agents and depending on the severity of the disease, long-acting bronchodilators, tiotropium soft mist preparations, and leukotriene receptor antagonists are used in combination [9]. In Step 1, low-dose inhaled corticosteroids are used, and in Step 2, low to moderate doses of inhaled corticosteroids are used, sometimes in combination with long-acting $\beta_2$-stimulants or tiotropium soft mist preparations. In Step 3, a long-acting $\beta_2$-stimulant is added to a moderate- to high-dose inhaled corticosteroids, and if symptoms are uncontrolled, a tiotropium soft mist, leukotriene receptor antagonist, or sustained-release theophylline is added. In Step 4, even with high-dose inhaled corticosteroids and the above concomitant medications, symptoms often worsen and daily life is restricted. Add-on treatment options that may be considered include anti-immunoglobulin-E (IgE), anti-interleukin (IL)-5 antibody, anti-IL-5 receptor $\alpha$-antibody, or oral corticosteroids. Short-acting $\beta_2$-stimulants are used for exacerbations [9].

### 3.9.2 During an Acute Attack

For mild exacerbations, inhaled short-acting $\beta_2$-stimulants should be administered. Patients with more than moderate exacerbations should be treated in the emergency room or hospitalized. In such cases, inhalation of short-acting $\beta_2$-stimulants, intravenous corticosteroids, and oxygen inhalation are used [9].

## 3.10 Complications

Asthma is often associated with other allergic diseases such as allergic rhinitis, eosinophilic sinusitis, nasal polyps, and atopic dermatitis. The combination of bronchial asthma and COPD is known as asthma-COPD overlap (ACO).

A severe asthma attack may occur 30 min to 2 h after taking acidic nonsteroidal anti-inflammatory drugs (NSAIDs) such as aspirin, and called aspirin-induced asthma. 5–10% of adult-onset asthma cases are observed, and nasal polyps and sinusitis are often associated. Because NSAIDs other than aspirin can cause asthma, administration of indomethacin, ibuprofen, naproxen, diclofenac sodium, ketoprofen, piroxicam, and mefenamic acid is contraindicated. In addition to oral medications, injections, suppositories, and transdermal patch containing similar ingredients may also cause this condition.

## 3.11 The Latest Therapeutic Drugs

A series of biologic agents have been introduced for the treatment of refractory/severe asthma: omalizumab, an anti-IgE antibody, was approved in 2009, followed by mepolizumab, an anti-IL-5 antibody, in 2016, and benralizumab, an anti-

IL-5 receptor alpha antibody, in 2018, and dupilumab, an anti-IL-4 receptor alpha antibody, was added in 2019. They provide exacerbation control, improved quality of life, and a reduction in the need for oral corticosteroids, expanding the range of options for the treatment of severe asthma, which has been difficult to treat.

Type II inflammation is an inflammation of the respiratory tract in which Th2 cells and type 2 innate lymphocytes (ILC2) are involved. Cytokines such as IL-4, IL-5, and IL-13 are secreted by Th2 cells and ILC2 upon antigen stimulation; IL-4 and IL-13 stimulate IgE production from B cells, and IL-5 induces eosinophilic inflammation.

## 3.12 Notes from Dentistry Perspective [9–14]

Hitoshi Miyashita, Tetsu Takahashi

### 3.12.1 Bronchial Asthma and Dentistry

Bronchial asthma is defined as "a disease characterized by chronic airway inflammation with variable symptoms of airway narrowing (wheezing, dyspnea) and cough."

In this section, we describe (essential) considerations and managements of bronchial asthma in dental treatment.

### 3.12.2 At the Time of Initial Examination

#### Interview and Examination

When patients with characteristic symptoms of bronchial asthma (Table 6.2) come to the hospital, you need to take medical history about the time of onset, symptoms, and treatment.

**Table 6.2** Typical symptoms of asthma (created based on [9])

- The recurrence of paroxysmal dyspnea, wheezing, and cough
- Exacerbations may be induced by a viral infection, exercise, allergen exposure, climate change, cold air, or cigarette smoking
- Asthma symptoms often vary with seasons and even with the time of the day; they may occur at night or early in the morning

#### Prevention

The prevention of bronchial asthma is described in terms of "high risk of the disease and primary prevention," "risk factors of asthma attack and secondary prevention," and "risk factors for exacerbations and tertiary prevention." Tertiary prevention includes preventing exacerbations after developing asthma and avoiding allergens and nonspecific factors for exacerbations. In addition to drug therapy, we need to recognize the importance of environmental improvement for avoidance of allergens and antigen removal.

#### Triggers for Asthma Attacks

(1) Allergens, (2) air pollution, (3) smoking, (4) weather changes, (5) food and food additives, (6) irritancy (odors, etc.), and (7) respiratory tract infections are considered as the environmental factors related to asthma and induced factors for attack.

Identify and understand every factor for each patient.

#### Aspirin-Induced Asthma (AIA)

Patients with AIA has been reported to be approximately 10% of those with adult asthma. It is more common in cases with severe asthma. The acute attack rapidly affects airways and total body. This disease is induced by oral administration of NSAIDs such as loxoprofen sodium, which is widely used. People who develop AIA likely have nasal polyps, sinusitis, olfactory dysfunction, recurring nasal congestion, and sensitivity to NSAIDs. It is important to check the history of developing drug-induced asthma attack and consult attending physicians to identify drugs available for each patient with AIA.

#### Severity

The severity of bronchial asthma should be assessed according to tables in [9].

#### Treatment

In addition to various long-term maintenance treatments, including inhaled corticosteroids, inhalation of inhalation of short-acting $\beta_2$-

stimulants is often prescribed to treat an acute attack. Refer to "9. Treatment" in 3. Bronchial Asthma section. Check these prescription drugs.

#### Management of Asthma Attacks

It is required to understand primary care management of asthma attacks. In cases with intermittent or mild asthma, short-acting bronchodilator, which is commonly called "relievers" or "rescue medications," provides fast relief of the attacks. However, in moderate or severe cases, patients should be treated at emergency hospitals immediately.

#### Consultation with Attending Physicians

It is important to get the information for taking asthma medications, severity, and control status and to make sure how we manage asthma attacks.

### 3.12.3 Dental Considerations in Patients with Bronchial Asthma

#### Before Starting Dental Treatment

Close cooperation with attending physicians is essential.

- In unstable cases or cases with moderate to severe disease, you should ask specialists of general or university hospital for their treatment.
- In intermittent or mild cases, if patients are appropriately treated and symptoms are well controlled, you should treat them with care.
- As a general rule, it is better to cancel or postpone the treatment if patients have symptoms such as wheezing or cough.
- There is a risk of another asthma attack in patients presenting attacks within a month.
- It is always necessary to prepare for oxygen therapy and check medical monitors.

#### Preventing Asthma Exacerbations

- Treat when the patient's condition is well.
- Be aware that asthma attacks commonly tend to occur in the early morning, at night, or during seasonal changes.
- Remove dust and clean the room.
- Make sure of the asthma control status, and confirm the patient has "a reliever" or "a rescue medication" when you treat.

#### During Treatment

- It is better to instruct patients that if they are aware of asthma symptoms, tell us as soon as possible.
- The treatment should be kept as short as possible.
- You should care of the patients' condition under treatments and take a break and gargle.
- Pay attention to the patient's position during treatment so that it is comfortable for the patient. Breathing may become difficult in the horizontal position. In this case, the patient should be examined in a semi-sitting position.
- Suction of cuttings during dental treatment should be performed, and dental laboratory operations should be avoided around the patient; also, be careful not to inhale irritating odors into the respiratory tract. Since many dental chemicals have a characteristic odor, it is necessary to prevent attacks. Extraoral suction systems can be effective for these.
- It is advisable to always use a pulse oximeter for monitoring $SpO_2$.
- You have to prepare for oxygen therapy.
- Try to avoid giving pain and to reduce stress as much as possible.
- Sedation may be effective if you are skilled. Unless you are a sedation expert, you should not administer sedation. Laughing gas may induce attacks, especially if airway hypersensitivity is increased.

#### Local Anesthetics in Dentistry

- Methyl parahydroxybenzoate, which is contained as antiseptics in some dental local anesthetics and surface ones, have been reported to impact asthma development. Use methyl parahydroxybenzoate acid-free local anesthetics.
- If patients use $\beta_2$-stimulants as bronchodilators, concomitant use with epinephrine contained in local anesthetics may cause arrhythmia because of the increasing adrenergic stimulation.

### 3.12.4 How to Manage Asthma Attacks

The management is needed in accordance with "Table in [9]. Severity and treatment of acute bronchial asthma attacks."

First, discontinue treatment immediately, and check the level of consciousness and respiratory status of the patient.

Next are the following:

1. Place the patient in a sitting position to relieve dyspnea, loosen their clothes, and instruct them to take a deep breath.
2. Use "a reliever" or "a rescue medication."
3. Administer oxygen to them, and measure $SpO_2$ and other vital signs.
4. In intermittent or mild asthma, these procedures may be able to provide relief of the attacks.
5. In moderate to severe or refractory asthma, the patient should be treated at emergency hospitals immediately.
6. Subcutaneous injection of 0.1–0.3 mg (0.1–0.3 mL) of Bosmin® (0.1% adrenaline) is recommended as an emergency treatment for patients with moderate disease or more. You can administer repeated doses every 20–30 min.[1] You should keep their pulse rate below 130 bpm.

### 3.12.5 How to Manage Patients with AIA

AIA is more common in patients with severe asthma.

1. Oral administration of acetaminophen is considered to be safer than regular NSAIDs. It has been reported that the administration of less than 500 mg, or preferably even less than 300 mg of acetaminophen, is relatively safe.
2. Selective COX-2 inhibitor, celecoxib, has been reported to be a safety profile.
3. Intramuscular injection of Bosmin® (0.1% adrenaline) is the first-choice treatment for symptoms induced by NSAIDs. Administering repeated doses of 0.1–0.2 mg Bosmin® always with oxygen administration is recommended.
4. Rapid injection of intravenous steroids is considered an absolute contraindication, as attacks tend to exacerbate and become severe. Administer a phosphate-type steroid preparation (Rinderon®, Decadron®, etc.) over 1–2 h or longer.

### 3.12.6 In Patients Taking Oral Steroids for a Long Time

- In such cases, asthma control is often inadequate.
- The adrenal glands may not secrete sufficient cortisol against the stress because of its dysfunction. Therefore, in cases needing invasive procedures such as oral surgical approach, it is important to consult with attending physicians about the dosage of steroids.
- Such patients are immune-compromised and already at risk of infectious complications. We have to work for preventing and controlling infections.

### 3.12.7 Bronchial Asthma Medications and the Oral Environment

- Oral symptoms sometimes occur as a side effect of bronchial asthma medications (e.g., $\beta_2$-stimulants and steroids). Inhaled $\beta_2$-stimulants are reported to decrease saliva secretion by 20–35%, and this leads to causing making dry mouth, dental caries, and periodontitis. In addition, patients using inhaled steroids may develop oral candidiasis. Therefore, the regular care for oral hygiene and dental treatment is necessary.

### 3.12.8 Summary

1. In general, it is important to build a good (trustful) relationship with patients and to provide careful treatment.
2. Always prepare for oxygen therapy and check medical monitors.
3. Understand asthma triggers and the details of the treatment. You need to beware of AIA.

[1]Administration is contraindicated in patients receiving some antipsychotic drugs, α-blockers, and catecholamine preparations and in patients with elevated intraocular pressure such as glaucoma. In addition, it is contraindicated in patients with arteriosclerosis, hyperthyroidism, diabetes, severe arrhythmia, and neuropsychiatric disorders.

4. Understand how to manage asthma attacks.
5. The first step is to prevent asthma attacks. So it is essential to take all necessary precautions.
6. Manage oral hygiene regularly.

## 4 Pulmonary Tuberculosis

Yasuhiro Gon, Tetsuo Shimizu

### 4.1 Epidemiology

In the past, there were many patients with pulmonary tuberculosis in Japan, but the number of patients decreased with postwar economic growth. However, about 20,000 cases of tuberculosis still occur every year, and it is a disease that always requires differentiation among respiratory infections. Tuberculosis (TB) is more prevalent in developing countries and less prevalent in developed countries, but the incidence rate is high in Japan among developed countries. The incidence of tuberculosis (TB) varies widely among regions, with higher incidence in urban areas. The risk factors include the elderly, diabetes mellitus, chronic kidney disease, steroid therapy, and low nutrition, but the disease can also occur in relatively healthy young people; if cough and sputum persist, suspect pulmonary tuberculosis.

### 4.2 *Mycobacterium tuberculosis*

*Mycobacterium tuberculosis* cannot be detected by conventional staining methods for bacteria and is classified as a mycobacteria using Ziehl-Neelsen stain. *Mycobacterium tuberculosis* can be transmitted from person to person, but mycobacteria other than *Mycobacterium tuberculosis* (nontuberculous mycobacteria) cannot be transmitted from person to person. The route of infection is airborne infection, and the lungs are infected by inhalation of *Mycobacterium tuberculosis* spewed with cough. Patients with pulmonary tuberculosis (TB) who detected *Mycobacterium tuberculosis* in their sputum are infectious, so they are usually admitted to a ward isolated from the general public (TB ward), and medical personnel who deal with them use N95 masks as a measure to prevent infection. *Mycobacterium tuberculosis* (TB) invades blood vessels and lymph vessels from the lungs and can infect cervical lymph nodes, larynx, intestines, urinary tract, bones, etc. as extrapulmonary TB.

### 4.3 Symptoms

Symptoms of pulmonary tuberculosis include low fever, cough, sputum, blood sputum, decreased appetite, and weight loss. If cough, sputum, or blood sputum persists for more than 2 weeks, a chest X-ray should be performed to confirm pulmonary tuberculosis.

### 4.4 Diagnostic Imaging

Because pulmonary tuberculosis forms foci in the lung, chest imaging such as chest X-ray and chest CT is important. Pathologically, pulmonary tuberculosis causes caseous necrosis inside the lesion, and cavity lesions are formed when the necrotic material is expelled from the bronchi. The cavity is a typical chest X-ray finding (Fig. 6.10) and the upper lung field is the most common site. If a cavity is found on chest X-ray, pulmonary tuberculosis must be differentiated. A chest computed tomography (CT) scan (Fig. 6.11) can reveal the nature of the shadows in more detail than a chest X-ray. Because *Mycobacterium tuberculosis* is spread through the respiratory tract, small nodules around the cavity and granular shadows along the bronchi are seen.

### 4.5 Examination of Sputum

Bacteriological examination of sputum includes general bacteriological examination and mycobacterium examination. Pulmonary tuberculosis belongs to mycobacteria, and therefore, mycobacterium test is performed. There are three types of mycobacterium tests: smear test, culture test, and PCR test (Table 6.3).

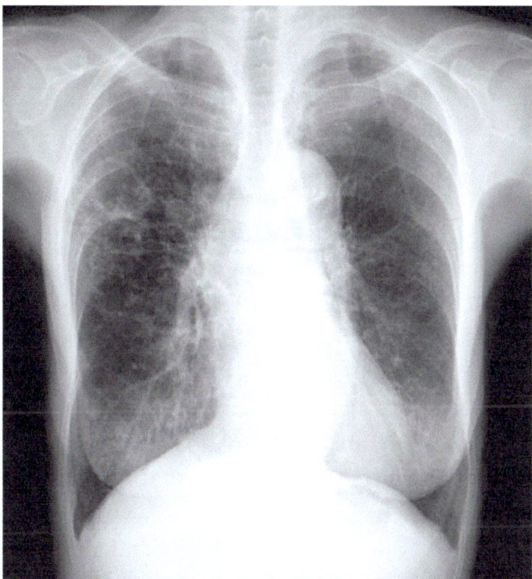

**Fig. 6.10** Chest X-ray. Chest X-ray showing a cavity in the right upper lung field is present

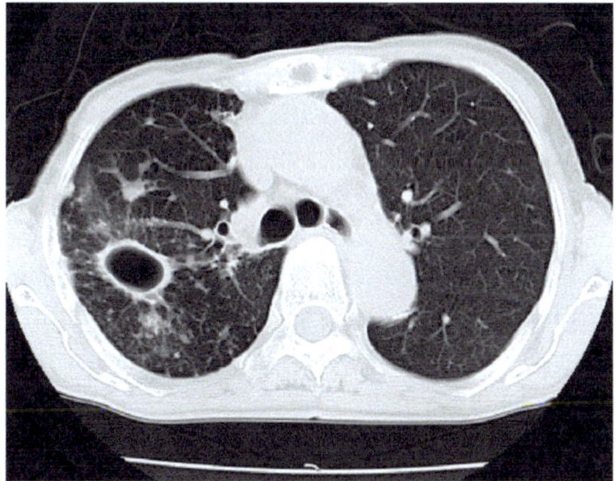

**Fig. 6.11** Chest CT. Chest CT showing a cavity in the right upper lobe with a small nodular and granular shadow around it

**Table 6.3** Methods of antimicrobial testing

| Antiacid bacteria test | Features |
|---|---|
| Smear test | Short time, positive for non-tuberculosis antimicrobial bacilli |
| Culture test | Time consuming, differentiation between viable and dead bacteria, and drug resistance test |
| PCR test | Differentiation of *Mycobacterium tuberculosis* and non-tuberculous mycobacteria |

A combination of smear test, culture test, and PCR test is used to diagnose pulmonary tuberculosis and to determine the effect of treatment after initiation. The smear test is rapid and gives results within a few hours, but it cannot diagnose pulmonary tuberculosis by smear test alone, because nontuberculous mycobacteria are also positive. Although it takes at least a week or more to obtain the results of the culture test, it is possible to determine whether the bacteria are viable or dead and to test for microbial sensitivity test. PCR test can be performed in 2–3 days and can differentiate between *Mycobacterium tuberculosis* and nontuberculous mycobacteria. Clinically, pulmonary tuberculosis is diagnosed when the smear test is positive and the PCR test is positive for *Mycobacterium tuberculosis*. During treatment with anti-tuberculosis drugs, sputum examination (smear test and culture test) should be performed periodically. If there are no symptoms of sputum and sputum examination cannot be performed, gastric juice examination (mycobacterium test in gastric juice) or bronchoscopy should be performed.

## 4.6 Treatment

Antituberculosis drugs such as isoniazid, rifampicin, ethambutol, streptomycin, and pyrazinamide are administered for treatment. Because single-agent antituberculosis drugs tend to develop resistance, the principle of TB treatment is multidrug therapy with antituberculosis drugs. Among antituberculosis drugs, isoniazid and rifampicin are the two main drugs, and the standard treatment for pulmonary tuberculosis is a combination of three to four antituberculosis drugs including these two drugs for more than 6 months (Fig. 6.12). Patients are discharged from the tuberculosis ward when sputum examination shows no evidence of *Mycobacterium tuberculosis* after treatment, and subsequent treatment is provided on an outpatient basis. After completion of the standard treatment, the patient should continue to visit the hospital for 2 years to check for recurrence of pulmonary tuberculosis by chest X-ray. Since each antituber-

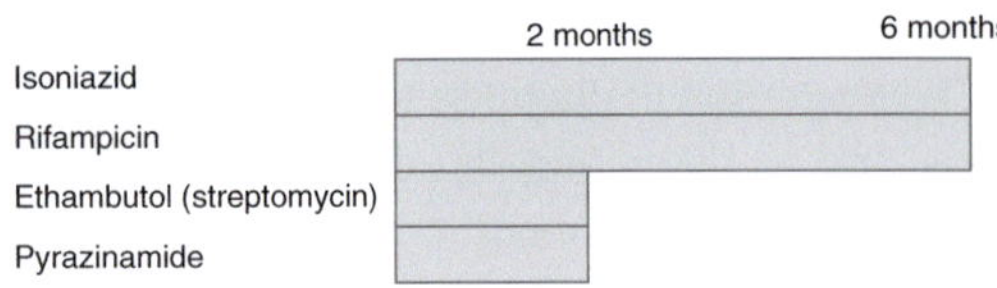


**Fig. 6.12** Standard treatment of tuberculosis

**Table 6.4** Side effects of antituberculosis drugs

| Anti-tuberculosis drugs | Side effect |
|---|---|
| Isoniazid | Peripheral neuropathy |
| Rifampicin | Liver dysfunction and skin rash |
| Ethambutol | Optic neuritis |
| Streptomycin | Hearing impairment |
| Pyrazinamide | Hyperuricemia and liver dysfunction |

culosis drug has its own characteristic side effects, it is important to check the side effects by periodic blood tests (Table 6.4).

It is necessary to instruct patients to take anti-tuberculosis drugs for a specified period of time even after symptoms disappear, because interruption of medication and irregular medication may cause *Mycobacterium tuberculosis* to become drug resistance.

## 4.7 Contact Medical Examination

When a case of infectious tuberculosis (TB) occurs, a contact examination is performed on family members and other contacts who live with the patient, mainly to determine the presence of TB infection. The interferon gamma release assay (IGRA), which is unaffected by BCG vaccination, is currently used to diagnose tuberculosis infection. IGRA includes QFT-3G, which measures interferon gamma in whole blood, and T-SPOT, which measures the number of interferon gamma-producing mononuclear cells.

Latent tuberculosis infection is a condition in which a person is infected with *Mycobacterium tuberculosis* but has not yet developed the disease. If a person is found to have latent tuberculosis infection during a contact examination, prophylactic medication should be considered to prevent the development of tuberculosis. Prophylaxis usually consists of isoniazid for 6 months.

## 4.8 Notes from Dentistry Perspective

Yu Ohashi

### 4.8.1 Pulmonary Tuberculosis and Dental Treatment

Tuberculosis (TB) is an infectious disease caused by *Mycobacterium tuberculosis* and spread by inhalation of droplet nuclei produced during coughing, sneezing, and talking [15]. Droplet nuclei can remain suspended in the air for several hours [16], so adequate infection controls are necessary when dental treatment is performed in patients with active *Mycobacterium tuberculosis* infection. Pulmonary and laryngeal tuberculosis are airborne, so care must be taken to avoid infection [17]. If symptoms such as prolonged coughing, general malaise, anorexia, weight loss, night sweats, bloody sputum, and low-grade fever are observed, pulmonary tuberculosis should be suspected, and the patient should be referred to a respiratory specialist or infectious disease specialist immediately. When a patient suspected of being infected with tuberculosis visits a dental clinic, the patient should be isolated from other patients in time and space and should wear a surgical mask, except when receiving treatment. Individuals at high risk for tuberculosis include older adults; those in precarious employment; civil engineering and construction workers; the homeless; short-term foreign residents from Southeast Asia and South America; refugees; those with HIV infection, diabetes mellitus, and collagen diseases; and regular users of steroids and immunosuppressive drugs [18]. Nonurgent dental treatment should be postponed until the specialist confirms that the patient does not have infectious tuberculosis or that the patient is no longer infectious with active tuberculosis. However, if urgent dental treatment is required for a patient with active TB, the healthcare worker should wear an N95-type mask and treat the patient in a negative pressure room or in a facility that purifies indoor air with a high efficiency particulate air (HEPA) filter [19]

There are many antituberculosis drugs available in Japan, but rifampicin, isoniazid, pyrazinamide, ethambutol, and streptomycin are most frequently used. These antituberculosis drugs are used in the initial standard treatment for tuberculosis [20]. Although the frequency is unknown, rifampicin, isoniazid, and pyrazinamide are likely to cause hepatic damage, and ethambutol may cause visual impairment in addition to hepatic damage. In addition, streptomycin is associated with deafness, tinnitus, and vertigo in the eighth cerebral nerve and numbness and tingling of the lips.

#### 4.8.2 Extrapulmonary Tuberculosis in Dentistry

Tuberculosis that develops outside the lungs, trachea, and bronchi is called extrapulmonary tuberculosis. In general, extrapulmonary tuberculosis can occur throughout the whole body and includes tuberculous pleurisy, lymph node tuberculosis, miliary tuberculosis, intestinal tuberculosis, spinal tuberculosis, tuberculous meningitis, renal and urinary tract tuberculosis, skin tuberculosis, tuberculous peritonitis, pharyngeal tuberculosis, laryngeal tuberculosis, genital tuberculosis, and ocular tuberculosis. In the dental and maxillofacial regions, tuberculous cervical lymphadenitis and oral tuberculosis may be encountered and require attention. In 2017, the total number of newly registered TB patients was 16,789, while the number of extrapulmonary TB patients was 3,599, of which 779 patients developed lymph nodes outside the hilar and mediastinal regions, including tuberculous cervical lymphadenitis. Because there is no category for oral tuberculosis, the number of cases is unknown [21]. Most extrapulmonary tuberculosis is caused by *Mycobacterium tuberculosis* disseminated hematogenously or lymphogenously from the lungs, when immunocompetence is impaired if *Mycobacterium tuberculosis* remain unsterilized by immune cells [22]. Tuberculous cervical lymphadenitis is staged by Jones and Campbell classification as the following:

- Stage 1: enlarged, firm, mobile, discrete nodes showing nonspecific reactive hyperplasia
- Stage 2: large rubbery nodes fixed to surrounding tissues owing to periadenitis
- Stage 3: central softening due to abscess formation
- Stage 4: collar-stud abscess formation
- Stage 5: sinus tract formation

The diagnostic criteria are (1) presence of a cervical mass, (2) positive tuberculin reaction, (3) presence of caseous granuloma in pathological tissue, (4) evidence of mycobacteria in biopsy material, (5) evidence of *Mycobacterium tuberculosis* in culture from biopsy material, and (6) response to chemotherapy with antituberculosis drugs [23]. In recent years, the usefulness of diagnostic methods such as T-SPOT® TB, which counts the number of interferon gamma-producing cells produced by isolating peripheral blood lymphocytes by blood sampling and culturing them with specific antigens (ESAT-6, CFP-10), has been recognized [24]. Oral tuberculosis causes ulcers on the oral mucosa, most of which are secondary infections from pulmonary tuberculosis foci. This is called ulcerative tuberculosis, and the symptoms are irregular, superficial, and perforated ulcers, with ulcer bases that are granular and covered with grayish-yellow coat, accompanied by marked contact pain, and no induration. Diagnosis is made by detection of *Mycobacterium tuberculosis* in cultures from sputum, saliva, or smears from local lesions and pathological examination by biopsy [25]. The treatment of extrapulmonary tuberculosis is the same as that of pulmonary tuberculosis and mainly consists of drug therapy by a respiratory specialist or an infectious disease specialist [26].

## 5 Sleep Apnea Syndrome

Shigeru Sakurai, Keisuke Hosokawa

### 5.1 Disease Overview (Definition)

Sleep apnea syndrome (SAS) is a chronic and persistent condition that causes repeated respiratory depression and cessation during sleep and sleep disturbance due to hypoxemia and frequent arousals (awakening).

At the time of the report in 1976 [27], hypopnea was defined as “more than 30 apneas lasting more than 10 s during 7 h of sleep, or more than 5 apneas per hour of sleep, with apneas also present during non-REM sleep." However, it was later added to the definition of hypopnea as "a phenomenon in which the respiratory airflow decreases by 30% or more from the baseline during wakefulness, and the oxygen saturation decreases by 3% or more, or is accompanied by an arousal response" (American Sleep Association, 1999) and is now called sleep apnea-hypopnea syndrome. Apnea and hypopnea during sleep are both described as respiratory events, and in adults, the apnea-hypopnea index (AHI), which is the total number of respiratory events divided by the sleep time based on the all-night electroencephalography (EGG), is defined as "the number of respiratory events per hour of sleep is 5 or more," as well as the number of sleep apnea and hypopnea. The latest International Classification of Sleep Disorders (ISDS) defines SAS as "a number of respiratory events per hour of sleep greater than or equal to 5" and daytime symptoms such as drowsiness and hypertension. In the latest International Classification of Sleep Disorders (ICSD-III), SAS is included in sleep-related breathing disorder (SRBD).

## 5.2 Pathophysiology

SAS is a syndrome and includes multiple pathophysiologies. However, both conditions are characterized by repeated respiratory depression and cessation during sleep and can be divided into two major groups: obstructive sleep apnea (OSA) and central sleep apnea (CSA) [28].

In OSA, the upper airway repeatedly collapses due to sleep-induced muscle tone loss, resulting in narrowing and complete obstruction. During the cessation of airflow, movement of the thoracoabdominal wall with respiratory effort is seen, and there is strong snoring when breathing resumes. Obesity is the most important factor associated with the onset of OSA, but maxillofacial morphology and otorhinolaryngological factors (e.g., enlarged tonsils) are also important, and many cases do not have obesity, especially Asian population. OSA is frequently complicated by glucose intolerance, hypertension, cardiovascular disorders (myocardial infarction), cerebrovascular disorders (cerebral infarction, cerebral hemorrhage), etc. Frequent awakenings during sleep disturb sound sleep, resulting in excessive daytime sleepiness and fatigue. In recent years, the relationship between sleep disorders and traffic accidents has become a social problem [29], and the Road Traffic Law has been revised in Japan, so that sleep-related disorders with drowsiness can be grounds for disqualification from driving.

In CSA, respiratory effort itself is lost due to dysfunction of the respiratory center. No movement of the thoracoabdominal wall is observed during airflow cessation, and snoring does not occur. There are several causes of CSA, including organic brain diseases, drug-induced diseases, and primary (idiopathic) CSA.

In addition, Cheyne-Stokes respiration (CSR), a type of CSA, is more common in patients with circulatory dysfunction such as congestive heart failure.

CSR is caused by hyperresponsiveness to partial pressure of carbon dioxide ($PaCO_2$), which leads to hyperventilation by some stimulus, followed by apnea due to the resulting $PaCO_2$ decrease. A gradual increase in respiration is followed by a gradual decrease and cessation of respiration. It is thought to be due to a delay in blood circulation time from the lungs to the chemoreceptors in the neck.

## 5.3 Epidemiology

In a large US survey [30], an AHI of 5 or more was reported in 24% of men and 9% of women, and an AHI of 5 or more with sleepiness was reported in 4% of men and 2% of women. In a subsequent survey report, an AHI of 15 or more was reported in 10% of men aged 30–49 years and 17% of those aged 50–70 years and in 3% of women aged 30–49 years and 9% of those aged 50–70 years [31].

### 5.4 Categories

In addition to the abovementioned classification of clinical classifications such as OSA and CSA, there is a severity classification by AHI obtained by polysomnography (PSG). The AASM (American Academy of Sleep Medicine) classifies AHI less than five times/hour as normal, 5–15 as mild, 15–30 as moderate, and 30 or more as severe [32].

However, diagnostic criteria may vary from country to country due to health insurance system, for example, in Japan 5 to less than 20 is classified as mild disease, 20 to less than 40 as moderate disease, and 40 or more as severe disease and 20 or more as subject to health insurance.

### 5.5 Symptoms

In many cases, patients are referred to a medical institution after being pointed out by others as having strong snoring, apnea, or gasping breathing. In some cases, patients fall asleep on the dental table and show symptoms of apnea and/or snoring or fall asleep in the waiting room while waiting for treatment. Subjective symptoms include midnight awakening, daytime drowsiness, headache and lightheadedness on waking, lack of sound sleep, and fatigue. Other symptoms include heartburn, cough, and nocturia. In addition, clinical symptoms and social problems vary with age.

In children, associations with cognitive-behavioral abnormalities such as attention deficits, hyperactivity, problem behaviors [33], learning disabilities [34], and developmental effects [35] have been reported, and the effects are severe even when the AHI is lower. In the elderly, cases of cognitive dysfunction and confusion with depression, as well as an association with verbal memory, have also been reported [36].

### 5.6 Clinical Examinations

For the definitive diagnosis of SAS based on the definition, it is essential to perform PSG, which can identify the sleep time on EEG, but a simpler diagnostic test is the out-of-center sleep test (OCST) using a portable monitor (PM).

PSG is the gold standard of sleep studies because it simultaneously records electroencephalography (EEG), electroretinography (EOG), nasal airflow, otogeal electromyography (EMG), snoring sounds, chest and abdominal wall movements, electrocardiography (ECG), oxygen saturation, and electromyography of the lower extremities. However, the number of facilities that can perform this test is limited because it requires a dedicated laboratory, testing equipment, and specialized technicians.

PM can be performed at home and can be worn by patients themselves in their usual sleeping environment. However, PM does not include electroencephalography (EEG), so it is difficult to evaluate sleep in terms of both quantity and quality. The results are expressed as the Respiratory Event Index (REI), which is the number of respiratory events divided by the time of the test, and may underestimate the severity of the disease compared with the AHI by PSG.

The Epworth Sleepiness Scale (ESS) is commonly used to evaluate daytime sleepiness, and the ESS scores the degree of sleepiness in situations where sleepiness is likely to occur. If daytime sleepiness is suspected based on the score, it is recommended to refer the patient to a medical institution that can perform an objective sleep test.

### 5.7 Treatment

The first-line treatment for OSA is continuous positive airway pressure (CPAP) therapy. This therapy maintains the patency of the upper airway, which tries to close during sleep, by adding positive pressure to the airway through a nasal mask and keeping it higher than atmospheric pressure. The therapeutic effect is high, and the suppression of complications and improvement of life prognosis have been confirmed. However, it requires a power supply and is not easy to carry. In Japan, the health insurance benefit standard (insurance coverage) is an AHI of at least 20 times/hour for PSG and an REI of at least 40 times/hour for PM.

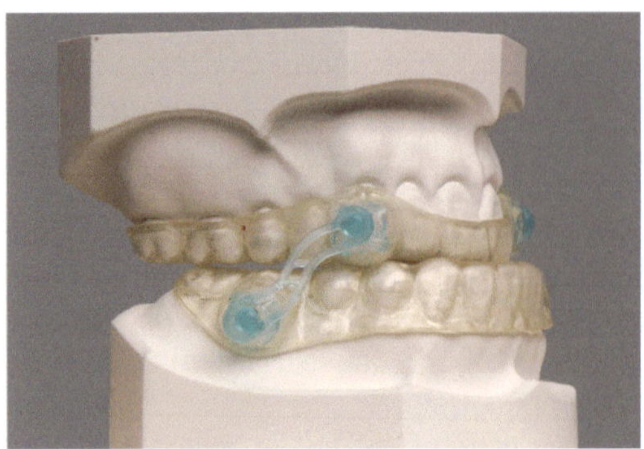

**Fig. 6.13** An example of an oral appliance (OA). Separate upper and lower jaw OA

In some cases, however, it is difficult to control apnea, and adjunctive ventilation such as Adaptive Servo-Ventilation (ASV) or bilevel-positive airway pressure (BiPAP) may be used.

The oral appliance (OA) or mandibular advancement device (MAD) is a dental treatment method (Fig. 6.13), which is more portable and easier than the CPAP device. Other treatments include weight loss and otorhinolaryngological treatment (pharyngoplasty), but in each case, the treatment effect depends on the patient, so it is essential to evaluate the treatment effect after intervention.

## 5.8 Prognosis

Although the severity of SAS is associated with mortality, sleep-disordered breathing is rarely a direct cause of death, and the development of various complications is problematic; when classified into AHI 5–15 (mild), 15–30 (moderate), and >30 (severe), the hazard ratios of death compared with subjects without SAS are 0.93, 1.17, and 1.46, respectively [37]. Furthermore, the hazard ratio for death in men aged 40–70 years with severe SAS is 2.09. In a long-term observational study, when compared with healthy subjects and mild and moderate SAS with AHI 5–30, SAS with AHI 30 or more have a higher incidence of cardiac disease [38]. Furthermore, SAS with an AHI of 15 or more has been reported to be associated with mortality, incidence of stroke, incidence of cancer, and mortality from cancer compared with healthy subjects [39].

## 5.9 Recent Findings

Continuation of treatment with CPAP and OA is essential. In a recent study, the incidence of cardiovascular disease was significantly lower in patients who continued CPAP therapy than in those who discontinued it [40]. The continuation rate of CPAP therapy is determined by checking the usage status recorded in the memory of the device and is judged to be good if it is more than 4 h per day and more than 70% of the treatment period. In general, it is difficult to objectively assess OA use, but recent studies that objectively assessed OA use rate reported that the continuation rate was not related to AHI or ESS at diagnosis but was related to a decrease in snoring and oral dryness [41].

## 5.10 Notes from Dentistry Perspective [42]

Kazuro Satoh

### 5.10.1 Indications for Dental Treatment

The most common type of OSA is sleep apnea Syndrome (SAS), which can be treated by dentistry, while central sleep Apnea (CSA) and mixed sleep apnea (MSA) cannot be treated by dentistry.

### 5.10.2 Dental Treatment Methods: Conservative and Surgical Treatment

In dental treatments, OA, which is regarded as a conservative treatment, is widely performed for OSA in most of the cases. There is also a method of sucking the tongue out of the oral cavity in OA; however, OA is widely used to physically open the airway by guiding the mandible forward in Japan (Figs. 6.13 and 6.14). The application of OA treatments is considered to be mild OSA patients ($5 \leq AHI < 15$), but various methods have been also considered such as combined use with CPAP

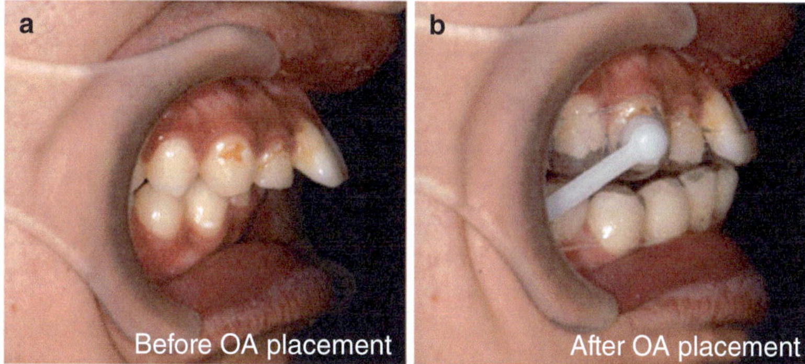


**Fig. 6.14** Oral cavity before (**a**) and after (**b**) OA placement. Forward guidance of the mandible in cases of mandibular recession

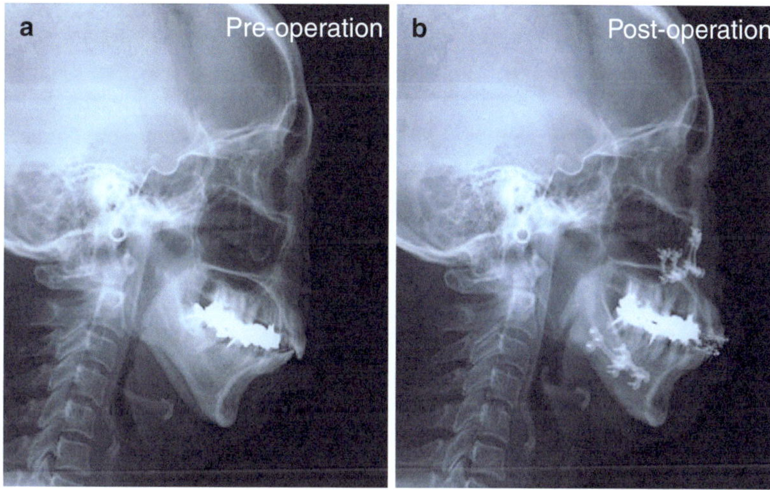


**Fig. 6.15** A case of skeletal type maxillary protrusion with simultaneous upper and lower jaw bone movement by surgical orthodontic treatment. The anterior and posterior diameters of the mesopharynx and inferior pharynx are widened by the upward movement of the maxilla and the forward movement of the mandible

therapy for patients with OSA in the moderate or higher disease. Although OA is relatively a simple treatment, it is difficult to apply to patients with edentulous jaws and complete dentures, whereas there is a risk of causing changes in jawbone position and occlusion by long-term application.

On the other hand, surgical treatments in the dental field include anterior displacement of the genioglossus muscle, partial tongue resection, and surgical orthodontic treatment to reconstruct the occlusion and change the position of the jawbone (Fig. 6.15).

OSA is frequently associated with Treacher Collins syndrome and Pierre Robin syndrome, which show mandibular hypoplasia; Crouzon syndrome, which shows maxillary hypoplasia; and acrocephaly. Although non-syndromic micrognathia can also cause OSA, from the standpoint of dentistry, surgical orthodontic treatment including jawbone movement with occlusal reconstruction may be applied in both symptomatic and non-symptomatic cases of jaw deformity with skeletal malocclusion (jaw deformity). In such patients, orthodontics, plastic surgery, and oral surgery work as a team to treat the jaw deformity and malocclusion.

## 6 Interstitial Lung Disease

Toshimi Chiba

It is a general term for diseases in which the interstitium, such as alveolar septa and interstitium in the broad sense (interlobular interstitium, bronchovascular bundles, pleural lamina propria), is the basic site of inflammation and fibrosis. Diffuse lung disease (interstitial lung disease) is defined as a disease in which diffuse shadows are seen in the bilateral lung fields on chest radiographs or CT images and includes (1) interstitial pneumonia of unknown cause (idiopathic interstitial pneumonias (IIPs)), (2) diseases of unknown cause other than IIPs (sarcoidosis, eosinophilic pneumonia, pulmonary alveolar proteinosis, etc.), and (3) diseases with known causes or underlying diseases [43].

In this section, we describe idiopathic pulmonary fibrosis (IPF), which accounts for more than half of the idiopathic interstitial pneumonia designated as an intractable disease by the Ministry of Health, Labour and Welfare (MHLW) and has a poor prognosis.

## 6.1 Idiopathic Pulmonary Fibrosis (IPF)

### 6.1.1 Disease Overview

It is a type of idiopathic interstitial pneumonia characterized by cryptogenic progressive fibrosis, eventually forming an irreversible honeycomb lung with severe restrictive ventilation and impaired pulmonary diffusing capacity.

### 6.1.2 Pathophysiology

Repeated damage to the alveolar epithelium and basement membrane and proliferation of fibroblasts and myofibroblasts during the repair process cause fibrosis of the interstitium and reconstruction of the alveolar structure. Progressive fibrosis causes respiratory dysfunction, and subpleural honeycomb lung is observed. The pathological diagnosis shows a usual interstitial pneumonia (UIP) pattern, with a complex distribution of fibrotic lesions of various degrees and normal areas adjacent to each other. Heterogeneity of fibrosis is observed and fibrosis progresses from the margin of the lobule.

1. Acute exacerbation of IPF: During the course of IPF, rapid respiratory failure develops on a daily basis, and bilateral diffuse and extensive ground glass appearance to infiltrating shadows newly appear. A decrease in $PaO_2$ and an increase in serum KL-6 are also observed. The prognosis is extremely poor, with a mortality rate of 80%, despite the use of steroid pulse therapy, immunosuppressive agents, anticoagulant therapy, and neutrophil elastase inhibitors. The pathophysiology of acute exacerbation of IPF is diffuse alveolar damage (DAD) which develops based on IPF.

### 6.1.3 Epidemiology

According to the epidemiological survey of IIPs in Japan (2010), the annual incidence rate was 2.65/100,000 and the prevalence rate was 11.8/100,000, of which IPF accounted for more than 90%. However, it is estimated that there is a considerable number of idiopathic nonspecific interstitial pneumonia (iNSIP) that does not appear in statistics, because the diagnosis of disease types other than IPF requires pathological diagnosis by surgical lung biopsy [44]. It is more common in middle-aged men, with a mean age at onset of 64–68 years.

### 6.1.4 Risk Factors

Risk factors for the onset and progression of the disease include smoking, dust exposure, and gastroesophageal reflux disease, with a possible genetic predisposition.

### 6.1.5 Symptoms

The initial symptoms are dry cough and dyspnea on exertion. Fine crackles are heard at the end of inspiration in the bilateral inferior lung fields in more than 90% of cases, and a clubbed finger is present in 30–60% of cases. With progression of the disease, cyanosis, pulmonary heart disease, and peripheral edema are observed.

### 6.1.6 Clinical Examination

1. Hematological and biochemical tests: Elevated levels of sialylated carbohydrate antigen KL-6 and surfactant proteins (SP-D and SP-A) are used as serum markers to monitor the presence of the disease, its pathogenesis, and response to treatment. Autoantibodies such as antinuclear antibodies and rheumatoid factor are found in 10–20% of patients with IPF, and high titers suggest the presence of collagen disease.

2. Plain chest X-ray examination: Reticular and ring-shaped shadows with bilateral inferior lung fields are seen.
3. High-resolution computed tomography (HRCT) of the chest: The findings of honeycombed lung with cystic structures in the bilateral lower lobes, dorsal side, and directly under the pleura (Fig. 6.16).
4. Respiratory function tests: This is a condition based on lung volume reduction, with restrictive ventilation impairment (decrease in total lung capacity and vital capacity (%VC < 80%)) and decreased pulmonary diffusing capacity.
5. Blood gases: Arterial partial oxygen pressure ($PaO_2$) and arterial blood oxygen saturation ($SpO_2$) decrease even at rest. The alveolar-arterial oxygen difference (A-aDo2) increases.

### 6.1.7 Treatment

1. Treatment of chronic stage
   (a) Pharmacotherapy: Recently, the antifibrotic agents pirfenidone (which inhibits the production of growth factors such as TGF-β and platelet-derived growth factor (PDGF)) and nintedanib (PDGF, fibroblast growth factor (FGF), vascular endothelial growth factor (VEGF) receptor antagonist, small molecule tyrosine kinase inhibitor) have been developed and shown to be effective in inhibiting fibrosis.
   (b) Home oxygen therapy (HOT): It is characterized by marked hypoxemia during exertion compared with rest, and HOT should be introduced when $SpO_2 < 90\%$ during ambulation.
   (c) Respiratory rehabilitation: It is recommended for patients in the chronic stable stage with moderate pulmonary function decline and effort lung capacity (FVC) of 60–80%.
2. Treatment of acute exacerbation
   (a) Pharmacotherapy: It has been reported that high-dose steroid therapy and combined use of steroids and immunosuppressive agents prolong survival. In addition, thrombomodulin, which neutralizes high mobility group box 1 protcin (HMGB-1) and has anti-inflammatory effects, and neutrophil elastase inhibitors have been reported to be effective.
   (b) Endotoxin adsorption therapy: PMX-DHP (direct hemoperfusion with a polymyxin B immobilized fiber column), which removes activated neutrophils, has been reported to improve the prognosis of acute exacerbations.

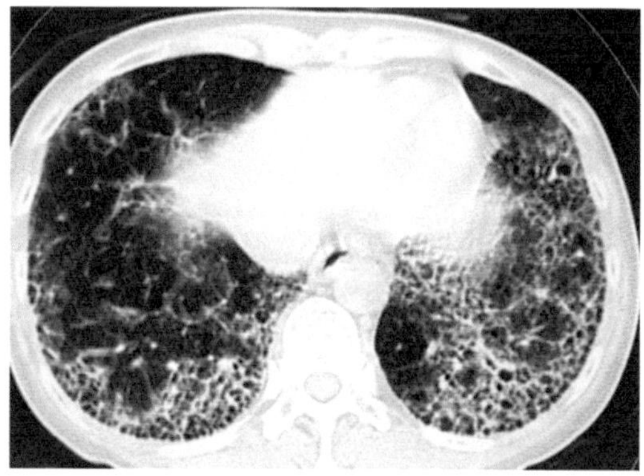

**Fig. 6.16** Chest CT finding shows idiopathic pulmonary fibrosis (IPF). The findings of honeycombed lung with cystic structures in the bilateral lower lobes, dorsal side, and just below the pleura are observed

### 6.1.8 Prognosis

The mean survival is 3–5 years, but individual differences are large and the prognosis is extremely poor. Poor prognostic factors include acute exacerbation, complication of lung cancer, and pulmonary hypertension.

### 6.1.9 Recent Findings

Lung transplantation: IIP is recognized as an indication for lung transplantation in Japan, and the median survival after transplantation is reported to be 4 years. The proportion of living-donor lung transplantation among lung transplantation cases in Japan is higher than in Europe and the United States.

## 6.2 Notes from Dentistry Perspective

Atsushi Ogawa

### 6.2.1 Cause of Interstitial Pneumonia and Its Relation to Dentistry

In Japan, there have been case reports of interstitial pneumonia caused by administration of Hanxia pharmaceutical for cheilitis [45] and tegafur, gimeracil, and oteracil potassium (S-1) for tongue cancer [46, 47]. Reports of interstitial pneumonia have been accumulated not only with anticancer drugs but also with relatively safe Kampo formula [45].

On the other hand, dental workers are 23 times more likely to suffer from idiopathic pulmonary fibrosis than other occupations. This may be due to exposure to infectious agents, chemicals, and fugitive dust in the work environment. It is important for us to note that inhalation exposure increases the risk of occupational respiratory diseases [48].

### 6.2.2 Dry Mouth Symptoms and Interstitial Pneumonia in Sjögren's Syndrome

Sjögren's syndrome is a chronic inflammatory disease of unknown etiology characterized by ocular dryness and xerostomia due to impaired secretion of the lacrimal and salivary glands. Although the clinical manifestations of Sjögren's syndrome are diverse, interstitial pneumonia is an important complication that requires special treatment. Hirohata et al. [49] reported that among 58 patients with Sjögren's syndrome, xerostomia was a glandular symptom in 43 patients (74.1%) and interstitial pneumonia was an extraglandular symptom in 11 patients (19.0%). Furthermore, the complications of interstitial pneumonia in Sjögren's syndrome were almost equal in the proportion of primary and secondary cases [49].

### 6.2.3 Dental Treatment of Patients with Interstitial Pneumonia

Although there are no oral symptoms characteristic of patients with lung diseases, but especially in patients with interstitial pneumonia, dental treatment is often unreasonable because of long-term steroid therapy or complications of lung cancer [50]. If the Fletcher, Hugh-Jones classification [8] (Table 6.1) for dyspnea is II or lower, normal outpatient dental treatment is possible, but if it is IV or higher, only emergency dental treatment is possible [50].

Asahi et al. [51] reported that a patient with idiopathic interstitial pneumonia corresponding to grade IV in the Fletcher, Hugh-Jones classification [8] underwent resin filling under systemic control and died 10 days later of respiratory failure, although no causal relationship to dental treatment was found. On the other hand, oral hygiene should be actively practiced to reduce the aggravating factors of interstitial pneumonia, such as prevention of aspiration pneumonia. Morita et al. [52] considered that professional oral care has a suppressive effect on further exacerbation of pneumonia, especially in patients who have been hospitalized for a long time and are in the terminal stage of severe pneumonia.

### 6.2.4 Home Oxygen Therapy and Dental Treatment and Oral Care

Regardless of whether a patient has interstitial pneumonia or is receiving home oxygen therapy, firework should be avoided near the patient because of the risk of ignition. It has been suggested that inadvertent use of semiconductor laser irradiation in patients receiving home oxygen therapy may result in ignition from the area around the nasal cannula during oxygen inhalation. With the social background of the promotion of home dental care, it is necessary to alert the public to such unexpected risks [53].

Patients receiving home oxygen therapy, especially those receiving oxygen by the mask method, often have dry oral cavity, resulting in viscous sputum and halitosis. In addition, the oral mucosa is easily damaged. Therefore, it is essential to take care of the oral cavity to keep it constantly moist [54].

### 6.2.5 Oral Adverse Events of Pirfenidone

Pirfenidone is an antifibrotic agent indicated for the treatment of idiopathic pulmonary fibrosis. The incidence of oral adverse events caused by this drug has been reported to be 1–5% for stomatitis, and the incidence of adverse events increases with dose escalation. Akiyama et al. [55] reported a case in which multiple painful ulcers appeared on the tongue at the initial dose. In this case, the pain subsided within 1 week after withdrawal of pirfenidone, and the ulcers healed within 2 weeks.

## References


1. The Japanese Respiratory Society. Guidelines for the treatment of adult pneumonia 2017. Tokyo: The Japanese Respiratory Society; 2017. (in Japanese).
2. Yoneyama T, et al. Oral care and pneumonia. Lancet. 1999;354:515.
3. The Japanese Respiratory Society Committee for the preparation of the 5th edition of the COPD guidelines. Guidelines for the diagnosis and treatment of COPD (Chronic obstructive pulmonary disease). 5th ed. 2018. (in Japanese).
4. Omori M, et al. Position paper: smoking and periodontal tissue. J Periodont J. 2011;53(1):40–9. (in Japanese).
5. Furukawa K, et al. Special issue: smoking and health disorders. Influence of tobacco on dental and oral diseases. Jpn J Clin Med. 2013;71(3):459–63. (in Japanese).
6. Kusama M, Kambe Y, et al. Atlas of oral mucosal lesions related to systemic diseases useful for daily clinical practice. Tokyo: Iryoubunkasha; 2011. p. 138. (in Japanese).
7. Kunugita N, et al. Issues surrounding new tobacco and related products such as smokeless tobacco and e-cigarettes. J Natl Inst Public Health. 2015;64(5):501–10. (in Japanese).
8. Fletcher CM. The clinical diagnosis of pulmonary emphysema; an experimental study. Proc R Soc Med. 1952;45:577–84.
9. Nakamura Y, Japanese Society of Allergology, et al. Japanese guidelines for adult asthma 2020. Allergol Int. 2020;69(4):519–48.
10. Committee for Preparing The JRS Guidelines 2019 for The Management of Refractory Asthma. In: The JRS guidelines 2019 for the management of refractory asthma. Tokyo: The Japanese Respiratory Society; 2018. (in Japanese).
11. Japanese Society of Allergology. Japanese guideline for the diagnosis and treatment of allergic diseases 2019. Tokyo: Kyowa Kikaku; 2019. (in Japanese).
12. Kaneko A, Tomino K, Aoki Y, Sano K, Shibahara T, Kawabe R, Shinohara M. Therapeutic agent for bronchial asthma: how to use drugs in dentistry 2019–2022. Tokyo: Dental Diamond; 2018. (in Japanese).
13. Azuma N, Mitsui C, Taniguchi M. Treatment of bronchial asthma advances in aspirin-exacerbated respiratory disease (AERD). Tokyo: Nihon Rinsho; 2016. (in Japanese).
14. Gon Y. Management of asthma and its complications. Tokyo: Nihon Iijishinposha; 2020. (in Japanese).
15. American Thoracic Society, CDC. Diagnostic standards and classification of tuberculosis in adults and children. Am J Respir Crit Care Med. 2000;161:1376–95.
16. Wells WF. Aerodynamics of droplet nuclei [Chapter 3]. In: Wells WF, editor. Cambridge, MA: Harvard University Press; 1955.
17. American Thoracic Society/Centers for Disease Control and Prevention. Diagnostic standards and classification of tuberculosis. Am Rev Respir Dis. 1990;142:725–35.
18. Takahashi T. Infection control in home and visiting dentistry. Monthly Hodanren. 2014;1175:21–6. (in Japanese).
19. Mitsuda T, et al. CDC guidelines for infection control in dentistry. Tokyo: Kokusai Igaku Shuppan; 2004. p. 43–5. (in Japanese).
20. Treatment Committee of the Japanese Society of Tuberculosis. Revision of the "standards of tuberculosis medicine". Kekkaku. 2018;93:61–8. (in Japanese).
21. Center for Epidemiological Information, Research Institute of Tuberculosis. Statistics on tuberculosis, annual report, overview of tuberculosis incidence trends, foreign-born tuberculosis. (2018.10.3) (in Japanese). http://www.jata.or.jp/rit/ekigaku/toukei/nenpou/. Accessed 11 Apr 2019.
22. Nagayama N. Tuberculosis Up to Date A. What are the extrapulmonary tuberculosis? Tokyo: Nankodo; 2013. p. 116–20. (in Japanese).
23. Cantrell RW, et al. Diagnosis and management of tuberculous cervical adenitis. Arch Otolaryngol. 1975;101:53–7.
24. Ohashi Y, et al. A case of tuberculous cervical lymphadenitis in which interferon gamma release assay (IGRA) was useful. J Stomatol. 2018;67:17–22. (in Japanese).
25. Kusama M. Oral mucosal diseases diagnosed by general practitioners: from diagnosis to treatment. Dental Diamond. 2010;35(10):92–3.
26. Treatment Committee of the Research Institute of Tuberculosis. Review of the "standards of tuberculosis care". Kekkaku. 2014;89:683–90. (in Japanese).
27. Guilleminault C, Tilkian A, Dement WC. The sleep apnea syndromes. Annu Rev Med. 1976;27:465–84.
28. American Academy of Sleep Medicine. International classification of sleep disorders. 3rd ed. Darien, IL: American Academy of Sleep Medicine; 2014.
29. Ward KL, Hillman DR, James A, et al. Excessive daytime sleepiness increases the risk of motor vehicle crash in obstructive sleep apnea. J Clin Sleep Med. 2013;9(10):1013–21.
30. Young T, et al. The occurrence of sleep-disordered breathing among middle-aged adults. N Engl J Med. 1993;328(17):1230–5.

31. Peppard PE, Young T, Barnet JH, et al. Increased prevalence of sleep-disordered breathing in adults. Am J Epidemiol. 2013;177(9):1006–14.
32. Sleep-related breathing disorders in adults. Recommendations for syndrome definition and measurement techniques in clinical research. Sleep. 1999;22(5):667–89.
33. Liukkonen K, et al. Symptoms at presentation in children with sleep-related. Int J Pediatr Otorhinolaryngol. 2012;76(3):327–33.
34. Urschitz MS, et al. Snoring, intermittent hypoxia and academic performance in primary school children. Am J Respir Crit Care Med. 2003;168(4):464–8.
35. Nieminen P, et al. Growth and biochemical markers of growth in children with snoring and obstructive sleep apnea. Pediatrics. 2002;109(4):e55.
36. Aloia MS, et al. Neuropsychological changes and treatment compliance in older adults with sleep apnea. J Psychosom Res. 2003;54(1):71–6.
37. Punjabi NM, et al. Sleep-disordered breathing and mortality: a prospective cohort study. PLoS Med. 2009;6(8):e1000132.
38. Marin JM, et al. Long-term cardiovascular outcomes in men with obstructive sleep apnoea-hypopnoea with or without treatment with continuous positive airway pressure: an observational study. Lancet. 2005;365(9464):1046–53.
39. Marshall NS, et al. Sleep apnea and 20-year follow-up for all-cause mortality, stroke, and cancer incidence and mortality in the Busselton Health Study cohort. J Clin Sleep Med. 2014;10(4):355–62.
40. Myllylä M, et al. Nonfatal and fatal cardiovascular disease events in CPAP compliant obstructive sleep apnea patients. Sleep Breath. 2019;23(4):1209–17.
41. Dieltjens M, Verbruggen AE, Braem MJ, et al. Determinants of objective compliance during oral appliance therapy in patients with sleep-disordered breathing: a prospective clinical trial. JAMA Otolaryngol Head Neck Surg. 2015;141(10):894–900.
42. Pirklbauer K, Russmueller G, Stieberlehner L, et al. Maxillomandibular advancement for treatment of obstructive sleep apnea syndrome: a systematic review. J Oral Maxillofac Surg. 2011;69(6):e165–76.
43. Japanese Respiratory Society Committee for the preparation of guidelines for the diagnosis and treatment of diffuse lung disease: guide to the diagnosis and treatment of idiopathic interstitial Pneumonia. Revised 3rd ed. Tokyo: Nankodo; 2016. (in Japanese).
44. Health and Labor Sciences Research Grants-in-Aid for Intractable Diseases Policy Research Project "Research Study on Diffuse Lung Diseases "Group, Committee for Preparation of Treatment Guidelines for Idiopathic Pulmonary Fibrosis, editor. Treatment guidelines for idiopathic pulmonary fibrosis. Tokyo: Nankodo; 2017. (in Japanese).
45. Kashima M, Matsuda M, et al. A case of interstitial pneumonia probably caused by Hanxia pharmaceutica prescribed for cheilitis. J Stomatol. 2012;61:265–70. (in Japanese).
46. Tada Y, Taguchi Y, et al. Pulmonary toxicity by cytotoxic agent, S-1. Intern Med. 2007;46:1243–6. (in Japanese).
47. Yokoe H, Watanabe N, et al. A case of S-1-induced interstitial pneumonia during tongue carcinoma treatment. J Jpn Soc Oral Med. 2012;58:576–80. (in Japanese).
48. Nett RJ, Cummings KJ, et al. Dental personnel treated for idiopathic pulmonary fibrosis at a tertiary care center-Virginia, 2000–2015. MMWR. 2018;67:270–3.
49. Hirohata T, Abe M, et al. Epidemiological analysis of patients with Sjogren's syndrome in Tokyo. Kitasato Igaku. 2016;46:19–23. (in Japanese).
50. Tominaga K. Each theory of patient management (points to be considered in dental treatment). In: Japanese Society of Dentistry for medically compromised patient ed. Dentistry for the sick. 1st ed. Kyoto: Nagasue Shoten; 2018. p. 142–6. (in Japanese).
51. Asahi Y, Kim Y, et al. Management of a patient with severe cardiac and pulmonary dysfunction. J Jpn Soc Dent Med Compromised Patient. 1998;6:60–3. (in Japanese).
52. Morita H, Yamaguchi M, et al. Investigation report of visiting dental managements by our college in the community-based acute hospital without dental unit. Geriatr Dent. 2015;30:337–42. (in Japanese).
53. Yoshida K. Medical safety—safety measures in the field of dentistry and oral surgery. JJSLSM. 2019;40:125–31. (in Japanese).
54. Yamada N. Oral care of patients on oxygen therapy. JIM. 1998;8:610–1. (in Japanese).
55. Akiyama H, Isuke A, et al. A case of pirfenidone-induced tongue ulcerations. J Jpn Soc Oral Med. 2014;27:142–5. (in Japanese).

# 7 Endocrine Diseases

Haruhiro Sato, Yoshiki Sugiyama, Tomoko Hashimoto, Toshie Segawa, and Hiroki Bukawa

## 1 Hyperthyroidism

Haruhiro Sato

### 1.1 Hyperthyroidism [1–5]

#### 1.1.1 Disease Overview

Hyperthyroidism is a condition in which the synthesis of thyroid hormones by the thyroid gland is increased. Therefore, some diseases are known to cause hyperthyroidism. The thyroid gland consists of a follicle and stroma surrounded by thyroid follicular epithelial cells, and thyroglobulin is stored in the follicle. The thyroid follicular epithelial cells produce and secrete thyroxine (T4) and triiodothyronine (T3). Parafollicular cells (C cells) are scattered in the stroma and produce calcitonin. In other words, the thyroid gland produces T4, T3, and calcitonin, but the term thyroid hormone usually refers to both T4 and T3.

#### 1.1.2 Pathophysiology

Hyperthyroidism is a condition in which thyroid hormone synthesis is increased, but thyroid hormones stored in the thyroid follicles leak into the blood and cause elevated blood T4 and T3 levels in conditions in which thyroid follicles are destroyed. On the other hand, the clinical symptoms based on high blood T4 and T3 levels are the same as those of hyperthyroidism, so that these conditions are sometimes referred to together as thyrotoxicosis and strictly distinguished from hyperthyroidism. The main effects of thyroid hormones are to promote growth and maturation and to increase basal metabolic rate, and hyperthyroidism is associated with increased basal metabolic rate.

#### 1.1.3 Epidemiology

The causes of hyperthyroidism vary widely and are thought to account for about 1% of the total population, depending on the region and the report.

#### 1.1.4 Classification

Hyperthyroidism can be classified into primary hyperthyroidism, which is caused by the thyroid gland, and secondary (central) hyperthyroidism, which is caused by extrathyroidal factors. Thyrotoxicosis is classified into primary hyperthyroidism, secondary (central) hyperthyroidism, thyroid destruction, and others (Table 7.1).

H. Sato
Department of Internal Medicine, Oji Seikyo Hospital, Kita-ku, Tokyo, Japan

Y. Sugiyama · T. Hashimoto
Iwate Medical University, Morioka, Iwate, Japan

T. Segawa (✉)
Division of Diabetes, Metabolism and Endocrinology, Department of Internal Medicine, Iwate Medical University, Yahaba, Iwate, Japan
e-mail: psegawa@iwate-med.ac.jp

H. Bukawa
Department of Oral and Maxillofacial Surgery, Institute of Medicine, University of Tsukuba, Tsukuba, Ibaraki, Japan



T. Chiba, H. Yamada (eds.), *Internal Medicine for Dental Treatments*,
https://doi.org/10.1007/978-981-99-3296-2_7

**Table 7.1** Classification of thyrotoxicosis

| |
|---|
| I. Hyperthyroidism |
| 1. Primary |
| Graves' disease |
| Thyroid hormone-producing thyroid tumor (Plummer's disease) |
| 2. Secondary (central) |
| TSH-producing pituitary adenoma |
| II. Due to destruction of the thyroid gland |
| Painless thyroiditis, subacute thyroiditis, etc. |
| III. Others |
| Thyroid hormone overdose |

Primary hyperthyroidism is characterized by autonomous production of T4 and T3 by the thyroid gland independent of thyroid-stimulating hormone (TSH) and is represented by Basedow's disease and thyroid hormone-producing thyroid tumors (Plummer's disease). Secondary (central) hyperthyroidism is represented by pituitary adenomas that produce TSH. Painless thyroiditis and subacute thyroiditis are disorders in which the thyroid follicles are destroyed and blood thyroid hormone levels are elevated. In these diseases, thyroid hormone production is impaired due to the destruction of thyroid follicles. Excessive intake of thyroid hormone preparations also causes symptoms of high blood thyroid hormone levels.

The most frequent cause of hyperthyroidism is primary hyperthyroidism due to Graves' disease.

### 1.1.5 Symptoms

The increased basal metabolic rate causes palpitations, hyperhidrosis, weight loss, general malaise, hand tremors, and tachycardia. When high thyroid hormone levels cause high output heart failure, edema may be observed.

### 1.1.6 Clinical Examination

Blood tests may show low cholesterol, elevated ALP (alkaline phosphatase), AST (aspartate transaminase), ALT (alanine transaminase), and hyperglycemia. Electrocardiography may show sinus tachycardia or atrial fibrillation.

Most of T4 and T3 are bound to serum thyroxine binding globulin, but free T4 and T3 are not bound to thyroxine binding globulin and are biologically active. In hyperthyroidism, high free T4 and high free T3 levels are commonly observed. The diagnosis of primary hyperthyroidism is made when TSH levels are low due to negative feedback, and high TSH levels are diagnosed secondary (central) hyperthyroidism, and hypothalamic and pituitary abnormalities should be investigated. Free T4 and free T3 are also elevated in conditions in which thyroid follicles are destroyed, and TSH is low due to negative feedback.

### 1.1.7 Treatment

In principle, treatment of the causative disease of hyperthyroidism is essential. Therefore, treatment differs depending on the cause of each disease. The treatment of Graves' disease, the most common cause of hyperthyroidism, will be described later. Thyroid hormone-producing thyroid tumor (Plummer's disease) and TSH-producing pituitary adenoma are treated by tumor removal surgery in principle. In principle, beta-blockers are used to treat tachycardia and hypertension caused by high thyroid hormone levels.

### 1.1.8 Prognosis

The causes of hyperthyroidism vary widely, but the prognosis is generally good with appropriate diagnosis and treatment. However, the mortality rate is high in cases of thyroid crisis as described below.

### 1.1.9 Recent Findings

Subclinical hyperthyroidism is a condition in which free T4 and free T3 are within the reference level, but TSH is suppressed and lower than the reference level. It has been suggested that subclinical hypothyroidism may increase the risk of cardiovascular disease and osteoporosis. However, because of the wide variety of causes of hyperthyroidism, it is controversial whether it should be treated or not, and no conclusion has been reached.

## 1.2 Basedow's Disease

### 1.2.1 Disease Overview

It is a thyroid organ-specific autoimmune disease caused by persistent stimulation of the TSH receptor by anti-TSH receptor antibodies, which are autoantibodies against the TSH receptor expressed on the surface of thyroid follicular epithelial cells, resulting in excessive production of T4. It is the most common cause of hyperthyroidism.

#### 1.2.2 Epidemiology

It is more common in women aged 15–50 years, with a male to female ratio of approximately 1:7 to 10.

#### 1.2.3 Symptoms

Palpitation, hyperhidrosis, weight loss, general malaise, hand tremor, and tachycardia are common symptoms of high thyroid hormone levels.

Graves' disease is characterized by (1) goiter, (2) tachycardia, and (3) ocular proptosis, which are collectively referred to as the Merseburg triad. Ocular protrusion is a symptom of the autoimmune mechanism of Graves' disease.

#### 1.2.4 Clinical Examination

A diagnosis of primary hyperthyroidism caused by Graves' disease can be made if blood tests show high free T4, high free T3, low TSH, and positive anti-TSH receptor antibody.

When the radioactive iodine ($^{123}I$) uptake rate test of nuclear medicine is performed, a diffuse increase in the uptake of $I^{123}$ in the thyroid gland is observed.

#### 1.2.5 Treatment

There are three treatment methods for Graves' disease: (1) medical treatment with oral antithyroid medication, (2) isotope therapy, and (3) surgical treatment. In Japan, medical treatment with antithyroid medication is often chosen.

Two types of antithyroid drugs, thiamazole and propylthiouracil, have pharmacologic effects that inhibit the synthesis of thyroid hormones. Severe side effects include leukopenia and hepatic dysfunction.

Isotope therapy is a treatment that takes radioiodine ($^{131}I$); $^{131}I$ destroys follicular epithelial cells in the thyroid gland. It is not indicated for pregnant women, lactating women, and growing children.

In recent years, total thyroidectomy is the most common surgical treatment. Although the thyroid hormone-lowering effect is reliable, postoperative hypothyroidism occurs, and lifelong oral thyroid hormone therapy is required.

### 1.3 Thyroid Crisis

#### 1.3.1 Disease Overview

Thyroid crisis is a life-threatening condition requiring urgent medical treatment in which the body's compensatory mechanism for excessive thyroid hormone action fails and multiple organs become dysfunctional when some kind of severe stress is applied in the presence of untreated or poorly controlled underlying thyroid disease that causes thyrotoxicosis. The clinical symptoms of thyroid crisis are as follows: The clinical manifestations of thyroid crisis include disturbance of consciousness, cardiac failure, shock, tachycardia, high body temperature, diarrhea, and jaundice. Graves' disease is the most common cause.

### 1.4 Thyroid Hormone Regulation [6–8]

Yoshiki Sugiyama

Thyroid hormones consist of thyroxine (T4), triiodothyronine (T3), and reverse T3 (rT3), which are derived from iodine. More than 99% of thyroid hormones in the blood are bound to thyroxine binding globulin, but free thyroid hormones (FT4 and FT3) exert their biological effects. T4 is secreted in larger amounts than T3, but T3 exerts its effects more rapidly and is more active than T4.

The synthesis and secretion of these thyroid hormones are mainly regulated by the hypothalamic-pituitary-thyroid system. In other words, thyrotropin-releasing hormone (TRH) secreted from the hypothalamus stimulates the synthesis and secretion of thyroid-stimulating hormone (TSH) in the anterior pituitary gland and thyroid hormones (T3 and T4) in the thyroid gland. T3 and T4 have a negative feedback mechanism against TRH and TSH, and their blood levels are regulated.

### 1.5 The Action of Thyroid Hormones [6]

1. Heat-producing effect: It increases oxygen consumption and promotes calorie consumption by increasing basal metabolic rate.

2. Effects on growth: It is essential for brain development and bone development.
3. Effect on lipid metabolism: It lowers serum cholesterol level.
4. Actions related to glucose metabolism: It increases absorption of sugar from the intestinal tract and raises blood glucose levels.
5. Actions related to protein metabolism: It plays an important role in the maintenance of protein synthesis.
6. Effect on autonomic nervous system: It has a potentiating effect on beta-adrenergic receptors and increases the heart rate.
7. Effect on the skin: It suppresses subcutaneous tissue deposition of glycosaminoglycan (mucopolysaccharide). In hypothyroidism, myxedema-like facial appearance and edema of the anterior neck that do not leave indentation when compressed (non-pitting edema) are observed.

## 1.6 Notes from Dentistry Perspective

Hyperthyroidism is a condition in which the thyroid gland itself is hyperactive, resulting in increased thyroid hormone synthesis and secretion. On the other hand, thyrotoxicosis, which is often confused with hyperthyroidism, is a condition in which thyroid hormone action is exaggerated due to an excess of thyroid hormones in the body, regardless of the cause. Therefore, it includes not only hyperthyroidism but also cases in which excessive hormones are released due to destruction of the thyroid gland, excessive intake of thyroid hormones, or ectopic thyroid tissue.

### 1.6.1 Diseases Indicative of Hyperthyroidism [6–9]

#### Basedow's Disease (or Graves' Disease)

It is caused by a disruption of immune regulatory mechanisms with the involvement of multiple environmental and genetic factors.

The clinical manifestations include goiter, thyrotoxic symptoms, ocular symptoms, and cutaneous symptoms such as myxedema. As mentioned above, goiter, tachycardia, and ocular proptosis are known as the Merseburg triad. Excessive thyroid hormone action is a symptom of thyrotoxicosis. Thyrotoxic symptoms include palpitations, fatigue, excessive sweating, hand tremors, weight loss, mental instability, tachycardia, increased systolic blood pressure, decreased diastolic blood pressure, and atrial fibrillation. Complications include periodic tetraplegia and myasthenia gravis.

Oral manifestations include tremor of the tongue, early eruption and early loss of deciduous teeth, early eruption of permanent teeth, osteoporosis of the jawbone and skull, and periodontal disease.

#### Hyperthyroidism Other Than Basedow's Disease

There are functional adenomas, toxic multinodular goiter, TSH-producing tumors, hydatidiform moles, and malignant chorioepitheliomas.

#### Thyroid Crisis

Thyroid crisis occurs in patients with untreated or poorly controlled hyperthyroidism who are subjected to severe stress, such as infection, trauma, surgery, or overwork. Thyroid crisis is caused by the failure of the body's compensatory function against excessive thyroid hormone secretion, resulting in the dysfunction of multiple organs. Symptoms include fever and sweating, sinus tachycardia, atrial fibrillation, gastrointestinal symptoms such as vomiting and jaundice, and disturbance of consciousness such as excitement and confusion.

### 1.6.2 Dental Treatment of Patients with Hyperthyroidism [7, 9]

1. In principle, dental treatment should be performed once thyroid function is normalized and cardiac complications are under control. Specifically, if the blood levels of T4, T3, FT4, FT3, and TSH are within the normal range and there are no complications, normal dental treatment can be performed.
2. The severity of the disease and the medications should be checked before treatment. If

necessary, consult a physician. The patient may have been prescribed beta-blockers, anti-arrhythmic agents, or anti-thrombotic agents, and these should be checked. In dental treatment, regular medications should be continued. In addition, hyperthyroidism is a cause of secondary hypertension, and if the patient has hypertension, treatment should be based on the severity of the hypertension. Furthermore, oral surgery, such as tooth extraction, can cause thyroid crisis, so it should be performed only after normalization of thyroid function and confirmation that there are no cardiac complications.

3. During dental treatment, local anesthesia and sedation should be used to reduce stress. A monitor should be attached during treatment. The use of adrenaline-containing local anesthetics should be determined after checking for normal function and the presence of cardiac complications. If necessary, a local anesthetic with felypressin can be used for local anesthesia. In the case of tachycardia or atrial fibrillation, a heart rate of more than 100 beats per minute is associated with high risk [6].

## 2 Hypothyroidism [1, 2, 10–12]

Haruhiro Sato

### 2.1 Hypothyroidism

#### 2.1.1 Disease Overview

Hypothyroidism is a condition in which the synthesis of thyroid hormones by the thyroid gland is decreased. There are diseases that cause hypothyroidism. The thyroid gland consists of a follicle and stroma surrounded by thyroid follicular epithelial cells, and thyroglobulin is stored in the follicle. The thyroid follicular epithelial cells produce and secrete thyroxine (T4) and triiodothyronine (T3).

Chronic thyroiditis is the most common cause of hypothyroidism, but chronic thyroiditis may be associated with normal thyroid function, so chronic thyroiditis and hypothyroidism are not necessarily the same.

#### 2.1.2 Pathophysiology

However, in thyroid hormone resistance syndrome, in which cells cannot respond to T3 due to a loss-of-function mutation in the thyroid hormone receptor in the cell nucleus, the clinical symptoms may be the same as those of hypothyroidism, even if the thyroid T4 and T3 synthetases are normal.

The major actions of thyroid hormones are to promote growth and maturation and to stimulate basal metabolic rate, and these actions are reduced by hypothyroidism.

#### 2.1.3 Epidemiology

Hypothyroidism has a wide range of causes and is thought to affect approximately 3–7% of the population, depending on the region and reports. The male to female ratio is about 1:5 to 10.

#### 2.1.4 Classification

There are three types of hypothyroidism: primary hypothyroidism, in which the thyroid gland itself is injured and the production of T4 and T3 is decreased; secondary (central) hypothyroidism, in which hypothalamic and pituitary gland injury such as tumor, inflammation, circulatory disorders, and so on is observed (with the decrease of the thyroid-stimulating hormone (TSH) or TSH-releasing hormone (TRH), as a result, thyroid hormone secretion is decreased); and, as mentioned above, thyroid hormone resistance syndrome (Table 7.2).

Primary hypothyroidism is caused by chronic thyroiditis (Hashimoto's disease), total thyroidectomy, radiation therapy, or iodine deficiency.

**Table 7.2** Classification of hypothyroidism

| |
|---|
| I. Primary hypothyroidism |
| Chronic thyroiditis (Hashimoto's disease), after total thyroidectomy, after thyroid exposure by radiotherapy, iodine deficiency, cretinism (congenital), etc. |
| II. Secondary (central) hypothyroidism |
| Hypothalamic and pituitary diseases (tumor, inflammation, circulatory disorders, etc.) |
| III. Others |
| Thyroid hormone resistance syndrome |

Primary hypothyroidism is caused by chronic thyroiditis (Hashimoto's disease), total thyroidectomy, thyroid exposure due to radiation therapy, or iodine deficiency. Chronic thyroiditis is the most common cause of hypothyroidism.

### 2.1.5 Symptoms

A decrease in basal metabolic rate due to low thyroid hormone levels causes general malaise, coldness, weight gain, constipation, muscle stiffness, dry skin, bradycardia, hypotension, cardiac failure due to decreased cardiac output, slow movements, somnolence, memory loss, and depression. In the elderly, memory loss and depression worsen, and dementia may be diagnosed.

Edema of the face and lower extremities may occur due to mucopolysaccharide deposition caused by decreased mucopolysaccharide metabolism. Unlike edema caused by water retention in the interstitium due to cardiac failure, this type of edema is characterized by the absence of indentation even when pressure is applied and is called myxedema. Myxedema is characterized by an enlarged lip and a giant tongue due to the deposition of mucopolysaccharide and is called a myxedema-like face. When myxedema caused by hypothyroidism is accompanied by consciousness disorder, it is called myxedematous coma.

### 2.1.6 Clinical Examination

Anemia due to hematopoietic disorders of the bone marrow, high cholesterol and triglyceride levels, and elevations of AST, ALT, and CK (creatine kinase) may be observed. The electrocardiogram may show bradycardia and hypotension.

Most of the blood T4 and T3 are bound to the serum protein thyroxin binding globulin, but free T4 and T3 are more bioactive than free T4 and T3. In hypothyroidism, low free T4 and low free T3 are commonly observed in blood tests. A high level of TSH due to negative feedback is diagnosed as primary hypothyroidism, and a low level of TSH is diagnosed as secondary (central) hypothyroidism.

To diagnose secondary (central) hypothyroidism, a TRH stress test may be performed to stimulate thyrotrophs in the anterior pituitary gland and confirm decreased TSH secretion.

When the radioactive iodine ($^{123}$I) uptake rate test of nuclear medicine is performed, a decrease in $^{123}$I uptake into the thyroid gland is observed.

### 2.1.7 Treatment

In hypothyroidism, appropriate doses of thyroid hormone replacement therapy (levothyroxine sodium) are administered regardless of the causative disease. The dose is gradually increased starting with a small dose, and the maintenance dose is the dose at which TSH, free T4, and free T3 are within the reference values. If the dose is higher than the initial dose, there is a risk of inducing ischemic heart disease because the workload of the heart increases rapidly and the oxygen requirement of the myocardium increases.

Secondary (central) hypothyroidism may be associated with secondary (central) hypoadrenocorticism due to decreased adrenocorticotropic hormone (ACTH) secretion. In this case, adrenocorticotropic hormone should be administered first. In such cases, adrenocortical hormones should be administered first, because prior administration of thyroid hormone may cause metabolic degradation of adrenocortical hormones and exacerbate hypoadrenocorticism.

### 2.1.8 Prognosis

The causes of hypothyroidism vary widely, but the prognosis is generally good with appropriate diagnosis and thyroid hormone replacement therapy. However, myxedematous coma has a high mortality rate and requires prompt diagnosis and treatment.

### 2.1.9 Recent Findings

Subclinical hypothyroidism is a condition in which free T4 and free T3 are within the reference values but TSH is higher than the reference value. It has been suggested that subclinical hypothyroidism may be associated with an increased risk of cardiovascular disease, but whether or not it should be treated has been controversial and inconclusive.

## 2.2 Chronic Thyroiditis (Hashimoto's Disease)

### 2.2.1 Disease Overview

Histopathological examination shows a high lymphocytic infiltration of the thyroid gland, formation of lymphatic follicles, atrophy of the thyroid follicles, and fibrosis of the stroma. It is a thyroid organ-specific autoimmune disease in which the thyroid-specific autoantibodies, anti-thyroid peroxidase antibody, and anti-thyroglobulin antibody are positive. Hashimoto's disease was first reported by Dr. Hakaru Hashimoto. It is the most common cause of primary hypothyroidism, but normal thyroid function is also common.

### 2.2.2 Epidemiology

It is more common in women aged 20–50 years and increases with age. The male to female ratio is 1:10 to 20.

### 2.2.3 Symptoms

A diffuse, firm, and painless goiter is often palpable. When thyroid follicular epithelial cell injury due to autoimmune mechanisms progresses, thyroid hormone production capacity decreases, and clinical symptoms and abnormal laboratory findings common to hypothyroidism due to other causes appear.

### 2.2.4 Clinical Examination

Blood tests are positive for anti-TPO (thyroid peroxidase) and anti-Tg (thyroglobulin) antibodies. Thyroid cytology shows lymphocytic infiltration. In cases of primary hypothyroidism due to atrophy and destruction of thyroid follicles caused by chronic thyroiditis, free T3 and free T4 are low and TSH is high, and the findings are the same as those in primary hypothyroidism due to other causes.

### 2.2.5 Treatment

If thyroid function is normal, observation is sufficient. In the case of primary hypothyroidism, appropriate doses of thyroid hormone (levothyroxine sodium) should be administered.

### 2.2.6 Prognosis

The prognosis is good with proper diagnosis and thyroid hormone replacement therapy, but caution is required because the disease may be complicated by Sjögren's syndrome or malignant lymphoma.

## 2.3 Cretinism

### 2.3.1 Disease Overview

Primary congenital hypothyroidism with a giant tongue that protrudes from the mouth due to mucopolysaccharide deposits, a peculiar facial appearance, short stature especially in the limbs, and decreased intelligence. Treatment consists of prompt administration of appropriate doses of thyroid hormones.

## 2.4 Notes from Dentistry Perspective

Yoshiki Sugiyama

### 2.4.1 Diseases Indicating Hypothyroidism with Visiting of Dentistry

#### Chronic Thyroiditis (Hashimoto's Disease) [7–9]

Thyroid hormone (T4, FT4, T3, FT3) levels in the blood are low, and thyroid-stimulating hormone (TSH) levels increase due to negative feedback. This disease is an organ-specific autoimmune disease in which autoantibodies against thyroglobulin (anti-Tg antibodies) and thyroid peroxidase (anti-TPO antibodies) are found in the blood.

Symptoms include decreased metabolism and myxedema. Diffuse goiter is present in more than 90% of patients.

Systemic symptoms include general malaise, weight gain, decreased body temperature, lethargy, and decreased thinking ability. Cardiovascular symptoms include bradycardia, a decrease in systolic blood pressure, and a decrease in pulse pressure due to an increase in diastolic blood pressure. Gastrointestinal symptoms include decreased peristalsis, decreased appetite, and constipation. Other symptoms include a myxedema-like face, thick lips, macroglossia, dry skin, alopecia, and hoarseness. In severe cases, edema without indentation (non-pitting edema due to myxedema) is seen in the extremities. It is also frequently associated with autoimmune diseases such as Sjögren's syndrome and rheumatoid arthritis. It is treated with thyroid hormone replacement therapy.

**Cretinism [6]**

Cretinism is a congenital form of hypothyroidism. In Japan, the frequency of cretinism is 1 in 6000–7000. Thyroid hormones play an important role during development, and cretinism is associated with short stature, retardation of intellectual and mental development, eyelids with edematous swelling, and a peculiar facial appearance such as a giant tongue from the neonatal period.

#### 2.4.2 Dental Treatment of Patients with Hypothyroidism [7–9]

Oral manifestations of hypothyroidism include delayed tooth eruption, enamel hypoplasia and serrated teeth, plexus and malocclusion due to mandibular dysplasia, and periodontal disease. Because the clinical course of the disease progresses slowly, it is often undiagnosed and requires attention.

If the blood levels of T4, T3, FT4 (free T4), FT3, and TSH are within normal limits, normal dental treatment can be performed.

Patients with hypothyroidism have increased cholesterol levels, which promotes atherosclerosis and may be complicated by atherosclerotic diseases such as angina pectoris, myocardial infarction, and cerebral infarction. Dental treatment should be started only after these cardiac complications are under control. In addition, Schmidt's syndrome, which presents with complications of chronic thyroiditis and Addison's disease, may cause adrenal insufficiency during tooth extraction and oral surgery, and steroid coverage is necessary.

In patients taking thyroid hormone preparations, T4 (Thyradin S®) potentiates the effects of adrenaline and warfarin, so caution should be exercised in the case of local anesthetics and hematological procedures.

In actual dental treatment, consideration should be given to the following: (1) confirming that the patient is taking thyroid hormone preparations on the day of treatment, (2) preventing the room temperature from becoming too low, (3) wearing a monitor to prevent bradycardia and hypotension, and (4) using surface anesthesia and sedation to avoid stress during treatment.

## 3 Adrenal Gland Hyperfunction

Toshie Segawa, Tomoko Hashimoto

### 3.1 Structure and Function of the Adrenal Gland

The adrenal glands are 2–3 cm in diameter and 5–6 g in weight, located at the upper pole of the left and right kidneys, and consist of a cortex and medulla.

The cortex produces aldosterone, cortisol, and adrenal androgens, and the medulla produces catecholamines (dopamine, epinephrine, and norepinephrine).

Aldosterone secretion is regulated by the renin-angiotensin-aldosterone (RAA) system, which promotes reabsorption of sodium and water in the renal collecting ducts and is responsible for elevated blood pressure and increased circulating plasma volume. Cortisol is secreted from the adrenal cortex by ACTH, which is secreted from the anterior pituitary gland. Cortisol regulates glucose, protein and lipid metabolism, immune function, anti-inflammatory activity, and blood pressure. Furthermore, as a stress-responsive hormone, secretion increases during physical, mental, and physiological stress (trauma, surgery, anxiety, etc.), and it is an important hormone that protects the body from stress. Adrenal androgens are involved in the development and maintenance of reproductive organs and the development of pubic and axillary hair. On the other hand, catecholamines secreted from the adrenal medulla have potent hypertensive effects by vasoconstriction, increased heart rate and cardiac contractility, lipolysis, and increased blood glucose.

## 3.2 Adrenal Gland Hyperfunction

We describe primary aldosteronism (PA), an aldosterone excess from the adrenal cortex; Cushing's syndrome, a cortisol excess; and pheochromocytoma, a catecholamine excess from the adrenal medulla.

### 3.2.1 Primary Aldosteronism

1. Definitions and Pathophysiology

   Excess aldosterone produced autonomously by adrenal adenomas or hyperplasia acts on the distal tubule and renal collecting ducts to reabsorb sodium and excrete potassium in the urine, resulting in hypertension and hypokalemia.
2. Epidemiology

   It accounts for more than 5% of all hypertension [13] and is slightly more common in women between 30 and 50 years of age.
3. Classification

   Unilateral aldosterone-producing adenomas account for 80% of cases, and idiopathic aldosteronism due to bilateral adrenal hyperplasia accounts for about 20%.
4. Symptoms

   Almost all patients have hypertension and may complain of lightheadedness and dizziness. Hypokalemia may cause muscle weakness, weakness attacks, and tetany and polyuria and polydipsia due to impaired urine concentration.
5. Clinical Examination

   It is characterized by high blood aldosterone levels, low plasma renin activity, and hypokalemia. The electrocardiogram may show QT prolongation and U waves due to hypokalemia. CT and adrenal scintigram are useful to evaluate adrenal lesions, and selective adrenal vein sampling is performed to collect aldosterone from the right and left adrenal veins for localization.
6. Treatment

   Patients with unilateral disease are treated with adrenalectomy, whereas patients with inoperable or bilateral disease are treated with pharmacotherapy. The first choice of drug therapy is aldosterone antagonists such as spironolactone and eplerenone, with the goal of suppressing direct organ damage caused by aldosterone (Fig. 7.1). If blood pressure is difficult to control with aldosterone antagonists, calcium channel blockers should be used in combination. For hypokalemia, potassium supplementation may be used.
7. Prognosis

   After adrenalectomy, the blood pressure improved to less than 140/80 mmHg in 28–56% of patients. Patients with curable hypertension have a short history of hypertension (less than 5 years) and tend to be younger than 50 years of age. Early diagnosis and treatment are important.
8. Latest Findings

   In addition to hypertension-mediated organ damage, direct aldosterone-induced cerebral and cardiovascular damage has attracted attention, and it has been reported that patients with PA have a sixfold higher incidence of cardiovascular disease and a fourfold higher incidence of stroke than patients with essential hypertension [14]. Therefore, it is important not only to control blood pressure but also to suppress aldosterone action.

### 3.2.2 Cushing's Syndrome

1. Definition and Pathophysiology

   It is a general term for conditions that cause hypersecretion of cortisol due to adrenal tumors, adrenal hyperplasia, ACTH-producing pituitary adenomas, etc. and results in characteristic symptoms and metabolic abnormalities.
2. Epidemiology/Classification

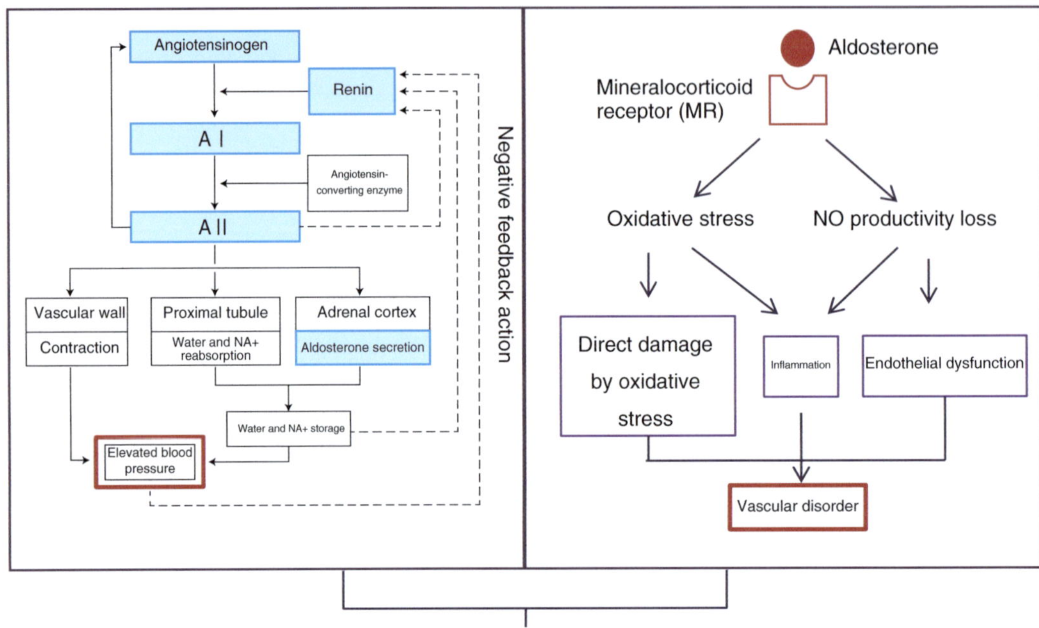


**Fig. 7.1** Elevated blood pressure and vascular damage caused by aldosterone

Cushing's syndrome is rare, with an incidence of 0.7–2.4 per million population per year. The ACTH-dependent form includes a pituitary ACTH-producing adenoma (Cushing's disease) and ectopic ACTH-producing tumors such as small cell lung cancer. ACTH-independent tumors include adrenal adenomas, adrenal carcinomas, and adrenal hyperplasia. Treatment with long-term administration of glucocorticoid causes iatrogenic Cushing's syndrome (Fig. 7.2). ACTH-dependent Cushing's syndrome accounts for 80–85% of cases. Of these, 75–80% are due to Cushing's disease and 15–20% are due to ectopic ACTH syndrome. Adrenal adenomas are responsible for about 10–15% of cases and carcinoma for less than 5%.

3. Symptoms

Most symptoms are due to excess cortisol, and hypertension, hyperglycemia, and lipid abnormalities may occur, as well as ringworm, candidiasis, and other serious infections due to impaired immunity. Physical characteristics include a moon face, central obesity characterized by fat deposition in the trunk and atrophy of the skeletal muscles of the extremities, and thinning of the skin (Fig. 7.3) [16].

4. Clinical Examination

Excessive autocrine secretion of cortisol is diagnosed by the absence of nocturnal diurnal variation in cortisol (it does not decrease even at midnight) and the absence of suppression of cortisol in the low-dose dexamethasone suppression test. Leukocytes are increased in peripheral blood, and biochemical tests show glucose intolerance and lipid abnormalities. In addition to high cortisol levels, high or normal ACTH levels suggest ACTH dependence, and low ACTH levels suggest ACTH independence. In the case of iatrogenic Cushing's syndrome, endogenous ACTH secretion is suppressed by external corticosteroid administration. Imaging studies include CT and adrenal scintigram to confirm adrenal tumor and MRI to confirm pituitary adenoma.

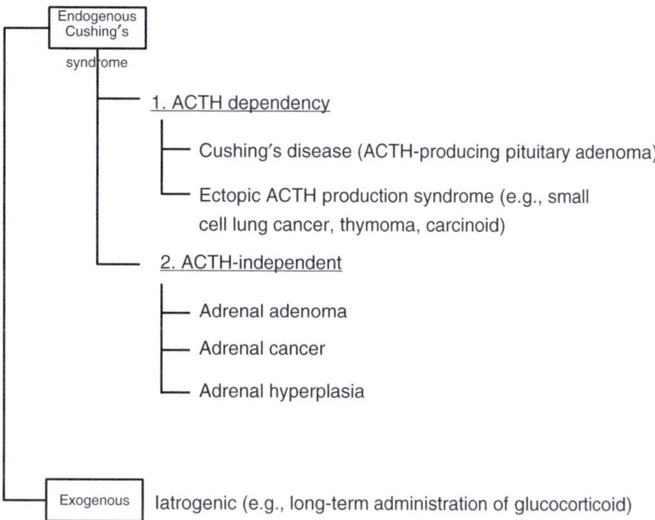


**Fig. 7.2** Classification of Cushing's Syndrome

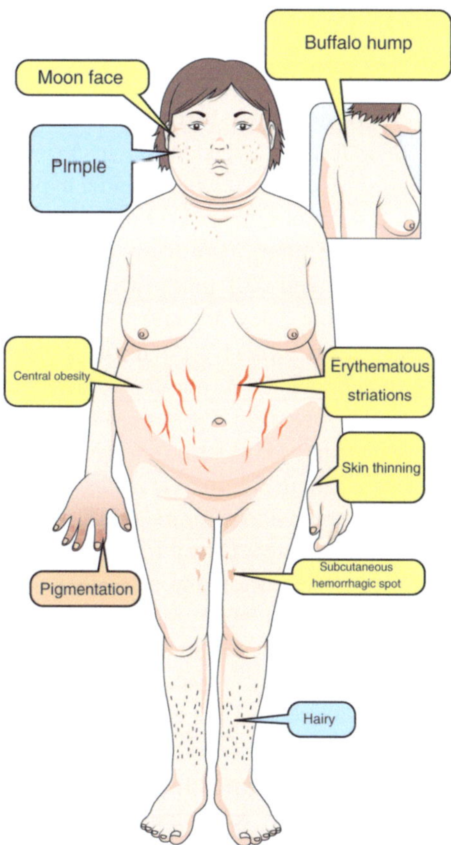


**Fig. 7.3** Symptoms of Cushing's Syndrome. (Modified from [15] with Permission)

5. Treatment

   Adrenal adenomas and adrenal carcinomas are treated with adrenalectomy on the diseased side. Pituitary adenomas are usually treated with surgery and stereotactic radiation (gamma knife) or a combination of these therapies, and it is widely accepted that removal of the primary tumors is the first-choice treatment for ectopic ACTH-producing tumors. In all cases, the original physiological secretion of cortisol is suppressed due to long-term cortisol excess, and cortisol replacement is required for 6 months to 1 year after surgery until adrenocortical function is restored. In inoperable patients, pharmacotherapy with adrenal steroid synthase inhibitors is indicated.

6. Prognosis

   Depending on the primary disease, normalization of cortisol can be expected to improve quality of life.

7. Latest Findings

   Adrenal subclinical Cushing's syndrome, which does not show typical Cushing's signs, is also known to cause lifestyle diseases such as hypertension, obesity, diabetes mellitus, and osteoporosis [15]. This should be kept in mind in patients at multiple risks of developing cardiovascular diseases.

### 3.2.3 Pheochromocytoma

1. Definitions and Pathophysiology

   A catecholamine-producing tumor arising from the adrenal medulla or paraganglionic tissue, presenting as hypertension and hypermetabolism.
2. Epidemiology

   There is no gender difference, and it is more common in people aged 20–50 years. It is estimated to account for 0.5% of hypertension.
3. Classification

   There are two types of pheochromocytoma: pheochromocytoma in the narrow sense, which originates from the adrenal medulla, and extra-adrenal pheochromocytoma (paraganglioma), which originates from the extra-adrenal paraganglia. They are collectively referred to as pheochromocytoma.
4. Symptoms

   The symptoms include fluctuating hypertension, hyperglycemia, tachycardia, emaciation, headache, and excessive sweating. Paroxysmal elevation of blood pressure is known to be induced by abdominal pressure, defecation, and iodine contrast media.
5. Clinical Examination

   Blood catecholamines and their metabolites, urinary metanephrines and normetanephrines, are elevated. Pheochromocytoma is a relatively large tumor, and CT, MRI, and scintigram are useful for diagnosis.
6. Treatment

   Tumor resection is the first choice, but medical management is necessary before surgery. It is important to administer sufficient doses of $\alpha_1$-adrenergic receptor blockers to control vasoconstriction and stabilize blood pressure before surgery. In addition, the circulating blood volume is generally low due to vasoconstriction, and adequate fluid replacement should be given to correct this.
7. Prognosis and Latest Findings

   Although about 90% of cases can be cured by surgical treatment, there is no way to reliably diagnose benign, even if it is solitary, and the 2017 WHO classification of endocrine tumors defines "all pheochromocytomas and paragangliomas are tumors with the potential to metastasize (malignant)" [17]. Therefore, long-term follow-up is necessary with the possibility of metastasis in the mind even after surgery.

## 3.3 Notes from Dentistry Perspective

Hiroki Bukawa

The adrenal cortex synthesizes steroid hormones. The spheroid layer synthesizes mineralocorticoids (aldosterone), the bundle layer synthesizes glucocorticoids (cortisol), and the reticular layer synthesizes androgens. The adrenal medulla also synthesizes catecholamines. Hyperadrenalism is a condition in which each steroid hormone or catecholamine is overproduced. Therefore, it is necessary to plan dental treatment according to each adrenal hyperfunction.

### 3.3.1 Primary Aldosteronism (PA)

PA is the cause of hypertension in 5–10% of hypertension. Compared with essential hypertension, PA is 4.2 times more likely to be associated with stroke, 6.5 times more likely with myocardial infarction, and 12.1 times more likely with atrial fibrillation. They are also more likely to have renal impairment. Hypertension, hypokalemia, metabolic alkalosis, muscle weakness, and tetany may be observed. Plasma renin activity is decreased and plasma aldosterone is increased. If the patient is taking aldosterone antagonists (spironolactone, eplerenone) for treatment, hyperkalemia should be noted. Dental treatment requires attention to hypertension and relaxation of tension. Laughing inhalation sedation should be used if necessary. Local anesthesia can be administered with any local anesthetic if the PA has been adequately treated.

### 3.3.2 Cushing's Syndrome

It is a general term for conditions that cause excessive cortisol secretion, such as ACTH-producing pituitary tumors (Cushing's disease), adrenal adenomas, and adrenal hyperplasia.

The most common cause is the administration of exogenous steroids. Cortisol has a 1:1 ratio of glucocorticoid to mineralocorticoid activity, resulting in an increase in the effects of both. Moon face, central obesity, buffalo-like shoulders, red skin streaks, thinning of the skin, subcutaneous hemorrhage due to vascular fragility, hypertension, hyperglycemia, osteoporosis, renal urinary calculi, hypernatremia, hypokalemia, peptic ulcer, easy infection, hypercoagulability, dyslipidemia, muscle weakness, depression, hypertrichosis, and acne are observed. Dental treatment should be planned taking into account the presence of treatment-resistant hypertension, hyperglycemia, osteoporosis, coronary artery disease, easy infection, and deep vein thrombosis. Antimicrobial agents should be administered for hematological procedures. There is no problem with local anesthesia, but if hypertension is significant, be careful about the amount of adrenaline added.

In Cushing's disease, pituitary tumors induce the excessive secretion of ACTH, resulting in pigmentation of the skin and oral mucosa.

#### 3.3.3 Congenital Adrenocortical Hyperplasia and Adrenogenital Syndrome

This condition is caused by an excess of adrenal-derived male hormones (androgens), resulting in abnormal sexual characteristics. The symptoms of masculinization (hypertrophy of clitoris) are observed from birth in girls and from infancy to early puberty (hypertrophy of the penis and appearance of pubic hair) in boys. The most common form of congenital adrenocortical hyperplasia is 21-hydroxylase ($P450_{c21}$) deficiency, which results in adrenal insufficiency due to the lack of aldosterone and cortisol production. In dentistry, androgen excess is usually not a problem, but the possibility of adrenal insufficiency should be considered (see the sect. 7).

#### 3.3.4 Pheochromocytoma

It is a catecholamine-producing tumor arising from the adrenal medulla or paraganglionic tissue. The five major signs are hypertension, headache, hypermetabolism, hyperglycemia, and hyperhidrosis. Other sympathomimetic symptoms include palpitations, tachycardia, nausea, vomiting, and weight loss. The patient is usually dehydrated and the blood is concentrated. Urinary and plasma catecholamines (adrenaline, noradrenaline) are elevated. Elevation of metanephrine and normetanephrine in urine is observed. The degree of catecholamine-induced damage to target organs should be assessed during dental treatment. Catecholamine-induced dilated cardiomyopathy and hypertrophic cardiomyopathy occur in 20–30% of patients. Congestive heart failure, decreased circulating blood volume, intracranial hemorrhage, hyperglycemia, and renal failure may occur, requiring minimally invasive dental treatment and antimicrobial therapy for hematologic procedures. Sympathetic nervous system tension should be avoided as much as possible because of the large blood pressure fluctuation caused by catecholamines. Local anesthetics without adrenaline should be used. During invasive treatment, blood pressure should be measured over time. Laughing inhalation sedation is also effective.

## 4 Adrenal Insufficiency

Toshie Segawa, Tomoko Hashimoto

### 4.1 Introduction

Hypoadrenalism (adrenal insufficiency) is a condition in which adrenal cortical hormones are insufficient. It is classified into primary adrenal insufficiency and secondary adrenal insufficiency according to the location of the lesion. Primary hypoadrenalism (Addison's disease) is caused by chronic bilateral adrenal lesions (Table 7.3). Secondary hypoadrenalism results from decreased level of ACTH released from the pituitary gland. Acute adrenal insufficiency (adrenal crisis) is caused by rapid adrenocortical hormone deficiency. Iatrogenic hypoadrenocorticism is a condition in which endogenous cortisol secretion is decreased by long-term treatment with exogenous glucocorticoid.

**Table 7.3** Causes of hypoadrenocorticism

| |
|---|
| 1. Primary hypoadrenalism (PA) |
| (a) Addison's disease |
| • Autoimmunity |
| • Infectious diseases (such as adrenal tuberculosis) |
| (b) Adrenal hemorrhage |
| • Traumatic, anticoagulant, etc. |
| (c) Adrenal metastasis of cancer |
| (d) Bilateral adrenalectomy |
| (e) Congenital adrenal cortical hyperplasia |
| 2. Secondary hypoadrenalism |
| (a) Panhypopituitarism |
| • Tumor, postoperative, trauma, postpartum pituitary apoplexy, etc. |
| (b) Isolated ACTH deficiency |
| (c) Postoperative Cushing's syndrome |
| (d) Iatrogenic |
| • Long-term high-dose administration of adrenal corticosteroids |

## 4.2 Primary Hypoadrenalism (Addison's Disease)

### 4.2.1 Definitions and Pathophysiology

Chronic hypoadrenocorticism occurs when the adrenal cortex is more than 90% destroyed in a primary adrenal gland lesion, and the clinical manifestations are a comprehensive depletion of cortisol, aldosterone, and adrenal androgens. Specific symptoms include skin and mucosal hyperpigmentation caused by increased ACTH from the pituitary gland due to cortisol deficiency.

### 4.2.2 Epidemiology

The incidence of primary hypoadrenalism is estimated 0.8 cases per 10,000 person years. Autoimmune destruction of the adrenal cortex (autoimmune adrenalitis) accounts for 49%, infectious diseases for 27%, and others for 11% of cases. The proportion of idiopathic autoimmune adrenalitis is increasing with the decrease of tuberculosis.

### 4.2.3 Classification

The most common cause is autoimmune adrenalitis, and other causes include tuberculosis, bacterial, fungal, and AIDS infections, adrenal metastases from cancer, traumatic adrenal hemorrhage, and postoperative Cushing's syndrome.

### 4.2.4 Symptoms

Cortisol deficiency causes fever, weight loss, anorexia, fatigue, nausea and vomiting, hypoglycemia, and psychiatric symptoms, and aldosterone deficiency causes hypotension. Adrenal androgen deficiency causes loss of pubic and axillary hair and menstrual irregularities in women. Hyperpigmentation due to elevated ACTH is characteristic of a wide range of areas, including the face, oral mucosa, gingiva, tongue, fingers, and nails.

### 4.2.5 Clinical Examination

Adrenocortical hormones such as cortisol, aldosterone, and adrenal androgens are low and ACTH level is high. CT scan shows calcification of the adrenal glands in tuberculosis, enlargement of the adrenal glands in hemorrhage or cancer metastasis, and atrophy of the bilateral adrenal glands in autoimmunity.

### 4.2.6 Treatment

The principle of treatment is the replacement of deficient adrenal corticosteroids. Hydrocortisone is administered orally at a dose of 10–20 mg/day to match the daily cortisol secretion of normal subjects. Because cortisol requirements increase during stress, such as fever, tooth extraction, and surgery, the dose should be increased 2–3 times to prevent relative adrenal insufficiency. It is important to instruct patients not to stop taking the drug at their own discretion and to cope with stress.

### 4.2.7 Prognosis

The prognosis is good if cortisol is adequately supplemented.

### 4.2.8 Recent Findings

In a nationwide survey, 60% of the triggers of acute adrenal insufficiency were reported to be infectious diseases [18], and it is important to provide guidance on how to respond during infectious diseases such as influenza.

### 4.3 Acute Adrenal Insufficiency (Adrenal Crisis)

#### 4.3.1 Definitions and Pathophysiology

It is a condition that is mainly caused by circulatory failure due to a rapid decrease in the function of the adrenal cortex and can be fatal if left untreated.

#### 4.3.2 Epidemiology

The incidence of adrenal crisis in patients with adrenal insufficiency is estimated to be 6–8 per 100 patient years. Adrenal crisis occurs in primary as well as secondary adrenal insufficiency.

In epidemiological studies in Japan, infections and surgery or trauma were responsible for inducing acute adrenal insufficiency in 63% and 6% of patients, respectively.

#### 4.3.3 Classification

It is most commonly seen in patients with chronic hypoadrenalism when stress, such as infection, increases cortisol demand or when long-term glucocorticoids are inappropriately reduced or discontinued for therapeutic purposes. It can also occur after Cushing's syndrome surgery, such as after removal of a cortisol-producing adenoma or ACTH-producing adenoma.

#### 4.3.4 Symptoms

Fever, hypotension, abdominal pain, vomiting, diarrhea, and arthralgia are the most common symptoms. As the disease progresses, shock, impaired consciousness, and convulsions may occur.

#### 4.3.5 Clinical Examination

Cortisol and aldosterone are low, and there is hypoglycemia, hyponatremia, and eosinophilia.

#### 4.3.6 Treatment

If the syndrome is suspected, a 100 mg dose of hydrocortisone should be administered intravenously immediately after ACTH and cortisol collection, if possible, followed by 100–200 mg of hydrocortisone over the next 24 h. At the same time, hypotension and electrolyte correction should be initiated by infusion of fluids.

#### 4.3.7 Prognosis

The prognosis is good if appropriate treatment is given. Patient education, such as not interrupting treatment and coping with stress, is important.

#### 4.3.8 Recent Findings

In recent years, many cases of hypopituitarism induced by immune checkpoint inhibitors have been reported. When the diagnosis is made, immediate treatment is required in parallel with a thorough examination, and it is desirable to take prompt action in cooperation with related departments [19].

### 4.4 Notes from Dentistry Perspective

Hiroki Bukawa

Hypoadrenalism is a condition in which the adrenal cortical hormones (steroid hormones) are insufficient. Primary hypoadrenalism (Addison's disease) is caused by damage to the adrenal glands, and secondary hypoadrenalism is caused by damage to the hypothalamus and pituitary gland.

#### 4.4.1 Addison's Disease: Primary Hypoadrenalism

Cortisol deficiency symptoms include weight loss, hypoglycemia, and psychiatric symptoms, and aldosterone deficiency symptoms include hyponatremia, hyperkalemia, and hypotension. Androgen deficiency symptoms include menstrual irregularities and loss of pubic and axillary hair in women. Hyperpigmentation of the face, neck, gingiva, tongue, lips, and fingers is a symptom of ACTH excess. There is a decrease in blood cortisol and an increase in blood ACTH.

The treatment of Addison's disease involves physiologic cortisol secretion (10–20 mg) and replacement therapy (morning/evening = 15 mg:5 mg) that approximates diurnal variation. In dental treatment, especially in minor surgery such as tooth extraction, hydrocortisone (cortisol) should be administered in two- to threefold doses (30–50 mg) preoperatively and returned to the original dose on the first postoperative sick day. In middle surgery (surgery for jaw deformities and oral cancer), 50–75 mg is given preoperatively, 50 mg every 8 h during surgery, and 20 mg every 8 h on the first postoperative day. The dose is returned to the original level on the second postoperative day. In major surgery (extended surgery for oral cancer), hydrocortisone is administered at 100 mg at the start of surgery, followed by a continuous infusion of 200 mg in 24 h, 50 mg every 8 h until the second or third postoperative day, and then the dose is reduced by 50% daily until it returns to the preoperative dose. Because patients with hypoadrenalism are sensitive to sedatives, anesthetics, and vasodilators, the dose should be carefully adjusted in small doses to avoid circulatory depression.

### 4.4.2 Secondary Hypoadrenalism

Secondary cases include pituitary tumors and Sheehan's syndrome (pituitary dysfunction caused by heavy bleeding during childbirth), which is a steroid hormone deficiency caused by decreased secretion of ACTH. Therefore, similar to Addison's disease, the patient presents with cortisol deficiency symptoms such as weight loss, hypoglycemia, and psychiatric symptoms but without the hyperpigmentation of the skin and oral mucosa that is characteristic of ACTH excess symptoms. In many cases, aldosterone deficiency symptoms (hyponatremia, hyperkalemia, and metabolic acidosis) are not seen.

### 4.4.3 Iatrogenic Adrenal Hypofunction

There is a meta-analysis showing that the most common type of adrenal insufficiency is iatrogenic (drug-induced). First of all, the physiological secretion of steroids is 5 mg of prednisolone per day, and in principle, it is safe to discontinue up to 5 mg suddenly. In addition, if a patient is taking prednisolone 30 mg due to asthma and autoimmune disease and so on, there would be safe to discontinue prednisolone immediately within 2 weeks. If a patient has been taking prednisolone for more than 2 weeks, it is necessary to gradually decrease the dose without stopping abruptly. Inhalation of fluticasone propionate for asthma has been associated with adrenal insufficiency when stopped abruptly. Adrenal insufficiency should be suspected in patients with general malaise, weight loss, and hyponatremia.

### 4.4.4 Adrenal Crisis (Acute Adrenal Insufficiency)

Adrenal crisis is a life-threatening condition due to a marked decrease in adrenal function. Adrenal crisis is caused by severe stress such as trauma, infection, or surgery during the course of chronic adrenal insufficiency, sudden bilateral adrenal hemorrhage, decreased ACTH secretion due to pituitary gland damage, or sudden discontinuation of medication in patients on long-term steroids. The frequency of adrenal crisis in Addison's disease is 6.6/100 patients per year. The most common triggers are gastrointestinal diseases (32.6%) and infections other than those of the gastrointestinal tract (24.3%). Rapidly progressive hypoglycemia leads to impaired consciousness, shock due to hypotension, nausea, vomiting, diarrhea, and dehydration, which can be fatal if appropriate treatment is not given immediately. In the basal state, hydrocortisone should be administered at a dose of 10–20 mg daily (15 mg in the morning and 5 mg at 4 pm) or prednisolone at a dose of 5–7.5 mg once daily. The dose of hydrocortisone should be increased in times of stress. Treatment of adrenal crisis includes intravenous fluids (saline with 5% dextrose), steroid replacement (hydrocortisone 100 mg IV or dexamethasone 6 mg IV, plus hydrocortisone 50 mg

**Table 7.4** Glucocorticoid activity and mineralocorticoid activity

| Steroid | Relative efficacy<br>Glucocorticoid activity | Mineralocorticoid activity | Equivalent dose (mg) |
|---|---|---|---|
| **Short-acting (8–12 h)** | | | |
| Cortisol[a] | 1.0 | 1.0 | 20 |
| Cortisone | 0.8 | 0.8 | 25 |
| Aldosterone | 0.3 | 3000 | – |
| **Intermediate-acting (12–36 h)** | | | |
| Prednisolone | 4.0 | 0.8 | 5 |
| Methylprednisolone | 5.0 | 0.5 | 4 |
| Fludrocortisone | 10.0 | 125 | – |
| **Long-acting (>24 h)** | | | |
| Dexamethasone | 25–40 | 0 | 0.75 |

[a]The relative activity of each steroid is shown when the activity of cortisol is set at 1

IV every 8 h or continuous IV), positive inotropic agents, and electrolyte correction as needed. The dose of hydrocortisone is reduced by 50% every 1–2 days according to clinical symptoms (Table 7.4).

## References

1. Yazaki Y. (supervised). IV Renal and urinary tract system, endocrine system, metabolism and nutrition hyperthyroidism. In: Yazaki Y (supervised). ASAKURA internal medicine. 11th ed. Tokyo: Asakura Shoten; 2017. p. 1576–9. (in Japanese).
2. Nishida J, Kojima T, Okubo N. Thyroid diseases. In: Nishida J, Kojima T, Okubo N, editors. Internal medicine for the odontology. Revised 4 ed. Tokyo: Nankodo; 2018. p. 205–10. (in Japanese).
3. Braverman LE, et al. Thyroid disieases: thyrotoxicosis. In: Cooper DS BLE, editor. Werner & Ingbar's the thyroid. 10th ed. Philadelphia: Lippincott Williams & Wilikins; 2013. p. 354–522.
4. Japan Thyroid Association. Guidelines for the diagnosis of Graves' disease. Tokyo: Japan Thyroid Association; 2013. (in Japanese). http://www.japanthyroid.jp/doctor/guideline/japanese.html#basedou. Accessed 28 Feb 2022.
5. Japan Thyroid Association. Guidelines for the treatment of Graves' disease with antithyroid drugs. Tokyo: Nankodo; 2019. p. 36–71. (in Japanese).
6. Sugimoto H, Yazaki Y. III: Renal and urinary system, endocrine system, metabolism and nutrition, 12-4 thyroid. In: Sugimoto H, Yazaki Y, editors. ASAKURA internal medicine. 9th ed. Tokyo: Asakura Shoten; 2007. p. 1337–65. (in Japanese).
7. Sugiyama K. Chapter 15: Dental treatment of patients with hypothyroidism. In: Nishida M (supervised). Guidelines for dental treatment of the prevalent elderly. Tokyo: Quintessence Publishing; 2013. p. 32–42. (in Japanese).
8. Ida K, Dozen H, Nishida J. Thyroid diseases. In: Ida K, Dozen H, Nishida J, editors. Internal medicine for the odontology. 3rd ed. Tokyo: Nankodo; 2016. p. 181–4. (in Japanese).
9. Shirakawa M, Furuya H, Japanese Society of Dentistry for Medically Compromised Patient. 8. Endocrine disorders. In: Shirakawa M, Furuya H, Japanese Society of Dentistry for Medically Compromised Patient, editors. Handbook of dental treatment for the medically compromised patient. Tokyo: Quintessence Publishing; 2001. p. 115–127, 244–245. (in Japanese).
10. Braverman LE, et al. Thyroid Disieases: Hypothyroidism. In: Braverman LE, Cooper DS, editors. Werner & Ingbar's the thyroid. 10th ed. Philadelphia: Lippincott Williams & Wilikins; 2013. p. 523–634.
11. Japan Thyroid Association. Guidelines for the diagnosis of hypothyroidism. Tokyo: Japan Thyroid Association; 2013. (in Japanese). http://www.japanthyroid.jp/doctor/guideline/japanese.html#teika. Accessed 28 Feb 2022.
12. Japan Thyroid Association. Guidelines for the diagnosis of chronic thyroiditis (Hashimoto's disease). Tokyo: Japan Thyroid Association; 2013. (in Japanese). http://www.japanthyroid.jp/doctor/guideline/japanese.html#teika. Accessed 28 Feb 2022.
13. Gordon RD, et al. Primary aldosteronism: are we diagnosing and operating on too few patients? World J Surg. 2001;25:941–7.
14. Milliez P, Girard X, et al. Evidence for an increased rate of cardiovascular events in patients with primary aldosteronism. J Am Coll Cardiol. 2005;45:1243–8.

15. Otsuki M. Diagnosis and treatment of Cushing's syndrome and adrenal subclinical Cushing's syndrome. J Jpn Soc Intern Med. 2018;107:674–80. (in Japanese).
16. Morino K, et al. Supervised. Byouki ga mieru, vol. 3: Diabetes, metabolism and endocrinology. 4th ed. Tokyo: Medic Media Co., Ltd. p. 257. (in Japanese).
17. Naruse K, Hirata Y, Tanabe M, et al. Manual of Pheochromocytoma treatment. Revised 2 ed. Tokyo: Shindanto Chiryou-sha; 2012. (in Japanese)
18. Yanase T, et al. Addison's disease and adrenal subclinical Cushing's syndrome: a nationwide survey. Research on adrenal hormone production abnormality, research group on adrenal hormone production abnormality, research report 2010; 2011. p. 139–146. (in Japanese).
19. Fukushima S. A review of adverse events caused by immune checkpoint inhibitors. Jpn J Clin Immunol. 2016;39:30–6. (in Japanese).

# Cardiovascular Diseases

# 8

Genzou Takemura, Izumi Yoshioka, Shinichiro Tanaka, Masayo Fukuhara, Masayuki Fukuda, Tatsuaki Matsubara, Shigeo Ishikawa, Mitsuyoshi Iino, Hiromi Mitsubayashi, Hiroki Miyate, Akihiko Hasegawa, Kenichi Sato, Shin Inoue, and Masahito Sato

## 1 Myocardial Infarction

Genzou Takemura

### 1.1 Disease Overview

Coronary artery occlusion is a disease that causes irreversible necrosis of the myocardium in the dominant territory. The primary cause of occlusion is coronary thrombus. Thrombi are mainly formed by the disruption of plaques in atherosclerotic lesions but can also be caused by coronary spasm, coronary arteritis, or embolization.

### 1.2 Pathophysiology

Necrosis of the myocardium is associated with a variety of complications, including the following:

The original version of the chapter has been revised. A correction to this chapter can be found at https://doi.org/10.1007/978-981-99-3296-2_21

Genzou Takemura was deceased at the time of publication.

G. Takemura
Asahi University, Mizuho, Gifu, Japan

I. Yoshioka · M. Fukuhara
Division of General Internal Medicine, Kyushu Dental University Faculty of Dentistry, Kitakyushu, Fukuoka, Japan

S. Tanaka
Department of Cardiology, Asahi University Hospital, Gifu, Japan

M. Fukuda
Dentistry and Oral Surgery, Akita University, Akita, Japan

T. Matsubara
Department of Physical and Mental Health Sciences, Faculty of Human Science, Aichi Mizuho College, Nagoya, Aichi, Japan

S. Ishikawa · M. Iino
Department of Dentistry, Oral and Maxillofacial Plastic and Reconstructive Surgery, Faculty of Medicine, Yamagata University, Yamagata, Japan

H. Mitsubayashi
School of Life Dentistry at Tokyo, The Nippon Dental University, Chiyoda-ku, Tokyo, Japan

H. Miyate
Dental and Oral Surgery, Hakodate Goryoukaku Hospital, Hakodate, Hokkaido, Japan

A. Hasegawa
Division of Internal Medicine, Department of Comprehensive Medical Sciences, Meikai University School of Dentistry, Sakado, Saitama, Japan

K. Sato · M. Sato
Division of Dental Anesthesiology, Department of Reconstructive Oral and Maxillofacial Surgery, School of Dentistry, Iwate Medical University, Morioka, Iwate, Japan

S. Inoue (✉)
Department of Internal Medicine, Showa University Dental Hospital, Ota-ku, Tokyo, Japan
e-mail: inoues@med.showa-u.ac.jp



T. Chiba, H. Yamada (eds.), *Internal Medicine for Dental Treatments*,
https://doi.org/10.1007/978-981-99-3296-2_8

1. Arrhythmia: 65% of deaths due to acute myoc ardial infarction occur within the first hour of onset and are mainly due to ventricular fibrillation. Other arrhythmias such as ventricular tachycardia and atrioventricular block also occur.
2. Shock to heart failure: The larger the area of myocardial necrosis, the more pump malfunction occurs, resulting in shock to severe heart failure. In other words, when 20% of the left ventricular myocardium is necrotic, symptoms of heart failure occur, and when the percentage is nearly 50%, cardiogenic shock occurs.
3. Cardiac rupture causes immediate death. It is difficult to save the patient.
4. Ventricular septal perforation: Prone to anterior wall septal infarction.
5. Papillary muscle rupture causes mitral regurgitation.
6. Ventricular aneurysm: A thinning of the ventricular wall caused by infarction, which expands outward due to pressure from the lumen of the heart. Mural thrombus tends to form.
7. Post-myocardial infarction syndrome (Dressler's syndrome): Epicarditis caused by an autoimmune reaction in transmural infarction.

## 1.3 Epidemiology

The annual incidence of acute myocardial infarction is estimated to be 75 per 100,000 population (approximately 150,000 per year) in Japan. Myocardial infarction is rarely observed in premenopausal women because of the antiatherosclerotic effect of female hormones. Because aging is the most important risk factor for atherosclerosis, the number of patients with acute myocardial infarction is increasing with the relative growth of the elderly population.

## 1.4 Categories

### 1.4.1 Classification by the Passage of Time

1. Acute myocardial infarction: Within 1 month of onset.
2. Old myocardial infarction: 1 month or more has passed since onset

### 1.4.2 Classification by the Depth of the Lesion

1. Transmural myocardial infarction: All layers from endocardium to epicardium are infarcted. In myocardial infarction, necrosis progresses from the endocardium to the epicardium.
2. Nontransmural myocardial infarction: Infarction of only a part of the myocardial layer is infarcted. Subendocardial infarction, in particular, is an infarction confined to the subendocardium.

### 1.4.3 Classification by Infarction Site

Anteroseptal infarction, extensive anterior infarction, inferior wall myocardial infarction, lateral myocardial infarction, high posterior infarction, right ventricular infarction, etc.

## 1.5 Symptoms

### 1.5.1 Subjective Symptoms

It is typically a sudden onset of severe chest pain lasting more than 30 min and is not relieved by nitroglycerin. Chest pain is characterized by constriction in chest, pressure, burning, and radiating pain (in the left shoulder, upper limbs, neck, and mandible) and may be accompanied by cold sweat. An anginal attack may be recognized as a premonitory symptom. In elderly patients and those with inferior wall myocardial infarction, chest pain is not typical and only gastrointestinal symptoms such as epigastric pain, nausea, vomiting, diarrhea, and defecation desire may be present. Diabetic patients may have no chest pain (painless myocardial infarction). If the infarct area is large, patients may present with symptoms of left heart failure such as respiratory distress, dyspnea on exertion, palpitations, and orthopnea and may go into shock. If fatal arrhythmias appear, cardiopulmonary arrest and death may result.

### 1.5.2 Objective Findings

1. Visual observation: Facial pallor, cold sweat, and anguish-like expression
2. Palpation: Tachycardia, arrhythmia, and weak pulse in shock

3. Auscultation: Excess heart sounds such as sounds III and IV in heart failure and pansystolic murmur in case of mitral regurgitation due to papillary muscle dysfunction caused by infarction or ventricular septal perforation are heard

## 1.6 Examinations

1. Electrocardiogram (ECG): This is the most important test in the diagnosis of myocardial infarction (No ECG, No MI!). ECG changes over time from the early stage of myocardial infarction, but the key point is ST elevation, and the infarcted area is identified by the ST elevation.
2. Echocardiography: Decreased wall motion in the infarcted area is observed.
3. Chest X-ray: Pulmonary congestion and pleural effusion may be seen. Enlargement of the cardiac shadow is seen when the infarct size is large.
4. Blood test: Necrosis of myocardial cells releases myocardial enzymes into the blood, resulting in increases in AST (aspartate aminotransferase) (GOT), LDH (lactate dehydrogenase) (type I), and CK (creatine kinase) (type MB). The total amount of CK is useful in estimating the size of infarction. CK increases from about 3 h after the onset of symptoms and usually reaches its peak in 24 h, but if the occluded vessel is successfully reperfused, the release accelerates and the peak time is shortened. Troponins T and I (TnT, TnI), myoglobin, heart type fatty acid-binding protein (H-FABP), leukocytosis, CRP, and erythrocyte sedimentation rate are also elevated. Recently, high-sensitivity TnT and H-FABP, which can be measured easily and released into the blood faster than CK, are useful for early diagnosis.
5. Myocardial scintigraphy: Thalliun-201 ($^{201}$Tl) shows a perfusion defect cold spot, and technetium-99m ($^{99m}$Tc) shows a hot spot in necrotic myocardium.
6. Cardiac catheterization: An urgent coronary angiogram is performed. After confirming the occlusion of the coronary artery (culprit lesion), reperfusion therapy is performed to rescue the ischemic myocardium that has not fallen into necrosis and to reduce the infarct volume. Left ventriculography confirms contractile dysfunction of the left ventricular myocardium.

## 1.7 Treatment

The optimal treatment is to revascularize the occluded artery as soon as possible. Treatment for various complications is then performed, followed by rehabilitation.

### 1.7.1 General Treatment

Analgesia with morphine hydrochloride should be administered, and the ECG should be monitored continuously. When ventricular fibrillation occurs, direct current defibrillation should be attempted. Diuretics and nitrites should be administered to treat heart failure. In cases of cardiogenic shock, cardiotonic agents, intra-aortic balloon pumping (IABP), and percutaneous cardiopulmonary support (PCPS) should be used. For persistent hypertension, β-blockers are mainly used to control systolic blood pressure to 100–120 mmHg to prevent cardiac rupture.

### 1.7.2 Reperfusion Therapy

1. Percutaneous coronary intervention (PCI): It takes 6 h for myocardial necrosis to complete even if the coronary artery is completely occluded and blood flow is interrupted. Successful reperfusion of the coronary artery responsible for the infarction within 6 h leads to a reduction in infarct size, preservation of left ventricular function, and mortality. PCI is a procedure in which a balloon is attached to the tip of a cardiac catheter to dilate the occluded coronary artery from the inside to achieve reperfusion. In many centers, revascularization is achieved with a success rate of more than 95%.
2. Intravenous thrombolytic therapy: In facilities without cardiac catheters, intravenous thrombolysis may be used. Intravenous administration of thrombolytic agents (mainly tissue plasminogen activator (tPA)) can achieve a

reperfusion rate of 70–80%. When administering this treatment, the presence of bleeding tendency should be confirmed, and it is important that patients with a history of peptic ulcer or cerebral hemorrhage should not be treated with this therapy.

### 1.7.3 Daily Life Management

1. Diet therapy: After fasting for 1–2 days at the onset of symptoms, patients should be shifted to a liquid diet, congee diet, or regular diet every 1–2 days. Salt content should be limited to 8 g/day or less or 5 g/day or less in patients with heart failure.
2. Exercise therapy: Acute rehabilitation begins 2–3 days after the onset of acute myocardial infarction, and the amount of exercise load is increased step by step while confirming that there are no symptoms, electrocardiographic abnormalities, or large fluctuations in blood pressure. Patients are discharged when they are able to take a bath alone. The purpose of rehabilitation after discharge from the hospital is to facilitate the patient's return to society, reduce coronary risk factors, and prevent recurrence of myocardial infarction. As a general rule, exercise is performed three times a week for 1–2 h at an intensity of 70–80% of the maximum heart rate during the exercise tolerance test.
3. Pharmacotherapy: Pharmacotherapy is administered for the following three purposes:
   (a) Prevention of recurrent myocardial infarction: Beta-blockers and antiplatelet agents are effective. MG-CoA reductase inhibitors (statins) are effective in preventing recurrent myocardial infarction in patients with high LDL cholesterol due their ability to stabilize atherosclerotic plaques and to reduce the migration of smooth muscle that may cause restenosis.
   (b) Management of heart failure associated with reduced left ventricular function: Angiotensin II receptor blockers (ARBs), angiotensin-converting enzyme inhibitors, β-blockers, and diuretics are mainly selected for use.
   (c) Prevention of sudden death due to fatal arrhythmias: Implantable cardioverter-defibrillators (ICDs) are effective.

## 1.8 Prognosis

The mortality rate of acute myocardial infarction is still 20–40%, and about 10% of patients who reach the hospital die. The recurrence rate of myocardial infarction is high, and the incidence rate is 4–6 times higher than that of patients without myocardial infarction, so secondary prevention such as reduction of risk factors should be strictly implemented.

## 1.9 Recent Findings

If the infarcted area is large, the patient suffers from heart failure even in the chronic phase, which is a serious problem. In recent years, the effectiveness of cardiac rehabilitation for heart failure has been recognized, and its effect is comparable to that of one drug used for treating heart failure.

## 1.10 Notes from Dentistry Perspective

Izumi Yoshioka

Patients with ischemic heart disease may develop angina attacks or myocardial infarction based on increased blood pressure and tachycardia due to stress during dental treatment.

The American College of Cardiology/American Heart Association (ACC/AHA) has developed "Guidelines for the Perioperative Cardiovascular Evaluation of Patients Undergoing Noncardiac Surgery." This guideline includes information on the risk of perioperative myocardial infarction (PMI) and methods of assessing cardiac function for noncardiac surgery, but there is little information on low-risk surgery and no mention of dental treatment [1]. The European Society of Cardiology's "Risk classification of non-cardiac surgery based on cardiac complication rate" also classifies dental surgery as a low-risk group and does not describe it in detail [2]. Thus, there are no guidelines for dental treatment of patients with ischemic heart disease. However, the mortality rate of PMI is 3.5–25%, and avoidance of myocardial infarction during or after dental treatment is a critical issue.

It is important to discuss the risk of ischemic heart disease and the need for dental treatment (urgency and degree of invasiveness) with the cardiologist to determine the timing and method of dental treatment.

### 1.10.1 Risk Assessment

It is important to share information about the risk assessment of ischemic heart disease with cardiologists. When assessing risk, it is important to understand not only cardiac disease but also other medical history and systemic diseases.

#### Myocardial Infarction

Previously, dental treatment was contraindicated in the first 6 months after myocardial infarction; the ACC/AHA guidelines state that "the incidence of PMI and mortality following myocardial infarction with surgery of intermediate risk or greater does not change significantly after approximately 60 days."

However, there is no clear evidence on when dental treatment can be safely performed after the onset of myocardial infarction. For each case, obtain information from the cardiologist about the medication, treatment, and complications. The timing and method of dental treatment should be determined in consideration of the need for dental treatment, urgency, and degree of invasiveness.

### 1.10.2 Perioperative Management

#### Before Treatment (Surgery)

Stress and mental excitement associated with dental treatment can trigger an anginal attack. Make sure that the patient has nitrates and is ready to take them. If the patient does not have nitrates, make sure that they are stored in the treatment room. If the patient is receiving an isosorbide dinitrate patch (e.g., Frandol®tape), apply it 2 h before the procedure.

#### During Dental Treatment (Surgery)

During dental treatment, blood pressure and ECG should be monitored. It is important to reduce the increase in myocardial oxygen demand and the decrease in myocardial oxygen supply. As a rule of thumb, RPP (rate pressure product; systolic blood pressure × heart rate) should be maintained below 12,000.

Stress caused by fear and pain should be minimized as much as possible, and the patient should be treated under sedation if necessary.

#### Local Anesthetics

Dental local anesthetics are widely used in cartridges to which vasoconstrictors have been added (Table 8.1). Adrenaline and adrenaline hydrogen tartrate are added to lidocaine hydrochloride preparations to enhance the anesthetic effect, prolong the duration of action, and achieve local hemostasis. These vasoconstrictors may cause circulatory disturbances, especially in patients with cardiovascular disease. The use of adrenaline-containing lidocaine hydrochloride products is contraindicated in patients with hypertension, arteriosclerosis, heart failure, hyperthyroidism, diabetes mellitus, and a history of vasospasm. Therefore, systemic diseases other than ischemic heart disease and the patient's medical history should be fully understood.

For patients with cardiovascular disease, there is no clear criterion for limiting the amount of local anesthetics to which adrenaline is added; there are reports of adrenaline doses of up to 45 μg (two cartridges) for grades I and II in the NYHA (New York Heart Association) classification (Table 8.2) and up to 22.5 μg (one cartridge) for grade III (Table 8.3) [3]. Although this criterion is simple, other systemic diseases and medical history should be considered.

**Table 8.1** List of local anesthetics for dental use

| Generic name | Concentration | Trade (brand) name | Vasoconstrictor | Concentration |
|---|---|---|---|---|
| Lidocaine hydrochloride preparation | 2% | ORA Injection Dental Cartridge | Adrenaline hydrogen tartrate | 0.025 mg/mL (0.0137 mg as adrenaline) |
| | | Xylocaine Cartridge for Dental Use | Adrenaline | 0.0125 mg/mL |
| | | EPILIDO CARTRIDGE | Adrenaline | 0.0125 mg/mL |
| | | INJ. XYLESTESIN-A (CARTRIDGE) | Adrenaline | 0.0125 mg/mL |
| Propitocaine hydrochloride preparation | 3% | Citanest-Octapressin Cartridge for Dental Use | Felypressin | 0.03 units/mL |
| Mepivacaine hydrochloride preparation | 3% | Scandonest Cartridge | – | – |

**Table 8.2** New York Heart Association (NYHA) cardiac function classification and dental treatment

| |
|---|
| Class 1: Patients who do not experience fatigue, palpitations, shortness of breath, or angina pectoris with daily physical activity |
| Class 2: No symptoms at rest, but fatigue, palpitation, shortness of breath, and angina pectoris occur even with daily physical activity |
| Class 3: No symptoms at rest, but fatigue, palpitation, shortness of breath, angina pectoris, and even with light daily physical activity or less |
| Class 4: Heart failure or anginal symptoms even at rest |

**Table 8.3** Criteria for the use of local anesthetic added adrenaline in patients with cardiac disease. (Created based on [3])

| Up to 45 μg (up to two cartridges) | Up to 22.5 μg (up to one cartridge) |
|---|---|
| NYHA classification: Class 1 and Class 2 | NYHA classification: Class 3 |
| | β-blocker addict |

Cartridge: Lidocaine 1.8 mL with adrenaline 0.0125 mg/mL

Some reports recommend felypressin, which has been shown to have little effect on the heart. However, the onset of the anesthetic effect of propitocaine hydrochloride with felypressin is slower, and the duration of action is shorter than that of lidocaine hydrochloride with adrenaline.

In local anesthesia for patients with ischemic heart disease, the type and amount of local anesthetic should be determined by evaluating the patient's cardiac condition. In addition, it is important to provide sufficient analgesia considering the content of the dental treatment, the treatment site, and the time required for treatment.

#### Antithrombotic Therapy

Antithrombotic therapy is often used in patients with ischemic heart disease. The antithrombotic agent depends on the nature of the cardiac surgery and the cardiac disease. When antithrombotic therapy is used, intraoperative and postoperative bleeding should be considered. The treatment should be performed in collaboration with a cardiologist in accordance with "Clinical practice guideline for tooth extraction in patient on antithrombotic therapy (2020 edition)" [4].

#### Postoperative Management

The majority of cardiac complications in noncardiac surgery patients occur postoperatively, and aggressive postoperative analgesia is important [5].

### 1.10.3 In Case of Chest Pain Attack

Acute coronary syndrome (ACS) is an acute course of ischemic heart disease caused by occlusion or severe narrowing of the coronary arteries. When a patient complains of chest pain, dental treatment should be stopped immediately, and the patient should be placed in a comfortable position for rest. If the symptoms persist despite nitrates, the patient should be seen by a specialist.

# 2 Angina Pectoris [6–8]

Shinichiro Tanaka

Angina pectoris is a transient myocardial ischemia caused by abnormalities (arteriosclerosis, spasm, etc.) in the coronary arteries that supply oxygen to the myocardium, resulting in chest pain and sense of oppression in the chest. It can be classified according to the pathogenesis, mode of onset, and course.

## 2.1 Classification by Developmental Mechanism

1. Organic angina: Angina pectoris is mainly caused by atherosclerotic stenosis of the coronary arteries.
2. Coronary spastic angina: Coronary artery spasm is the cause of stenosis and causes symptoms.

## 2.2 Classification by Mode of Onset

1. Angina of effort: Angina that presents during physical activities (e.g., during exercise) and is common in organic angina pectoris.
2. Angina at rest: Symptoms occur at rest and are common in coronary spastic angina.

## 2.3 Classification by Clinical Course

1. Stable angina: Angina pectoris with stable symptoms and no attacks in the past 3 weeks.
2. Unstable angina: Angina of new onset within the last 3 weeks or worsening attacks. Unstable angina is treated as an acute coronary syndrome because it can progress to myocardial infarction.

The term "angina pectoris" generally refers to organic, effort, and stable angina pectoris.

**Table 8.4** Coronary heart disease risk factors

| |
|---|
| 1. Age (45 years old or older for men, 55 years old or older for women) |
| 2. Family history |
| 3. Smoking |
| 4. Dyslipidemia |
| 5. Hypertension |
| 6. Glucose intolerance |
| 7. Obesity |
| 8. Metabolic syndrome |
| 9. Chronic kidney disease |
| 10. Stress |

## 2.4 Causes

It is caused by inadequate blood supply to the myocardium due to atherosclerotic stenosis or spasm of the coronary arteries. In particular, there are factors that promote coronary atherosclerosis (coronary risk factors) as shown in Table 8.4.

## 2.5 Symptoms

Sixty to eighty percent of cases can be diagnosed on the basis of symptoms alone. Sudden onset, anterior chest pain, vague sensation, effort participation, nitroglycerin effectiveness, and short duration are well-known symptoms and are referred to as the "SAVENS" of angina pectoris. They are often reproducible.

Sometimes there is radiating pain from the epigastric region to the neck and left shoulder. Other symptoms include palpitations, arrhythmias, dyspnea, headache, and vomiting. If the symptoms are left untreated, critical adverse events such as myocardial infarction and ventricular fibrillation may occur.

## 2.6 Examinations

### 2.6.1 Electrocardiogram

The ECG is within the normal range in the absence of an attack (or at rest), but ST depression is seen during an attack (Fig. 8.1).

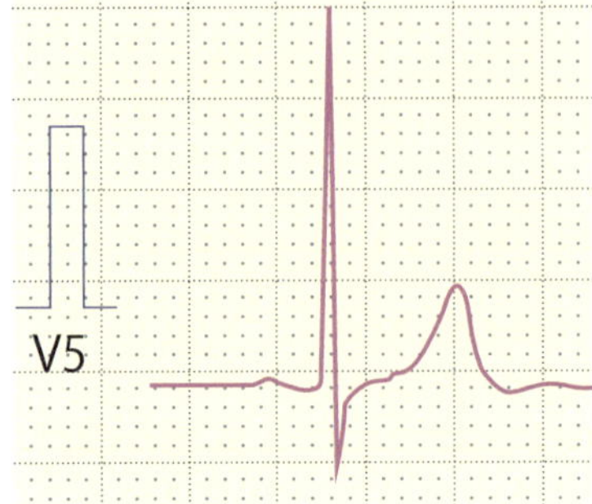


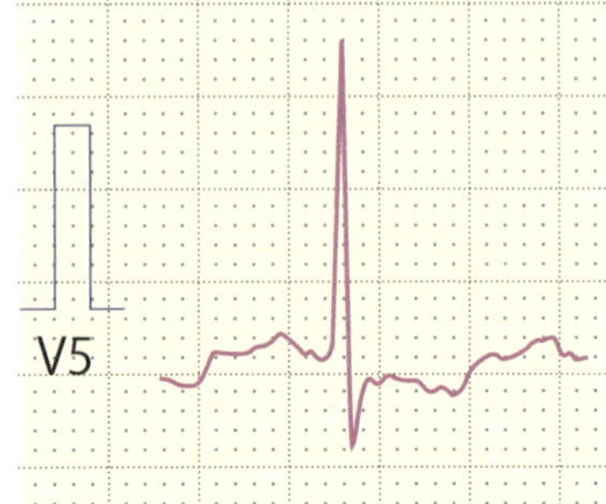


**Fig. 8.1** ECG of a patient with angina pectoris at rest (left) and during an attack (right), showing ST depression

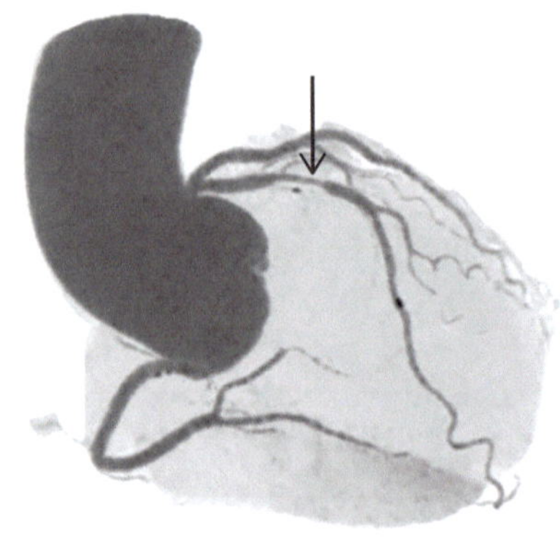

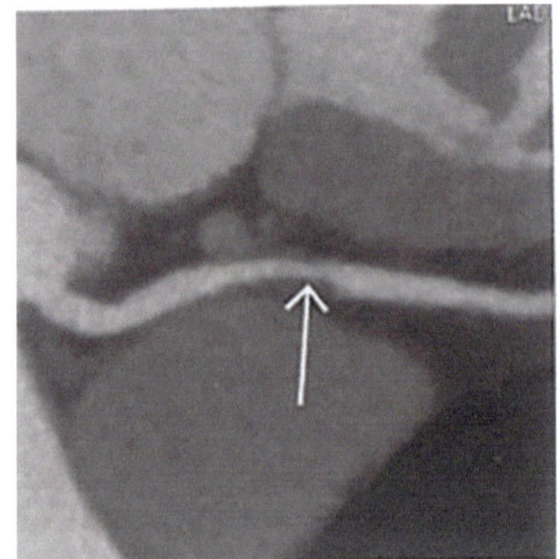

**Fig. 8.2** Example of coronary CT. This is a same case in Fig. 8.1. There is a plaque-induced stenosis in the left anterior descending branch

#### 2.6.2 Load Electrocardiogram

ST depression was observed in the master two step test, bicycle ergometer, and treadmill (walking) test.

#### 2.6.3 Holter Electrocardiogram

A small electrocardiographic recorder is carried 24 h a day for examination. ST segment depression can be seen during ischemic attacks. Coronary spastic angina with ST segment elevation observed from midnight to early morning is called variant angina pectoris.

#### 2.6.4 Blood Test

Enzymes that are elevated in myocardial infarction, such as troponin T, H-FABP (heart-type fatty acid-binding protein), leukocytes, CRP (C-reactive protein), CK, CK isozyme, AST, and LDH, are often not elevated because of the absence of myocardial necrosis.

#### 2.6.5 Echocardiography

Wall motion is normal at rest. Regional wall motion abnormalities are seen with exercise or drug (dobutamine, dipyridamole, etc.) loading.

#### 2.6.6 Myocardial Perfusion Scintigraphy

A radioisotope (RI) such as thallium is used, which is taken up by the myocardium. It accumulates in the presence of blood flow. It accumulates at rest, but accumulation decreases in the ischemic region after exercise or drug (adenosine, dipyridamole, etc.) loading. Diagnosis of angina pectoris is made by comparing the mismatch between the resting state and the stress state.

#### 2.6.7 Coronary Angiography CT (Fig. 8.2)

Synchronize the imaging with ECG. It can evaluate the tissue characteristics of coronary artery stenosis and plaque. It is less invasive and useful for exclusion diagnosis in screening.

#### 2.6.8 Coronary Angiography (CAG)

It is useful in the definitive diagnosis of coronary artery disease. In coronary spastic angina pectoris, drug (such as acetylcholine and ergonovine) stress test can be used to induce spasm and confirm the diagnosis. In addition, percutaneous coronary intervention can be performed consecutively.

## 2.7 Treatment

The main objectives are to prevent progression of stenosis and attacks due to atherosclerosis and to prevent the development of acute coronary syndromes. ABCDE is an important factor in the management of stable angina pectoris (Table 8.5). Risk factors should be controlled (smoking cessation, blood pressure control, correction of glucose intolerance, correction of dyslipidemia, etc.), drug therapy should be continued, and invasive treatment (PCI, CABG [coronary artery bypass graft surgery]) should be performed if necessary.

## 2.8 Drug Therapy

Aspirin and other antiplatelet agents for prevention of thrombogenesis are considered essential.

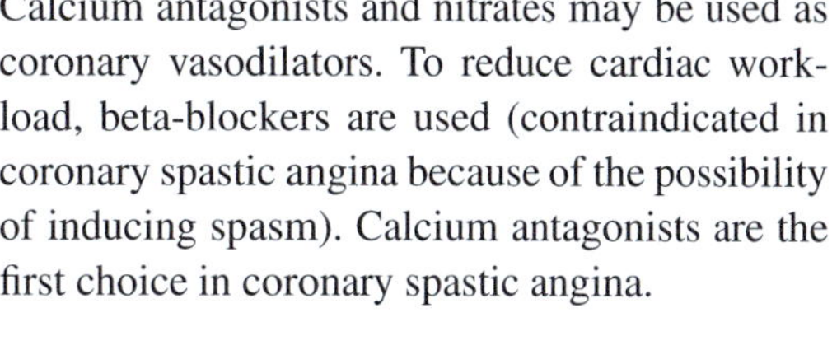

Calcium antagonists and nitrates may be used as coronary vasodilators. To reduce cardiac workload, beta-blockers are used (contraindicated in coronary spastic angina because of the possibility of inducing spasm). Calcium antagonists are the first choice in coronary spastic angina.

**Table 8.5** ABCDE of angina pectoris management

| |
|---|
| A: Aspirin and antianginal |
| B: β-blocker and BP control |
| C: Cholesterol and cigarette smoking |
| D: Diabetes and diet |
| E: Exercise and education |

## 2.9 Invasive Treatment

### 2.9.1 Percutaneous Coronary Intervention (PCI)

A guidewire is passed through the stenotic lesion, and a balloon catheter is inserted into the stenotic area along the guidewire for dilation. A stent (metal lining) is often implanted in the dilated area (Fig. 8.3).

The risk of restenosis is dramatically reduced with the use of drug-eluting stents (DES) because of inhibiting neointimal proliferation (Fig. 8.4), and mTOR (mammalian target of rapamycin) inhibiters (macrolide compound) impede proliferation of the smooth muscle.

### 2.9.2 Coronary Artery Bypass Graft Surgery (CABG)

It is a surgical procedure to bypass the stenosis and maintain coronary blood flow by anastomosing a graft from the aorta (or internal thoracic artery) to the periphery of the stenotic coronary artery and bypassing the stenotic area. It is mainly

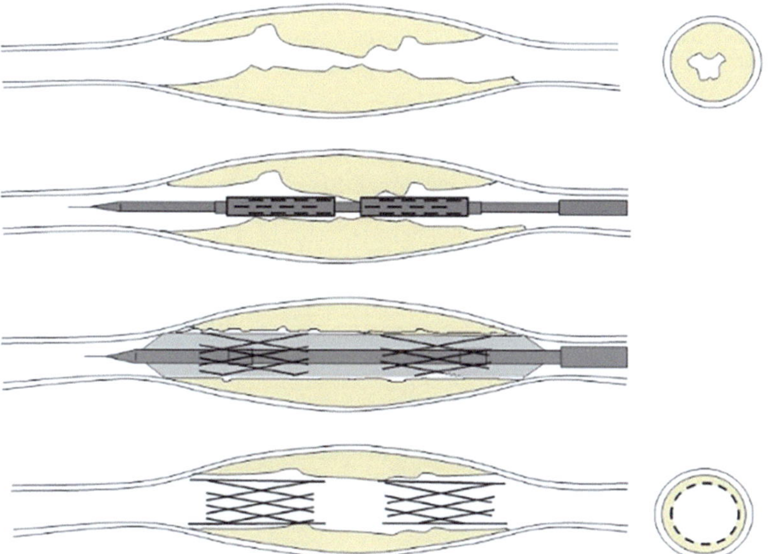

**Fig. 8.3** Schematic diagram of stent implantation in percutaneous coronary intervention (PCI). Stenting and dilate the balloon catheter at the site of stenosis. Implant the stent and remove the balloon catheter

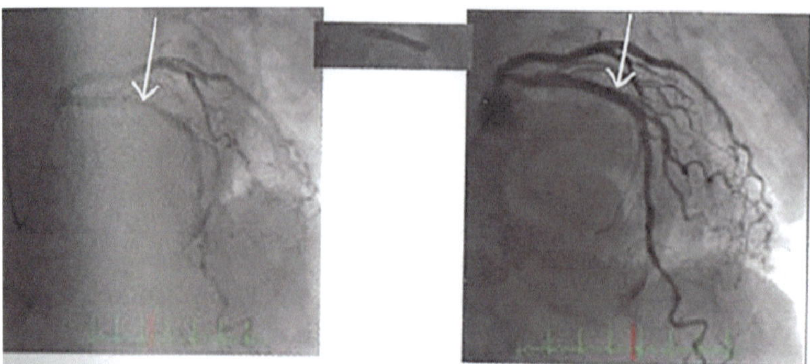

**Fig. 8.4** A case of coronary angiography and drug-eluting stent implantation. This is the same case as Figs. 8.1 and 8.2. A drug-eluting stent was implanted in the left anterior descending branch

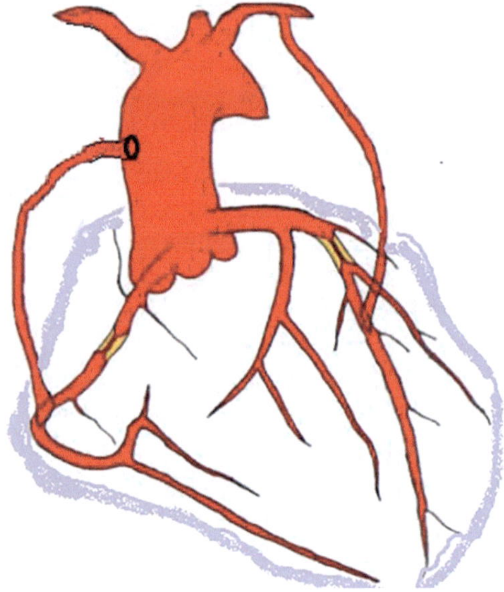

**Fig. 8.5** Coronary artery bypass graft surgery (CABG). The schematic diagram shows the internal thoracic artery bypassed to the left anterior descending branch and the aorta bypassed to the right coronary artery using a venous graft

indicated for left main coronary artery lesions and advanced three-vessel lesions (Fig. 8.5).

### 2.10 Notes from Dentistry Perspective

Izumi Yoshioka

If the patient has been treated for angina pectoris and has not had an angina pectoris attack in the last month or has had one or two mild attacks, dental treatment is often possible. For unstable angina, dental treatment should be avoided except for emergency treatment, and cardiac treatment should be given priority. Perioperative management should be in accordance with the description in the "Myocardial Infarction" section.

## 3 Heart Failure

Masayo Fukuhara

### 3.1 Concepts and Definitions

The functions of the heart include (1) pumping (sending blood to the whole body and supplying oxygen) and (2) controlling rhythm (automaticity).

Heart failure is defined as "a clinical syndrome in which some cardiac dysfunction, i.e., organic and/or functional abnormality of the heart that disrupts the compensatory mechanism of the cardiac pump function, results in the appearance of dyspnea, malaise, and edema, and a concomitant decrease in exercise tolerance" [9]. Simply, it is a life-shortening condition caused by abnormalities in the pumping function of the heart, resulting in shortness of breath and swelling.

### 3.2 Epidemiology, Causes, and Pathogenesis

Heart disease is the second common cause of death for 2019 in Japan. Of these, heart failure is the most common. Heart failure is caused by a variety of diseases. As shown in Table 8.6, many cardiac diseases cause heart failure, among which ischemic heart disease (especially myocardial infarction), hypertension, and valvular heart disease are common [9].

In myocardial infarction and cardiomyopathy, the myocardium is directly damaged, resulting in heart failure. In hypertension and valvular heart disease, the myocardium is subjected to long-term stress resulting in heart failure from dysfunction. In arrhythmia, heart failure occurs due to hemodynamic deterioration.

Heart failure might be caused by pulmonary diseases. Heart failure may appear as one symptom of endocrine and metabolic diseases and collagen diseases (autoimmune diseases). In addition, heart failure may be caused by excessive fluid volume, such as renal failure or excessive fluid transfusion.

In most cases of heart failure, cardiac output is decreased, but there are exceptions. In hyperthyroidism and severe anemia, cardiac output increases, the heart is overloaded, and the compensatory function fails, resulting in heart failure. This is called high cardiac output heart failure.

**Table 8.6** Causes of heart failure

| Causes of heart failure |
|---|
| Cardiac disease: various cardiac diseases |
| Ischemic heart disease |
| Hypertension: hypertensive heart disease |
| Valvular heart disease |
| Cardiomyopathy: hypertrophic cardiomyopathy and dilated cardiomyopathy |
| Congenital heart disease |
| Arrhythmia: tachyarrhythmia (atrial fibrillation, supraventricular tachycardia, ventricular tachycardia) and bradyarrhythmia (sick sinus syndrome, atrioventricular block) |
| Myocarditis and pericarditis |
| Lung disease |
| Chronic obstructive pulmonary disease (COPD) |
| Pulmonary thromboembolism |
| Others |
| Endocrine and metabolic diseases: diabetes mellitus, thyroid disease, and beriberi |
| Collagen disease (autoimmune disease) |
| Blood disease: severe anemia |
| Cardiotoxic substances: alcohol, drugs, and radiation |
| Renal failure |
| Excess infusion |

## 3.3 Classification

Heart failure is staged according to the American College of Cardiology Foundation (ACCF)/American Heart Association (AHA) heart failure stage classification. There is also the New York Heart Association (NYHA) heart function classification, which uses exercise tolerance (the limit of how much exercise a patient can tolerate) as an index (Table 8.7) [10]. The NYHA cardiac function classifica-

**Table 8.7** Comparison of ACCF/AHA stages of HF and NYHA functional classification. (Reproduced with permission from [10])

| ACCF/AHA stages of HF [11] | | NYHA functional classification [12] |
|---|---|---|
| A. At high risk for HF but without structural heart disease or symptoms of HF | None | |
| B. Structural heart disease but without signs or symptoms of HF | I | No limitation of physical activity. Ordinary physical activity does not cause symptoms of HF |
| C. Structural heart disease with prior or current symptoms of HF | I | No limitation of physical activity. Ordinary physical activity does not cause symptoms of HF |
| | II | Sight limitation of physical activity. Comfortable at rest, but ordinary physical activity results in symptoms of HF |
| | III | Marked limitation of physical activity. Comfortable at rest, but less than ordinary physical activity causes symptoms of HF |
| | IV | Unable to carry on any physical activity without symptoms of HF, or symptoms of HF at rest |
| D. Refractory HF requiring specialized interventions | IV | Unable to carry on any physical activity without symptoms of HF, or symptoms of HF at rest |

ACCF indicates American College of Cardiology Foundation, *AHA* American Heart Association, *HF* heart failure, *NYHA* New York Heart Association

tion is easy to use. Class I has no limitation in ordinary physical activity. Class II is mild to moderate limitation of physical activity. In Class III, there is marked limitation of physical activity, and symptoms appear with mild physical activity. In Class IV, symptoms are present even at rest.

## 3.4 Symptoms

The most common symptoms are palpitation, shortness of breath, dyspnea, and edema. When divided into left and right heart failure, the symptoms of left heart failure are all congestion of the lungs in front of the left heart system. The symptoms of left heart failure include shortness of breath, dyspnea, tachypnea, and orthopnea. In the early stages, shortness of breath occurs during exertion. In advanced stages, shortness of breath appears with light exertion, and in severe cases, it also appears at rest. Right heart failure is a sign of systemic congestion and includes jugular venous distention, edema, weight gain, and hepatomegaly. The edema is bilateral, tends to occur inferiorly, and leaves digital impression when pressed (pitting edema). The edema tends to be located in the extremities, but if the edema extends to the intestinal tract or liver, anorexia (loss of appetite) and abdominal fullness may occur [9].

Symptoms of decreased cardiac output include fatigability, decreased ability to concentrate, disturbance of memorization, and disturbance of consciousness [9].

## 3.5 Examination and Diagnosis

In the diagnosis of heart failure, the possibility of heart failure is considered based on subjective symptoms, medical history, physical examination, ECG, and chest X-ray findings [9].

On chest X-ray, the size of the heart should be noted. If there is an enlarged cardiac shadow, heart failure is suspected. The cardiothoracic ratio (normal is less than 50%) should be evaluated. Other findings include dilated pulmonary vasculature (edema around pulmonary vessels), butterfly shadow (butterfly-shaped alveolar congestion centered on the pulmonary hilum), and pleural effusion (Fig. 8.6).

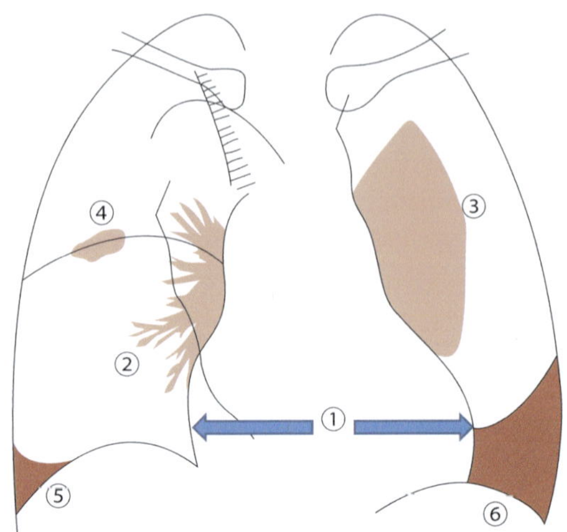


**Fig. 8.6** Chest X-ray of heart failure. (Created based on [9]). (1) Enlargement of cardiac shadow. (2) Enhancement of pulmonary vascular shadows: edema around pulmonary vessels. (3) Butterfly shadow: butterfly-shaped alveolar congestion centered on the hilum of the lung. (4) Vanishing tumor: pleural effusion accumulated in the interlobar pleura of the lung looks like a mass. (5, 6) Dulled costophrenic angle and pleural effusion

Echocardiography allows the evaluation of structural abnormalities (valve abnormalities, congenital abnormalities), size (lumen diameter), and properties, thickness, and movement of the myocardial wall. The contractility of the entire left ventricle is indicated by the ejection fraction (EF) (%). Cardiac output can be estimated.

Brain natriuretic peptide (BNP) or the N-terminal prohormone of BNP (NT-proBNP) is a biomarker that reflects the degree of ventricular load. BNP is useful not only in diagnosing the presence of heart failure but also in diagnosing the severity of the disease.

## 3.6 Treatment

Heart failure is the name of a condition, and there is an underlying disease that causes it. The principles of treatment for heart failure are (1) treatment of the underlying disease, (2) treatment of the heart failure itself, and (3) elimination of the triggers of heart failure. The triggers of heart failure include infections (respiratory tract infections, etc.), excessive fluid and salt intake, overwork, and self-discontinuation of medications.

- Considering treatment of heart failure itself, dietary guidance such as salt reduction should be given. Exercise should be limited depending on the patient's condition, but too much restriction of physical activity may decrease exercise tolerance. Exercise tolerance should be maintained by moderate exercise.

Angiotensin-converting enzyme (ACE) inhibitors, angiotensin II receptor blockers (ARBs), β-blockers, and diuretics are used as drug therapy. Cardiotonic agents (digitalis, adrenergic agonists, etc.) and vasodilators (nitrate medicines, hydralazine, etc.) are used in combination as needed. For more information on the effects of each drug, please refer to Sect. 7 in this chapter.

Patients with persistent ventricular tachycardia or ventricular fibrillation associated with heart failure are at high risk of arrhythmia recurrence and should receive an implantable cardioverter defibrillator (ICD) to prevent sudden death. In addition, cardiac resynchronization therapy (CRT) is used to treat severe cases of heart failure. In rare cases, an artificial heart or heart transplantation may be required.

## 3.7 Point[1] of Dental Treatment for Patients with Heart Failure (from the Viewpoint of Cardiologist)

It is important to understand the degree of heart failure and underlying disease, including NYHA cardiac function classification, cardiothoracic ratio on chest X-ray, echocardiographic findings (especially EF), and blood BNP or NT-proBNP. In addition, there are various underlying diseases, which should be understood, including therapeutic drugs.

[1] For reducing patient's discomfort under dental procedure and preventing lethal arrhythmia or sudden death due to local anesthesia including catecholamine.

At the time of medical consultation, the attending physician would like to know the outline of dental treatment, including the anesthesia method, the time required, and whether there is bleeding.

On the day of the dental examination, check for (1) symptoms of heart failure, (2) vital signs, and (3) transcutaneous arterial blood oxygen saturation ($SpO_2$). If necessary, monitor the electrocardiogram.

## 3.8 Notes from Dentistry Perspective

Masayuki Fukuda

In patients with heart failure, the stage of heart failure should be determined before treatment, because the stage determines whether dental treatment is appropriate. The ACCF/AHA heart failure stage classification is often used to determine the stage of heart failure, but it is useful to compare it with the NYHA Functional Classification, which is a classification of severity based on the ability to perform physical activities of daily living and is simple and reflects the patient's QOL (quality of life) (Table 8.7) [10].

Exogenous adrenaline is only one factor when considering blood catecholamine levels, and it would be less stressful and safer to obtain reliable pain relief with adrenaline-containing local anesthetics. However, there is an acceptable dose of adrenaline so that cardiac function is not affected. There are two ways to reduce the dose of adrenaline: 1:80,000 adrenaline-doped lidocaine and 0.03 U/mL of 3% propitocaine with felypressin or adrenaline diluted to 1/200,000 from a lidocaine ampule. The latter may be difficult to use in general dental clinics.

If the patient has a class I NYHA Functional Classification, normal dental treatment can be performed under monitoring. The tolerable amount of adrenaline that does not significantly affect cardiac function is about 40 μg [13]. One 1/80,000 adrenaline-doped lidocaine cartridge (1.8 mL, 22.5 μg adrenaline) can be administered, and if there is no significant change in circulatory dynamics, up to half a cartridge (0.9 mL, 11.25 μg adrenaline) can be administered.

Additional doses are administered with 0.03 U/mL of 3% propitocaine with felypressin.

In class II, the duration of treatment should be kept as short as possible to avoid psychological stress on the patient under monitoring. The tolerable dose of adrenaline is about 20 μg. One-half adrenaline lidocaine cartridge with 1/80,000 adrenaline (0.9 mL, 11.25 μg adrenaline) can be administered, and up to one-half cartridge with 0.9 mL adrenaline (11.25 μg adrenaline) can be administered if there is no significant change in circulatory status. Additional doses are administered with 0.03 U/mL of 3% propitocaine with felypressin.

In case of class III, keep first-aid and conservative therapy under monitoring and reduce treatment time as much as possible. The use of 1/2 lidocaine cartridge with 1/80,000 adrenaline (0.9 mL, 11.25 μg adrenaline) and 0.03 U/mL of 3% propitocaine with felypressin should be used.

In class IV, basically no dental treatment is performed.

Although felypressin is considered safe and has less effect on circulatory status than adrenaline, it may cause myocardial ischemia when used in large doses or in patients with severe coronary artery stenosis. The use of 0.03 U/mL of 3% propitocaine with felypressin is considered to be clinically safe for no more than three cartridges.

In all cases, referral to the attending physician in internal medicine is necessary, and depending on the severity of the disease, referral to the oral surgery department of a nearby general hospital or university hospital should be considered.

## 4 Infective Endocarditis

Tatsuaki Matsubara

### 4.1 Disease Overview

Infective endocarditis (IE) is a systemic septic disease accompanying generation of vegetations containing bacterial aggregation on the valve, endocardium, and intima of large vessels and showing a variety of clinical manifestations such as bacteremia, vascular embolism, and cardiac disorders. It is not a very common disease, but once it occurs, it can cause many complications and be fatal if not properly diagnosed and treated.

### 4.2 Pathophysiology

Non-bacterial thrombotic endocarditis (NBTE), which is caused by abnormal blood flow associated with valvular disease, congenital heart disease, or foreign bodies after valve replacement, is considered important in the development of IE. When transient bacteremia occurs in a patient with NBTE after dental or otolaryngology procedures, bacteria adhere to a NBTE site, growing to generate a vegetation. Therefore, vegetations are often found on the atrial side of atrioventricular valves; on the ventricular side of semilunar valves, where regurgitant blood flow strikes; or on the endocardial surfaces of abnormal jets such as shunt or stenotic blood flow.

### 4.3 Epidemiology

The incidence of IE in the general population is estimated to be 3 to7/100,000 person years.

It is often seen in patients with underlying cardiac diseases, but it may also occur in patients without a history of cardiac diseases. The predisposing event is unclear in many cases. It is important to always keep the possibility of IE in mind when making a differential diagnosis. In recent years, IE due to hemodialysis and lead infection of pacemakers has been increasing.

### 4.4 Classification

1. Pathogenesis: acute (causative microorganism: *Staphylococcus aureus*, *β*-Hemolytic streptococci, etc.), subacute (causative microorganism: Viridans group streptococci, Coagulase-negative staphylococci, Enterococcus species, etc.)
2. Affected valve: native and prosthetic
3. Infection status: community-acquired, nosocomial, healthcare-associated

## 4.5 Symptoms (Table 8.8) [14–16]

Fever is present in most cases, accompanied by chills, anorexia, weight loss, and fatigue. If the patient has already undergone treatment at a medical institution, the fever is often less than 38 °C.

Erythematous painless macules of the palms and soles (Janeway's lesions), Osler's nodules, a painful rash, and petechial hemorrhage, subungual hemorrhage, and retinal hemorrhage (Roth's spots) may be present. A heart murmur is audible in more than 80% of cases.

As a vascular complication, embolism is evident in about 30% of IE patients. Cerebral infarction can have a serious outcome, but many cases are asymptomatic. Acute myocardial infarction due to coronary embolism, splenic or renal infarction, and pulmonary embolism may also occur. Another vascular complication is infected aneurysms of the cerebral arteries, which can cause rupture even after prescribed treatment with antimicrobial agents.

Heart failure is often associated with valvular disease of the left heart system, inducing acute valve regurgitation and worsening hemodynamics.

**Table 8.8** Diagnostic criteria for infective endocarditis (IE). (Modified from the Duke Criteria) (Created based on [14–16])

| | |
|---|---|
| Definite IE | Pathological criteria |
| | 1. Microorganisms demonstrated by culture or on histologic examination of a vegetation, a vegetation that has embolized, or an intracardiac abscess specimen |
| | 2. Pathological lesions: vegetation or intracardiac abscess confirmed by histologic examination showing active endocarditis |
| | Clinical criteria |
| | 1. Two major criteria |
| | 2. One major criterion and three minor criteria |
| | 3. Five minor criteria |
| Possible IE | 1. One major criterion and one 1 minor criterion |
| | 2. Three minor criteria |
| Rejected | 1. Firm alternate diagnosis explaining evidence of IE |
| | 2. Resolution of syndromes suggesting IE with antibiotic therapy for ≦4 days |
| | 3. No pathological evidence of IE at surgery or autopsy, with antibiotic therapy for ≦4 days |
| | 4. Does not meet criteria for possible IE, as above |
| Definition of criteria | |
| Major criteria | • Blood culture positive for IE |
| | – Typical microorganisms consistent with IE from two separate blood cultures |
| | *Streptococcus viridans*, *Streptococcus bovis*, HACEK group, and *Staphylococcus aureus* |
| | Community-acquired enterococci, in the absence of primary focus |
| | – Microorganisms consistent with IE from persistently positive blood cultures, defined as follows: |
| | At least two positive cultures of blood samples drawn >12 h apart |
| | All of three or a majority of >4 separate cultures of blood (with first and last sample drawn at least 1 h apart) |
| | – Single positive blood culture for *Coxiella burnetii* or phase I IgG antibody titer >1:800 |
| | • Evidence of endocardial involvement |
| | – Echocardiogram positive for IE (transesophageal echocardiography recommended in patients with prosthetic valves, related at least "possible IE" by clinical criteria, or complicated IE [paravalvular abscess], transthoracic echocardiography at first test in other patients, defined as follows: |
| | Oscillating intracardiac mass on valve or supporting structures, in the path of regurgitant jets, or on implanted material in the absence of an alternative anatomic explanation |
| | Abscess |
| | New partial dehiscence of prosthetic valve |
| | – New valvular regurgitation (worsening or changing of pre-existing murmur not sufficient) |

(continued)

**Table 8.8** (continued)

| | |
|---|---|
| Minor criteria | 1. Predisposition, predisposing heart condition, or injection drug use |
| | 2. Fever, defined as temperature >38 °C |
| | 3. Vascular phenomena: major arterial emboli, septic pulmonary infarcts, infectious (mycotic) aneurysm, intracranial hemorrhage, conjunctival hemorrhages, and Janeway's lesions |
| | 4. Immunological phenomena: glomerulonephritis, Osler's nodes, Roth's spots, and rheumatoid factor |
| | 5. Microbiological evidence: positive blood culture but does not meet a major criterion as noted above or serological evidence of active infection with organism consistent with IE |

## 4.6 Clinical Examinations (Table 8.8) [14–16]

### 4.6.1 Blood Culture

Blood culture is very important in the diagnosis of IE, and once the causative microorganism is isolated, bacterial species identification and drug susceptibility tests can be performed. However, if antimicrobial agents have already been administered, the blood culture positive rates may decrease significantly depending on the bacterial species. Therefore, temporary drug withdrawal may be performed in patients with a subacute course, with a period of 2–3 days considered appropriate. However, treatment should not be discontinued in patients with respiratory and circulatory instability, such as those with heart failure and advanced infection or at high risk for embolism. At least three sets of specimens should be submitted for blood culture. The interval for collection of blood specimens has not been established, although there have been some recommendations such as collection of every 30 min, the interval of 1 h between the first and last collection, and 6 h or more. There is no difference in the detection rate between arterial and venous blood, and it is unnecessary to collect blood specimens at the time of fever.

For patients with positive blood cultures, blood cultures should be submitted within a few days (approximately 3 days, 48–72 h) after the start of antimicrobial therapy to check the effect of the treatment. Although it is not necessary to discontinue antimicrobial therapy at the time of specimen collection, it is reasonable to collect specimens immediately before administration of antibacterial agents when antimicrobial blood concentrations are low.

### 4.6.2 Echocardiographic Examination

Echocardiography plays the most important role in the diagnosis, treatment, follow-up, and estimation of prognosis of IE and should be performed in all patients with suspected IE, including those with negative blood cultures.

The major echocardiographic findings of Duke diagnostic criteria include (1) vegetation, (2) abscess, (3) new partial dehiscence of the prosthetic valve, and (4) new valvular regurgitation (worsening or changing of the pre-existing murmur not sufficient).

Transthoracic echocardiography (TTE) is noninvasive and repeatable and should be performed as soon as possible in all patients with suspected IE (Fig.8.7). Transesophageal echocardiography (TEE) should be performed when TTE cannot be diagnosed because of poor imaging, when there is clinical suspicion of IE even if TTE is negative, or when IE is suspected in patients with prosthetic valves or other devices (Fig. 8.8). If TTE and TEE are both negative, but IE is clinically suspected, repeat testing after 3–7 days is recommended.

## 4.7 Treatment

### 4.7.1 Medical Treatment

The choice of antimicrobial agent and treatment period are mainly based on the type of causative microorganism, antimicrobial susceptibility results, and valve type (native or prosthetic). Examples of targeted therapy prescriptions when the causative organism is known are presented in Tables 8.9 and 8.10 [14, 15, 17].

When antimicrobial treatment is started before the results of blood culture are known,

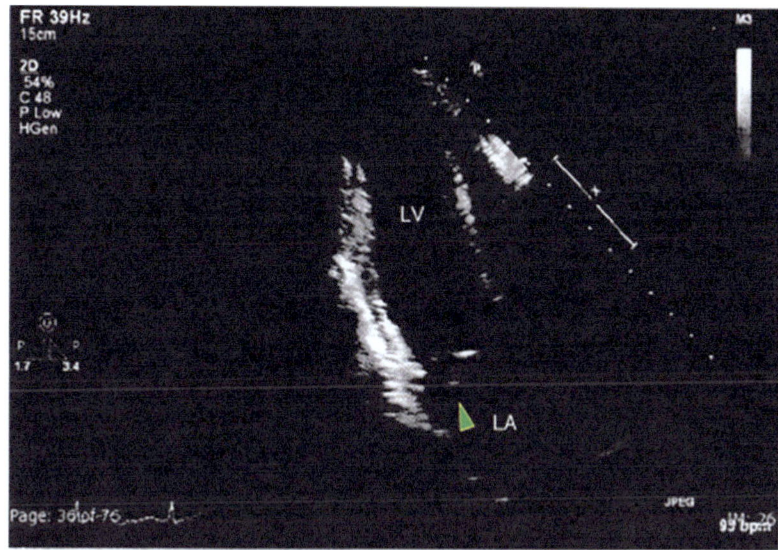


**Fig. 8.7** Transthoracic echocardiogram. A 55-year-old woman with persistent fever for 2 weeks was found to have *Streptococcus agalactiae* on blood culture. A mass is evident at the anterior mitral valve leaflet (green arrowhead). *LA* left atrium, *LV* left ventricle

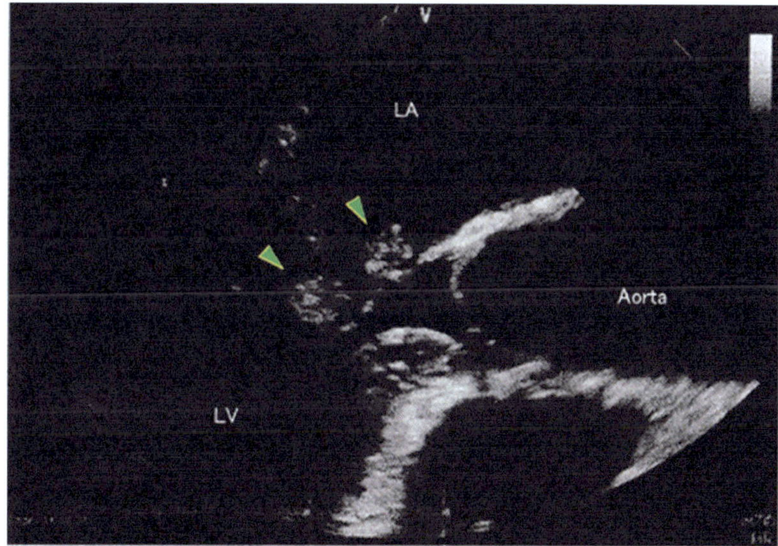


**Fig. 8.8** Transesophageal echocardiogram. Same case as Fig. 8.7. The round masses on the anterior leaflet of the mitral valve (green arrowhead) were judged to be vegetations. *LA* left atrium, *LV* left ventricle

so-called empirical treatment, agents should be selected according to the frequency of causative microorganisms, patient background, and clinical course.

The efficacy of the drug should be judged on the basis of a negative blood culture, with reference to symptoms such as fever and echocardiographic findings.

#### 4.7.2 Surgical Treatment

Indications for surgical treatment should be considered when congestive heart failure, uncontrolled infection, and infectious embolism are confirmed or anticipated (Table 8.11) [14, 15, 18].

### 4.8 Prognosis

The main factors associated with the prognosis of IE are patient background, complications of IE such as heart failure, causative organisms, and echocardiographic findings. The mortality rate during hospitalization for IE is high, ranging from 15 to 30%. When staphylococci are the

**Table 8.9** Recommendations of targeted therapy for native valve infective endocarditis. (Created based on [14, 15, 17])

| Antibiotics | Dosage | Duration (weeks) | Remarks |
|---|---|---|---|
| 1. Penicillin G-sensitivity (MIC ≤ 0.12 μg/mL) *Streptococcus (Streptococcus viridans), Streptococcus gallolyticus, Streptococcus gallolyticus,* and other *Streptococci)* | | | |
| Penicillin G | 24 million units/day in six divided doses or continuously | 4 | |
| Ampicillin | 8–12 g/day in 4–6 divided doses or continuously | 4 | |
| Ceftriaxone | 2 g, once daily | 4 | Patients allergic to penicillin, elderly patients, and patients with decreased renal functions |
| Penicillin G | 24 million units/day in six divided doses or continuously | 2 | |
| + Gentamicin | 3 mg/kg, once daily | 2 | |
| Vancomycin | 1 g, twice daily, or 15 mg/kg, twice daily | 4 | Patients allergic to β-lactams |
| 2. *Streptococcus* nonsensitivity to penicillin G (MIC ≥ 0.25 μg/mL) | | | |
| Penicillin G | 24 million units/day in six divided doses or continuously | 4 | Gentamicin can be administered at a dose of 1 mg/kg, 2–3 times daily |
| + Gentamicin | 2–3 mg/kg, once daily | 2 | Not recommended in the case of MIC > 1.0 μg/mL for penicillin G |
| Ampicillin | 8–12 g/day in 4–6 divided doses or continuously | 4–6 | Gentamicin can be administered at a dose of 1 mg/kg, 2–3 times daily |
| + Gentamicin | 2–3 mg/kg, once daily | 2–6 | |
| Vancomycin | 1 g, twice daily, or 15 mg/kg, twice daily | 4 | Patients allergic to penicillin |
| 3. Enterococci | | | |
| Ampicillin | 8–12 g/day in 4–6 divided doses or continuously | 4–6 | Gentamicin can be administered at a dose of 1 mg/kg, 2–3 times daily |
| + Gentamicin | 2–3 mg/kg, once daily | 4 (2)–6 | |
| Ampicillin | 8–12 g/day in 4–6 divided doses or continuously | 6 | Should not be administered for elderly patients and patients with decreased renal functions and *Enterococcus faecium* infection |
| + Ceftriaxone | 2 g, twice daily | 6 | |
| Vancomycin | 1 g, twice daily, or 15 mg/kg, twice daily | 4–6 | Patients allergic to β-lactams |
| + Gentamicin | 2–3 mg/kg, once daily | 4–6 | Not allowed for strains highly resistant of gentamicin |
| 4. Methicillin-susceptible *Staphylococcus aureus* | | | |
| Cefazolin | 2 g, three times daily | 4–6 | Cefazolin can be replaced with sulbactam/ampicillin |
| 5. Methicillin-resistant *Staphylococcus aureus* | | | |
| Daptomycin ± β-lactams, panipenem, betamipron, etc. | 8–10 mg/kg, once daily | 4–6 | Daptomycin can be administered at a dose of ≥10mg/kg, once daily |
| Vancomycin | 1 g, twice daily, or 15 mg/kg, twice daily | 4–6 | Vancomycin dose should be adjusted to trough serum concentration of 15–20 μg/mL |
| | | | Teicoplanin can be used (therapeutic drug monitoring is necessary) |

**Table 8.10** Recommendations of targeted therapy for prosthetic valve infective endocarditis. (Created based on [14, 15, 17])

| Antibiotics | Dosage | Duration (weeks) | Remarks |
|---|---|---|---|
| 1. *Streptococcus (Streptococcus viridans, Streptococcus gallolyticus,* and other *Streptococci)* | | | |
| Penicillin G | 24 million units/day in six divided doses or continuously | 6 | Monotherapy is permitted for the cases susceptible to penicillin G (MIC ≤ 0.12 μg/mL) |
| ± Gentamicin | 2–3 mg/kg, once daily | 2–6 | Gentamicin can be administered at the dose of 1 mg/kg, 2–3 times daily |
| Ampicillin | 8–12 g/day in 4–6 divided doses or continuously | 6 | Gentamicin can be administered at the dose of 1 mg/kg, 2–3 times daily |
| ± Gentamicin | 2–3 mg/kg, once daily | 2–6 | |
| Vancomycin | 1 g, twice daily, or 15 mg/kg, twice daily | 6 | Patients allergic to β-lactams |
| 2. Enterococci | | | |
| Ampicillin | 8–12 g/day in 4–6 divided doses or continuously | 6 | Not allowed for strains highly resistant of gentamicin |
| + Gentamicin | 2–3 mg/kg, once daily | 6 | Gentamicin can be administered at the dose of 1 mg/kg, 2–3 times daily |
| Ampicillin | 8–12 g/day in 4–6 divided doses or continuously | 6 | Should not be administered for *Enterococcus faecium* infection |
| + Ceftriaxone | 2 g, twice daily | 6 | |
| 3. Methicillin-susceptible *Staphylococcus aureus* | | | |
| Cefazolin | 2 g, three times daily | 6–8 | Cefazolin can be replaced with sulbactam/ampicillin |
| + Gentamicin | 2–3 mg/kg, once daily | 2 | Gentamicin can be administered at the dose of 1 mg/kg, 2–3 times daily |
| ± Rifampicin | 450–600 mg/day in 1–2 divided doses | 6–8 | |
| 4. Methicillin-resistant *Staphylococcus aureus* | | | |
| Daptomycin + β-lactams, panipenem, betamipron, etc. | 8–10 mg/kg, once daily | 6–8 | Daptomycin can be administered at a dose of ≥10mg/kg, once daily. Additional antibiotics are the following: *β*-lactams such as panipenem/betamipron 2.0 to 3.0g/day and sulbactam/ampicillin 9g/day, gentamicin at 2 to 3mg/kg/day, rifampicin at 450 to 600mg/day, fosfomycin at 6.0g/day, and sulfamethoxazole/trimethoprim such as trimethoprim at 5 to 8mg/kg/day |
| Vancomycin | 1 g, twice daily, or 15 mg/kg, twice daily | 6–8 | Vancomycin dose should be adjusted to trough serum concentration of 15–20 μg/mL |
| + Gentamicin | 2–3 mg/kg, once daily | 2 | Teicoplanin can be used (therapeutic drug monitoring is necessary) |
| ± Rifampicin | 450–600 mg/day in 1–2 divided doses | 6–8 | Gentamicin can be administered at the dose of 1 mg/kg, 2–3 times daily |

causative organisms, the risk of death from heart failure or cerebral embolism is elevated, and IE caused by gram-negative bacillus other than the HACEK (*Haemophilus* species, Aggregatibacter actinomycetemcomitans, *Cardiobacterium hominis*, *Eikenella corrodens*, and *Kingella kingae*) group bacilli is difficult to treat and can be severe. Prosthetic valve infection has a poor prognosis.

## 4.9 Recent Findings

Diagnosis of IE is based on clinical symptoms associated with sepsis, confirmation of a causative organism in the blood, and observation of destruction of intracardiac structures associated with infection, including vegetation, and therefore blood cultures and echocardiography are empha-

**Table 8.11** Indications and timing of early surgery for infective endocarditis. (Created based on [14, 15, 18])

| Situation | Indication/recommendation | Timing |
|---|---|---|
| Heart failure | Refractory pulmonary edema and cardiogenic shock due to acute severe valve dysfunction or fistula formation | Emergency |
| | Heart failure due to severe valve dysfunction or rapidly progressive perivalvular regurgitation | Urgent |
| Uncontrolled infection | Annulus abscess, pseudoaneurysm formation, fistula formation, increasing size of vegetation, and atrioventricular conduction disturbance | Urgent |
| | Persistent infection despite appropriate antibiotic therapy (persisting positive blood cultures or fever lasting >3–5 days after onset of therapy), with no presence of other infections | Urgent |
| | Infection caused by fungi or multiresistant organisms | Urgent/elective |
| | Prosthetic valve endocarditis caused by multiresistant staphylococci, non-HACEK gram-negative bacteria | Urgent/elective |
| Prevention of embolism | Infective endocarditis with persistent vegetations >10 mm after one or more embolic episode despite appropriate antibiotic therapy | Urgent |
| | Native valve endocarditis with mobile vegetations >10 mm and severe valve dysfunction | Urgent |
| | Infective endocarditis with isolated very large vegetations >30 mm | Urgent |
| Timing of surgery in patients with neurological complications | In patients of concomitant cerebral infarction, surgery for infective endocarditis should not be postponed if indicated | |
| | Note: Except for cases with coma, brain herniation, cerebral hemorrhage, and extensive neurological damage | |
| | In patients with intracranial hemorrhage, open heart surgery should be postponed for at least 4 weeks | |
| | Note: Except for cases with cerebral microbleeds | |

sized. However, identification of causative organisms by genetic analysis, detection of perivalvular abnormalities by cardiac computed tomography (CT), and the ability of positron emission tomography (PET) to depict inflammation sites have been reported to be useful. The latest European guidelines incorporate new imaging criteria into the Duke diagnostic criteria.

## 4.10 Notes from Dentistry Perspective

Shigeo Ishikawa, Mitsuyoshi Iino

Since it has long been reported that IE is induced by transient bacteremia associated with dental treatment, all dentists involved in clinical dentistry should be aware of dental treatments that can cause IE and their prevention methods. In order to contribute to the prevention of IE as a dentist, it is essential to recognize the risk groups for IE, to be familiar with the dental procedures that have a high risk of causing bacteremia, and to administer appropriate antimicrobial agents within 30 min to 1 h before the high-risk dental procedures. This chapter focuses on the dental treatments that may cause infective endocarditis, the risk groups for infective endocarditis, and the measures to be taken.

### 4.10.1 Dental Treatment at High Risk of Causing Bacteremia

Bacteremia associated with dental treatment has been shown in many reports to occur in almost all procedures that involve bleeding. In particular, not only major oral surgical procedures, which are highly invasive, but also minor procedures such as tooth extraction and dental implants and periodontal surgery and treatment are known to be dental procedures with a high risk of bacteremia. In addition, procedures that do not involve clinically obvious bleeding, such as root canal procedures, as well as oral surgical procedures for local infected sites, such as intraoral anti-inflammatory surgery for dental infections, are also included in dental procedures that cause bacteremia. Bacteremia has also been reported with minor invasive procedures such as suture removal, local anesthesia to the periodontal ligament, and brushing, which can cause bleeding in daily life. On the other hand, the risk of bacteremia is considered to be low in filling and restorative procedures and in noninfectious pulpectomy.

#### 4.10.2 Risk Groups for Infective Endocarditis and Appropriate Administration of Antimicrobials

At this stage, for patients at risk of IE, a single oral dose of amoxicillin 2 g, a penicillin antimicrobial agent, is recommended within 1 h before the procedure in patients who can be administered orally [14]. For patients who are allergic to penicillin or who cannot be administered orally, the use of alternative drugs such as those listed in Table 8.14 is recommended [14].

According to the guidelines for the prevention and treatment of infective endocarditis, antimicrobial prophylaxis is "strongly recommended" for patients in the high-risk group and "weakly recommended" for patients in the moderate-risk group. Considering that there are not many complications associated with antimicrobial prophylaxis [20], it is considered practical to actively administer prophylaxis to patients in the moderate-risk group. However, it is not practical to administer antimicrobial agents to all dental procedures for which the possibility of bacteremia has been reported, as shown in Table 8.12. Therefore, it is presumed that many facilities consider the major surgeries in oral surgery, minor surgeries such as tooth extractions and implants, and periodontal surgery, periodontal procedures such as scaling and root planing (SRP), and infected root canal therapy such as dental treatment with high risk of bacteremia and subject to antimicrobial prophylaxis. In addition, local anesthesia for dental treatment and procedures is based on infiltration anesthesia in the mucobuccal fold, avoiding infiltration anesthesia in the periodontal ligament space, which is considered to have a high risk of bacteremia, and in the gingiva, which may have gingivitis.

**Table 8.12** Incidence of bacteremia in dental treatments and procedures. (Modified from [19])

| Dental procedures | Incidence rate (%) |
|---|---|
| Extraction | 0–85 |
| Scaling | 8–79 |
| Periodontal surgery | 36–88 |
| Infected root canal | 42 |
| Ligament injection | 97 |
| Rubber dam device | 29 |
| Removal of thread | 5 |
| Brushing | 7–50 |
| Chewing | 0–51 |

#### 4.10.3 Current Status and Future

Although the incidence of IE due to dental treatment has been known for a long time, it is difficult to say that all dentists are aware of these facts. It has been reported that many dentists who do not major in oral surgery examine only a few IE risk group patients per year, and that about 30% of dentists use penicillin antibiotics for IE prevention [21, 22]. It will be important to continue to educate dentists about IE, dental treatment, and its prevention.

## 5 Hypertension

Hiromi Mitsubayashi

### 5.1 Abnormal Blood Pressure

#### 5.1.1 Essential Hypertension and Secondary Hypertension

1. Outline

   Blood pressure is the pressure in the arterial vasculature and is one of the vital signs. It is the physical pressure that occurs when the left ventricle of the heart repeatedly contracts and expands. It is called systolic (blood) pressure (SBP) and diastolic (blood) pressure (DBP), respectively. Persistent hypertension causes organic changes in the heart and vessel walls, resulting in organ damage/cardiovascular disease. High blood pressure is distinguished from hypertension. High blood pressure is a transient elevation of blood pressure that returns to normal when the cause of the elevated pressure is eliminated. Hypertension, on the other hand, is a persistent elevation of blood pressure that progresses to cause secondary organ damage/cardiovascular disease. Hypertension caused by other diseases is called secondary hypertension, and hypertension caused by etiologies other than secondary hypertension is called essential hypertension (primary hypertension).

2. Epidemiology

   According to the 2010 National Health and Nutrition Examination Survey, 60% of Japanese men and 45% of Japanese women aged 30 years or older were judged to have hypertension (systolic blood pressure of 140 mmHg or higher, diastolic blood pressure of 90 mmHg or higher, or taking antihypertensive medication). The prevalence of hypertension (same definition as above) increased with age, exceeding 60% in men aged 50 years and older and in women aged 60 years and older, with the highest prevalence in both men and women in their 60s.

3. Pathophysiology

   There is a relationship between "blood pressure and cardiac output x total peripheral vascular resistance. In order for blood pressure to increase, either an increase in cardiac output or an increase in total peripheral vascular resistance is required. Factors that increase blood pressure include a complex combination of chemical substances (vasoactive substances, hormones, etc.), nerves, vascular elasticity, cardiac output, blood viscosity, circulating blood volume, blood vessel diameter, and vascular reactivity (Page's mosaic theory). More recently, racial differences, salt intake and sensitivity, presence of comorbidities, gender, body mass index, age, smoking, cold, alcohol, mental stress, physical inactivity, and hyperinsulinemia have also been implicated. Season, temperature, humidity, weather, time of the day, mental tension, exercise, diet, excretion, and bathing are also factors that affect blood pressure.

4. Symptoms

   The progression of hypertension is gradual, and there are no subjective symptoms in the early stages. Headache, cloudiness, dizziness, ringing, stiff shoulders, palpitations, and shortness of breath may occur. However, these symptoms are not specific to hypertension.

   Hypertension leads to complications such as organ damage and cardiovascular disease. In such cases, the symptoms of organ damage/cardiovascular disease appear.

5. Diagnosis

   (a) Blood Pressure Measurement in the Examination Room

      The blood pressure and pulse should be measured in the resting position, averaged over two visits, and based on blood pressure values on at least two different occasions. At the first visit, the patient should be examined for left-right differences in blood pressure, orthostatic variations in blood pressure and pulse, and the presence of arrhythmia. The face and neck are examined for the presence of anemia, jaundice, ocular fundus findings, goiter, carotid murmur, and jugular vein engorgement. The chest should be examined for the location of the apex beats, presence of thrill, murmur, third and fourth tones, and irregularities. In the lung field, examine for rhonchus. In the abdomen, examine for vascular murmurs and hepatorenal tumors, and in the extremities, examine for arterial pulsations, left-right differences, coldness, edema, motor and sensory disturbances, and tendon reflexes.

   (b) Secondary Hypertension

      Secondary hypertension is caused by renal disease (chronic renal parenchymal disease, renal vascular disease), endocrine disease (pheochromocytoma, primary aldosteronism, Cushing's syndrome), aortic stenosis, brain tumors, and sleep apnea syndrome. Among these, renal disease is the most common, followed by primary aldosteronism, Cushing's syndrome, and pheochromocytoma.

(c) Findings Suggestive of Secondary Hypertension

Cushing's syndrome should be suspected in the presence of abdominal wall skin linear atrophy lesions and hypertrichosis. Paroxysmal elevation of blood pressure, palpitations, sweating, and headache are indicative of pheochromocytoma; weakness, periodic paralysis of limbs, polyuria, and hypokalemia are indicative of primary aldosteronism; and an abdominal vascular murmur is suspicious of renal vascular hypertension. Daytime drowsiness and snoring are suspicious for sleep apnoea syndrome, and drug-induced hypertension is suspected if the patient is taking nonsteroidal anti-inflammatory drugs (NSAIDs), herbal medicines, or oral contraceptives.

6. Examinations

The purpose of the examination is to assess the presence and extent of secondary hypertension and organ damage/cardiovascular disease. The examination includes general tests (general blood, urine, liver function, renal function, lipids, electrolytes, blood glucose, chest X-ray, and electrocardiogram) and recommended tests (ocular fundus examination, cognitive function test, depression assessment, head MRI, and MR angiography). Detailed examinations include microalbuminuria excretion, echocardiography, carotid echocardiography, ankle/brachial blood pressure ratio, pulse wave velocity, and 24-h ambulatory blood pressure monitoring. To screen for secondary hypertension, plasma renin activity, blood aldosterone, cortisol, catecholamine three fraction, urinary metanephrine fraction at any time, 24-h urinary catecholamine, and nocturnal transcutaneous oxygen partial pressure measurement are performed. Abdominal echocardiography (kidney and adrenal gland) is also performed. Special tests include adrenal CT, renal blood flow echography and scintigraphy, adrenal vein sampling, and polysomnography. If secondary hypertension can be ruled out, the possibility of essential hypertension is high.

7. Classification [23–33]

A systolic blood pressure of less than 130 mmHg and a diastolic blood pressure of less than 85 mmHg are considered normal. Hypertension is defined as systolic blood pressure of 140 mmHg or more, diastolic blood pressure of 90 mmHg or more, or home blood pressure of 135 mmHg or more or diastolic blood pressure of 85 mmHg. The higher the blood pressure value, the more severe the disease.

8. Treatment

(a) Antihypertensive target: Less than 130/80 mmHg in young- and middle-aged patients; less than 140/90 mmHg in patients aged 75 years or older; less than 130/80 mmHg in diabetic patients, patients with renal impairment, and patients after myocardial infarction; and less than 140/90 mmHg in patients with cerebrovascular disease.

(b) General therapy: Modification of lifestyle. Restriction of salt (≤6 g/day), encouragement of vegetable and seafood intake, restriction of fat (cholesterol, saturated fatty acid), maintenance of appropriate body weight (BMI ≤25 kg/m$^2$), moderate intensity aerobic exercise, restriction of alcohol, and smoking cessation.

(c) Pharmacotherapy (antihypertensive drugs): Calcium (Ca) channel blockers, angiotensin II receptor blockers (ARBs), angiotensin-converting enzyme (ACE) inhibitors, diuretics, beta-blockers, and alpha-blockers. If an adequate effect is not obtained, other drugs should be added or the patient should be switched to another drug. Periodic follow-up should be performed with attention to side effects.

(d) Side effects of major antihypertensive drugs: Beware of side effects of antihypertensive drugs, and the following drugs should be administered with caution: (1) Ca antagonists (bradycardia, heart failure, gingival hyperplasia), (2) ARBs (pregnancy, renal artery stenosis, hyperpotassemia), (3) ACE inhibitors (pregnancy, renal artery stenosis, angioneurotic edema, hyperpotassemia), (4) diuretics (pregnancy, gout, hyperpotassemia, glucose intolerance), and (5) beta-blockers (obstructive pulmonary disease, peripheral artery disease, asthma, severe bradycardia, impaired glucose intolerance).

9. Prognosis

   The prognosis of essential hypertension is relatively good if there are no cerebral or renal organ complications with controlled blood pressure. Complications such as organ damage and cardiovascular disease worsen the prognosis and result in loss of quality of life (QOL).

### 5.1.2 Hypertensive Emergency: Hypertensive Urgency

1. Malignant Hypertension

   It is a condition in which organ damage/cardiovascular disease progresses acutely due to a severe increase in blood pressure (≥180/120 mmHg). These include hypertensive encephalopathy, acute aortic dissection with hypertension, left heart failure with hypertension and pulmonary edema, acute coronary syndrome with hypertension, pheochromocytoma crisis, and eclampsia. Under these conditions, the prognosis is poor and the risk of death is great. These diseases require hospitalization and transvenous antihypertensive therapy. Patients with severe hypertension with nonprogressive organ damage, however, should be treated as hypertensive urgency with oral medication.

2. Morning Hypertension

   Early morning, post-awakening home blood pressure is specifically higher than the night blood pressure (≥135/85 mmHg). High risk of organ damage/cardiovascular complications (stroke, myocardial infarction, etc.).

3. White Coat Hypertension: White Coat Phenomenon

   In untreated patients, blood pressure measured by a physician is hypertensive (≥140/90 mmHg), but home blood pressure (≤135/85 mmHg) or 24-h blood pressure (≤130/80 mmHg) is normal. In a patient undergoing treatment, transient elevation of blood pressure observed by physician is called the white coat phenomenon. In these conditions, transient elevation of sympathetic nerve activity possibly due to anxiety disorder should be considered.

4. Reversal White Coat Hypertension (Masked Hypertension)

   It is the opposite of white coat hypertension. This is a case in which the blood pressure measured by the doctor in the examination room is normal, but the blood pressure measured at home is hypertensive. It is also called "masked hypertension" in the sense that the hypertension is concealed. Masked hypertension is often associated with organ damage and cardiovascular disease.

5. Obstructive Sleep Apnea Syndrome

   Obstructive sleep apnea syndrome (OSAS), which has attracted attention in recent years for its association with hypertension, has been described in the section on secondary hypertension. Fifty to 60% of patients with OSAS have hypertension, and 30–40% of patients with hypertension have OSAS. A transient increase in blood pressure is observed during sleep apnea or hypopnea immediately after resumption of breathing.

## 5.2 Notes from Dentistry Perspective

Hiroki Miyate

It is extremely important to take the patient's medical history before dental treatment. Blood pressure is always measured at the first visit, because many patients have high blood pressure but are unaware of their hypertension. If the blood pressure is 180/110 mmHg or higher, the patient should be referred to a physician. If the patient is under medical management for hypertension, ask the physician in charge about the severity of the condition, medications, and complications. In particular, if an oral surgical procedure is necessary, consult with the doctor as early as possible. Blood pressure should always be measured before any surgical procedure; if the patient's blood pressure is over 180/110 mmHg, the patient should be treated for only emergency procedures, and if the patient's blood pressure is over 160/85 mmHg, invasive and difficult extractions and extractions of impacted teeth should not be performed; the patient should be referred to a hospital or university dental clinic.

Elevated blood pressure may cause serious symptoms such as heart failure, myocardial infarction, and cerebral hemorrhage, so it is necessary to prevent abnormal blood pressure elevation. Elevated blood pressure during dental treatment is caused by psychological stress such as anxiety and nervousness, pain from treatment and local anesthesia, and physical stress from prolonged time of open mouth, which results in the release of endogenous catecholamines. During treatment, blood pressure fluctuates constantly due to stress. In principle, blood pressure should be measured continuously in hypertensive patients and the elderly.

To prevent psychological and physical stress, avoid surgical and/or lengthy procedures at the time of initial examination. Maintain a calm atmosphere in the examination room. Do not fill the mouth with water during treatment. It is important to provide painless treatment.

Laughing gas inhalation sedation and intravenous sedation are effective when the patient is very nervous or when the procedure is highly invasive. If the facility is not skilled in sedation, it is advisable to request hospital dentistry. Patients should be asked to urinate before the procedure and to check whether or not they have the urge to urinate during the procedure, especially if the patient is elderly and the procedure takes a long time.

The most common cause of elevated blood pressure is treatment-induced pain. Although epinephrine contained in dental local anesthetics may cause an increase in blood pressure, it does not particularly affect blood pressure up to about two cartridges, and endogenous catecholamines caused by pain have a greater effect on blood pressure. Therefore, it is important to obtain sufficient anesthetic effect by infiltration anesthesia up to two cartridges, with sufficient surface anesthesia to avoid pain at the time of insertion and slow injection of the drug solution.

If intraoperative blood pressure increases to 180/110 mmHg or more, discontinue the procedure. If the increase in blood pressure persists after discontinuation, a Ca antagonist such as nifedipine 5 mg should be administered orally. If chest pain, palpitations, headache, nausea, or other symptoms suggest a heart attack or cerebrovascular accident, consult a physician or request emergency medical assistance.

In hypertensive patients, hemostasis after tooth extraction or hemostatic procedures may be difficult, so suture hemostasis should be considered even for normal extractions. In addition, abnormal bleeding from the periodontal pocket may be observed, and suturing of the interdental papillae may be necessary.

When Ca antagonists are administered for the treatment of hypertension, gingival hyperplasia may be observed (Fig. 8.9), and gingival bleeding may occur from the same area. The gingival hyperplasia may disappear with periodontal therapy such as scaling and brushing, but excision of the proliferated area is necessary. If the antihypertensive drug can be changed, ask the physician to switch to another type of applicable drug.

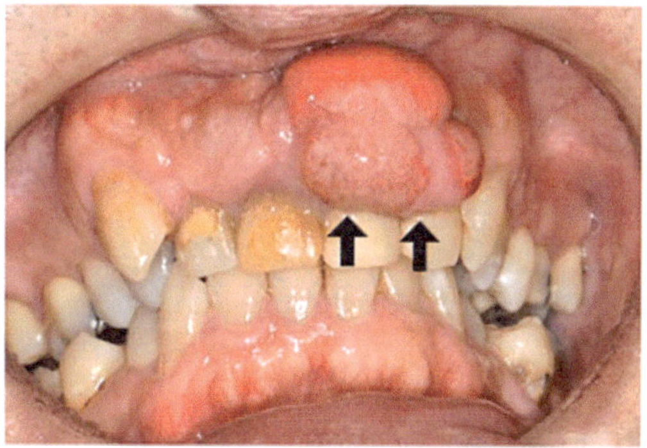

**Fig. 8.9** Gingival hyperplasia induced by calcium channel blocker

Besides the association between periodontal disease and systemic diseases such as cardiovascular disease and diabetes has been reported before, it was recently reported that edentulous jaws are a risk factor for hypertension. In postmenopausal women, the risk of developing hypertension is increased by about 20% in edentulous jaw individuals compared with toothed jaw individuals [24].

# 6 Cardiac Arrhythmias

Akihiko Hasegawa

## 6.1 Mechanism of Development

The sinoatrial (SA) node (also known as the sinus node) is in the wall of the right atrium at the entrance of the superior vena cava. The SA node cells produce an impulse (electrical impulse) that travels through the impulse conducting system to the ventricular muscle, causing the heart to contract.

Cardiac arrhythmias are abnormalities of cardiac rate and/or rhythm that result from disorders of impulse formation and/or impulse conduction. Mechanisms responsible for disorders of impulse formation include enhanced normal automaticity, abnormal automaticity, and triggered activity, while those responsible for disorders of impulse conduction include conduction block and reentry.

## 6.2 Tachyarrhythmias

### 6.2.1 Sinus Tachycardia

Sinus tachycardia refers to a condition in which the sinus rate is regularly increased to ≥100 beats per minute (beats/min) and is caused by enhanced normal automaticity (ability of impulse generation) of the SA node. Factors that trigger enhanced normal automaticity include physical exercise, excitement, anemia, pyrexia, dehydration, mental stress, intense pain stimuli, shock, and hyperthyroidism.

### 6.2.2 Premature Atrial Contraction (PAC) (Fig. 8.10)

A PAC is caused by a premature impulse generated in the atrium (not by the SA node). On an electrocardiogram (ECG), a PAC manifests as a premature P wave with a different form from that observed under normal sinus rhythm, while the QRS complex remains unaffected. The primary mechanism involved is abnormal automaticity. PACs are also common in those who are healthy and have a favorable prognosis. Persons with PACs often require no specific treatments if they remain asymptomatic (e.g., free of palpitations).

### 6.2.3 Atrial Fibrillation (AF) (Fig. 8.11)

ECG features of AF include a loss of P wave, a continuous baseline oscillation (referred to as fibrillation waves), and a variable R-R interval. AF is caused by multiple reentrant circuits generated in both atria. AF is a type of arrhythmia

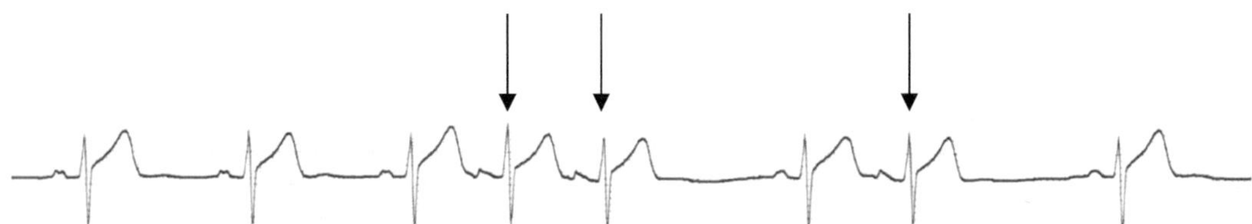

**Fig. 8.10** Premature atrial contraction. Three premature atrial contractions (arrows) are present. The shape of the P waves is different from that of the normal sinus rhythm, but the QRS complexes are almost the same shape as the normal sinus rhythm

whose prevalence increases with aging. AF commonly occurs with conditions such as mitral stenosis, mitral regurgitation, heart failure, acute myocardial infarction, and hyperthyroidism but can also occur without any such underlying conditions. Treatments used for AF include rate control agents, antiarrhythmic agents, and catheter ablation. Of note, patients with AF are at risk of developing an intra-atrial thrombus, which can be a source of cerebral embolism. Anticoagulation treatment to prevent this complication has conventionally been oral warfarin potassium but has recently been replaced by direct oral anticoagulants (DOACs: direct inhibitors of thrombin or activated factor X [Xa]).

### 6.2.4 Atrial Flutter (AFL) (Fig. 8.12)

ECG features of AFL include a loss of P wave and the appearance of regular serrated atrial waves (referred to as flutter waves) at 240–440 beats/min. Heart rate is often accelerated. The primary mechanism involved is reentry generated in the atrium. Treatments for AFL include rate control agents, antiarrhythmic agents, and catheter ablation. As for AF, people with AFL are treated with oral warfarin potassium or DOAC for anticoagulation to prevent cerebral embolism.

### 6.2.5 Paroxysmal Supraventricular Tachycardia (PSVT) (Fig. 8.13)

PSVT refers to an episode of tachycardia with a regular heart rate of 100–240 beats/min that starts and stops abruptly. The most prominent ECG feature of PSVT is a hardly discernible P wave often superimposed on a QRS complex. Reentry is the primary mechanism of PSVT. Treatments for PSVT include vagal nerve stimulation (e.g.,

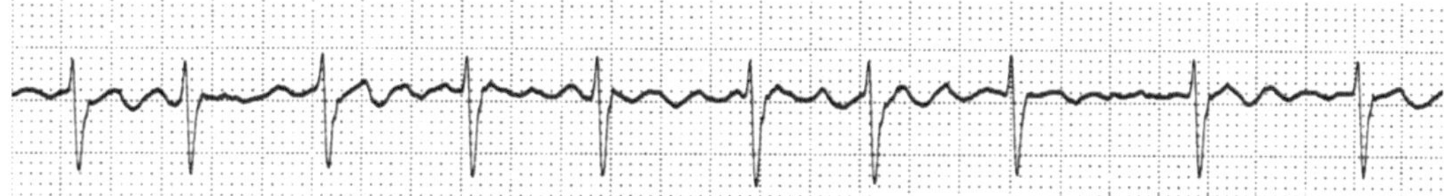

**Fig. 8.11** Atrial fibrillation. The baseline shows a continuous oscillation (fibrillation waves) with no P waves. The R-R intervals are variable

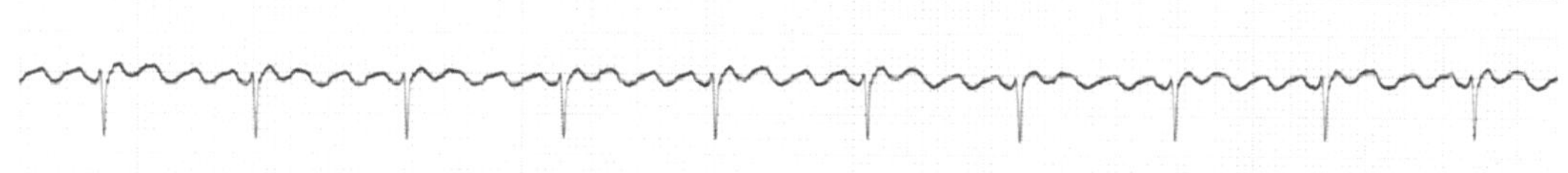

**Fig. 8.12** Atrial flutter. There are serrated waves referred to as flutter waves. In this case, one QRS complex appears after every four flutter waves (conduction ratio 4:1)

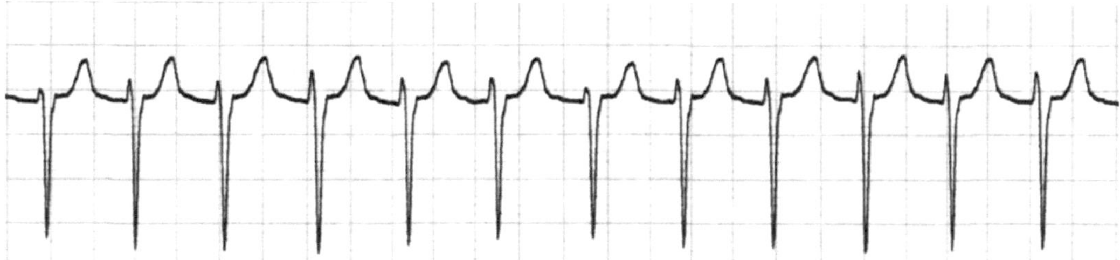

**Fig. 8.13** Paroxysmal supraventricular tachycardia. A recording of paroxysmal supraventricular tachycardia with a rapid regular heart rate of 140 beats/min

breath holding, carotid sinus compression), pharmacological therapy, and catheter ablation.

### 6.2.6 Wolff-Parkinson-White (WPW) Syndrome (Fig. 8.14)

WPW syndrome refers to a condition in which a sinus impulse travels prematurely from the atrium to the ventricle through a congenital accessory pathway (Kent bundle) that has more rapid conduction than the normal atrioventricular (AV) node. This premature ventricular stimulation generates a Δ (delta) wave, resulting in a shortened PQ interval and a prolonged QRS duration. The reentrant circuit generated between the Kent bundle and the AV node occasionally causes PSVT. If AF coexists, the rapid AV impulse conduction via the Kent bundle may induce pseudo ventricular tachycardia, potentially leading to ventricular fibrillation. Treatments for WPW syndrome include antiarrhythmic agents and catheter ablation.

### 6.2.7 Premature Ventricular Contraction (PVC) (Fig. 8.15)

A PVC occurs with premature impulse generated in the ventricle and on an ECG manifesting early wide deformed QRS complex without preceding P wave. The most common mechanism involved is abnormal automaticity. PVCs may appear after myocardial infarction and in patients with cardiomyopathy but are also observed frequently in healthy individuals. PVCs are often asymptomatic, although some are recognized as temporary palpitations or pulse deficits. Treatments

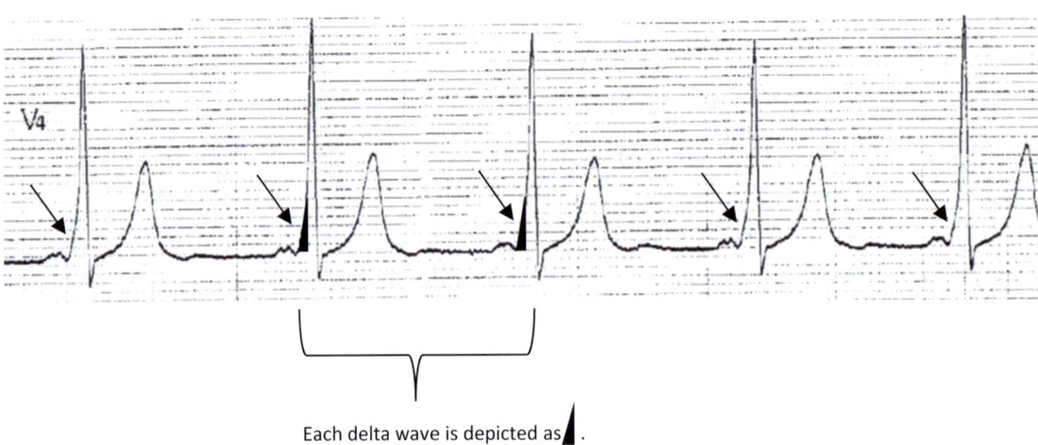


**Fig. 8.14** Wolff-Parkinson-White (WPW) syndrome. Δ (delta) waves (arrows) are observed, accompanied by short PQ intervals and wide QRS complexes

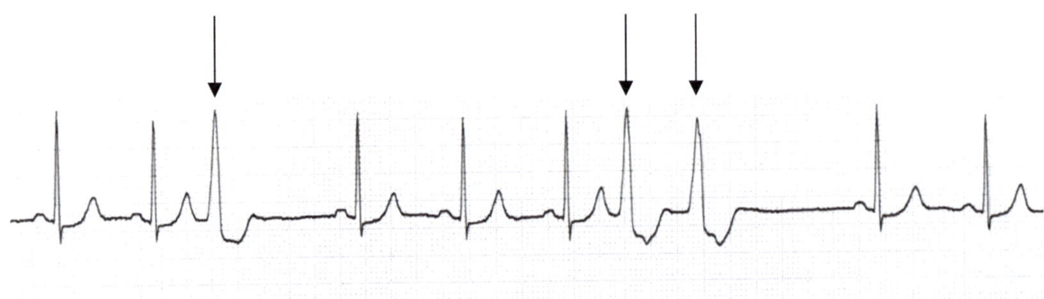

**Fig. 8.15** Premature ventricular contraction. There are three premature ventricular contractions (arrows), with wide deformed QRS complexes appearing prematurely without preceding P waves

used for PVCs include β-blockers and antiarrhythmic agents. In principle, specific treatments are not required in healthy, asymptomatic persons.

### 6.2.8 Ventricular Tachycardia (VT) (Fig. 8.16)

VT is defined as a series of three or more successive PVCs at a rate of ≥100 beats/min. VT is referred to as sustained VT if each series of successive PVCs lasts for ≥30 s; it is referred to as nonsustained VT if each series of successive PVCs lasts for <30 s. The primary mechanism responsible for sustained VT is reentry, while those responsible for nonsustained VT are abnormal automaticity and triggered activity. The most common underlying conditions are myocardial infarction and cardiomyopathy. VT may lead to ventricular fibrillation. Pulseless VT, which is associated with decreased blood pressure and a decreased level of consciousness, requires cardiopulmonary resuscitation and direct current cardioversion. Treatments used for VT include antiarrhythmic agents, catheter ablation, and implantable cardioverter-defibrillator (ICD) implantation.

### 6.2.9 Ventricular Fibrillation (VF) (Fig. 8.17)

VF is the most serious type of arrhythmia. On an ECG, VF manifests as irregular undulations of the baseline with no discernible QRS complexes or T waves. VF is caused by multiple reentrant circuits connected in a deregulated manner. The deregulated excitation of ventricular myocytes results in a loss of ventricular contraction, leading to syncope and cardiac arrest within a few seconds. VF should therefore be immediately treated by cardiopulmonary resuscitation and electrical defibrillation using an automated external defibrillator (AED). After resuscitation from VF, patients are usually treated with antiarrhythmic agents and ICD implantation. Underlying conditions include acute myocardial infarction, cardiomyopathy, and Brugada syndrome.

## 6.3 Bradyarrhythmias

### 6.3.1 Sick Sinus Syndrome (SSS)

SSS refers to a condition in which impaired function of the SA node (natural pacemaker) or impaired impulse conduction to the atria results in sustained sinus bradycardia, sinus arrest, sino-

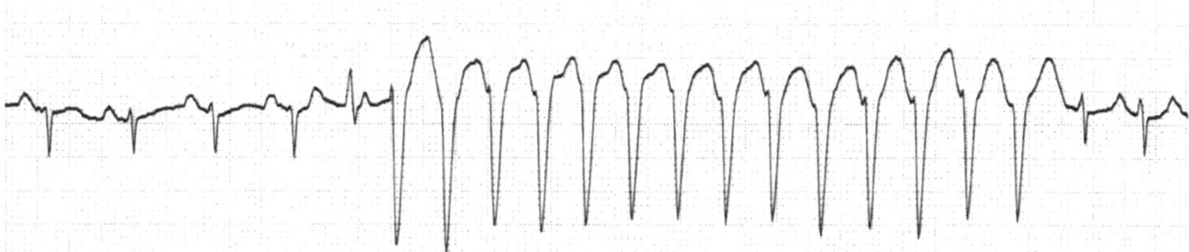

**Fig. 8.16** Ventricular tachycardia. There are 14 consecutive wide QRS complexes

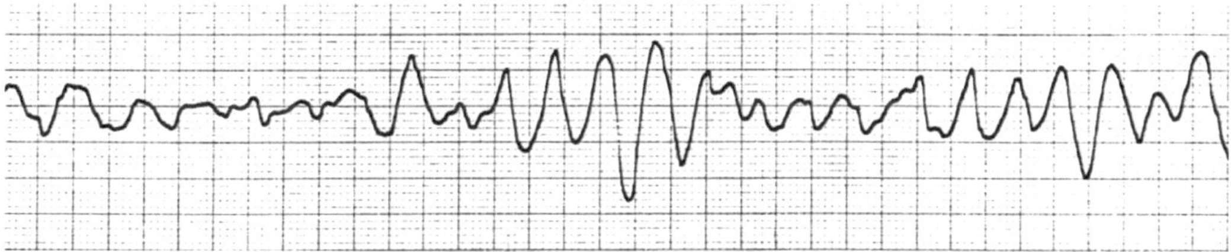

**Fig. 8.17** Ventricular fibrillation. Irregular undulations of the baseline are observed. QRS complexes and T waves cannot be distinguished

atrial block, or bradycardia-tachycardia syndrome, in which any of these types of bradycardia alternates with paroxysmal AF or AFL. Sinus bradycardia refers to a sustained regular bradycardia with a sinus rate of ≤50 beats/min (Fig.8.18). Sinus arrest occurs with an abrupt loss of P waves and QRS complexes and a prolonged P-P interval whose length is not a whole number multiple of its previous length (Fig. 8.19). If the length of a prolonged P-P interval is a whole number multiple of its previous length, the condition is referred to as sinoatrial block (Fig. 8.20). Underlying conditions include ischemic heart disease, although SSS of unknown etiology is the most common. Symptoms associated with bradycardia are dizziness, syncope, and shortness of breath. Treatments for SSS include pharmacological treatment (e.g., atropine sulfate) and permanent pacemaker implantation.

### 6.3.2 Atrioventricular Block (AV Block)

AV block refers to a condition in which impulse conduction from atria to the ventricle is delayed or disrupted and is categorized by severity into first-degree, second-degree, and third-degree AV block. Underlying conditions include parasympathetic hypertonia, fibrosis of the impulse conducting system, and acute inferior myocardial infarction; some cases of AV block are drug-induced.

First-degree atrioventricular block (Fig. 8.21): Impulse conduction from atria to the ventricle is delayed, resulting in a prolonged PQ interval of

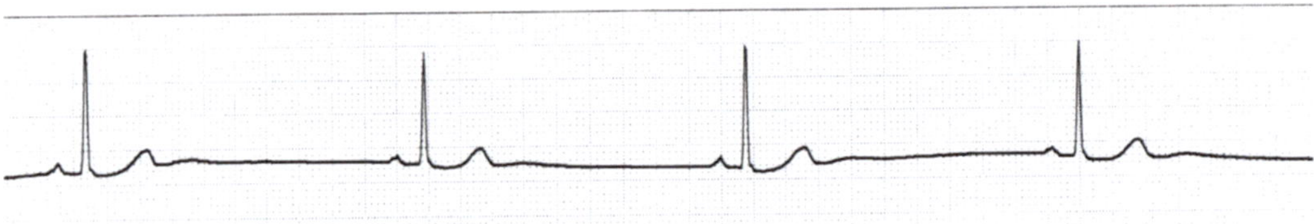

**Fig. 8.18** Sinus bradycardia. The heart rate is 29 beats/min in this case

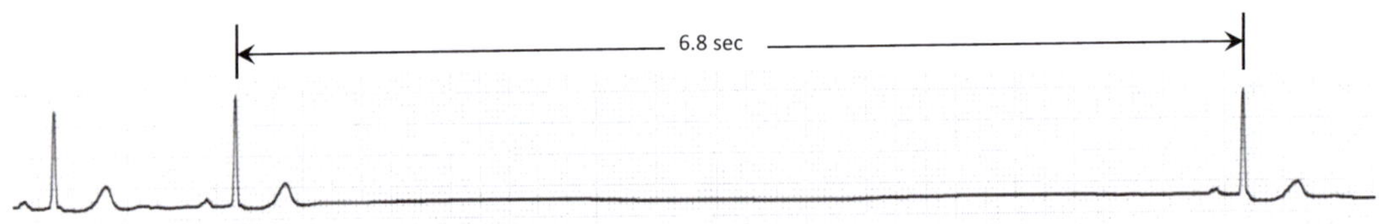


**Fig. 8.19** Sinus arrest. Sinus arrest for 6.8 s is apparent

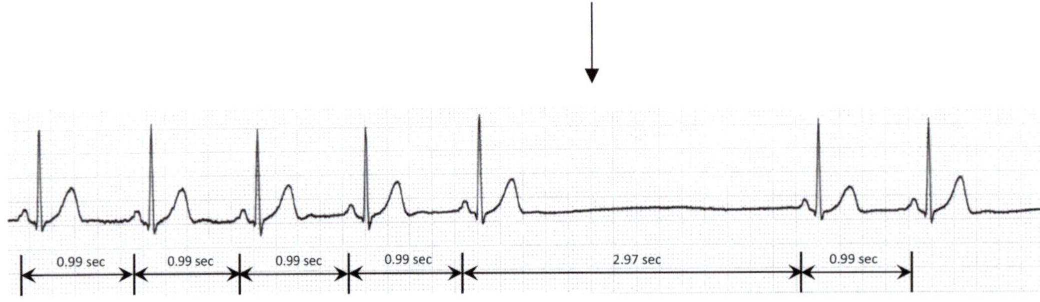


**Fig. 8.20** Sinoatrial block. The P wave and QRS complex are abruptly lost (arrow), and prolonged P-P interval (2.97 s) is observed. Prolonged P-P interval is three times longer than the P-P interval immediately before the loss (0.99 s)

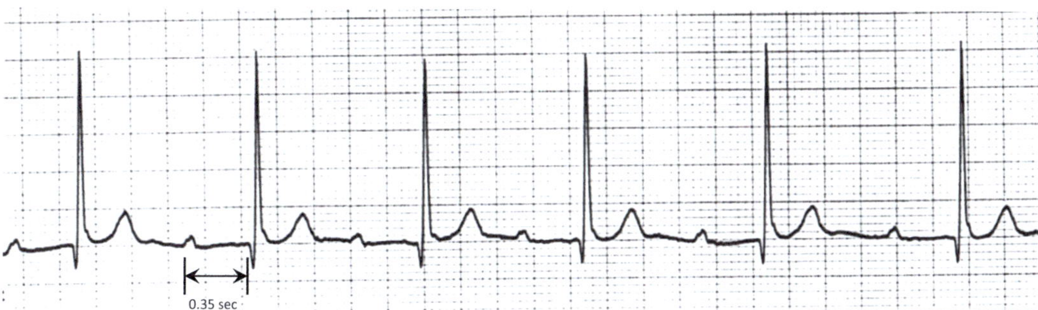


**Fig. 8.21** First-degree atrioventricular block. The PQ intervals are prolonged to 0.35 s without losing QRS complexes

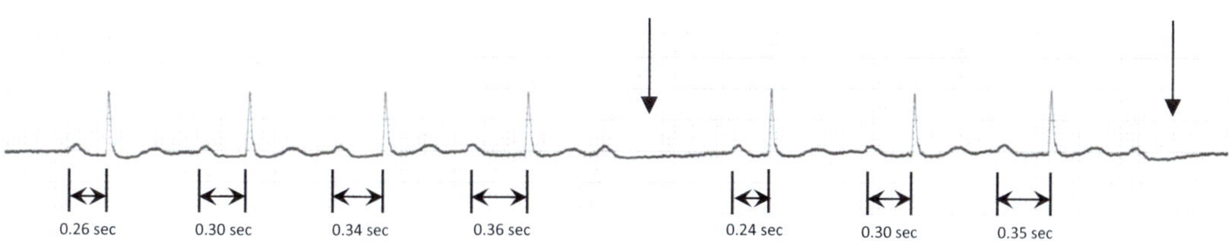


**Fig. 8.22** Second-degree atrioventricular block (Wenckebach type). Progressive prolongation of PQ interval and eventual loss of QRS complex (arrows) are shown

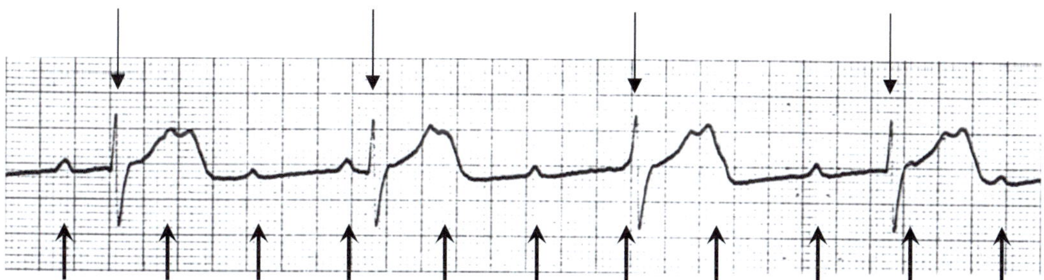

**Fig. 8.23** Third-degree atrioventricular block (complete atrioventricular block). P waves (↑) and QRS complexes (↓) appear at independent (mutually unrelated) frequencies, resulting in bradycardia in heart rate of 40 beats/min

≥0.21 s without losing QRS complexes. No specific treatment is needed.

Second-degree atrioventricular block (Fig. 8.22): Impulse conduction from atria to the ventricle is occasionally disrupted. Wenckebach type second-degree atrioventricular block, characterized by a progressive prolongation of PQ interval and eventual loss of QRS complex, needs no treatment in most cases. In contrast, Mobitz type II second-degree atrioventricular block, characterized by an abrupt loss of QRS complex with an unaltered PQ interval, is an organic block and a more severe type.

Third-degree atrioventricular block (complete AV block) (Fig. 8.23): Impulse conduction from atria to the ventricle is constantly disrupted, and P waves and QRS complexes appear at independent (mutually unrelated) frequencies. Hence, third-degree atrioventricular block is often associated with severe bradycardia and syncope, requiring permanent pacemaker implantation.

## 6.4 Notes from Dentistry Perspective

Kenichi Sato

During dental treatment, mental and physical stress may induce arrhythmias and increase the frequency of arrhythmias.

Arrhythmias that are problematic during treatment include abnormalities in pulse rate, such as tachycardia and bradycardia, and rhythm irregularities, such as extrasystoles [25, 26]. Patients with arrhythmias often have underlying conditions such as ischemic heart disease (angina pectoris, myocardial infarction), atrial fibrillation, or valvular disease, so the patient should be referred to an attending physician in internal medicine to confirm whether there is an underlying disease causing the arrhythmia and, if so, what kind of disease it is and to discuss the relationship between the underlying disease and dental treatment [27].

The causes of arrhythmia include anxiety and stress in the patient, pain during injection of the local anesthetic, and pain associated with treatment. The adrenaline added to dental local anesthetics may also induce arrhythmia. In order to reduce such mental and physical stress, the use of sedation is very effective [25]. In this chapter, we describe atrial fibrillation, one of the most common arrhythmias, and patients with pacemakers (PMs), who are expected to be seen more frequently by dentists as the aging population.

In patients with non-valvular atrial fibrillation (AF), warfarin-based anticoagulation has been used to prevent cerebral infarction due to thromboembolism. In recent years, direct oral anticoagulant (DOAC), including direct thrombin inhibitors (dabigatran) and factor Xa inhibitors (rivaroxaban, apixaban, and edoxaban), have been administered to prevent thromboembolic stroke [28]. It is considered that tooth extraction is possible even with continued administration of DOACs, both direct thrombin inhibitors and factor Xa inhibitors. It is recommended that extraction be performed after 6 h of oral administration of anticoagulant or after 12 h if possible. Concomitant medications that require caution in patients taking warfarin include macrolides, NSAIDs, and COX-2 inhibitors, which increase the PT-INR (prothrombin time-international normalized ratio) and increase bleeding complications. Acetaminophen is thought to be relatively safe to use because of its low antiplatelet effect, but the maximum daily dose in Japan is currently 4 g (previously 1.5 g), so care should be taken when administering large doses [4].

As the aging population, the number of fatal arrhythmias and severe heart failure cases is increasing, and the number of patients with PM is increasing. Dental treatment must be performed after obtaining the severity of the underlying disease, the pacing style and status, and other information from the physician in charge or the patient's own PM handbook [29]. Although there are no particular restrictions on the daily life of PM patients, electromagnetic interference (EMI) is a problem. When a PM is subjected to electromagnetic interference, the following reactions are observed: (1) fixed rate, (2) change or loss of programming, and (3) induction of tachycardia due to malfunction. The causes of EMI include external leakage electromagnetic field leaking from the device and direct internal current from the oral cavity [30]. Devices that generate external electromagnetic field leakage include visible light irradiators and dental laser devices (carbon dioxide, semiconductor, and YAG lasers), and the power supply and rectifier circuit must be separated from the patient (more than 30 cm). The direct electric current includes electric root canal length measuring instruments, electric pulp diagnostic instruments, fluoride ion injectors, and monopolar electrocautery (the counter-electrode plate is attached to the body, so the body is energized); these devices are usually contraindicated. The use of ultrasonic instruments (scalers, root canal cleaners) is also contraindicated. Bipolar electrocautery (the counter-electrode is not attached to the body), which is used only in the cavity, can be used [31].

If there is an underlying disease, dental local anesthetics for patients with arrhythmia should be selected based on the severity of the disease determined by the New York Heart Association (NYHA) classification of cardiac disease severity (see Table 8.2).

The criteria for the use of adrenaline-containing local anesthetics are 45 μg or less in mild to moderate disease and 22.5 μg or less in severe disease. In patients with nonselective beta-blockers, the dose should be 22.5 μg or less because adrenaline may cause an increase in blood pressure. As for propitocaine-containing felypressin, a large dose of felypressin causes coronary artery constriction and depression of cardiac function, which worsens the oxygen demand balance, and therefore, no more than two cartridges are safe for patients with ischemic heart disease [23]. In any case, monitoring of blood pressure and pulse rate is essential during dental treatment, and it is important to minimize mental and physical stress.

## 7 Cardiovascular Medicine

Shin Inoue

### 7.1 Antithrombotic Drugs

As people live longer, the incidence of atherosclerosis and atrial fibrillation is increasing, and the number of prescriptions of antiplatelet and anticoagulant drugs is increasing dramatically.

#### 7.1.1 Anticoagulants

With the increase in non-valvular atrial fibrillation, warfarin (Warfarin®), a conventional vitamin K inhibitor (coumarin type), has been replaced by direct oral anticoagulants (DOACs), which do not require monitoring of prothrombin time and can easily maintain blood levels [31]. The DOACs include the direct Xa inhibitors, edoxaban (Lixiana®), rivaroxaban (Xarelto®), and apixaban (Eliquis®), and the direct thrombin inhibitor, dabigatran (Prazaxa®). With the exception of dabigatran, there are no monitoring indices for the hemorrhagic coagulation system, but unlike warfarin, dabigatran has a short half-life, making it easy to control bleeding complications. General dental procedures, such as tooth extraction, can be performed with continued treatment. Warfarin has many contraindications such as vitamin K-containing drugs and miconazole, while DOACs have only contraindications such as HIV protease inhibitors in rivaroxaban and itraconazole in dabigatran. However, concomitant use of NSAIDs and antiplatelet agents increases the risk of bleeding in the gastrointestinal tract, so caution is required.

#### 7.1.2 Antiplatelet Agents

Aspirin (Biaspirin®, Bufferin 81mg®) is the most common antiplatelet agent, but with the increase in the use of drug-eluting stents (DES) in coronary arteries, dual antiplatelet therapy (DAPT) is now being used. DAPT is performed for 6–12 months after stent insertion, after which the patient is switched to aspirin or a single agent of the P2Y12 inhibitors clopidogrel (Plavix®) and prasugrel (Effient®). If antiplatelet agents are prescribed, the administration of NSAIDs should be kept to a short period (less than 1 week) to be careful of gastrointestinal bleeding.

### 7.2 Antihypertensive Drug

The most common antihypertensive drugs are Ca antagonists with vasodilator effects, thiazides with diuretic effects, angiotensin-converting enzyme (ACE) inhibitors and angiotensin II receptor blockers (ARBs) with both effects, angiotensin II receptor blockers (ARBs), and β-blockers with sympathetic depressant effects. Their indications, contraindications, and cases of cautious use are described by the "Guidelines for the Management of Hypertension, 2019" by the Japanese Society of Hypertension [32]. The indications for the treatment of hypertension are discussed in a separate section, but the active indications for various drugs are listed in Table 8.13, and the contraindications or cases of cautious use are listed in Table 8.14.

**Table 8.13** Active indications for major antihypertensive drugs

| | | Ca antagonist | ARB/ACE inhibitor | Thiazide diuretic | β-Blocker |
|---|---|---|---|---|---|
| Left ventricular hypertrophy | | • | • | | |
| Heart failure | | | • | • | •[a] |
| Tachycardia | | •[b] | | | • |
| Angina pectoris | | • | | | •[c] |
| After myocardial infarction | | | • | | • |
| Chronic kidney disease (CKD) | (Proteinuria−) | • | •[a] | • | |
| | (Proteinuria+) | | •[a] | | |
| Chronic cerebrovascular disease | | • | • | • | |
| Diabetes/MetS[d] | | | • | | |
| Osteoporosis | | | | • | |
| Aspiration pneumonia | | | •[e] | | |

[a]Start with a small dose and titrate carefully
[b]Non-dihydropyridines
[c]Beware of coronary vasospastic angina
[d]Metabolic syndrome
[e]AEC inhibitors

**Table 8.14** Contraindications or cases of cautious use of major antihypertensive drugs

| Antihypertensive drug | Contraindication | Examples of prudent use |
|---|---|---|
| Ca antagonist | Bradycardia (non-dihydropyridine) | Heart failure |
| ARB | Pregnancy and hyperkalemia | Renal artery stenosis[a] |
| ACE inhibitor | Pregnancy, angioneurotic edema, hyperkalemia, and apheresis/hemodialysis with specific membranes | Renal artery stenosis[a] |
| Thiazide diuretic | Hypokalemia | Gout, pregnancy, and glucose intolerance |
| β-Blocker | Asthma and severe bradycardia | Glucose intolerance, obstructive pulmonary disease, and peripheral arterial disease |

[a]Contraindicated in cases of bilateral renal artery stenosis

## 7.3 Antianginal Drugs

The current main treatment for angina pectoris is percutaneous coronary intervention (PCI) with drug-eluting stent (DES) implantation. Since prevention of restenosis is important after PCI, cholesterol-lowering statins are administered to suppress smooth muscle proliferation in addition to the antiplatelet therapy described above. The main purpose of nitrates is to reduce the preload by vasodilation (dilation of the venous system) and to improve circulatory dynamics. Nitroglycerin (NTG) is the most common nitrate drug and is administered sublingually in the oral cavity to rapidly increase blood concentration, and sprays and patches are also available. β Blockers are effective in effort angina, and Ca antagonists are effective in coronary spastic angina; Ca antagonists are dihydropyridines and produce hypotension, and verapamil (Vasolan®) and diltiazem (Herbesser®) may produce cardiac depression and bradycardia. Especially caution should be noted in the concomitant use of these drugs and β-blockers.

## 7.4 Antiarrhythmic Drugs

Outlined according to the Vaughan Williams classification, Na channel blockers (class I) are associated with electrocardiographic QT prolongation and resulting polymorphic ventricular tachycardia especially in group Ia patients. In particular, quinidine is contraindicated in combination with antimicrobial agents, antifungal agents, antiviral agents, and antineoplastic agents. β-Blockers (class II) are associated with bradycardia and decreased cardiac function and blood pressure. k-Channel blockers (class III) have much evidence of efficacy but are contraindicated in combination with antiviral agents, antineoplastic agents, and antifungal agents. Ca antagonists (class IV) also require attention to QT prolongation with bepridil (Bepricor®) and have contraindications with antivirals and antifungals.

## 7.5 Heart Failure Drugs/ Hypertensive Drugs

Acute heart failure is mainly treated with loop diuretics (furosemide, Lasix®) and nitrates but also with alpha-human atrial natriuretic peptide (Carperitide®) and tribaptan (Samsca®), a selective competitive vasopressin receptor antagonist. In the former, hypotension and, in the latter, electrolyte abnormalities should be noted. Digitalis is used in patients with atrial fibrillation, and antialdosterone agents are used in patients with low potassium levels. Catecholamines, such as dopamine and dobutamine, are used to increase pressure in patients with low cardiac output such as cardiogenic shock. On the other hand, in chronic heart failure, evidence is lacking except for β-blockers and ACE inhibitors/ARBs. In acute heart failure, respiratory management with various devices and assisted circulation devices are used because of the limitation of drug therapy.

## 7.6 Assisted Circulatory Devices Mainly Used in Acute Heart Hailure

An assisted circulation system is used in heart failure or cardiogenic shock refractory to drugs.

### 7.6.1 Intra-aortic Balloon Pumping (IABP)

For the purpose of assist impaired circulation, this device inserts a catheter with a balloon into the descending aorta with a balloon and inflates and deflates it with helium gas in synchronization with the heartbeat. Mainly it is used for myocardial infarction and is expected to increase cardiac output.

### 7.6.2 Extra Corporeal Membrane Oxygenation (ECMO)/ Percutaneous Cardiopulmonary Support (PCPS)

An artificial heart and lung apparatus is used during acute heart failure. ECMO is a general term for extracorporeal circulation using a membrane artificial lung, and PCPS accounts for the majority of ECMO. After blood is removed from the right atrium, blood is oxygenated by a machine and pumped through the femoral artery to support heart and lung functions.

### 7.6.3 Ventricular Assist Device (VAD)

A VAD is a device that is surgically attached directly to the heart to assist blood circulation in place of the heart in heart failure. When the patient's condition recovers, he or she can move freely to some extent. There are two types of VADs, one is installed outside the body and the other is implanted inside the body, and they are used according to the severity of the disease and the underlying disease.

## 7.7 Other Latest Cardiovascular Medicine

Catheter technology has led to the development of a variety of implantable devices to assist cardiac function.

### 7.7.1 Biventricular Pacing (Cardiac Resynchronization Therapy: CRT)

The left and right ventricles contract within 0.1 s, but in myocardial infarction and dilated cardiomyopathy, there is a "gap" between the left and right ventricles; CRT uses a pacemaker to resynchronize the motion of both ventricles and improve pump function.

### 7.7.2 Catheter Treatment of Atrial Septal Defect (ASD)

As an alternative of open heart surgery to close the foramen ovale with thoracotomy under general anesthesia, catheter-based device therapy under local anesthesia and guide by intracardiac echocardiography has been introduced. Implantable closure plugs include the Amplatzer Septal Occluder® and the Occlutech Figulla® Flex II.

### 7.7.3 Transcatheter Aortic Valve Implantation (TAVI)

Aortic valve stenosis is increasing in recent years, associated with chest pain, syncope, and heart failure with poor prognosis. For the reason, there has been an increase in the number of atherosclerotic patients with aortic valve sclerosis. An invasive technique using a catheter to implant a bioprosthetic valve has been developed, which improves life expectancy compared with drug therapy and has shown results comparable to open heart aortic valve replacement in patients with high surgical risk. Edwards' Sapien3®, Medtronic's Evolut®, and others are available as artificial valves.

### 7.7.4 Transcatheter Mitral Valve Clipping

A catheter-based clipping technique was introduced to treat mitral regurgitation. The catheter is inserted from the right atrium to the left atrium under intracardiac echocardiography of the beating heart, and the anterior and posterior leaflets of the mitral valve are clipped together to reduce regurgitation. The device system is Abbott's MitraClip®NT.

## 7.8 Notes from Dentistry Perspective

Masahito Sato

The purpose of perioperative management, including that for patients with cardiovascular diseases, is to ensure the safety of the patient and to prevent deterioration of the patient's general condition and the development of accidental diseases, despite the invasive nature of surgery and dental treatment. In order to achieve this, it is essential that the disease is properly controlled by the physician before surgery. For example, in the case of grade III hypertension, various guidelines state that referral to a physician should be prioritized except for emergency treatment. In addition, it is necessary to know the main effects, side effects, and interactions of commonly used drugs. Intraoperative monitoring is necessary to monitor the general condition of the patient during dental treatment. Noninvasive blood pressure measurement, transcutaneous oxygen saturation, electrocardiographic waveform, and pulse rate should be monitored. Painless treatment is a prerequisite for procedures under local anesthesia. The dosage of vasoconstrictors in dental local anesthetics should not be reduced because of concern about the effect of vasoconstrictors, which may cause endogenous catecholamine secretion due to pain stimulation, resulting in altered or disrupted circulation. In addition, since many patients have some anxiety or fear of dental treatment, it is necessary to take measures to reduce this anxiety, especially in patients with cardiovascular disease. The combined use of intravenous sedation is a reliable method for this purpose.

Naturally, drug therapy is the mainstay of control by physicians. Appropriate control by the physician does not only mean, for example, that the blood pressure is in the normal range in hypertension. It also means that the side effects of antihypertensive drugs are not occurring or are under control. In dentistry, adverse effects that should be noted include gingival hyperplasia with Ca antagonists, cough and taste abnormalities with ACE inhibitors, cough and pharyngeal edema with ACE inhibitors and ARBs, and dry mouth with alpha-blockers. In terms of interactions, renal impairment has been reported due to concomitant use of three medicines such as NSAIDs which are frequently used in dentistry, diuretics, and ARBs or ACE inhibitors. In perioperative systemic management, orthostatic hypotension due to various antihypertensive drugs, hyperpotassemia, renal dysfunction, and asthma caused by beta-blockers should be considered. In recent years, compounding drugs are often prescribed to simplify prescription and improve adherence. It is necessary to be familiar with each of the ingredients included.

The package insert for lidocaine hydrochloride-containing adrenaline, a local anesthetic for dental use, states that it should not be administered to patients with hypertension, arteriosclerosis, cardiac insufficiency, hyperthyroidism, and diabetes mellitus and patients with a history of vasoconstriction. In patients with cardiovascular disease, the recommended adrenaline dose is 45 μg in mild to moderate disease and 22.5 μg in severe disease (equivalent to one 1.8-mL dental cartridge) or less. It should not be used in patients with obstructive hypertrophic cardiomyopathy.

Sympatholytic agents are cardiovascular agents that should be used with caution, particularly with regard to interactions with vasoconstrictors in dental local anesthetics. When adrenaline-containing local anesthetics are used in patients receiving nonselective beta-blockers, the alpha effect of adrenaline may predominate, resulting in increased blood pressure and reflex bradycardia. The use of adrenaline-containing local anesthetics in alpha-blocker users may result in a decrease in total peripheral vascular resistance and hypotension due to the predominance of adrenergic beta action. Since many antipsychotic drugs have alpha-blocking effects, the same consideration should be given.

Propitocaine hydrochloride-containing felypressin can be used relatively safely in patients with cardiovascular disease. However, the anesthetic effect may be reduced and the duration of anesthesia may be shorter than with adrenaline-containing lidocaine hydrochloride, so more care is needed to ensure and maintain a pain-free state. It has been suggested that large doses of felypressin may cause coronary artery constriction, and caution should be exercised in the use of felypressin in patients with ischemic heart disease. A maximum of two 1.8-mL cartridges for dental use is recommended. Another local anesthetic for dental use is mepivacaine hydrochloride, which does not contain vasoconstrictors and is therefore relatively safe to use in patients with cardiovascular disease. However, since mepivacaine hydrochloride has a short duration of anesthesia, pay close attention to the duration of painlessness.

## References


1. Fleisher, et al. ACC/AHA Guideline on perioperative cardiovascular evaluation and management of patients undergoing noncardiac surgery. J Am Coll Cardiol. 2014;64(22):e77–e137.
2. European Society of Cardiology (ESC), Poldermans D, et al. Task Force for Preoperative Cardiac Risk Assessment and Perioperative Cardiac Management in Non-cardiac Surgery. Guidelines for pre-operative cardiac risk assessment and perioperative cardiac management in non-cardiac surgery. Eur Heart J. 2009;30(22):2769–812.
3. Kaneko Y. Vasoconstrictors (with a local anesthetic) and their usage. (Kekkan Shushukuyaku; Kyokushomasui Tenkabutsu; to sono Tsukaikata). J Jpn Dent Assoc. 1996;48(12):4–48. (in Japanese).
4. Japanese Society of Dentistry for Medically Compromised Patient, Japanese Society of Oral and Maxillofacial Surgeons, and Japanese Society of Gerodontology. Clinical practice guideline for tooth extraction in patient on antithrombotic therapy. (Kagakuteki Konkyo nimotoduku Koukessenyouhou Kanjya no Basshi nikansuru Guideline). Revised in 2020. Tokyo: Gakujyutsu-sha. p. 2020. (in Japanese).
5. Hiraoka E, et al. JCS 2022 guideline on perioperative cardiovascular assessment and management for non-cardiac surgery. https://www.j-circ.or.jp/cms/wp-content/uploads/2022/03/JCS2022_hiraoka.pdf. Accessed 20 Nov 2022.
6. Yoshio Y, supervisor. ASAKURA internal medicine. (Naikagaku). 12th edn. Tokyo: Asakura Shoten; 2022. (in Japanese).
7. The Japanese Circulation Society, et al. Guidelines for diagnosis and treatment of patients with vasospastic angina (coronary spastic angina) (JCS2013) (in Japanese). https://www.j-circ.or.jp/cms/wp-content/uploads/2020/02/JCS2013_ogawah_h.pdf. Accessed 24 May 2022.
8. The Japanese Circulation Society, et al. Guidelines for the primary prevention of ischemic heart disease revised version (JCS 2012) (in Japanese). https://www.j-circ.or.jp/cms/wp-content/uploads/2020/02/JCS2012_shimamoto_h.pdf. Accessed 24 May 2022.
9. Tsutsui H, et al.; on behalf of the Japanese Circulation Society and the Japanese Heart Failure Society Joint Working Group, JCS 2017/JHFS 2017. Guideline on diagnosis and treatment of acute and chronic heart failure —— digest version. Circ J. 2019;83(8):1767–809.

https://www.jstage.jst.go.jp/article/circj/83/8/83_CJ-19-0549/_article/-char/ja. Accessed 1 Feb 2022.
10. Yancy CW, et al. 2013 ACCF/AHA guideline for the management of heart failure: a report of the American College of Cardiology Foundation/American Heart Association Task Force on Practice Guidelines. J Am Coll Cardiol. 2013;62:e147–239.
11. Hunt SA, et al. 2009 Focused update incorporated into the ACC/AHA 2005 guidelines for the diagnosis and management of heart failure in adults: a report of the American College of Cardiology Foundation/American Heart Association Task Force on Practice Guidelines. J Am Coll Cardiol. 2009;53:e1–e90.
12. The Criteria Committee of the New York Heart Association. Nomenclature and criteria for diagnosis of diseases of the heart and great vessels. 9th ed. Boston: Little & Brown; 1994.
13. Sugiyama K. Local anesthetics and vasoconstrictors in dentistry. Ann Kagoshima Univ Dent Sch. 1996;16:1–11. (in Japanese).
14. Nakatani S, et al. JCS 2017 guideline on prevention and treatment of infective endocarditis. Circ J. 2019;83:1767–809.
15. Habib G, et al. 2015 ESC guidelines for the management of infective endocarditis. The Task Force for the Management of Infective Endocarditis of the European Society of Cardiology (ESC). Eur Heart J. 2015;36:3075–123.
16. Nishimura RA, et al. 2014 AHA/ACC guideline for the management of patients with valvular heart disease. A report of the American College of Cardiology/American Heart Association Task Force on Practice Guidelines. J Am Coll Cardiol. 2014;63:e57–e185.
17. Baddour LM, et al. Infective endocarditis in adults: diagnosis, antimicrobial therapy, and management of complications. A scientific statement for Healthcare Professionals from the American Heart Association. Circulation. 2015;132:1435–86.
18. Otto CM, et al. 2020 ACC/AHA guideline for the management of patients with valvular heart disease. A report of the American College of Cardiology/American Heart Association Joint Committee on Clinical Practice Guidelines. J Am Coll Cardiol. 2021;77:e27–e197.
19. Hall G, Heimdahl A, Nord CE. Bacteremia after oral surgery and antibiotic prophylaxis for endocarditis. Clin Infect Dis. 1999;29(1):1–8.
20. Thornhill MH, Dayer MJ, Prendergast B, et al. Incidence and nature of adverse reactions to antibiotics used as endocarditis prophylaxis. J Antimicrob Chemother. 2015;70:2382–8.
21. Nomura R, Kokomoto K, Ohara T, et al. Current knowledge among Japanese experienced general dentists regarding prevention of infective endocarditis. Odontology. 2018;106:297–305.
22. Nakano K, Ooshima T. Common knowledge regarding prevention of infective endocarditis among general dentists in Japan. J Cardiol. 2011;57:123–30.
23. Ichinohe T. Chapter 3 Local Analgesic. (Kyokusyo Masuiyaku). In: Fukushima K, supervisor. Dental anesthesiology. 8th edn. Tokyo: Ishiyaku Shuppann; 2019. p. 126–40. (in Japanese).
24. Gordon JG, et al. Association of periodontal disease and edentulism with hypertension risk in postmenopausal women. Am J Hypertens. 2019;32(2):193–201.
25. Niwa H. Chapter 13 Systemic accidents in dentistry. (Shikachiryou niokeru Zenshinteki Guhatsushou). In: Fukushima K, supervisor. Dental anesthesiology. 8th edn. Tokyo: Ishiyaku Shuppann; 2019. p. 506–21. (in Japanese).
26. Noguchi I. Essence of the chairside care for medically compromised elderly; cardiac dysrhythmia. (Yuubyou Koureisha no chairside essence; Koureisya Fuseimyaku), vol. 40(2). Tokyo: Dental Diamond; 2015, p. 162–4. (in Japanese).
27. Sugiyama K. General care in dentistry. (Shin Shika Zenshinkanrigaku). Tokyo: Nihon Shika Shinbunsya; 2004. p. 88–101. (in Japanese).
28. The Japanese Circulation Society. Guidelines for pharmacotherapy of atrial fibrillation (JCS 2013) (in Japanese). https://www.j-circ.or.jp/cms/wp-content/uploads/2020/02/JCS2013_inoue_d.pdf. Accessed 1 Feb 2022.
29. Sakurai M. Chapter 5 general anesthesia. (Zenshinmasui). In: Fukushima K, supervisor. Dental anesthesiology. 8th edn. Tokyo: Ishiyaku Shuppann; 2019. p. 204–17. (in Japanese).
30. Kudo Y, et al. Use of an Apex locator and ultrasonic irrigation for patients with implanted cardiac PAcemaker or cardiovascular defibrillator: two case reports. Jpn J Conserv Dent. 2015;58:331–7.
31. The Japanese Circulation Society. Guidelines for rehabilitation in society, attending school and working in patients treated with pacemaker, ICD and CRT (JCS 2013). (in Japanese). https://www.j-circ.or.jp/cms/wp-content/uploads/2020/02/JCS2013_okumura_h.pdf. Accessed 1 Feb 2022.
32. Committee for Guidelines for the Management of Hypertension, editor. Guidelines for the management of hypertension 2019 (JSH 2019). Tokyo: Lifescience Shuppan; 2019. (in Japanese).
33. Urabe A, et al., editors. Therapeutic medicine today; handbook in 2020. (Konnichi no Chiryouyaku; Kaisetsu to Binran 2020). Nanko-do: Tokyo; 2020. (in Japanese).

# Cerebrovascular Diseases

# 9

Hiroaki Ooboshi and Takahiro Kanno

## 1 Intracranial Hemorrhage

Hiroaki Ooboshi

Brain hemorrhage refers to intracerebral hemorrhage in a narrow sense, but in a broader sense, intracranial hemorrhage, that is, all hemorrhages occurring within the skull, may be collectively referred to. In this article, among intracranial hemorrhage, we describe intracerebral hemorrhage, subarachnoid hemorrhage, and chronic subdural hemorrhage, excluding emergency diseases caused by trauma [1].

### 1.1 Brain Hemorrhage

Brain hemorrhage or intracerebral hemorrhage is caused by bleeding in the brain parenchyma and accounts for 20% of cerebrovascular disorders. Hypertensive cerebral hemorrhage accounts for 70% of hemorrhage. Hypertension causes arteriolosclerosis in cerebral arterioles with a diameter of 100–200 μm, and prolonged hypertension causes vascular lesions pathologically called lipohyalinosis or fibrinoid necrosis (Fig. 9.1a–c), which may lead to the formation of microaneurysms (Charcot-Bouchard aneurysms). These vascular lesions with hypertensive changes are believed to rupture when blood pressure rises, resulting in intracerebral hemorrhage. Hematomas occur most frequently in the putamen and thalamus, followed by the subcortical region, cerebellum, and pons. Special vascular abnormalities include amyloid angiopathy and moyamoya disease in the elderly and vascular malformations and cerebral venous sinus thrombosis in the young.

The clinical manifestations include neurological symptoms in the injured area depending on the site of onset. If the hematoma is markedly enlarged, vomiting, elevated blood pressure, and disturbance of consciousness may occur with increased intracranial pressure, and the symptoms of cerebral herniation characteristic of the compression site, such as Horner's sign and oculomotor paralysis, may appear, leading to decerebrate rigidity and respiratory failure and death. In the most common form of putaminal hemorrhage (Fig. 9.2a), contralateral motor paralysis (pyramidal tract lesion) often occurs because the pyramidal tract runs in the immediate vicinity.

When the lesion expands, the neural pathway for lateral gaze to the opposite side is impaired, and the both eye positions are often deviated toward the lesion (Fig. 9.3a), called conjugate deviation.

H. Ooboshi (✉)
Department of Internal Medicine, Fukuoka Dental College, Fukuoka, Japan
e-mail: ooboshi@fdcnet.ac.jp

T. Kanno
Department of Oral and Maxillofacial Surgery, Shimane University Faculty of Medicine, Izumo, Shimane, Japan



T. Chiba, H. Yamada (eds.), *Internal Medicine for Dental Treatments*,
https://doi.org/10.1007/978-981-99-3296-2_9

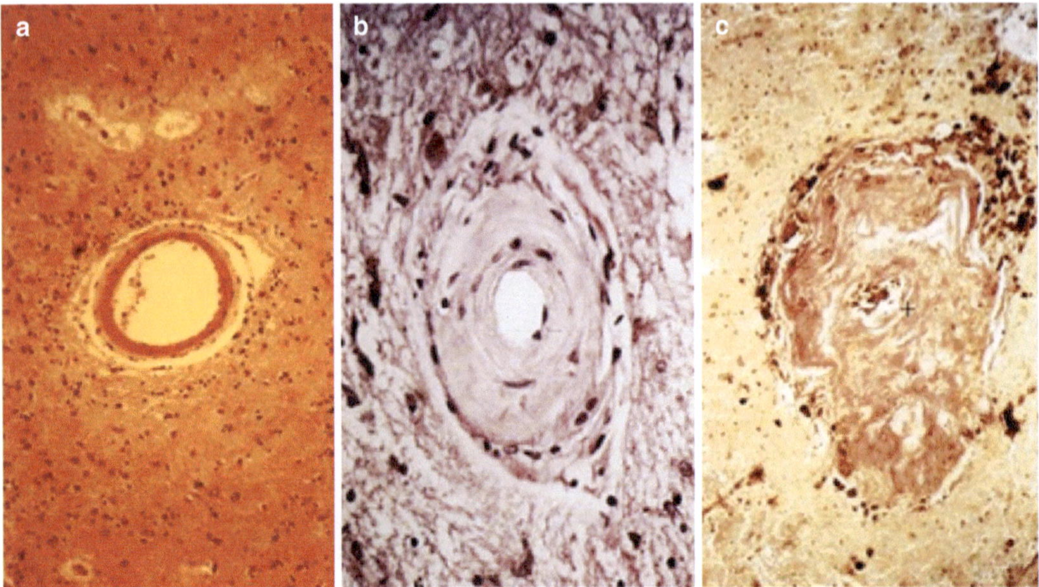

**Fig. 9.1** Hypertensive changes in cerebral arteries. (**a**) Normal intraparenchymal arteries. (**b**) Hypertension-induced arteriolosclerosis. (**c**) Hypertension-induced fibrinoid necrosis (lipohyalinosis) of intraparenchymal arteries. Hemorrhage is present in some cases

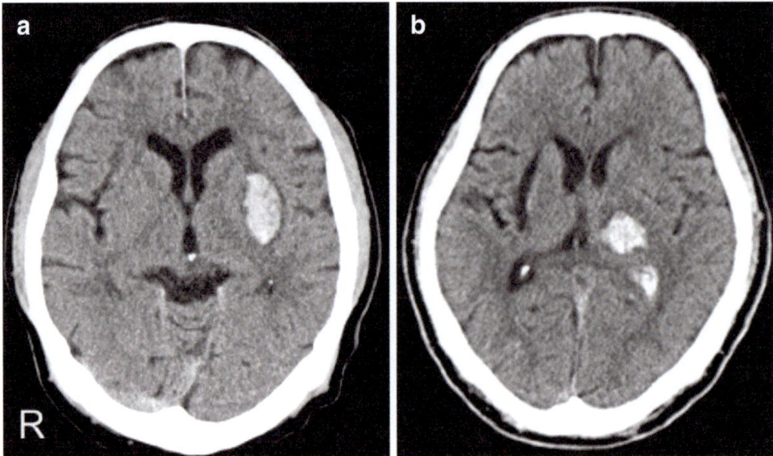


**Fig. 9.2** Head CT of cerebral hemorrhage. (**a**) High-density area observed in left putaminal hemorrhage. (**b**) High-density area observed in left thalamic hemorrhage. Perforation of the left lateral ventricle is observed. A slit-shaped low-density area in the right putamen is also seen, indicating an old brain hemorrhage

In thalamic hemorrhage (Fig. 9.2b), sensory deficits are prominent, but the proximity of the thalamus to the cerebral ventricles often causes ventricular perforation, which may lead to disturbance of consciousness and acute hydrocephalus. Although motor paralysis is also present, paralysis of the fingers tends to be milder [2]. It presents with miosis on the lesion side due to sympathetic nerve disorder (Horner's syndrome). Patients with intraventricular hemorrhage show characteristic downward gaze in addition to anisocoria (Fig. 9.3b). Cerebellar hemorrhage causes ataxic symptoms, but because the cerebellum is surrounded by the hard tent tissue, headache and vomiting due to increased cerebral pressure are more likely to occur. Cerebellar hemorrhage is also prone to cerebral herniation due to rapid obstructive hydrocephalus caused by compression of the fourth ventricle. Pontine hemorrhage has the highest mortality rate and is likely to cause tetraplegia. The prognosis is especially poor if the patient has severe disturbance of

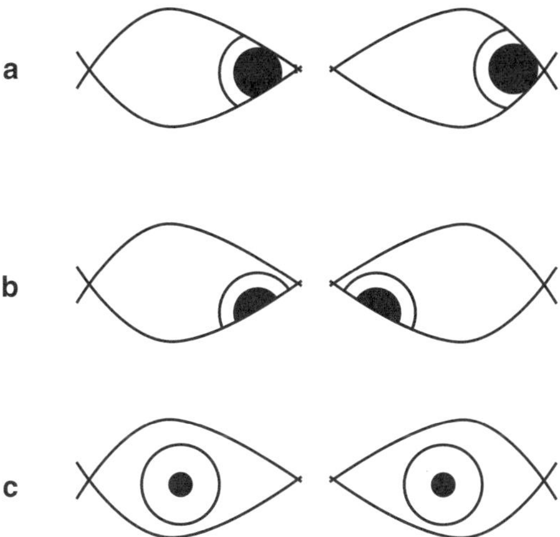


**Fig. 9.3** Characteristic eye position of cerebral hemorrhage. (**a**) Conjugate deviation to the side of the lesion in putaminal hemorrhage. (**b**) Medial downward eye position in thalamic hemorrhage. (**c**) Marked miosis and midline fixation in pontine hemorrhage

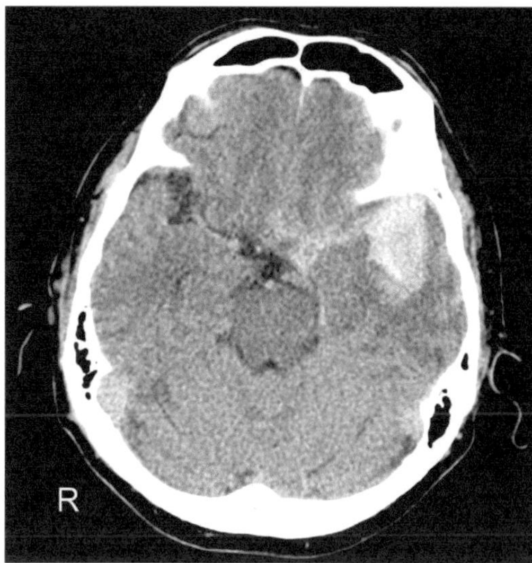


**Fig. 9.4** Head CT image of subarachnoid hemorrhage. The left temporal lobe around the left middle cerebral artery bifurcation and the subarachnoid space around the left middle cerebral artery show a high-density area. Low density in the left temporal lobe around the hematoma shows edema

consciousness, decerebrate rigidity, marked miosis (Fig. 9.3c), midline fixation of the eye position, and respiratory impairment.

Surgical hematoma removal is most effective for subcortical hemorrhage and cerebellar hemorrhage. In elderly patients with subcortical hemorrhage, however, repeated subcortical hemorrhage due to amyloid angiopathy may occur, and surgical indication should be carefully considered. For putaminal hemorrhage, which is most common, the indication for surgery is considered according to the amount of hematoma and the degree of consciousness disorder [3].

## 1.2 Subarachnoid Hemorrhage (SAH)

Although subarachnoid hemorrhage can be caused by traumatic events such as traffic accidents, most cases are caused by rupture of a cerebral aneurysm in the subarachnoid space between the meninges (arachnoid membrane and soft membrane). The cause of the aneurysm is not fully understood, but genetic factors may play a role. It develops with a sudden and severe headache (see the article on headache). The mortality rate is high (30–60%), and only 25% of patients are able to return to society. A CT scan of the head shows a high density zone around the brain (Fig. 9.4), and hematoma may also form in the brain parenchyma. In addition, vasospasm often occurs within 1–2 weeks after hemorrhage, and cerebral infarction is associated in one-third of cases. The rebleeding of a ruptured cerebral aneurysm is often seen within 24 h, and the mortality rate is high in that case; if subarachnoid hemorrhage is suspected, urgent medical treatment by neurosurgery is required. Clipping or endovascular treatment is performed for ruptured aneurysms. In the case of hydrocephalus, shunting is performed.

## 1.3 Chronic Subdural Hemorrhage

In the elderly, the bridging veins in the subdural space, between the dura mater, the outermost meninges, and the underlying arachnoid membrane, are easily damaged by minor trauma, resulting in formation of a subdural hematoma after hemorrhage. In elderly patients with cerebral atrophy, subdural hematoma can be caused

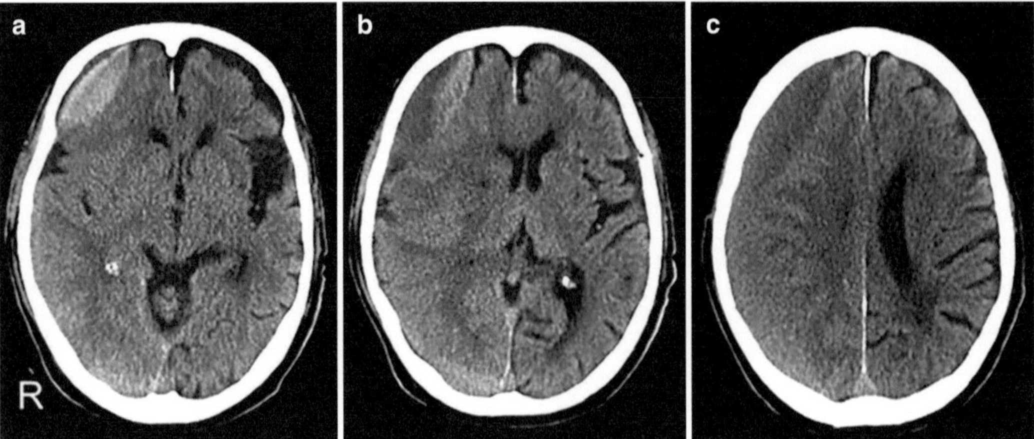


**Fig. 9.5** Head CT image of chronic subdural hematoma. (**a**, **b**) In the right frontal region, there is a spindle-shaped subdural hematoma with mixed high and low density. (**c**) In the right occipital region, the border of the brain surface is obscured, and there is a hematoma with a high-density area outside the border. The right cerebral hemisphere is shifted to the left

by head shaking to the level of a slump (Fig. 9.5). The hematoma gradually increases in size, causing neurological symptoms 3 weeks to 2 months after injury. Ten to 15% of cases are bilateral.

## 1.4 Notes from Dentistry Perspective

Takahiro Kanno

### 1.4.1 Clinical Consideration in Dentistry

Intracranial hemorrhage is a condition in which cerebral blood vessels in the skull collapse and bleed. Intracranial hemorrhage is divided into brain (intracerebral) hemorrhage and subarachnoid hemorrhage according to the site of bleeding. Intracerebral hemorrhage is hypertensive or non-hypertensive, with the former accounting for approximately 70% of all cases. Non-hypertensive causes include cerebral arteriovenous malformation, antithrombotic medication, amyloid angiopathy, and bleeding in brain tumors. When hypertension persists, arteriolosclerosis and fibrinoid necrosis occur, leading to aneurysm formation and hemorrhage.

In the perioperative period of dental and oral-maxillofacial treatment, the risk of intracerebral hemorrhage should be taken into consideration in the case of abnormal elevation of blood pressure due to the pain and discomfort before treatment, the image of treatment, and the invasion and stress during treatment. In particular, it should be noted that there is a gap between the dentist's and the patient's perception of invasiveness of the same dental and oral treatment procedures and that the patient feels a high stress during dental and oral-maxillofacial procedures even when the dentist considers the procedure to be noninvasive. It is known that adrenaline, which is added to dental local anesthetics, exerts a beta effect. The increase in heart rate due to this effect and the increase in cardiac output due to the increase in myocardial contractility cause an increase in blood pressure, which may pose a risk of brain hemorrhage. Therefore, it is necessary to refer to various guidelines for adrenaline dosage, etc. [4] and to take sufficient care.

### 1.4.2 Treatment Planning and Treatment Considerations in Dentistry

Patients should be carefully interviewed prior to dental and oral-maxillofacial treatment, and the aforementioned risks of intracerebral hemorrhage should be thoroughly discussed with the attending physician in order to understand the medical condition and prepare for treatment. Within 6 months after the onset of cerebrovascular disorders such as brain hemorrhage, symptoms and dynamics are not stable, and the risk of recurrence is high. Therefore, stress loading and surgical dental and oral-maxillofacial treatment should be postponed and avoided as much as possible.

On the other hand, the patient may not be aware of the risk. Therefore, in the case of invasive procedures, such as tooth extraction and pulpectomy under anesthesia, or painful dental treatment requiring local anesthesia or when the patient shows anxiety (such as treatment phobia), the patient's vital signs, especially blood pressure, should be checked, and continuous monitoring of the patient is needed during the treatment. In brain hemorrhage, a sudden increase in blood pressure during dental treatment is a serious risk, and a sustained elevation of blood pressure can cause dizziness, palpitations, headache, nausea, sweating, tinnitus, and bleeding from the wound. In addition, diabetes mellitus, dyslipidemia, ischemic heart disease, and aneurysms increase the risk of serious damage to the heart, cerebral vessels, kidneys, and other vital organs. When the systolic blood pressure (maximum blood pressure) is 160 mmHg or diastolic blood pressure is 100 mmHg or higher, the procedure may be posed, and the patient should be relieved by talking, followed by the adequate rest. Administration of high concentration of oxygen, peripheral venous line, electrocardiographic monitoring, continuous noninvasive blood pressure monitoring, and oxygen saturation ($SpO_2$) measurement may be performed. If the blood pressure is higher than 180 mmHg, antihypertensive drugs are considered. If blood pressure control is poor, collaboration with a medical or higher medical institution is essential. Although mental and physical stress can increase blood catecholamines, dental treatment with intravenous sedation is very useful to suppress the increase of blood catecholamines.

While the symptoms of brain hemorrhage vary depending on the location and amount of hemorrhage, most patients present with various symptoms such as headache, nausea, vomiting, motor paralysis of one side of the mouth and limbs, sensory disturbance, and inability to speak. In most cases, the symptoms occur suddenly, and depending on the amount of bleeding and the location of the bleeding, the patient may become unconscious and fall into a coma. If similar symptoms occur during dental treatment, an emergency response is required.

Because a 2% lidocaine hydrochloride anesthesia cartridge for dental and oral-maxillofacial treatment contains 1/8 million adrenaline, 22.5–25 μg of adrenaline per 1.8 mL/unit of cartridge is added to a 2% lidocaine hydrochloride anesthesia cartridge for dental and oral-maxillofacial treatment. For patients at risk of brain hemorrhage, it is important to administer the proper dose according to the guidelines (see below). Alternatively, adrenaline-free mepivacaine hydrochloride (Scandonest® Cartridge 3%) may be considered, but the duration of effect is short, and pain and stress reliefs are essential.

### 1.4.3 Safe Use of Local Anesthesia in Patients with Hypertension to Reduce the Risk of Brain Hemorrhage: With Special Attention to the Dose of the Vasoconstrictor Adrenaline

1. Grade I hypertension [systolic blood pressure (SBP) 140–159 mmHg or diastolic blood pressure (DBP) 90–99 mmHg]: Up to 45 μg. This means up to two regular (1.8 mL) dental cartridges (lidocaine preparations contain 1/8 million adrenaline: 12.5 μg or 25 μg adrenaline hydrogen tartrate: 13.7 μg adrenaline equivalent in 1 mL of 2% lidocaine hydrochloride).
2. Grade II hypertension (SBP 160–179 mmHg or DBP 100–109 mmHg): Similarly, up to two regular dental cartridges.
3. Grade III hypertension (SBP 180 mmHg or greater or DBP 110 mmHg or greater): 22.5 μg of adrenaline or up to one regular dental cartridge.

Adrenergic effects: (1) peripheral vasoconstriction; (2) increased cardiac output, increased blood pressure, and increased heart rate; (3)

increased blood glucose level; (4) bronchodilatation; etc. [5]

## 2 Brain Infarction and Transient Ischemic Attack (TIA)

Hiroaki Ooboshi

### 2.1 Brain Infarction

Brain infarction accounts for 70% of cerebrovascular diseases. In Japan, brain infarction is classified into the following clinical types according to the US National Institutes of Health (NIH) criteria: lacunar infarction due to hypertensive arteriolosclerosis, atherothrombotic infarction due to atherosclerotic lesions, cardioembolic infarction due to heart disease, brain infarction due to other causes, and brain infarction of unknown cause [6]. The reason for using this classification is that brain infarction is caused by different pathophysiological mechanisms, and it is necessary to perform proper treatment according to each type in both acute and chronic phases to prevent recurrence. In particular, antithrombotic drugs used in the chronic phase is important for medical and dental cooperation in dentistry.

### 2.2 Characteristics of Clinical Types

#### 2.2.1 Lacunar Infarction

The main pathogenesis of lacunar infarction is occlusion of the perforating artery which is damaged by hypertension-induced arteriolosclerosis. The perforating artery branches off from the origin of the middle cerebral artery or basilar artery and feeds the deep brain. Lacunar infarction is diagnosed when a small infarction of less than 15 mm in diameter (Fig. 9.6) is found in the territory of the perforating artery on CT/MRI images.

Although most recurrences of cerebrovascular diseases are homotypic recurrences, brain hemorrhage is the second most common recurrence type of lacunar infarction (homotypic lacunar infarction 35% and brain hemorrhage 18%), which is worthy of attention [7]. This is because arteriolosclerosis caused by hypertension is the common pathological basis of lacunar infarction and brain hemorrhage (Fig. 9.1c), and management of hypertension is the most important factor in preventing recurrence not only in patients with brain hemorrhage but also in patients with lacunar infarction. In addition, cilostazol, which has a low risk of brain hemorrhage, is used because the use of conventional antiplatelet agents such as aspirin for the prevention of recurrent lacunar infarction causes hematoma expansion at the onset of brain hemorrhage [8].

#### 2.2.2 Atherothrombotic Infarction

Brain infarction caused by a thrombus originating from an atherosclerotic lesion in the carotid artery or major artery of the brain is a type of systemic atherothrombosis (atherosclerosis) that occurs as a complication of high LDL cholesterol or diabetes rather than hypertension (Fig. 9.7). Atherosclerotic lesions occur most frequently at the origin of the internal carotid artery, and plaque rupture in this area can lead to rapid occlusion or artery-to-artery embolism, in which generated thrombi flow to the distal portion and cause occlusion.

Surgical treatment, such as carotid endarterectomy, may be performed if the main artery lesion is severe. Because platelet thrombi mainly occur in arteries, antiplatelet agents such as aspirin and clopidogrel are used as antithrombotic agents in the chronic phase. In addition, the evaluation and treatment of ischemic heart disease and arteriosclerosis obliterans are also important for prognosis.

#### 2.2.3 Cardioembolic Infarction

Atrial fibrillation, valvular abnormalities, presence of foreign bodies, and other cardiac diseases that produce fibrin thrombi in the heart can cause embolism throughout the body, but emboli are particularly likely to target the brain, which receives a large blood flow. Bacterial endocarditis, which is important in the dental field, also causes cardioembolic infarction with high frequency. In Japan, the most common cause of cardioembolic infarction is the atrial fibrillation without valvular disease (non-valvular atrial fibrillation). Neurological symptoms such as disturbance of consciousness, conjugate deviation

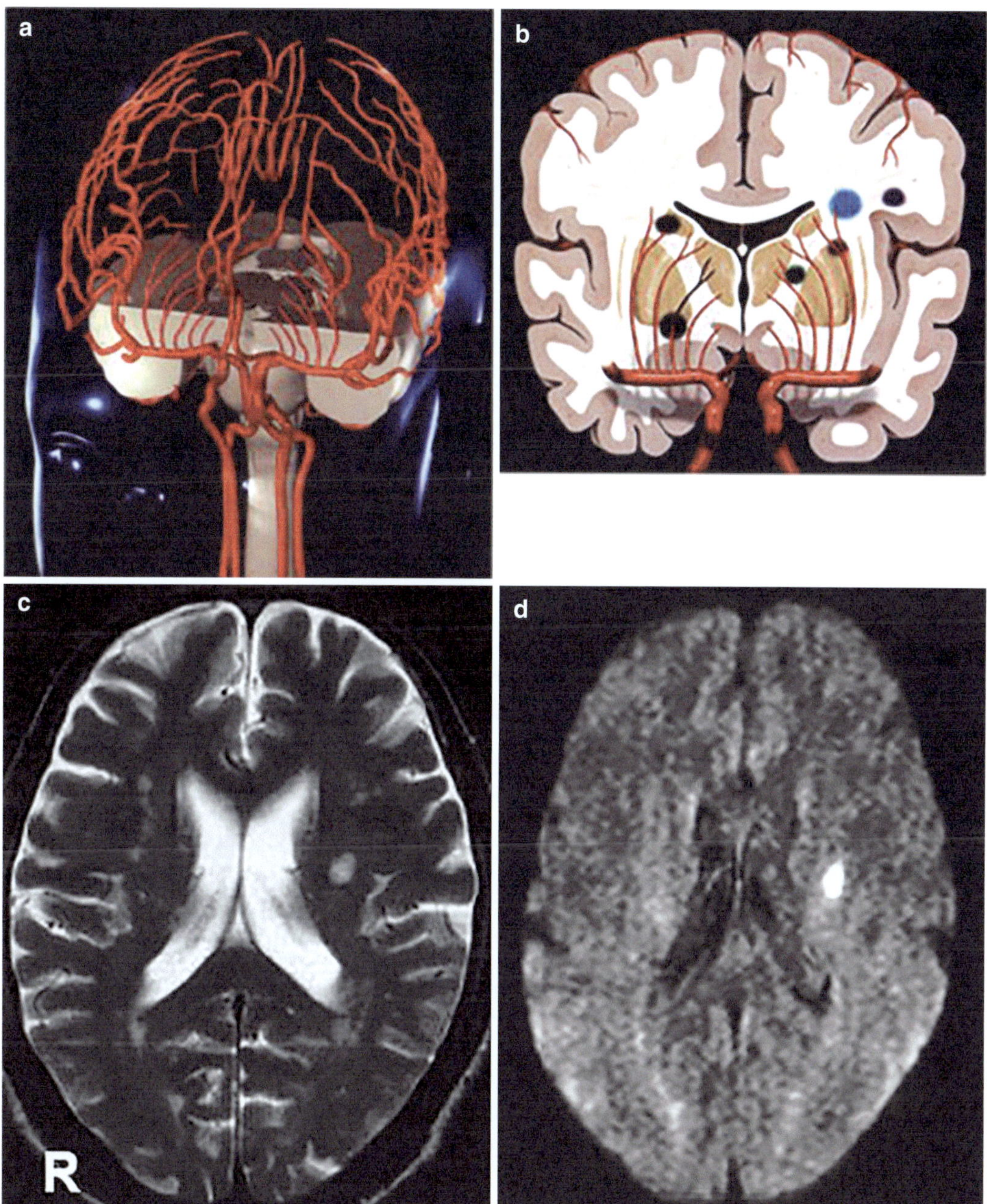


**Fig. 9.6** Relationship between perforating artery and lacunar infarction. (**a**) A small perforating artery branches from the origin of the middle cerebral artery to the deep brain. (**b**) A small infarction occurs due to occlusion of the perforating artery caused by hypertensive arteriolosclerosis, resulting in lacunar infarction. (**c**, **d**) MRI T2-weighted images (**c**) and diffusion-weighted images (**d**) show a small infarction of less than 15 mm in diameter in the left corona radiata. On diffusion-weighted images, only fresh infarcts show high signal

(Fig. 9.3a), and hemiplegia suddenly emerge during activity, presenting in a sudden completion manner. The lesions are often extensive, involving the cortex (Fig. 9.8), and multiple lesions are not uncommon. Hemorrhagic infarction occurs in half of the cases. It is the most common type of brain infarction with the highest mortality rate and the most severe sequelae.

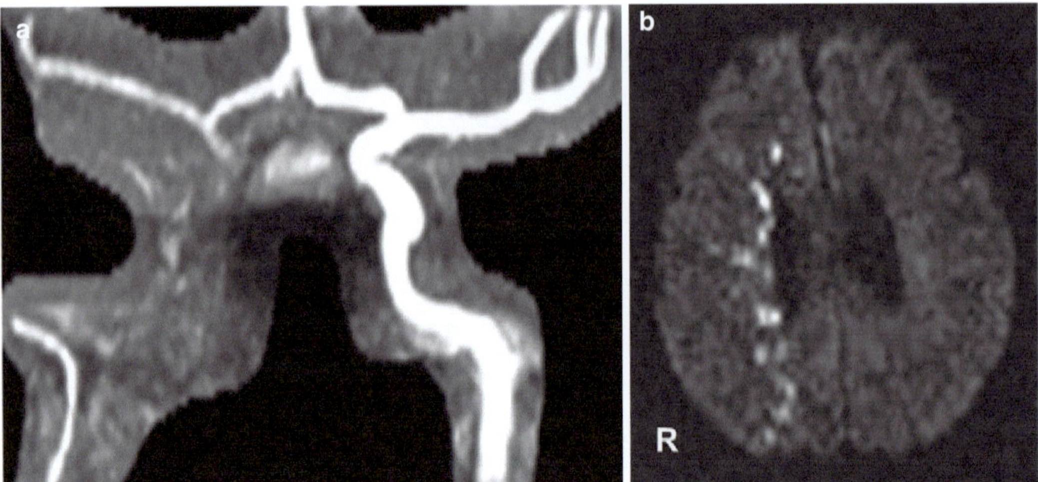


**Fig. 9.7** MR image of atherothrombotic brain infarction. MR angiogram (**a**) shows poor delineation of the right internal carotid artery; MRI diffusion-weighted image (**b**) shows linear high signal along the border of the middle cerebral artery and the anterior cerebral artery

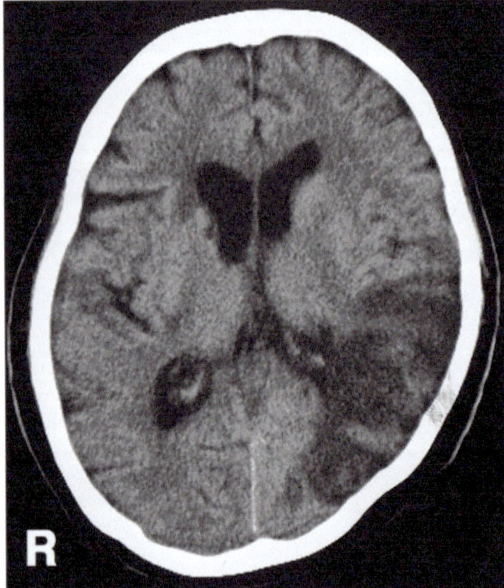


**Fig. 9.8** CT image of cardioembolic infarction. Head CT image shows a wedge-shaped low-density area in the left middle cerebral artery territory from the temporal lobe to the occipital lobe

## 2.3 Treatment of Brain Infarction

### 2.3.1 Acute Phase Treatment

In the acute treatment of brain infarction, various antithrombotic agents are used to reduce the size of thrombi in cerebral vessels. Injectable agents such as thromboxane A2 synthase inhibitor (Ozagrel) and antithrombin agent (Argatroban) are used for brain infarction other than cardioembolic infarction in Japan. The combination of aspirin and clopidogrel, oral antiplatelet agents, is also used in the acute phase of noncardioembolic infarction. For cardioembolic infarction with strong brain edema, the anti-edema drug glycerol and edaravone, which removes reactive oxygen species, are also useful.

Alteplase, a recombinant tissue plasminogen activator (rtPA), has fibrinolytic activity against local thrombus. The efficacy of intravenous administration of rtPA in the hyperacute phase of brain infarction within 3 h of onset was demonstrated in 1995. Although its approval in the United States was the following year, it was approved in Japan in 2005. Intravenous administration of rtPA is often very effective, and it was approved for use within 4.5 h of onset of stroke in 2012.

In recent years, endovascular devices have advanced, and since 2010, it has been possible to remove thrombus in the major artery by endovascular therapy. After the successful results of stent-type devices were reported in international trials in 2015, the endovascular treatment is recommended for cases of main trunk artery occlusion within 6–8 h of onset. In 2018, endovascular treatment has been shown to be effective within 16–24 h of onset when cell-damaged areas are smaller than perfusion-damaged areas (diffusion-perfusion mismatch) [9], and the treatment is strongly recommended in such occasions.

### 2.3.2 Chronic Phase Drug Treatment

Although control of concomitant hypertension, diabetes mellitus, and high LDL cholesterol is fundamental, it is important to select an anti-thrombotic agent according to the clinical type of brain infarction. In other words, cilostazol is used for lacunar infarction, antiplatelet agents for atherothrombotic stroke, and anticoagulants for cardioembolic infarction (Table 9.1). For a long time, warfarin has been used as one and only oral anticoagulant, and the prothrombin time (PT-INR) has to be monitored regularly to achieve an optimal PT-INR (usually 2–3, but 1.6–2.6 in patients older than 70 years with nonvalvular atrial fibrillation). In 2010, the first new oral anticoagulant in 50 years, dabigatran (factor II inhibitor), was introduced, followed by the development of three Xa inhibitors (rivaroxaban, apixaban, and edoxaban).

The new oral anticoagulants have been recognized for their advantages in reducing bleeding complications such as brain hemorrhage.

### 2.3.3 Surgical Treatment of Chronic Brain Infarction

Carotid endarterectomy (CEA) is considered as a surgical treatment for internal carotid artery stenosis that causes atherothrombotic stroke or transient ischemic attack. CEA is a surgical procedure to remove the stenotic intimal portion of the carotid artery. It is recommended when the diameter of the stenosis is more than 50% in symptomatic stenosis and more than 60% in asymptomatic stenosis. With recent advances in devices, carotid artery stenting (CAS) is also performed for difficult-to-treat cases. CAS is performed in symptomatic stenoses with a diameter of 50% or more and in asymptomatic stenoses with a diameter of 80% or more.

## 2.4 Transient Ischemic Attack

The diagnosis of transient ischemic attack (TIA) is made when brain ischemia causes a transient focal neurological syndrome that recovers in a short time. TIA is often associated with carotid plaque, microemboli from the heart, or early lacunar infarction. In the acute phase of TIA, brain infarction is seen on diffusion-weighted images in about 50% of cases. Even if symptoms have disappeared, evaluation of risk factors for atherosclerosis, imaging of major arterial lesions, and the presence of atrial fibrillation should be performed promptly.

It is estimated that 10–15% of patients develop brain infarction within 90 days, but most of them develop within 1 week. In recent years, the risk of occurrence of infarction within 2 days is evaluated by the ABCD2 score (Table 9.2). When embolization from the carotid artery or other sources occurs in the ophthalmic artery region,

**Table 9.1** Antithrombotic drugs used in the chronic phase of cerebral infarction according to disease type

| Type of disease | Antithrombotic agent |
|---|---|
| Lacunar infarction | Cilostazol |
| Atherothrombotic infarction | Antiplatelet agent |
| | Aspirin |
| | Clopidogrel |
| | Ticlopidine |
| | Cilostazol |
| Cardioembolic infarction | Anticoagulant |
| | Warfarin |
| | Dabigatran |
| | Rivaroxaban |
| | Apixaban |
| | Edoxaban |

**Table 9.2** ABCD2 scores

| Clinical findings | Category | Score |
|---|---|---|
| A Age | Over 60 years old | 1 |
| B Blood pressure | Systolic blood pressure >140 or diastolic blood pressure >90 | 1 |
| C Clinical symptom | Unilateral muscle weakness | 2 |
| | Dysarthria without paralysis | 1 |
| D Duration | 60 min or more | 2 |
| | 10–59 min | 1 |
| D Diabetes mellitus | Existence (at the present moment) | 1 |

Score indicates the risk of stroke within 2 days of the onset of transient ischemic attack
Scores 0–3, 1.0%; 4–5; 4.1%; and 5–7, 8.1%

which is a branch of the internal carotid artery, there may be a transient lack of the unilateral visual field. The condition is diagnosed as transient monocular blindness (amaurosis fugax) and treated similar to transient ischemic attack.

## 2.5 Notes from Dentistry Perspective

Takahiro Kanno

### 2.5.1 Clinical Consideration in Dentistry

Brain infarction is a condition in which the brain parenchyma perfused by a cerebral blood vessel becomes necrotic due to stenosis or occlusion of the vessel. There are two main mechanisms of brain infarction: thrombosis, in which the blood vessel is gradually clogged due to arteriosclerosis, and embolization, in which the blood vessel is suddenly clogged by a thrombus. At present, dental and oral-maxillofacial treatment and oral care by dentists in the acute stage of brain infarction and hemorrhage are regarded as important. In such treatment, it is necessary to fully understand the pathology and symptoms of stroke through medical and dental cooperation.

The typical sequelae of brain infarction and hemorrhage are paralysis and/or sensory impairment of limbs. In addition, the disorder also causes oral manifestations such as sensory and/or motor, and decreased salivary secretion, resulting in limited self-cleaning and delay of professional intervention, with the progressed oral pathology. Lower lip ptosis on the paralyzed side, incomplete lip closure, deviation of the tongue protrusion, poor movement of the cheek mucosa, and deviation of the uvula can be seen. In particular, impaired movement of the arm and fingers makes it difficult to brush, which leads to poor oral (including the teeth and periodontium) hygiene. In addition, dysphagia, which is often observed in stroke patients, increases the risk of aspiration pneumonia. Therefore, it is important for dentists to evaluate the swallowing function. Evaluation of swallowing function is particularly important in providing oral care "feeding function therapy" to patients with brain infarction, and "repetitive saliva swallowing test (RSST)" and "modified water swallowing test (MWST)" are performed as screening. Videoendoscopic evaluation of swallowing (VE) and videofluorographic evaluation of swallowing (VF) should be considered to examine the swallowing function for planning swallowing training. In cerebrovascular disease with unilateral lesion, which is overwhelmingly common, hemiparalysis is often observed, but dysphagia, dysarthria, and mastication disorders are limited in about 10% of patients. Although there are impairments in the oral preparatory and oral propulsive phases due to paralysis of the oral apparatus, the swallowing reflex is theoretically not directly affected because the medulla oblongata, the center of the swallowing reflex, is not impaired.

In the chronic phase of brain infarction, antiplatelet and anticoagulation therapy (Table 9.1) according to the stroke treatment guidelines [9] are used to prevent recurrence. Therefore, it is important to cooperate with the attending physician when invasive dental procedures, such as periodontal surgery and tooth extraction, are planned. If patients are prescribed with an anticoagulant, warfarin potassium, information about the coagulation status is essential. If the PT-INR [prothrombin time—international normalized ratio: a test to evaluate the function of prothrombin (a protein in plasma that functions as a blood clotting agent) with an internationally standardized value] is less than 3, it is possible to perform minor oral-maxillofacial surgery such as tooth extraction and periodontal surgery while continuing to take warfarin potassium. Since the amount of procedure-related bleeding inevitably increase by anticoagulation therapy, the patient should be treated with caution and cooperation with a higher-order medical institution should be considered. On the other hand, some new anticoagulants, such as dabigatran, a direct oral thrombin inhibitors, do not affect PT-INR values. Therefore, it is very important to confirm the medication history and to prepare for and respond to bleeding complications during dental treatment.

### 2.5.2 Treatment Planning and Treatment Considerations in Dentistry

In preparation for the dental and oral-maxillofacial treatment, it is necessary to cooperate with the attending physician. As with brain hemorrhage, symptoms and dynamics are not stable within 6 months after the onset of brain infarction, and the risk of recurrence is high. Therefore, stress load and open dental and oral-maxillofacial treatment should be postponed and avoided as much as possible. If it is urgent, the treatment needs cooperation with higher medical institutions. During dental and oral-maxillofacial treatment, panoramic radiographs are frequently performed, and carotid atherosclerotic lesions are often visualized on panoramic radiographs in elderly patients. Carotid atherosclerotic lesions are likely to cause serious complications by changing circulatory dynamics during invasive dental and oral-maxillofacial procedures. It is advisable to check the patient's condition by measuring vital signs before the dental and oral-maxillofacial procedure and to monitor the patient continuously during the procedure.

On the other hand, pneumonia, which is associated with medical treatment and sequelae of brain infarction, is one of the most serious complications. In addition to the direct causal relationship between periodontal disease and pneumonia, recent studies have revealed a causal relationship between periodontal disease and brain infarction as a risk factor. Therefore, avoidance of these diseases is an important issue, and deterioration of oral function and damaged conditions of the oral cavity, teeth, and periodontal environment are considered to be important risk factors for them. In particular, as stroke sequelae deteriorated, many patients become bedridden where seamless medical and dental collaboration is important. As a countermeasure, oral function management including oral care and swallowing assessment by dentists and dental hygienists has been shown to contribute greatly to the prevention of pneumonia and improvement of oral intake rate in both acute and chronic stages of brain infarction. In oral care, and dental and oral-maxillofacial treatment, it is necessary to understand the status of sensory and motor nerve paralysis. In particular, it is important to prevent procedure-associated aspiration. If possible, a sitting position is preferred. If sitting is difficult, the upper body should be raised to 45–60° and tilted toward the healthy side. To avoid the risk of aspiration, the patient should place the healthy side of the mouth downward when swallowing water. Paralysis and muscle weakness in the upper limbs make it difficult to perform oral care and brushing on one's own. Therefore, it may be necessary to change one's dominant hand and to use oral cleaning devices such as thicker toothbrush handles. Because patients are unable to perform oral care and brushing as they did in good health, they tend to be reluctant to do so. Through cooperation with family members and caregivers, it is essential for patients to understand the importance of eating, tasting, enjoying conversation, and cleaning and maintaining the oral cavity.

In addition, if the patient is to undergo anesthetic dental and oral-maxillofacial surgical procedures such as tooth extraction, pulpectomy under anesthesia, or periodontal treatment, vital signs should be measured, and the patient should be monitored continuously during the procedure. If the patient of brain infarction is treated according to the aforementioned guidelines, it is a principle to continue antiplatelet and anticoagulant medication without discontinuation and to perform dental and oral-maxillofacial procedures in cooperation with the attending physician. Depending on the content of treatment, the degree of invasion, and the patient's other complications such as circulatory, respiratory, metabolic, and endocrine conditions, patient's general status needs to be carefully evaluated in cooperation with the attending physician, and the dental and oral-maxillofacial priority and the cooperation with the higher institute should be planned and indicated.

## References

1. Kitazono T. Stroke science in clinical medicine. Part II: Cerebrovascular diseases. (Saishin Rinsyo Nousoccyu Gaku, Ge: Noukekkansyougai Kakuron). Nippon Rinsho: Osaka; 2014. (in Japanese).
2. Shizuka M. The relationship between clinical symptoms and extention of the hematoma on CT in patients with hypertensive thalamic hemorrhage. Jpn J Stroke. 1980;2(3):255–61. (in Japanese).
3. Committee for Stroke Guidelines in The Japan Stroke Society, editor. Japanese guidelines for the management of stroke 2021. Tokyo: The Japan Stroke Society; 2021. (in Japanese).
4. Committee for Guidelines for the Management of Hypertension in The Japanese Society of Hypertension, editor. Guidelines for the management of hypertension 2019 (JSH 2019). Tokyo: Lifescience Shuppan; 2019. (in Japanese).
5. Kanno T. Safe and skillful extraction for difficult cases. (Anzenni, sothite Jyouzuni Okonau Nanbasshi). Tokyo: Hyoron Publishers; 2019. (in Japanese).
6. Special report from the National Institute of Neurological Disorders and Stroke. Classification of cerebrovascular disease III. Stroke. 1990;21(4):637–76.
7. Hata J, et al. Ten year recurrence after first ever stroke in a Japanese community: the Hisayama study. J Neurol Neurosurg Psychiatry. 2005;76(3):368–72.
8. Shinohara Y, et al. Cilostazol for prevention of secondary stroke (CSPS 2): an aspirin-controlled, double-blind, randomised non-inferiority trial. Lancet Neurol. 2010;9(10):959–68.
9. Committee for Stroke Guidelines in The Japan Stroke Society, editor. Japanese Guidelines for the Management of Stroke 2015. Addendum 2019. Tokyo: Kyowa Kikaku; 2019. (in Japanese).

# Digestive Diseases

# 10

Takahiko Kudo, Hirotaka Sakaki, Shogo Ohkoshi, Akira Tanaka, Jiro Nishida, Takashi Muramatsu, Katsuhiko Hasegawa, Wataru Kobayashi, Hiroshi Kishikawa, Ryosuke Abe, Toshimi Chiba, and Seiji Nakamura

## 1 Gastric and Duodenal Ulcer [1–3]

Takahiko Kudo

### 1.1 Introduction

Gastric ulcers and duodenal ulcers are called peptic ulcers because they cause damage to their own tissues by the strong digestive effects of gastric acid and pepsin. Although peptic ulcer is a benign disease, the most serious problem is that patients have to be hospitalized for bleeding, perforation, and stricture and that the disease recurs even after healing. However, the involvement of *Helicobacter pylori (H. pylori) in* the pathogenesis of peptic ulcer and the fact that *H. pylori* eradication therapy almost completely suppresses ulcer recurrence have changed the concept of this disease. While *H. pylori* eradication therapy is widely used and the rate of *H. pylori* infection is decreasing, the use of non-steroidal anti-inflammatory drugs (NSAIDs) and low-dose aspirin has been increasing year by year, and these drugs have become an important cause of peptic ulcer in recent years.

### 1.2 Pathophysiology

#### 1.2.1 *H. pylori*

In 1982, Dr. Warren and Dr. Marshall in Australia succeeded in isolating and culturing

T. Kudo
Health Sciences University of Hokkaido, Sapporo, Hokkaido, Japan

H. Sakaki
Department of Oral and Maxillofacial Surgery, Hachinohe City Hospital, Hachinohe, Aomori, Japan

S. Ohkoshi · A. Tanaka · K. Hasegawa
School of Life Dentistry at Niigata, The Nippon Dental University, Niigata, Japan

J. Nishida (✉) · H. Kishikawa
Department of Gastroenterology, Tokyo Dental College, Ichikawa General Hospital, Ichikawa, Chiba, Japan
e-mail: nisida@tdc.ac.jp

T. Muramatsu
Department of Operative Dentistry, Cariology and Pulp Biology, Tokyo Dental College, Chiyoda-ku, Tokyo, Japan

W. Kobayashi
Department of Oral and Maxillofacial Surgery, Hirosaki University Graduate School of Medicine, Hirosaki, Aomori, Japan

R. Abe
Department of Dentistry and Oral Surgery, Iwate Prefectural Central Hospital, Morioka, Iwate, Japan

T. Chiba
Division of Internal Medicine of Dentistry, Department of Oral Medicine, Iwate Medical University, Morioka, Iwate, Japan

S. Nakamura
Faculty of Dental Science, Kyushu University, Fukuoka, Japan



T. Chiba, H. Yamada (eds.), *Internal Medicine for Dental Treatments*,
https://doi.org/10.1007/978-981-99-3296-2_10

*H. pylori* from biopsy material of the gastric mucosa, at a time when it was taken for granted that bacteria could not live in the strongly acidic environment of the stomach. In addition, Dr. Marshall drank the *H. pylori* culture and developed acute gastric mucosal lesions in his own stomach, which were subsequently cured by *H. pylori* eradication therapy, proving the relationship between *H. pylori* and peptic ulcer using his own stomach. In 2005, both doctors were awarded the Nobel Prize in Physiology or Medicine for this achievement.

*H. pylori is a* Gram-negative rod of about 4 μm in size (Figs. 10.1 and 10.2) and possesses strong urease activity. *H. pylori is* thought to protect itself from gastric acid by degrading urea in gastric mucus to ammonia and making the surrounding environment slightly alkaline. In addition to the peptic ulcer described in this section, other diseases caused by *H. pylori* infection include chronic gastritis, gastric cancer, gastric MALT (mucosa-associated lymphoid tissue) lymphoma, gastric hyperplastic polyps, functional dyspepsia, and idiopathic thrombocytopenic purpura.

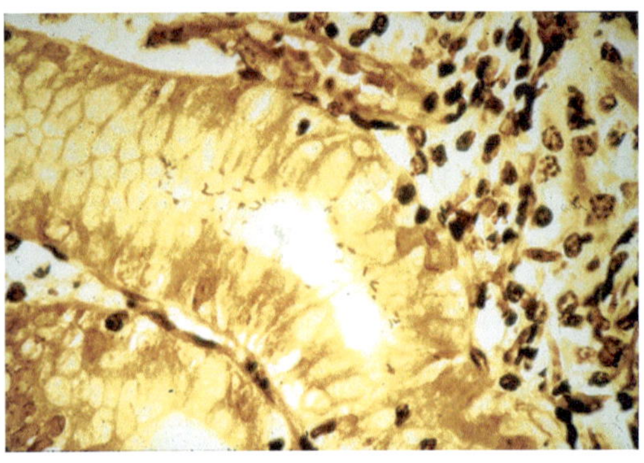

**Fig. 10.1** *H. pylori* light microscope image. (Courtesy of Dr. Masahiro Asaka)

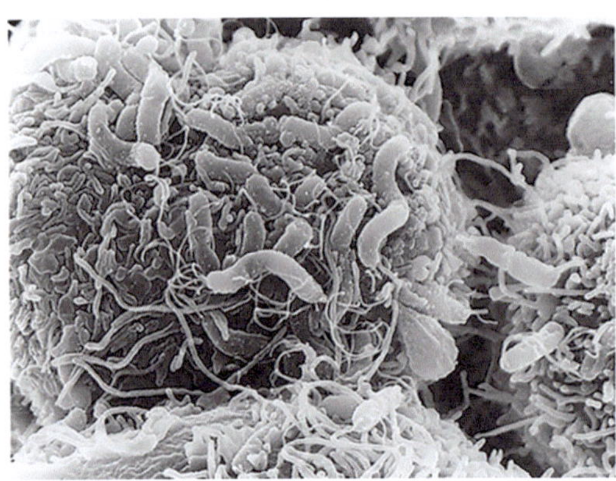

**Fig. 10.2** *H. pylori* electron microscopy image. (Courtesy of Dr. Masahiro Asaka)

### 1.2.2 NSAIDs and Low-Dose Aspirin

Drugs such as NSAIDs and low-dose aspirin are the second most common causes of peptic ulcers after *H. pylori*. NSAIDs are used as anti-inflammatory, analgesic, and antipyretic agents for a wide range of diseases such as common cold, headache, rheumatoid arthritis, osteoarthritis, and back pain, and low-dose aspirin is used to prevent recurrence of myocardial infarction and cerebral infarction. In Japan, the use of NSAIDs and low-dose aspirin is increasing year by year with the increase in the elderly population, and the number of peptic ulcers caused by these drugs is also increasing.

The pathogenesis of NSAIDs ulcers is thought to be the inhibition of cyclooxygenase (COX), a metabolic process of arachidonic acid, by NSAIDs, and the inhibition of prostaglandin synthesis, which has a protective effect on the gastric mucosa. There are two types of NSAIDs, oral and suppository, but the incidence of peptic ulcer is the same because both are absorbed into the bloodstream. It should be noted that the incidence of NSAIDs ulcers is higher in people with a history of ulcers, the elderly, users of high-dose or two or more NSAIDs, concomitant users of antithrombotic agents, *H. pylori*-positive patients, and users of bisphosphonates for the treatment of osteoporosis.

### 1.2.3 *Non-H. pylori* and Non-NSAIDs

*Non-H. pylori* and non-NSAID ulcers account for only a few percent of all cases. Stress, drugs other than NSAIDs, Zollinger-Ellison syndrome, Crohn's disease, and infections caused by *Helicobacter* or viruses other than *H. pylori* are thought to be responsible for these ulcers; these are sometimes called idiopathic ulcers. The term "stress ulcer" has been used in the past, but it has recently become clear that stress alone rarely leads to peptic ulcer. However, it is not true that stress does not trigger peptic ulcer at all, and it is correct to assume that peptic ulcer may develop in *H. pylori*-positive patients under strong stress. Carbohydrate steroids were also considered to be a causative agent of peptic ulcer in the past, but it is now concluded that they are not a risk factor for the development of peptic ulcer.

## 1.3 Symptoms

The most common subjective symptom of gastric and duodenal ulcer is abdominal pain, which is often dull and confined to the upper abdomen (epigastric region). In gastric ulcers, abdominal pain after eating or unrelated to eating may be observed, whereas in duodenal ulcers, abdominal pain during fasting or at night is common, and abdominal pain may be relieved when the acidity of gastric acid is weakened by eating. NSAID ulcers may occur suddenly with hematemesis, melena, or lightheadedness due to anemia, because symptoms such as abdominal pain are less likely to occur due to the effects of this drug, and many elderly and diabetic patients have few abdominal symptoms. Abdominal distension, anorexia, nausea and vomiting, and heartburn may also be reported. Sudden onset of severe upper abdominal pain should be as acute abdomen, such as gastric ulcer perforation or duodenal ulcer perforation.

## 1.4 Diagnosis

Esophagogastroduodenoscopy (EGD) is the most useful diagnostic tool for gastric and duodenal examination. In some cases, upper gastrointestinal radiography (gastric barium examination) performed during physical examinations can diagnose the disease, but in this case, repeat examination by EGD is recommended. Tissue biopsy can also be performed to differentiate peptic ulcer from cancer.

### 1.4.1 Endoscopic Diagnosis

In recent years, high-definition endoscopy has been widely used. Gastric and duodenal ulcers are divided into three stages: active stage, healing stage, and scar stage. In the active stage, the ulcer itself is deep and large, the peri-ulcer mucosa is edematous and subjective symptoms are strong, and complications such as bleeding and perforation may occur (Fig. 10.3).

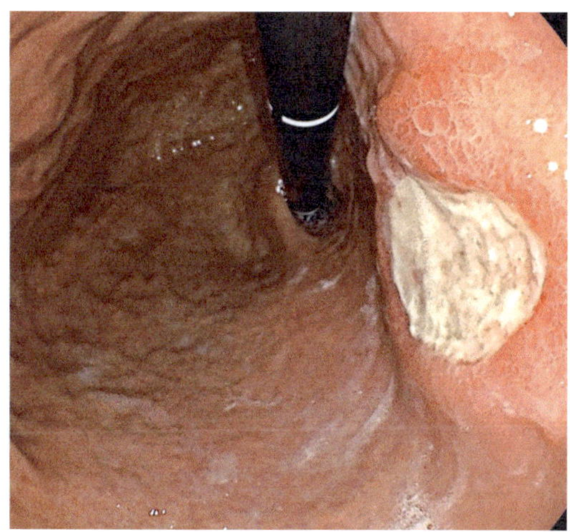

**Fig. 10.3** Gastric ulcer in active stage (gastric angle)

Regenerative epithelium appears around the ulcer, and when the mucosal defect gradually is reduced, it becomes a healing stage. When the ulcer itself is covered by the regenerating epithelium and the mucosal defect disappears, the disease shifts to the scarring stage. Gastric ulcers tend to be located in the lesser curvature of the gastric angulus, but in the elderly, ulcers are more common in the gastric body in the lesser curvature and posterior wall rather than in the gastric angulus. Duodenal ulcers tend to be located in the bulbus (Fig. 10.4), and NSAID ulcers tend to show multiple small ulcers and be located in the pyloric region of the anal side than in the gastric angulus.

### 1.4.2 Diagnosis of *H. pylori* Infection

The diagnosis of *H. pylori* infection can be classified into two categories: invasive tests using biopsy specimens obtained by endoscopy and noninvasive tests that do not require endoscopy. Invasive tests include the rapid urease test, histological examination, and bacterial culture from the gastric biopsy, while noninvasive tests include the urea breath test, measurement of *H. pylori*

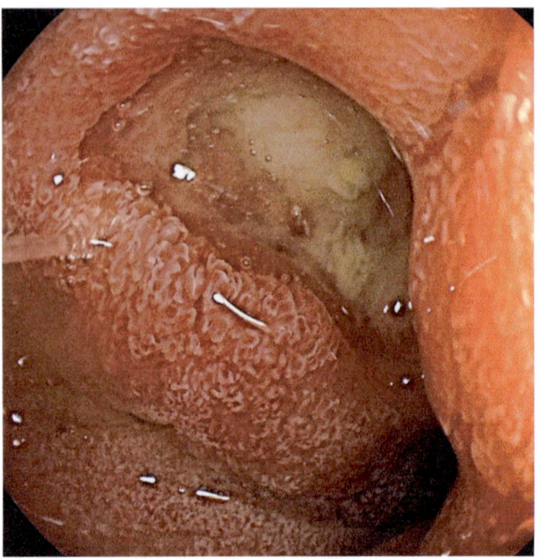

**Fig. 10.4** Active duodenal ulcer (bulb)

antigen in stool, and measurement of *H. pylori* antibody in serum or urine.

## 1.5 Treatment

Proton pump inhibitors (PPIs), potassium ion competitive acid blockers (P-CABs), and H2 receptor antagonists are used for the treatment of peptic ulcers. If the diagnosis of *H. pylori* infection is confirmed, eradication therapy is performed. Primary eradication consists of PPI or P-CAB plus amoxicillin and clarithromycin for 7 days. If the primary eradication is unsuccessful, the clarithromycin is replaced by metronidazole for 7 days as a secondary eradication. If eradication therapy is administered, eradication should be determined by urea breath test or stool antigen assay after 4 weeks of oral administration. The success rate of primary eradication is as high as about 90% because P-CAB is now used for eradication therapy.

In the case of peptic ulcer associated with oral administration of NSAIDs, it is advisable to discontinue NSAIDs, but if this is not possible, treatment with P-CABs, PPIs, or prostaglandins should be continued. Excessive alcohol consumption and smoking should be avoided.

## 1.6 Prognosis

In many cases, *H. pylori* infection is the main cause of peptic ulcer, so *H. pylori* eradication is important to prevent recurrence. In patients taking NSAIDs, PPIs and P-CABs should be used, because high healing rates of peptic ulcer have been observed. Even after successful eradication of *H. pylori,* patients are still at risk for gastric cancer, so it is important to explain to them that they should continue to undergo regular gastric cancer screening.

## 1.7 Notes from Dentistry Perspective

Hirotaka Sakaki

As a drug with a risk of gastrointestinal disorders, NSAIDs are prescribed for orthopedic diseases, and low-dose aspirin is prescribed as antiplatelet therapy for cerebrovascular and cardiovascular diseases. Since it is expected to increase in the future, it is essential to conduct an appropriate interview about the patient's medical history and confirm the medications they are taking even when visiting a dentist.

NSAIDs suppress the biosynthesis of prostaglandins (PGs) by inhibiting cyclooxygenase (COX) activity in the arachidonic acid cascade. Among PGs, it has anti-inflammatory, analgesic, and antipyretic effects by suppressing the synthesis of prostaglandin $E_2$($PGE_2$), which is a substance that enhances inflammation and pain. Therefore, NSAIDs are often used as symptomatic treatments for various diseases.

The arachidonic acid cascade is an important pathway in inflammatory reactions. Arachidonic acid synthesized from plasma membrane phospholipids consists of three main pathways: the COX pathway, which synthesizes PGs, the lipoxygenase pathway, which synthesizes leukotrienes, and the cytochrome P450 (CYP) pathway.

COX includes COX-1 distributed in systemic tissues and COX-2 expressed in inflamed areas. COX-1 is involved in the production of physiologically active PG in the gastrointestinal tract, platelets, kidneys, etc. and is important for maintaining homeostasis. COX-2 is induced by inflammation and synthesizes $PGE_2$, which is involved in the promotion of inflammatory reaction and pain.

NSAIDs show anti-inflammatory and analgesic effects mainly by COX-2 inhibition, but nonselective COX inhibitors, which are classical NSAIDs, have been considered to cause side effects such as gastrointestinal and renal disorders because they inhibit not only COX-2 but also COX-1. Although selective COX-2 inhibitors have been shown to reduce the frequency of gastrointestinal disorders compared with nonselective COX inhibitors [3], an increase in cardiovascular events has been a problem [4].

Low-dose aspirin inhibits platelet aggregation by inhibiting platelet COX-1 and thromboxane $A_2(TXA_2)$ production when aspirin is used at lower doses than those normally used for anti-inflammatory effects. This is because the use of aspirin at normal doses inhibits both COX-1 and COX-2, suppressing $PGI_2$ production in vascular endothelial cells and resulting in an aspirin dilemma where no antiplatelet effect is obtained.

In the field of general dentistry, acetaminophen (AAP), which is believed to cause less gastrointestinal damage than NSAIDs, can be used to relieve dental pain and post-extraction pain. However, AAP has little anti-inflammatory effect; NSAIDs are often used for anti-inflammatory purposes after oral surgery and for acute inflammation such as peri-jaw infection.

AAPs are safer than NSAIDs not only for children and pregnant women but also for patients at risk for renal, gastrointestinal, and cardiovascular dysfunction, although caution should be exercised in cases of hepatic dysfunction.

In addition, when NSAIDs are used for anti-inflammatory purposes, it is recommended that COX-2 selective inhibitors be combined with proton pump inhibitors (PPIs) in patients with a history of gastrointestinal disorders [5]. On the other hand, since COX-2 selective inhibitors increase the risk of cardiovascular events, the combination of naproxen and PPI is recommended for patients with high cardiovascular risk [6] (Fig. 10.5). When anti-inflammatory analgesics are used in the field of dentistry and oral sur-

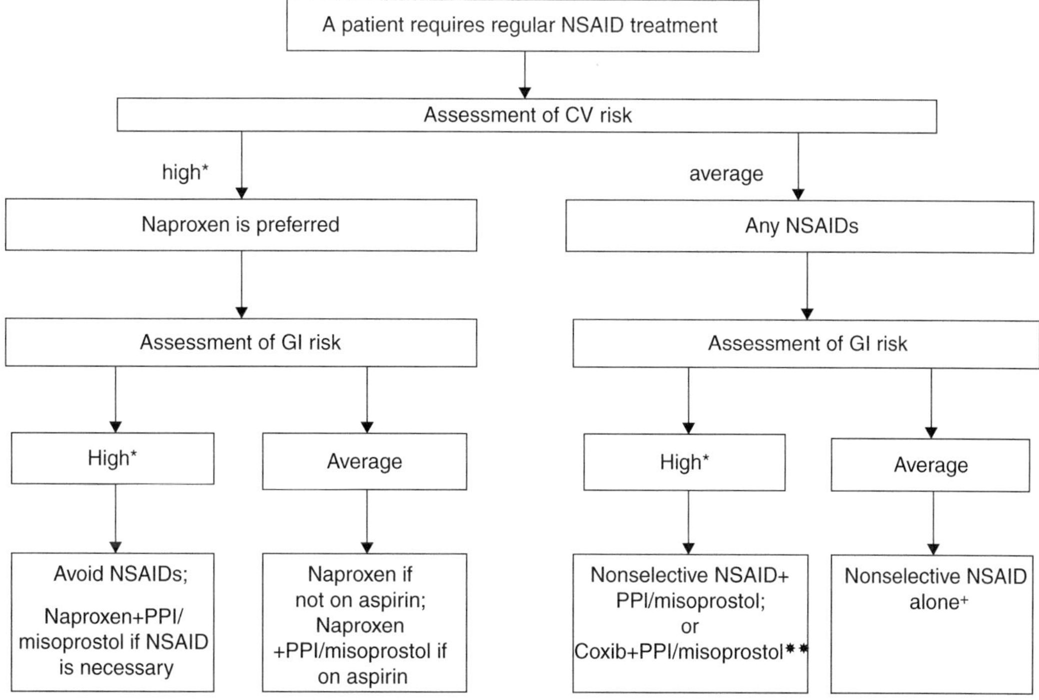


**Fig. 10.5** Management algorithm of patients on NSAIDs and aspirin. (Reproduced with permission from [6])

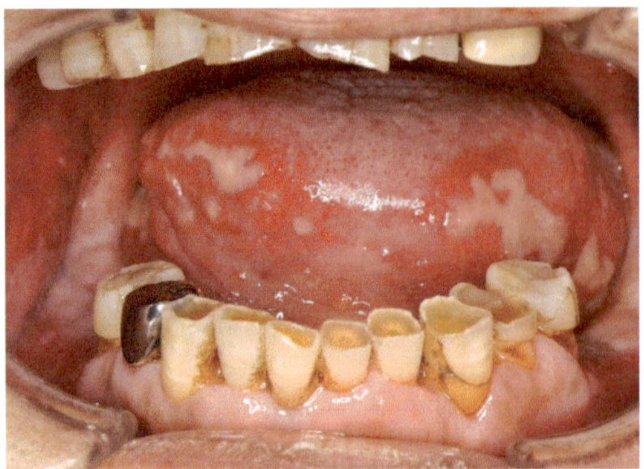

**Fig. 10.6** Oral mucositis caused by chemoradiation therapy for tongue cancer

gery, it is important to limit their administration to a short period of time and to select drugs with careful consideration of the patient's history.

Although the effects of peptic ulcer therapeutic agents on the oral cavity are limited, recent reports have shown that rebamipide gargling in addition to sodium azulene sulfonate, which has been used for oral mucositis associated with cancer chemotherapy (Fig. 10.6), has a certain effect [7], and further evaluation of effectiveness is desired in the future.

# 2 Acute/Chronic Hepatitis (Viral Hepatitis) [8, 9]

Shogo Ohkoshi

## 2.1 Disease Concept (Definition)

Viral hepatitis is a condition in which hepatocytes are destroyed by inflammation caused by a virus that specifically infects the liver (hepatitis A to E viruses). In hepatitis B virus (HBV) or hepatitis C virus (HCV) infection, if the virus cannot be eliminated, chronic hepatitis may develop after acute hepatitis. In general, it is defined as chronic hepatitis when liver dysfunction, such as abnormal ALT (alanine aminotransferase) levels, continues for more than 6 months. Chronic hepatitis is a cause of cirrhosis and liver cancer.

## 2.2 Pathophysiology

Acute hepatitis is often transient and curable. However, in rare cases, the disease becomes severe and is accompanied by loss of consciousness, which is called fulminant hepatitis. Fulminant hepatitis is often fatal and can only be saved by liver transplantation. On the other hand, patients who are persistently infected with HBV or HCV are collectively called "carriers."

Once a person becomes a carrier, it is rare for the virus to be eliminated spontaneously without treatment.

Chronic hepatitis causes persistent inflammation of the liver, and fibrosis of the liver occurs as a response. This is a characteristic reaction of the liver. As liver fibrosis progresses, the liver stiffness gradually increases. This reaction eventually leads to the transition from chronic hepatitis to liver cirrhosis.

## 2.3 Epidemiology

Among viral hepatitis, hepatitis A and E cause acute hepatitis but are not frequent diseases (class 4 infections). The main clinical problems in dentistry are HBV and HCV. The frequency of HBV and HCV carriers was about 1%, but now it has decreased to about 0.2% in blood donor data, which is related to vaccine prophylaxis (HBV), thorough infection prevention, and advances in treatment.

Mother-to-child transmission during childbirth was the most common source of HBV infection. Since 1986, when immunoglobulin (HBIG) and vaccines were started for children born to HBsAg-positive mothers, the frequency of carriers has decreased significantly. Since 2016, the vaccine has been given to all newborns. There is no vaccine for HCV, but transmission has decreased due to the elimination of transmission by blood transfusion and advances in safety management, including the elimination of reuse of used medical needles. HBV is a leading sexually transmitted disease, and its spread among young people is a problem.

## 2.4 Categories

There are five types of hepatitis viruses: hepatitis A to E (Table 10.1). Hepatitis A and E are orally transmitted viruses by food or other means, and the infection is acute and generally does not present as chronic hepatitis. HBV and HCV have both acute and chronic infection, as described above. Both are transmitted through blood and body fluids and cause cirrhosis and liver cancer. Hepatitis D (delta) is rarely seen in Japan.

## 2.5 Symptoms

The liver is known as the "silent organ," and it is difficult to show symptoms. However, in acute hepatitis, general malaise and fever may be observed. Jaundice (which tends to appear on the conjunctiva of the eyes) may also be observed because of the impaired metabolism of bilirubin in the liver. Chronic hepatitis causes only malaise at most, and many patients have no subjective symptoms.

## 2.6 Clinical Examination

The AST (aspartate aminotransferase) and ALT (alanine aminotransferase) values in biochemical tests are indicators of liver damage. These are sometimes referred to as GOT/GPT. These are cellular deviant enzymes that are involved in the metabolism of amino acids, and their levels increase when there is liver damage (the upper limit of the standard value is about 30 IU/L). In acute hepatitis, the level often rises above 1000, and jaundice (elevated bilirubin) may occur. In the case of chronic hepatitis, the level is generally less than 100, ranging 100–200 at the most. In patients with HBV and HCV, AST/ALT levels are often normal, and this condition is called asymptomatic carrier.

ALP (alkaline phosphatase) and gamma-GTP (gamma-glutamyltransferase) are biliary enzymes that indicate biliary stasis and are especially elevated in acute hepatitis.

The screening tests for HBV and HCV are HB antigen and HCV antibody, respectively (Table 10.2). Antibodies against HB antigen are HB antibodies; HB antibodies are protective antibodies induced by HBV vaccine; HBc antibodies indicate current or previous infection history. When a person becomes a carrier due to mother-to-child transmission or infection in infancy, most will remain HBsAg-positive for life, but some will become HBsAg-negative and HBs antibody-positive. HBeAg is positive in the early stages, and most carriers convert to HBe antibodies between their 10 s and 30 s. This is called seroconversion. In the HBeAg-positive period, the viral load (HBV DNA load) is high and the infectivity is high, but when anti-HBe is positive, the HBV DNA load decreases and the infectivity decreases. In acute hepatitis of HBV (mainly in adults), the HBV marker shows a similar pattern. In most cases, hepatitis ends within a few months with the acqui-

**Table 10.2** HBV and HCV markers

| | |
|---|---|
| HBs antigen | Screening of current infection |
| HBs antibody | After infection or vaccination |
| HBc antibody | Current or past infection |
| HBe antigen | First stage of infection (high viral load) |
| HBe antibody | Late stage of infection (low viral load) |
| HBV DNA | Nucleic acid test |
| HCV antibody | Screening for infection |
| HCV RNA | Nucleic acid test |

**Table 10.1** Hepatitis viruses (A–E)

| | Nucleic acid | Infection route | | Liver cirrhosis and liver cancer | Vaccine |
|---|---|---|---|---|---|
| HAV | RNA | Oral | Acute hepatitis | (−) | (+) |
| HBV | DNA | Blood and body fluid | Acute + chronic hepatitis | (+) | (+) |
| HCV | RNA | Blood and body fluid | Acute + chronic hepatitis | (+) | (−) |
| HDV | RNA | Blood and body fluid | Co-infection with HBV | (+) | |
| HEV | RNA | Oral | Acute hepatitis | (−) | (−) |

sition of anti-HBc and anti-HB antibodies. This pattern is recognized as pre-existing infection in later life; some acute hepatitis in adults become carriers as in mother-to-child transmission.

HCV antibody is a screening test for infection, and the presence of the virus is diagnosed by HCV RNA testing using PCR. When HCV antibody titer is low, HCV RNA is often undetectable by PCR. In this case, the patient may have had a false-positive reaction to the antibody or may reveal cured HCV infection.

## 2.7 Treatment

The treatment of both HBV and HCV has progressed in recent years, and both viruses can be effectively eliminated or suppressed for a long period of time by administration of oral medication with few side effects [9]. However, HBV and HCV are completely different viruses. HBV is DNA, whereas HCV is RNA. Therefore, the mechanisms of medicines that suppress viral replication are completely different. The therapeutic drugs for HBV and HCV are expensive but can be covered by the Japanese medical expense subsidies.

### 2.7.1 HBV

Because HBV uses reverse transcriptase for replication, oral reverse transcription inhibitors are the mainstay of therapy. The problem with these antiviral drugs is that during treatment, viruses with amino acid sequences that are ineffective against the drugs emerge (drug resistance). However, entecavir and tenofovir, and its derivative which have been used recently, may not develop resistance and can be administered safely for a long time. However, due to the nature of the virus, complete cure of HBV is difficult, and relapse often occurs if the therapy is discontinued, so the question as to how long the therapy should be continued remains.

### 2.7.2 HCV

The mainstay of HCV therapy had long been the interferon, an injectable drug with strong side effects, but as the mechanism of viral replication has become better understood, drugs that specifically inhibit individual viral proteins (direct-acting antivirals: DAA) have come into use. They are oral medicines, have few side effects, and can be used safely. HCV is different from HBV in that complete elimination of the virus can be achieved in a short time. For DAA treatment, the combination drug of pibrentasvir and glecaprevir can be used regardless of HCV genotype (there are two types, 1b and 2, in Japan), and complete elimination of the virus is achieved in almost 100% of cases after 2–3 months of treatment. Thus, the treatment of HBV and HCV has made epoch-making progress, but care must be taken because hepatocellular carcinoma can occur even when the virus is eliminated.

## 2.8 Prognosis

### 2.8.1 Acute Viral Hepatitis (HAV to HEV)

Most cases of acute viral hepatitis resolve spontaneously within 2–3 months of onset, unless they become fulminant. HBV is the most frequent cause of fulminant hepatitis among viral hepatitis, whereas HCV is far less likely to cause fulminant hepatitis.

### 2.8.2 Chronic Viral Hepatitis (HBV, HCV)

If the inflammation continues for more than 10 years, fibrosis of the liver progresses and the liver becomes cirrhotic. Cirrhosis literally means a state in which fibrosis of the liver has progressed and hardened. Most patients with cirrhosis have no subjective symptoms (compensated stage), but if the disease progresses to the uncompensated stage with symptoms such as jaundice, ascites, and hepatic encephalopathy, the prognosis can be several years. Complications of hepatocellular carcinoma also affect the prognosis.

## 2.9 Recent Findings

Reactivation is the process whereby infectious bacteria or viruses remain latent in the body for a long period of time (latent infection), even after they appear to be eliminated, but relapse with aging or immunity decline.

Reactivation of HBV is also known to occur, and this hepatitis is a major problem because it is generally severe and can be fatal. Reactivation occurs in patients treated with immunosuppressive drugs such as anticancer agents and steroids, because their immunity is severely weakened. Reactivation is less of a problem with HCV.

## 2.10 Notes from Dentistry Perspective [10–13]

Akira Tanaka

### 2.10.1 Associated with Hepatitis Occurring in the Jaw and Mouth Region: Signs of Liver Dysfunction

Patients with hepatitis may have jaundice associated with liver dysfunction. Jaundice appears on the ocular conjunctiva, facial skin, and oral mucosa, so it is important to observe the color of the face and mucosa during dental treatment. It may be accompanied by fever and malaise.

In patients with chronic hepatitis who have developed cirrhosis over a long period, symptoms such as spider angioma or palmar erythema, in which capillaries appear on the skin in the shape of the spider's feet, may be observed.

### 2.10.2 Points to Keep in Mind During Dental Treatment

#### General Considerations

In principle, dental treatment should be avoided in patients with acute hepatitis or active chronic hepatitis. If the patient reports viral hepatitis or hepatic dysfunction in the interview, the attending physician should be consulted regarding hepatic dysfunction and viral markers (antigen, antibody levels, etc.). If hepatic dysfunction is observed, hepatic excretion macrolides and tetracyclines should be avoided at the time of drug administration, and the dosage of acetaminophen, which can cause liver failure at high doses, should be carefully monitored.

#### Control of Hospital Infection

In the dental treatment of patients with viral hepatitis, hospital infection control of hepatitis virus is the most important issue. The main route of hepatitis virus infection is contact infection through blood, and it is not transmitted by droplet or airborne infection (droplet nuclei infection). Hepatitis B virus antibody tests are performed periodically for dental care workers, and vaccination is recommended for those who do not have antibodies.

In addition, it is important to conduct regular education and training on infection control and medical accidents among staff.

1. **Standard precautions:** Standard precautions are the basis of infection control. This concept, proposed by the Centers for Disease Control and Prevention (CDC) in 1996, states that all patients, regardless of whether they have hepatitis virus infection or not, should be treated as unidentified and potentially infectious, and measures should be taken to prevent needlestick accidents and blood exposure. Body fluids, excretions, blood (amniotic fluid, pericardial fluid, ascites, pleural fluid, joint synovial fluid, cerebrospinal fluid, semen, vaginal secretions, auricular secretions, wound exudates, urine, and stool), pathological tissues (biopsy materials, surgical resection materials, and autopsy organs), placenta, and extracted teeth are treated as potentially infectious. To protect patients from cross infection and health-care workers from infection in the course of their work, it is required to wear disposable protective equipment (gloves, aprons, masks, goggles) and to use medical instruments whenever possible, to handle infectious waste properly (sorting, storage, transport, and disposal), and to observe hygienic hand washing.
2. **Environmental infection control in the dental office:** It is important to adequately control environmental infection in an environment contaminated with body fluids (blood, saliva, etc.) from infectious viral hepatitis patients.

   For procedures that involve spattering of blood or saliva containing blood, it is recommended that an extraoral vacuum be used in combination with a face shield covering the face using standard precautions. It is also recommended that areas that are frequently touched with gloves or that are easily contaminated with blood be protected with disposable covers. In general dental treatment rooms, surfaces contaminated with blood or infectious biomaterials should be covered with protective equipment (gloves, disposable apron), wiped with disposable moisture-absorbent material to remove adhering material, and then dipped in sodium hypochlorite solution (effective concentration: 5500–1000 ppm) with a cloth or paper towel and wiped dry with a cloth or paper towel soaked in sodium hypochlorite solution.

3. **Countermeasures against hepatitis virus exposure (needlestick accident):** Many instruments used in dental treatment are sharp and small, such as injection needles. Exposure accidents can be transmitted not only by damage from sharp instrument, but also by exposure to blood on wounds, inflamed areas, and mucous membranes of the skin; therefore, it is essential to protect the skin surface with gloves and the eyes with goggles. The use of double gloves is recommended if necessary.

   As preventive measures against needlestick accidents involving injection needles (immersion needles), it is recommended that needle recapping be prohibited in principle and that the one-handed scoop-up recap method be used and that special disposal boxes be used when disposing of scalpels and injection needles that can be disposed of without using the hands.

4. **Response after exposure to hepatitis virus:** The most common type of exposure to hepatitis virus is a puncture injury caused by a sharp medical instrument such as an injection needle. When a person is aware of a needlestick, check for perforation of the glove and bleeding, and wash the area exposed to blood under running water thoroughly, regardless of the presence or absence of the hepatitis virus. In general, the infection rate for puncture wounds with medical instruments depends on the amount of virus (amount of blood) exposed, and the infection rate tends to increase for puncture wounds with hollow needles.

In the event of HBV exposure, the presence of HB antibodies in the injured person should be confirmed, and if the antibodies are negative or unknown, administration of high-titer human immunoglobulin (HBIG) and HBV vaccine is recommended.

When exposed to HCV, both the source (patient) and the injured person should be tested for HCV antibodies or HCV RNA, if possible. If the source is positive for HCV antibodies but negative for HCV RNA, HCV infection is unlikely to be established, and follow-up is not necessary except in special cases. If the source of the exposure is positive for HCV RNA, the injured person is considered infectious and requires care.

## 3 Liver Cirrhosis [14–16]

Jiro Nishida

### 3.1 Concept and Pathophysiology

Cirrhosis is the end stage of chronic hepatitis, which is caused by chronic inflammation caused by various factors-repeated hepatocyte necrosis, loss and regeneration, and advanced fibrosis. Histopathologically, the normal lobular structure is lost due to persistent inflammation, and a fibrous septum connecting the Gleason's sheath and central vein is formed, surrounded by pseudolobules. Additionally, nodules are formed grossly throughout the liver.

### 3.2 Epidemiology and Etiology

It is estimated that there are 400,000–500,000 patients with cirrhosis in Japan. Hepatocellular carcinoma accounts for approximately 70% of deaths from cirrhosis, but the annual number of deaths in patients with cirrhosis uncomplicated by hepatocellular carcinoma is approximately 17,000, and approximately 70% of these patients are male.

Cirrhosis can be classified according to its etiology, including viral hepatitis B and C, alcoholic liver disease, nonalcoholic steatohepatitis, autoimmune hepatitis, and primary biliary cholangitis. Cirrhosis caused by viral hepatitis B and C accounts for approximately 60% of all cases, followed by alcoholic hepatitis, which accounts for about 20%. In recent years, cirrhosis secondary to nonalcoholic steatohepatitis has been increasing, accounting for 5.8% of the cases in 2018, which is approximately three times higher than 10 years ago (Fig. 10.7).

## 3.3 Clinical Classification

In the compensated stage, the liver reserve is almost maintained, and the disease is almost asymptomatic, but in the decompensated stage, symptoms such as jaundice, ascites, and hepatic encephalopathy appear.

The Child-Pugh scoring system (Table 10.3) is often used to objectively assess the severity of cirrhosis and is divided into three grades (Grades A, B, and C). It is an important criterion in determining the treatment strategy for liver cancer and the indication for liver transplantation.

## 3.4 Clinical Symptoms

The liver is said to be a "silent organ," as patients with cirrhosis often show no subjective abnormalities during the compensated stage. In patients with cirrhosis in the decompensated stage, subjective symptoms such as general malaise, fatigue, decreased appetite, abdominal distension, and brown urine often appear.

In addition to physical findings such as jaundice, ascites, leg edema, gynecomastia, hepatic encephalopathy, and fluttering tremor, abnormal skin findings include palmar erythema (Fig. 10.8), which is found peripherally on the palms of the hands, and spider angioma (Fig. 10.9), which

**Table 10.3** Child-Pugh scoring system

| Score | One point | Two points | Three points |
|---|---|---|---|
| Hepatic encephalopathy | None | Minimal (I, II) | Advanced (III, IV) |
| Ascites | None | Slight | Moderate |
| Serum bilirubin (mg/dL) | <2.0 | 2.0–3.0 | >3.0 |
| Serum albumin (g/dL) | >3.5 | 2.8–3.5 | <2.8 |
| Prothrombin activity value (%) | >70 | 40–70 | <40 |

Scores 5–6, Grade A; scores 7–9, Grade B; scores 10–15 points, Grade C

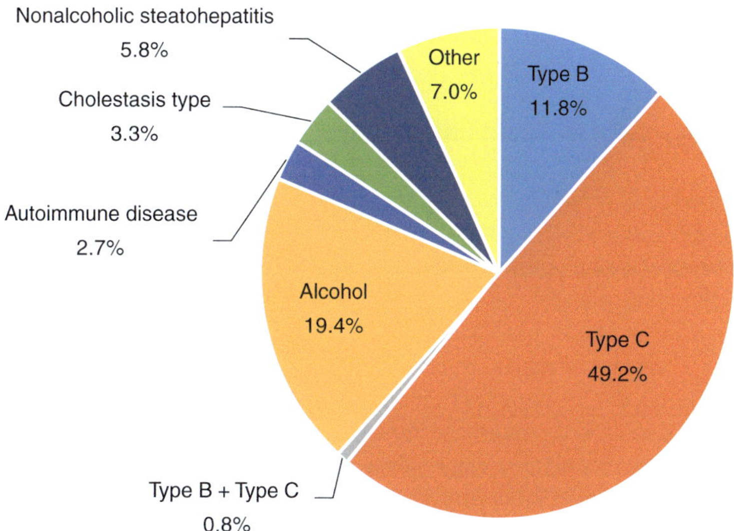


**Fig. 10.7** Classification of liver cirrhosis by etiology. (Created based on [14])

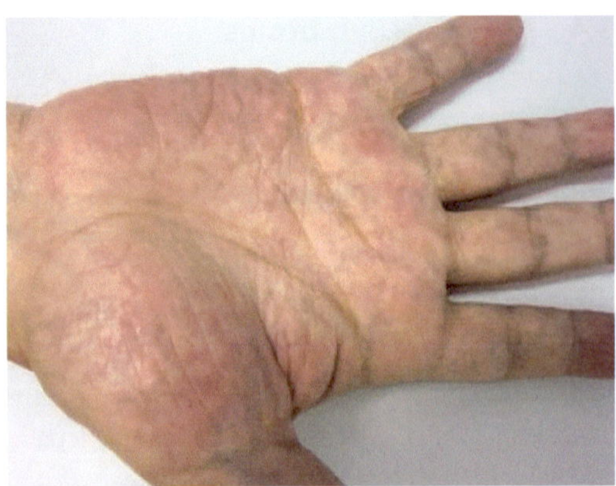

**Fig. 10.8** Palmar erythema in a patient with liver cirrhosis

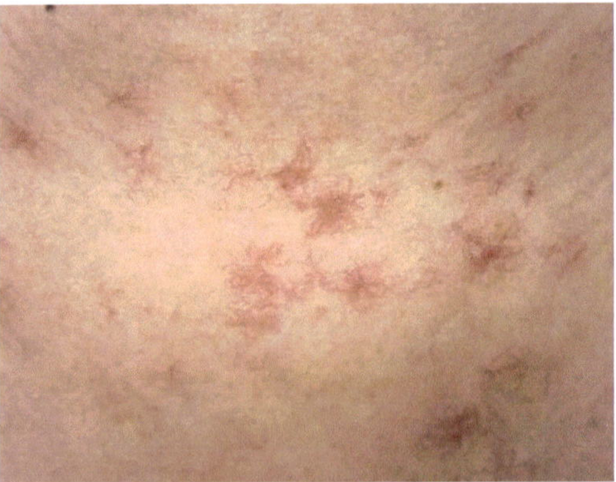

**Fig. 10.9** Spider angioma in the anterior chest of a patient with liver cirrhosis

appears on the neck and anterior chest. These findings are useful in diagnosing cirrhosis.

## 3.5 Clinical Examinations

Blood tests reveal thrombocytopenia and leukopenia in peripheral blood and a decrease in coagulation factors (prolongation of prothrombin time). Biochemical tests often show a mild increase in serum transaminases (AST > ALT) and a decrease in serum albumin and cholinesterase levels due to decreased protein synthesis in hepatocytes. Furthermore, the indocyanine green (ICG) test showed abnormal values. In patients with hepatic encephalopathy, high blood ammonia levels and abnormal amino acid balance are observed. α-Fetoprotein (AFP) and PIVKA-II are important tumor markers for the development of liver cancer.

A definitive diagnosis of cirrhosis requires a histopathological examination by liver biopsy. However, recently, cirrhosis is diagnosed using a combination of noninvasive imaging and blood tests without liver biopsy.

On abdominal ultrasonography, liver cirrhosis can be diagnosed based on findings such as abnormalities in liver size and shape, blunting of liver margins, and coarsening of liver parenchymal echogenicity. In addition, liver elastography using ultrasonography can be used to measure liver hardness and the degree of cirrhosis, making the diagnosis more accurate. Abdominal computed tomography (CT) and magnetic resonance imaging (MRI) can also be used to diagnose cirrhosis based on liver deformation, vascular changes, ascites, and splenomegaly. These imaging tests are useful in the diagnosis of cirrhosis, but they are very important in the search for the development of hepatocellular carcinoma secondary to cirrhosis.

Upper gastrointestinal endoscopy should always be performed to determine the presence of esophageal and gastric varices associated with cirrhosis and the risk of rupture.

## 3.6 Treatment and Prognosis

In the treatment of cirrhosis, the priority is to treat the etiology. For cirrhosis caused by hepatitis B or C viruses, antiviral therapy should be administered according to the respective treatment guidelines. Abstinence from alcohol is very important in the treatment of alcoholic cirrhosis, but these patients often have alcohol dependence and should consult with a psychiatrist.

Patients with advanced cirrhosis may develop esophageal varices due to portal hypertension, which can be diagnosed by upper gastrointestinal endoscopy and treated by endoscopic variceal ligation or sclerotherapy.

In patients with cirrhosis, in addition to splenomegaly induced thrombocytopenia, a tendency to bleed is often due to the reduced production of coagulation factors in the liver, and great care should be taken when performing surgical procedures such as tooth extraction.

Patients with hypoproteinemia should be treated with amino acid preparations and dietary therapy (1.2–1.3 g protein/standard weight kg/day). If ascites and leg edema occur, fluid and sodium restriction (3–6 g/day) should be indicated, and if symptoms persist, diuretics such as spironolactone or furosemide should be added. If the effects of these two drugs are inadequate, vasopressin V2 receptor antagonists should be considered. In end-stage cirrhosis, spontaneous bacterial peritonitis may occur as a complication, and ascites, fever, and abdominal pain are observed, requiring treatment with antimicrobial agents, but the prognosis is poor.

At the onset of hepatic encephalopathy, a low-protein diet is indicated. Synthetic disaccharides and nonabsorbable antibiotics are administered orally, and intravenous administration of branched-chain amino acid preparation is often used in refractory cases.

Although advances in the treatment of hepatic failure and gastrointestinal bleeding have reduced mortality in patients with cirrhosis, the incidence of hepatocellular carcinoma is extremely high (3–8% per year) and is a major cause of death in cirrhosis. Early detection of hepatocellular carcinoma is very important to reduce mortality in cirrhosis, and regular surveillance with tumor marker measurement and imaging examination every 3–4 months is strongly recommended in patients with cirrhosis.

## 3.7 Notes from Dentistry Perspective

Takashi Muramatsu

### 3.7.1 Gingival Bleeding Tendency

In the oral cavity, bleeding tendency from the gingiva may be observed (Figs. 10.10 and 10.11). In addition, hematomas may be formed when submucosal injury occurs not only in the gingiva but also in the buccal mucosa. Because gingival bleeding occurs easily, some patients avoid brushing for fear of bleeding, but the avoiding brushing promotes progression of periodontal disease and increases the risk of gingival bleeding.

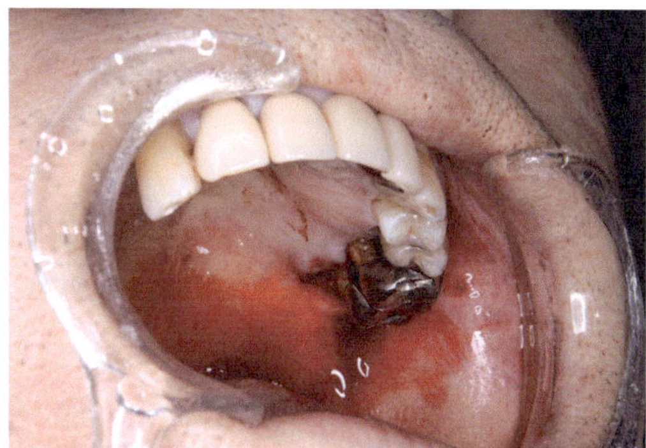

**Fig. 10.10** Cirrhotic patient with spontaneous bleeding from the gingiva. The patient was referred to the emergency room because of bleeding from the gingiva of the left maxillary second molar, but the bleeding was difficult to stop

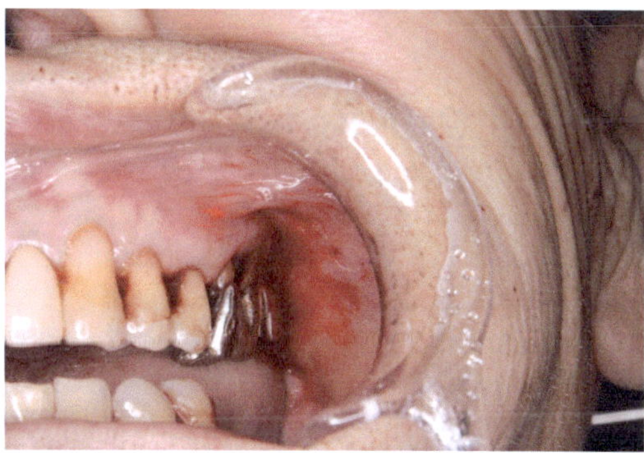

**Fig. 10.11** Same patient as Fig. 10.10. Laboratory results showed a platelet count of 55,000/μL, a clotting time of 15 s (reference value: 10–13 s), and a prothrombin time (PT) activity of 61% (reference value: 70–140%)

### 3.7.2 Dental Treatment Plan

Because many dental procedures involve bleeding, it is necessary to check the result of blood test before planning treatment. When invasive procedure is necessary, the bleeding time, platelet count, and prothrombin time (PT) should be measured before the procedure, so that the patient's condition can be assessed and measures can be taken to stop the bleeding. If the platelet count is more than 100,000/μL, the patient should be treated as usual. If the platelet count is 30,000/μL or higher, astriction and suturing can be used. However, if the platelet count is less than 30,000/

μL, hemostasis after tooth extraction is expected to be difficult, and platelet transfusion may be necessary in some cases.

When dental treatment is performed, each treatment should be short, and conservative treatment should be used as much as possible, with invasive procedure as the last option. Patients who avoid brushing for fear of bleeding have poor oral hygiene that leads to periodontal disease and cervical or root caries. When caries extends below the gingival margin, it is advisable to remove the gingiva with a gingival retraction cord containing a local hemostatic agent (adrenaline or aluminum chloride) and removing the dental caries (infected dentin).

Resin composite restorations are the main treatment for dental caries, but fluoride-releasing glass ionomer cement restorations are effective in preventing secondary caries in cervical and root surface caries due to the difficulty of moisture protection. If caries removal is difficult, or if the patient's condition is such that treatment cannot be performed for a while, application of a caries progression inhibitor (e.g., 38% silver diamine fluoride solution, Safolide®) is also effective. The basic treatment for periodontal disease is to improve cleaning of the oral cavity. However, when periodontal disease is advanced, spontaneous bleeding may occur, and patients may come to the dental office with a chief complaint of difficulty in stopping bleeding. The basic treatment is to use a local hemostatic agent and sutures, but in some cases, continuous bleeding from the insertion site of a suture needle may also be observed, so the use of a hemostatic bed is effective. If the situation of dental caries or periodontal disease is as bad as described above, tooth extraction should be considered, but if hemostasis is expected to be difficult in that case, it is necessary to refer the patient to a general hospital dental surgery department or university hospital and then hospitalize the patient for treatment.

#### 3.7.3 Complications

The rupture of esophageal varices may be caused by sudden pain or stress (insertion of a dental mirror into the soft palate, vacuuming, excessive movement of impression material to the pharynx during impression, etc.).

#### 3.7.4 Selecting a Safe Local Anesthetic

In liver cirrhosis, the decomposition (detoxication) in the liver is inhibited because of the decreased liver function, and the blood concentration of local anesthetics tends to increase. It is necessary to minimize the use of lidocaine hydrochloride (Xylocaine®), which has a strong anesthetic effect with a small amount.

## 4 Gastroesophageal Reflux Disease (GERD)

Katsuhiko Hasegawa

### 4.1 Concept of the Disease

Gastroesophageal reflux disease (GERD) is a disease caused by gastroesophageal reflux that results in either or both esophageal mucosal injury and bothersome symptoms and is classified as "erosive GERD" with esophageal mucosal injury or "nonerosive GERD" with only symptoms [17]. Gastroesophageal reflux (GER) is classified into "acid GER" and "nonacid GER" [17].

### 4.2 Pathophysiology

The lower esophageal sphincter (LES) functions as an anti-reflux mechanism for gastric contents [18]. The major causes of gastroesophageal reflux (GER) in GERD are hiatal hernia, transient LES relaxation, increased intra-abdominal pressure, and post-esophageal and gastric surgery. The aggravating factors of GERD are obesity, smoking, alcohol consumption, and aging [18].

### 4.3 Epidemiology

The prevalence of erosive GERD in Japan is approximately 10%. The prevalence of GERD is estimated to be about 20% when nonerosive GERD is included [17].

## 4.4 Categories

There are two types of GERD: erosive GERD (reflux esophagitis), in which endoscopy shows injury on the mucosal folds of the esophagus, and nonerosive reflux disease (NERD), in which endoscopy shows little or no change. The broad term nonerosive GERD (NERD) may include narrowly defined NERD involving gastric acid GER, reflux hypersensitivity not involving gastric acid GER, and functional heartburn; NERD has been suggested to involve hypersensitivity to gastric acid GER [19].

## 4.5 Endoscopic Classification

In Japanese gastrointestinal endoscopic practice, the revised Los Angeles Classification (LA Classification) is often used as the GERD classification [18]. In the LA Classification, esophageal mucosal injuries are classified into ABCD in order of severity.

(a) Length of mucosal injury is less than 5 mm.
(b) Length of mucosal injury is more than 5 mm.
(c) Two or more contiguous injuries on adjacent mucosal folds but not more than three-fourths of the total circumference.
(d) Mucosal injury of more than three-fourths of the total circumference.

The endoscopic findings of reflux esophagitis are shown in Figs. 10.12 and 10.13.

Endoscopic findings related to GERD are shown in Figs. 10.14 and 10.15.

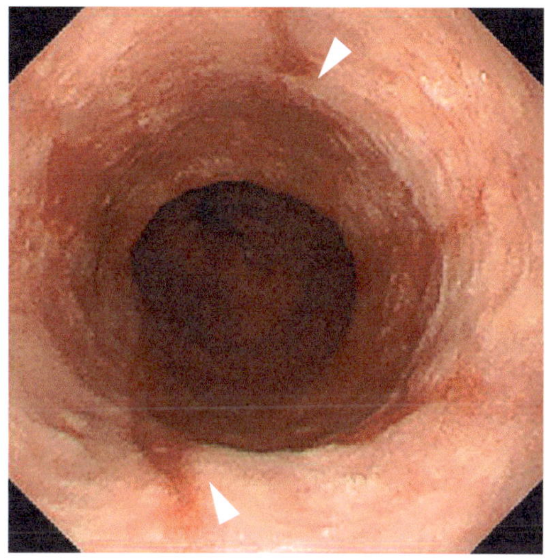

**Fig. 10.12** LA classification grade B. Multiple erosions larger than 5 mm on the lower mucosal folds of the esophagus

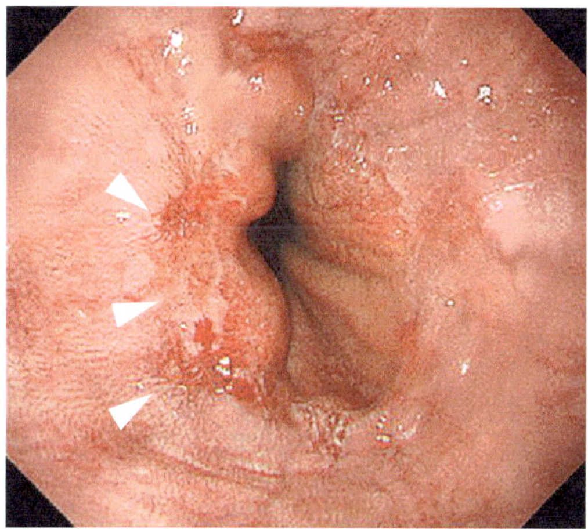

**Fig. 10.13** LA classification grade C. Mucosal injury is continuous at the esophagogastric mucosal border but does not exceed 3/4 of the total circumference

## 4.6 Clinical Symptoms

In addition to chest pain, heartburn, dyspepsia, epigastric pain, and acid regurgitation, extraesophageal symptoms include cough, laryngopharyngeal reflux disease, and acid erosion of the teeth. In severe cases of GERD, stenosis and bleeding may occur [17, 18].

## 4.7 Clinical Examination

The F scale is a diagnostic method based on a score using a questionnaire of subjective symptoms related to GERD.

Upper gastrointestinal endoscopy is useful in differentiating erosive GERD from NERD [17].

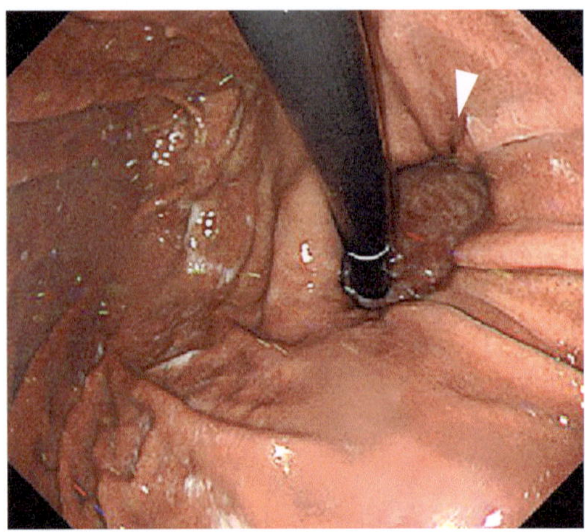

**Fig. 10.14** View of the esophageal hiatal hernia fossa from the inside of the stomach, with a gap at the side of the scope that allows reflux of gastric contents

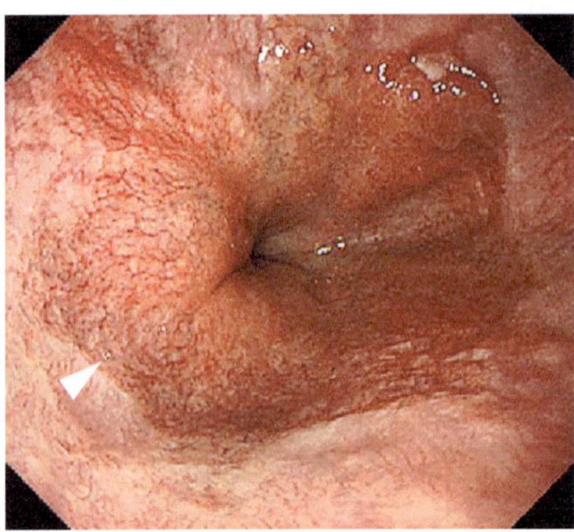

**Fig. 10.15** Barrett's esophagus. The lower esophageal palisade vessels are seen in the submucosal epithelium extending from the gastric side

Chest and abdominal X-rays are useful in differentiating esophageal diseases from those of adjacent organs. It may detect esophageal hiatal hernia. It can be used to differentiate constipation and ileus.

Esophageal and gastric radiography is useful in distinguishing GERD from esophageal cancer and gastric cancer. It can also differentiate primary esophageal motility disorders such as achalasia.

A 24-h esophageal pH impedance monitoring is a method that can detect reflux phenomena other than acid and can discriminate narrowly defined NERD caused by gastric acid GER from reflux hypersensitivity and functional heartburn [18].

## 4.8 Diseases That Need to Be Differentiated from GERD

Diseases showing chest pain, heartburn, dyspepsia and epigastric pain, esophageal cancer, gastric cancer, gastric and duodenal ulcer, acute and chronic gastritis, biliary tract disease, pancreatic disease, esophageal motility disorders such as esophageal achalasia, eosinophilic esophagitis, ischemic heart disease such as angina pectoris and myocardial infarction, and functional gastrointestinal disease (FGID) should be differentiated from GERD [19].

## 4.9 GERD Treatment

The initial treatment is proton pump inhibitor (PPI) for 8 weeks, and if the patient responds to PPI treatment for 8 weeks, maintenance therapy with PPI is performed for long term; if the patient does not improve after 8 weeks of PPI treatment, PPI double-dose divided dosing or using other drugs should be considered as PPI-resistant GERD [18].

Evidence-based clinical practice guidelines for GERD 2021 defined PPI-resistant as a condition in which (1) esophageal mucosal injury does not heal and/or (2) symptoms thought to be of GER origin do not improve sufficiently, even after 8 weeks of oral administration of a standard dose of PPI [18].

## 4.10 Prognosis

Surgical treatment may be considered in patients with PPI-refractory GERD that does not respond to other agents, repeated symptom flare ups, and advanced esophageal hiatal hernia [17, 18].

An association between GERD and Barrett's esophagus has been suggested, and the risk of esophageal adenocarcinoma from Barrett's esophagus has also been suggested, but the exact frequency of occurrence in the Japanese population is unknown [18].

In Evidence-based Clinical Practice Guidelines for GERD 2021, Barrett's esophagus is defined as "the esophagus with Barrett's mucosa, a columnar epithelium extending continuously from the stomach into the esophagus, with or without intestinal epithelialization."

## 4.11 Recent Findings

GERD is a disease that impairs the quality of life (QOL) due to persistent uncomfortable symptoms, and it is necessary to resolve the uncomfortable symptoms early by actively utilizing drugs with a high inhibitory effect on acid secretion. Recently, potassium-competitive acid blocker (P-CAB), a PPI with a novel mechanism of action, has been developed. P-CABs have the following characteristics: (1) rapid action, (2) sustained inhibitory effect on acid secretion, (3) stable to acid, and (4) less susceptible to genetic polymorphisms of drug-metabolizing enzyme CYP2C19.

Uncomfortable symptoms of GERD have been conditioned to be induced by the direct stimulation of esophageal sensory nerves with refluxed acids. However, it is now proposed that acid and pancreatic enzymes increase cytokine and chemokine production in esophageal mucosal epithelial cells and induce infiltration of inflammatory cells into the esophageal mucosa, thereby stimulating esophageal sensory nerves and contributing to symptoms such as heartburn [20].

## 4.12 Notes from Dentistry Perspective

Wataru Kobayashi

The backflow of highly acidic digestive juices from the esophagus to the oral cavity causes a variety of disorders, and in this section, we describe the relationship between the oral disease and gastroesophageal reflux disease.

### 4.12.1 Masticatory Dysfunction

Hyperphagia or eating quickly without chewing well can cause reflux due to transient relaxation of the lower esophageal sphincter, because a lot of air is swallowed with food. In the same way, when teeth are missing and the masticatory function has not been restored with prosthesis, the patient cannot chew well and gastric reflux is likely to occur.

### 4.12.2 Acid Erosion by Acid Regurgitation

Acid erosion (erosive disease) generally refers to defects of the hard tissue of the teeth caused by chemical action, especially acid action. One of the typical symptoms of gastroesophageal reflux disease is acid regurgitation that rises to the mouth. In addition to symptoms such as a sour or bitter taste caused by gastric juice, acid erosion occurs when the enamel and dentin are melted by the acid of digestive juice, and the lingual side of the anterior teeth and occlusal surfaces are demineralized by the hydrochloric acid of digestive juice. Unlike dental caries, which is caused by bacterial chemical action, acid erosion is caused by pure chemical action. Restorative dentistry and prosthetic treatment are necessary.

### 4.12.3 Salivary Hyposecretion and Gastroesophageal Reflux Disease

Saliva is always secreted in the oral cavity and moves from the esophagus to the stomach by swallowing. Saliva has a buffering effect and neutralizes acidity, so saliva raises the pH of refluxed gastric juice. Reflux of gastric juice is more likely to occur when the patient is lying down, and gastric juice is secreted more frequently around 2 a.m. Therefore, even if reflux of gastric juice occurs during sleep, saliva is reduced during sleep, which weakens the neutralizing effect of saliva on gastric juice, resulting in a vicious cycle that damages the esophageal mucosa and is likely to cause further acid erosion. Since most of the acid reflux occurs within

2–3 h after a meal, sleeping immediately after a meal should be avoided from the viewpoint of acid neutralization by saliva. In addition, in xerostomia, where saliva volume decreases with age, the buffering effect of saliva cannot be expected.

#### 4.12.4 The Relationship Between Brachycephaly and Gastroesophageal Reflux Disease

Sleep bruxism is the habit of unconsciously rubbing or clenching the upper and lower teeth together during sleep. Bruxism causes various problems such as tooth wear and fracture and temporomandibular joint symptoms, but no effective treatment has been established. Recently, the relationship between bruxism and GERD has attracted attention, and it has been reported that bruxism is frequently observed in patients with GERD [21, 22]. Mengatto et al. reported that bruxism is not significantly related to age, BMI, or stress and that bruxism is 6.58 times more common in patients with GERD. It has been experimentally confirmed that nocturnal gastroesophageal reflux and lowered pH in the esophagus can induce bruxism [23]. In other words, if bruxism is induced by gastroesophageal reflux disease, treatment of gastroesophageal reflux disease may be expected to improve bruxism. Kanematsu et al. [24] reported that 12 subjects who were aware of bruxism were divided into two groups and treated with proton pump inhibitor (PPI) or placebo; masseter muscle activity and rhythmic masticatory muscle activity (RMMA) related to bruxism were significantly suppressed in the PPI group. The results suggest that PPIs may be a new treatment for bruxism in patients with gastroesophageal reflux disease.

## 5 Inflammatory Bowel Disease [25–31]

Hiroshi Kishikawa

Nonspecific chronic inflammatory bowel diseases with unknown causes are often called "inflammatory bowel diseases." Representative diseases, including ulcerative colitis, Crohn's disease, and Behcet's disease, are described in this section.

### 5.1 Ulcerative Colitis

#### 5.1.1 Disease Overview

It is a diffuse, nonspecific inflammatory disease of unknown cause (not due to bacterial infection, radiation, or drugs) that affects the mucosa of the colon continuously from the rectum, forming erosions and ulcers. Remission and relapse occur in typical cases.

#### 5.1.2 Pathophysiology

It is thought to be caused by (1) abnormalities in the intestinal immune system, (2) genetics, and (3) environmental factors (microflora, smoking, etc.). However, the cause has not been elucidated.

#### 5.1.3 Epidemiology

The incidence of ulcerative colitis and Crohn's disease is increasing, especially in newly industrialized countries. The reported prevalence of ulcerative colitis is 505 per 100,000 in Europe and 208 per 100,000 in North America. In Japan, it is estimated that more than 220,000 people have this disease, and this number is also increasing. The median onset of ulcerative colitis is in the late 10 s to early 30 s, but it also has smaller peaks at 50 years of age.

#### 5.1.4 Classification

It is classified into three types according to the affected site: (1) proctitis, (2) left-sided colitis, and (3) total colitis. Disease is classified into four types: mild, moderate, severe, and fulminant. These classifications are important in deciding the treatment strategy. For example, suppositories are more effective in proctitis.

#### 5.1.5 Symptoms

Common symptoms include persistent diarrhea, recurrent bloody diarrhea, and abdominal pain, and systemic symptoms such as fever and weight loss may be observed in severe cases. Extraintestinal complications such as arthritis, skin lesions (erythema nodosum and pyoderma gangrenosum), and eye symptoms (episcleritis) may also occur.

### 5.1.6 Clinical Examinations

Examination of blood and stool specimens, endoscopy, and computed tomography (CT) were performed according to the disease activity and type. Blood tests are mainly used to evaluate activity and anemia, and stool cultures are used to exclude infectious enteritis. In ulcerative colitis, although blood tests are important as indicators to monitor disease activity, C-reactive protein CRP does not always reflect disease activity. Thus, leucine-rich alfa-2 glycoprotein can be used as a more specific serological disease marker. Endoscopic findings are characterized by loss of vascular pattern, granular mucosa, easy bleeding, erosions, and ulcers in a continuous pattern from the rectum (Fig. 10.16). The incidence of colorectal cancer is higher in patients with ulcerative colitis than in the general population; therefore, periodic endoscopic examinations are recommended. CT can also be used to evaluate activity. Recently, stool calprotectin, an inflammatory protein originating from neutrophils released from inflammation sites in the intestine, has been used as a diagnostic tool to predict disease activity in inflammatory bowel diseases.

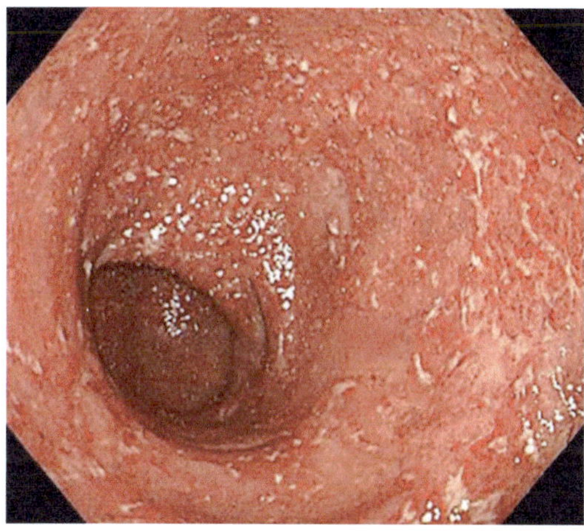

**Fig. 10.16** Colonoscopy image of ulcerative colitis. Loss of vascular markings, edematous mucosa, erythema, granular mucosa, and mucosal friability are observed

### 5.1.7 Treatment

Three types of treatments are known: drug therapy, leukapheresis, and surgical treatment.

It is important to balance the treatment for remission induction and relapse prevention.

5-Aminosalicylic acid (5-ASA) agents are the mainstay of treatment and are useful for remission induction and relapse prevention. In addition, steroids are used in cases refractory to 5-ASA or in severe or relapse cases. If the disease is poorly controlled with 5-ASA and steroids, other treatment strategies should be considered. Oral medications are candidates for steroid or steroid resistance. Tacrolimus is used for remission induction, azathioprine for relapse prevention, and tofacitinib for induction and relapse prevention. The injectable drugs, anti-TNF-α agents, including infliximab, adalimumab, golimumab, vedolizumab (anti-α4β7 integrin antibodies), and ustekinumab, (an anti-IL12/23p40 antibody), are effective for both induction and relapse prevention.

Leukapheresis (granulocyte/monocyte apheresis (GMA)) is a non-pharmacological therapeutic modality to taper or remove steroids and is used for remission and induction in relatively mild cases. In cases where inflammation is difficult to control or cancer or high-grade dysplasia has developed, surgery is often the treatment of choice, and total colorectal resection with ileal pouch-anal canal anastomosis (IACA) or ileal pouch-anal canal anastomosis (IPAA) is usually performed, which is a different treatment strategy from that of conventional colorectal cancer.

### 5.1.8 Latest Findings

Dysbiosis of the intestinal microflora is thought to be involved in the pathogenesis of ulcerative colitis, and fecal transplantation, in which feces from healthy individuals are administered to patients, has become a topic of discussion. However, there are positive and negative results regarding the therapeutic effects of fecal transplantation, and further studies are required.

## 5.2 Crohn's Disease

### 5.2.1 Disease Overview

It is a chronic inflammatory disease of unknown etiology, characterized by discontinuously distributed lesions (potentially involving the entire gastrointestinal tract) and transmural inflammation. Remission and relapse are repeated, as in other inflammatory bowel diseases.

### 5.2.2 Pathophysiology

As with ulcerative colitis, the cause of this disease has not been elucidated. Several factors, such as heredity, immune system, and environmental factors, play a role in its development; however, the involvement of heredity in Crohn's disease is stronger than in ulcerative colitis.

### 5.2.3 Epidemiology

It is estimated that more than 70,000 people have this disease in Japan, and this number is increasing. A recent systematic review reported that the highest prevalence was 322 per 100,000 in Europe and 319 per 100,000 in North America.

### 5.2.4 Classification

It is classified into ileitis, colitis, and ileocolitis types, according to the site of the lesion. Inflammation, fistula formation, and stenosis have been proposed as the disease patterns.

### 5.2.5 Symptoms

It presents with nonspecific recurrent symptoms such as chronic abdominal pain, diarrhea, fever, fatigue, and weight loss. Ulcers in the intestine can extend completely through the intestinal wall, creating a fistula in other organs, such as the intestine and skin. Fistula near the anus is also a common lesion; therefore, pain in the anus and perianal area should also be considered in cases suspected of this disease. Symptoms of bowel stenosis may also occur, including nausea and ileus-like symptoms. Cancer may develop in the affected lesion, and periodic surveillance by endoscopy, CT, and magnetic resonance imaging (MRI) should be performed.

### 5.2.6 Clinical Examinations

Endoscopy (colonoscopy and, in some cases, balloon enteroscopy) is important to diagnose this disease. Characteristic endoscopic findings include discontinuous skip lesions with normal intussusception mucosa, cobblestone appearance, longitudinal ulcers, multiple aphthae, strictures, fistulae, and anorectal lesions affecting any part of the gastrointestinal tract (Fig. 10.17). Similar lesions can also be observed in the X-ray contrast (Fig. 10.18). CT and MRI are particularly useful for evaluating fistula and abscess formation. Capsule endoscopy is used to evaluate small intestinal lesions, but clinicians should observe complications, including symptomatic retention of the capsule. To evaluate stenosis, the patency capsule should be considered. The clinical significance of the blood test results was almost the same as that of ulcerative colitis. Histopathology by endoscopic biopsy is characterized by the presence of granulomas, which are highly specific to this disease.

### 5.2.7 Treatment

Patients with mild-to-moderate active colorectal lesions are treated with 5-ASA and steroids. Patients with small intestinal lesions are also treated with nutritional therapy using Elental in

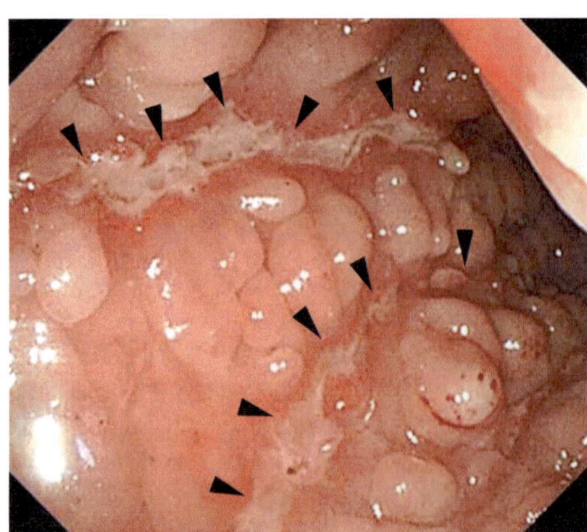

**Fig. 10.17** Colonoscopy image of Crohn's disease. A longitudinal ulcer (arrow) and a cobble stone appearance adjacent to it are recognized

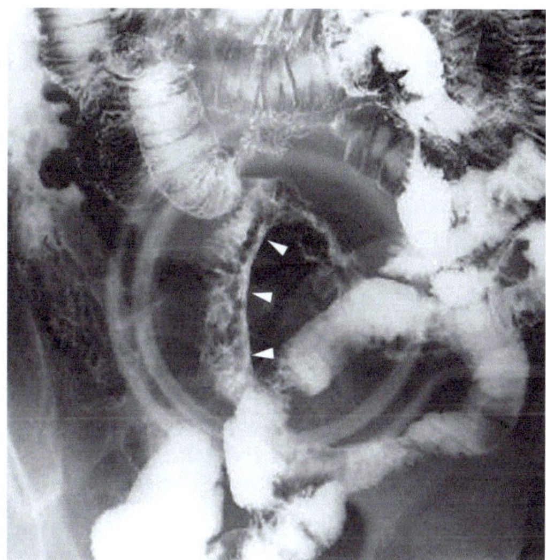

**Fig. 10.18** Small intestinal radiography for Crohn's disease. An active longitudinal ulcer (arrow) is seen in the distal ileum

Japan. Recently, budesonide, which has fewer systemic side effects, has been used for lesions in the ileum and right colon. In moderate to severe diseases, biologics, including anti-TNF-α antibodies (infliximab, adalimumab) and ustekinumab, an anti-IL12/23p40 antibody, are also used. However, "top-down therapy" by biologics is indicated from the early onset, especially in high-risk subjects such as broad small intestinal damages, severe and multiple endoscopic ulcers, stenosis or perforation, younger age, and multiple operation history. In intestinal stenosis cases, endoscopic dilatation or surgical resection may be performed. In fistulas, biologics and surgical treatments are used. It should be noted that as many as 70% of patients with Crohn's disease eventually require surgery, which is significantly higher than that of ulcerative colitis.

## 5.3 Intestinal Behçet's Disease

### 5.3.1 Disease Overview

Behçet's disease is a systemic inflammatory disease of unknown etiology, with recurrent oral and genital ulcerations, eye lesions, skin lesions, and a positive pathergy test. It is called "intestinal Behçet's disease" when gastrointestinal lesions are the main symptoms. This is a rare but the most common inflammatory bowel disease directly associated with oral lesions. Therefore, this disease is important to dentists, especially in the Middle East and Asia.

### 5.3.2 Epidemiology

It is also known as the "Silk Road" disease. It occurs frequently in the Middle East (ranging up to 240 per 100,000 in Turkey) and Asia, but it is a rare disorder in the USA and Europe (7.5, 7.1, and 1.1 per 100,000 population in Spain, France, and Germany). It is estimated that there are more than 20,000 patients with Behçet's disease in Japan, and about 20% of them are complicated with gastrointestinal lesions. The median age of onset is typically 30–40 years.

### 5.3.3 Symptoms

Various gastrointestinal symptoms have been observed, including abdominal pain, diarrhea, nausea, and melena. Right lower abdominal pain is common because the most commonly affected lesion is located in the ileocecal region. In some cases, intestinal perforation is the initial symptom of intestinal Behçet's disease; thus, it is important to suspect intestinal complications when sudden and severe abdominal pain is recognized in patients with Behcet's disease.

### 5.3.4 Clinical Examinations

On endoscopy, a deep, punched-out ulcer in the ileum is characteristic (Fig. 10.19) because the most commonly affected part of the lesion is the ileocecal lesion in intestinal Behçet's disease. Longitudinal ulcers or aphthae may also be present anywhere from the esophagus to the colon; however, the involvement of the esophagus, stomach, and rectum is rare. CT and MRI are useful for evaluating the affected lesions and complications, including perforation. As in other inflammatory bowel diseases, blood tests, including CRP, are also useful to evaluate the activity of this disease in some cases but are not specific.

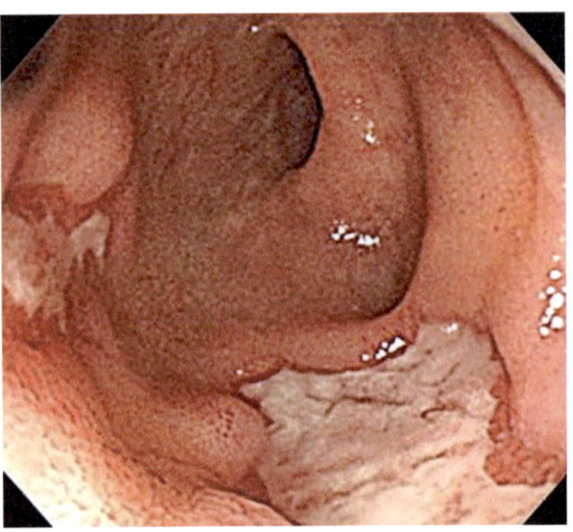

**Fig. 10.19** Colonoscopy for gastrointestinal Behçet's disease. Punched-like ulcers are seen in the ileocecal region

### 5.3.5 Treatment

In mild cases, 5-ASA agents are often used to treat ulcerative colitis and Crohn's disease. Steroids and anti-TNF-α antibody agents are used in severe cases. Immunomodulators may also be used in corticosteroid-dependent patients. The PDE4 inhibitor, apremilast, is covered by Japanese insurance for the treatment of oral ulcers caused by Behçet's disease after an inadequate response to topical therapy.

### 5.3.6 Latest Findings

In the general population, HLA-B51 positivity is 10–15%. In Behçet's disease, HLA-B51 positivity is as high as 50–60% and is considered to be one of the genetic factors that determine disease susceptibility. Therefore, HLA-B51 measurement is sometimes used as an adjunct diagnosis in Behçet's disease, although it is not covered by insurance.

## 5.4 Notes from Dentistry Perspective

Ryosuke Abe

Inflammatory bowel disease (IBD) is a disease that causes inflammation of the intestine due to an abnormality in the immune system that causes the immune cells to attack the intestinal cells and is accompanied by symptoms such as chronic diarrhea, bloody stools, and abdominal pain.

Dentists need to evaluate the general condition of patients with IBD. Patients with mild disease without symptoms such as bleeding, fever, and diarrhea can be treated with normal dental care. However, in patients with moderate to severe disease, dental treatment may not be indicated due to the various risks associated with bleeding, fever, and anemia and should be discussed with the attending physician.

Although it is a prerequisite to choose a complication-free period for dental treatment, it is important for the dentist to understand the patient's general condition, blood tests, and bleeding time before the surgical procedure such as tooth extraction. This is because the patient may have side effects such as hepatic, pulmonary, and renal dysfunction, anemia, and bone marrow suppression due to the administered drug.

Patients with IBD are often treated with immunosuppressive drugs and corticosteroids, and it is important to be aware of these factors in order to provide regular oral care. In such cases, it is also important to educate patients about oral care, including daily brushing instruction and cleaning of the oral mucosa, with in mind the possibility of worsening dental infections, and failure of healing after tooth extraction, as well as drug therapy-related oral candidiasis and gingival hypertrophy.

The use of anti-inflammatory drugs should be based on their impact on the intestinal tract and should avoid aspirin and other NSAIDs. The use of acetaminophen, COX-2 selective inhibitors, and proton pump inhibitors is also recommended.

Antimicrobial agents are given to patients with dental infections, but some types of antimicrobial agents promote the growth of clostridium and induce recurrence of symptoms and diarrhea. After prescribing an antimicrobial, the patient's condition should be carefully monitored, and if gastrointestinal symptoms are present, the patient's physician should be consulted.

There are also oral complications associated with IBD. Pemphigus, viral diseases, and Behcet's disease are among the diseases that cause stomatitis and oral mucosal ulcers, but the

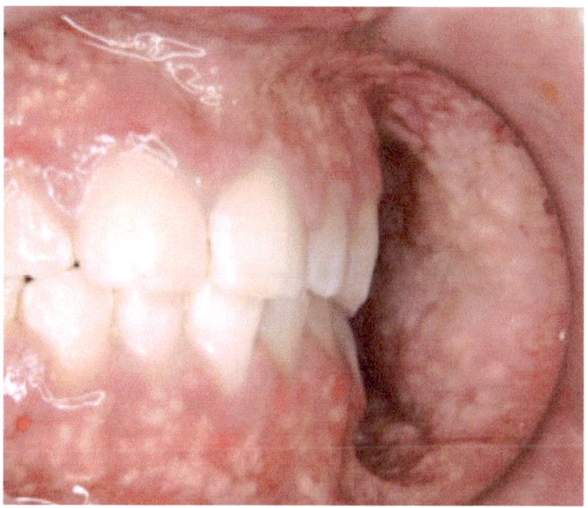

**Fig. 10.20** Intraoral photograph of proliferative pyogenic stomatitis. Involvement of the upper and lower gingiva and buccal mucosa. (By courtesy of Dr. Toyonori Suzuki, Azabu Kitami Triology Hospital)

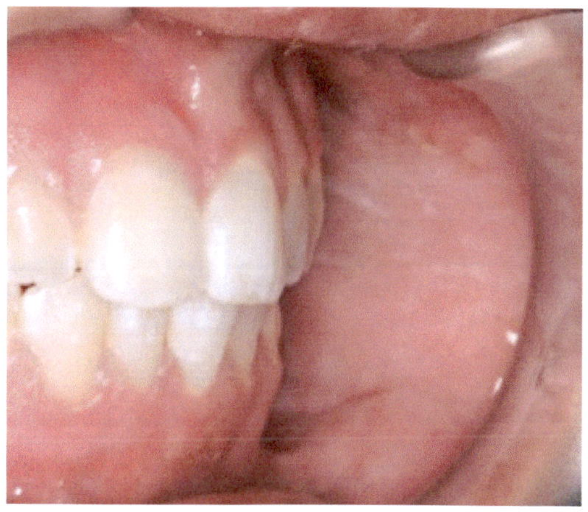

**Fig. 10.21** Intraoral photographs on day 7 after steroid administration. Disappearance of the lesion is observed. (By courtesy of Dr. Toyonori Suzuki, Azabu Kitami Triology Hospital)

possibility that some recurrent stomatitis may be associated with IBD should be kept in mind.

Pyostomatitis vegetans is a mucosal lesion characteristic of ulcerative colitis and was described by McCarthy in 1949 [28]. It affects the buccal gingiva, buccal mucosa, and oral mucosa and is often associated with contact and irritation pain (Fig. 10.20). The lesions are characterized by the formation of numerous papillary bumps with small abscesses on the oral mucosa with erythematous changes and cobblestone appearance. Histologically, it forms microabscesses with infiltration of numerous inflammatory cells under the mucosal epithelium [29]. Systemic administration of steroids has been reported to be more effective than local administration (Fig. 10.21).

Crohn's disease is a disease of unknown etiology that affects the entire gastrointestinal tract from the oral cavity to the anus, with the small and large intestines being the predominant sites. In the oral cavity, aphthous stomatitis and oral ulcers occur in about 20% of patients, and oral symptoms may precede the diagnosis for several years before it is confirmed. Oral symptoms are characterized by the chronic appearance of the lips, buccal mucosa, and tongue, which often appear when the primary disease worsens, and the oral cavity improves when the symptoms improve. Local application of steroid ointment is effective in treating oral lesions.

## 6 Gastrointestinal Polyposis

Toshimi Chiba

### 6.1 Concept

Gastrointestinal polyposis is a disease characterized by multiple polyps (usually ≥100) with a similar histology in the gastrointestinal tract and is classified according to hereditary status and histological findings (Table 10.4).

This section describes familial colorectal adenomatosis, which is relatively common, and Peutz-Jeghers syndrome, Cronkhite-Canada syndrome, and Cowden's disease, which are more likely to be associated with symptoms in the oral region.

### 6.2 Familial Adenomatous Polyposis (FAP)

#### 6.2.1 Disease Overview

Familial adenomatous polyposis (FAP) is a disease that is inherited in an autosomal dominant manner and is caused by mutations in the

**Table 10.4** Classification of gastrointestinal polyposis

| Type | Histopathological findings | Name of disease | Inheritance pattern | Causative gene | Gastrointestinal lesion location | Lesions other than gastrointestinal tract | Malignant tumor |
|---|---|---|---|---|---|---|---|
| Hereditary | Adenomatous | Familial adenomatous polyposis | Autosomal dominant inheritance | *APC* | Stomach to colon (hundreds to thousands), attenuated FAP: Less than 100 polyps | Gardner syndrome: Osteoma and soft tissue tumor<br>Turcot syndrome: Brain tumor (medulloblastoma, glioma, etc.) | Colorectal cancer, gastric cancer, and duodenal cancer |
| | Hamartomatous | Peutz-Jeghers syndrome | Autosomal dominant inheritance | *STK11/ LKB1* | Stomach to colon (several to several hundred) | Mucocutaneous pigmentation | Colorectal cancer, gastric cancer, cancer of other organs (gynecologic cancer, breast cancer, etc.) |
| | Hamartomatous | Cowden's disease | Autosomal dominant inheritance | *PTEN* | Esophagus to colon (multiple) | Multiple papules on the face, papilloma of the oral mucosa, and keratotic papules in the ends of extremities | Colorectal cancer, breast cancer, and thyroid cancer |
| | Hamartomatous | Juvenile polyposis | Autosomal dominant inheritance | *SMAD4, BMPR1A* | Stomach to colon (5–200 polyps) | Malformation of the heart and mental retardation | Colorectal cancer and gastric cancer |
| Nonhereditary | Others | Cronkhite-Canada syndrome | None | None | Stomach to colon (multiple) | Skin pigmentation, alopecia, and nail atrophy | Colorectal cancer |

*APC* tumor suppressor gene that result in multiple adenomatous polyps in the colon. Patients with FAP have a high incidence of colorectal cancer.

### 6.2.2 Pathophysiology

FAP is characterized by the development of 100 or more adenomatous polyps in the colon. It most commonly arises in patients with a family history of FAP who carry a germline *APC* variant [32]. Neoplastic and nonneoplastic lesions are present not only in the colon but also in the stomach, duodenum, small intestine, and organs outside the gastrointestinal tract.

### 6.2.3 Epidemiology

The frequency of FAP in the Japanese population is estimated to be 1/174,000; thus, FAP represents <1% of all colorectal cancer patients in Japan [32].

### 6.2.4 Classification

FAP is subdivided into a profuse phenotype and a sparse phenotype. In addition, subtypes include Gardner syndrome (associated with osteoma and soft tissue tumors), Turcot syndrome (associated with malignant tumors of the central nervous system, such as medulloblastoma), and attenuated FAP (characterized by <100 polyps).

### 6.2.5 Symptoms

Bloody stools from colorectal polyps or colorectal cancer are frequently observed, and diarrhea, abdominal pain, and anemia may be found.

### 6.2.6 Clinical Examination

Colonoscopy and barium enema may reveal multiple adenomatous polyps (Figs. 10.22 and 10.23), and upper gastrointestinal endoscopy may show fundic gland polyps or duodenal papillary tumors. The presence of congenital hypertrophy of the retinal pigment epithelium, osteoma of the gnathic bone or cranial bone, dental anomalies (e.g., impacted teeth, supernumerary teeth, and odontoma), and soft tissue tumors should also be confirmed.

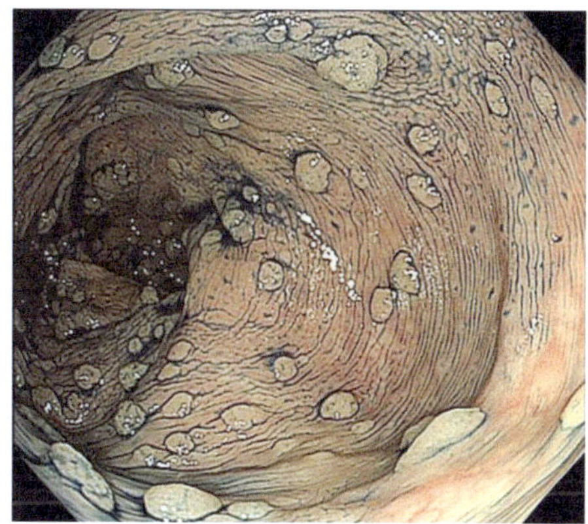

**Fig. 10.22** Colonoscopy finding of gastrointestinal polyposis. Multiple colonic polyps are observed

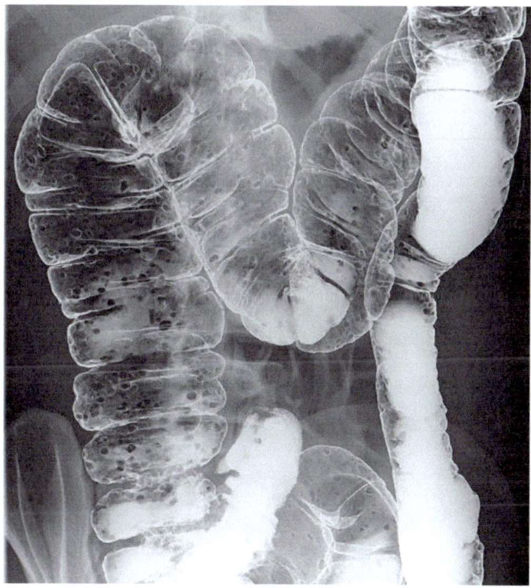

**Fig. 10.23** Barium enema finding of gastrointestinal polyposis. Multiple small elevated lesions are seen in the colon

### 6.2.7 Treatment

For FAP patients, prophylactic colorectal resection is performed, with total colectomy with ileal pouch anal (anal canal) anastomosis (IA(C)A) being the first choice.

### 6.2.8 Prognosis

The prognosis of FAP depends on the presence of colorectal cancer and the accuracy of cancer surveillance; >60% of deaths are colorectal cancer-related.

### 6.2.9 Recent Findings

1. ***MUTYH*-associated polyposis:** FAP caused by *MUTYH* gene mutations, which are inherited in an autosomal recessive pattern, is characterized by a relatively small number of colorectal polyps. Patients tend to be older at disease onset (range, 45–56 years) compared with patients with conventional FAP, and the cumulative morbidity rate of colorectal cancer in patients ≤70 years is reported to be about 80%.
2. **Counseling:** Genetic testing should be performed in children with a family history of FAP. For families with confirmed or suspected gene abnormalities, screening by colonoscopy is required beginning at age 10 years. Education about the risk of hepatoblastoma, retinal disease, and desmoid tumors is also necessary.

## 6.3 Peutz-Jeghers Syndrome

### 6.3.1 Disease Overview

Peutz-Jeghers syndrome is an autosomal dominant inherited disorder characterized by multiple hamartomatous polyps in the gastrointestinal tract and pigmentation of the lips, oral mucosa, and fingers.

### 6.3.2 Pathophysiology

The *STK11/LKB1* gene has been identified as a causative gene in 70–80% of cases [33]. In addition, two of three following criteria must be fulfilled for a diagnosis of Peutz-Jeghers syndrome: characteristic mucocutaneous pigmentation, multiple hamartomatous polyps in the small intestine, and a family history of the syndrome.

### 6.3.3 Epidemiology

The incidence of Peutz-Jeghers syndrome is 1 in 25,000–300,000; more than 600 cases have been reported in Japan.

### 6.3.4 Symptoms

Intussusception and ileus caused by small intestinal polyps are often observed, and bloody stools, abdominal pain, and prolapse of polyps from the anus may be seen. In addition, pigmentation of the lips, oral mucosa, palms of the hand, and soles of the feet beginning in childhood are characteristic of this disease (Fig. 10.24).

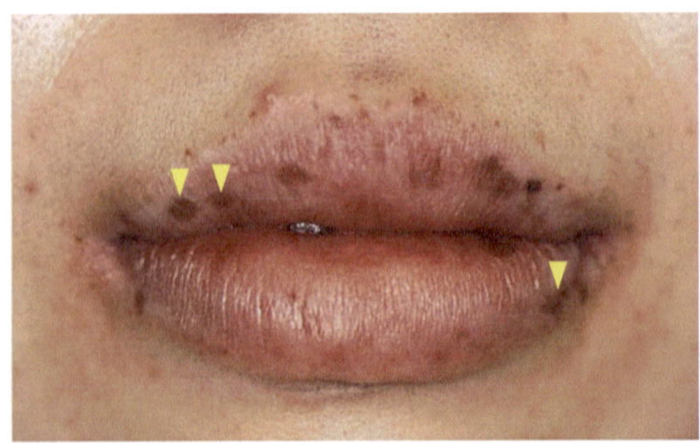

**Fig. 10.24** Lips of a patient with Peutz-Jeghers syndrome. Pigmentation of the lips is observed

### 6.3.5 Clinical Examination

Polyps range in size from a few millimeters to >5 cm, and 64% are found in the small intestine; therefore, gastrointestinal radiography and gastrointestinal endoscopy are the main diagnostic methods. With the development of endoscopic equipment, capsule endoscopy and enteroscopy have been useful for diagnosis. Pathologically, hamartomatous polyps are characterized by a hyperplastic mucosal layer and tree-like proliferation of the lamina muscularis mucosae. Affected individuals frequently have colorectal cancer, gastric cancer, and/or cancers of other organs (e.g., breast cancer, gynecologic cancer, and pancreatic cancer).

### 6.3.6 Treatment

Polypectomy is performed endoscopically for large polyps. Surgical treatment is required for intussusception and malignant tumors.

### 6.3.7 Prognosis

Adenoma presents in a hamartoma, which is associated with a risk of adenocarcinoma. Prognosis depends on the development of adenocarcinoma.

### 6.3.8 Recent Findings

If there is a family history, the presence of pigmented spots and testicular or ovarian tumors should be checked beginning at birth due to the high malignancy rate.

## 6.4 Cronkhite-Canada Syndrome

### 6.4.1 Disease Overview

Cronkhite-Canada syndrome (CCS) is a nonhereditary disorder of unknown etiology with gastrointestinal polyposis accompanied by ectodermal abnormalities, such as skin pigmentation, alopecia, and nail atrophy.

### 6.4.2 Pathophysiology

Symptoms of CCS include diarrhea, dysgeusia, and nutritional deficiency due to protein leakage from the gastrointestinal tract.

### 6.4.3 Epidemiology

The incidence of CCS is estimated to be 1/1,000,000. The disease develops in individuals in their 50 s and 60 s and is more common in males, and 70% of cases are reported from Japan.

### 6.4.4 Classification

The distribution of polyps varies from dense to scattered, with dense polyps being more common.

### 6.4.5 Symptoms

Frequent diarrhea is observed, and weight loss, abdominal pain, dysgeusia, and anorexia are seen. Alopecia, skin pigmentation, and nail atrophy are also common.

### 6.4.6 Clinical Examination

Hypoproteinemia, hypoalbuminemia, anemia, and electrolyte abnormalities are observed. Polyposis is found throughout the gastrointestinal tract, albeit rarely in the esophagus. Polyps of sessile to sub-pedunculated elevated lesions are densely present, and inflammatory changes in the intervening mucosa are observed. Pathologically, the lesions are nonneoplastic and are characterized by cystically dilated glands, hyperplasia, edema of the lamina propria, and inflammatory cell infiltration.

### 6.4.7 Treatment

An elemental diet or parenteral nutrition is administered to improve nutrition; if these strategies are ineffective, short-term administration of adrenocorticosteroids, 5-ASA (aminosalicylic acid), and antiplasmin agents may be effective.

### 6.4.8 Prognosis

The polyps shrink with treatment, and the prognosis is relatively good. Although the polyps themselves are not neoplastic, CCS is associated with a high risk of colorectal cancer or adenoma.

### 6.4.9 Recent Findings

This disease has been reported to be less common in the small intestine; however, advances in enteroscopy may lead to an increase in the reported incidence of CCS in the small intestine.

## 6.5 Cowden's Disease

### 6.5.1 Disease Overview

Cowden's disease is an autosomal dominant inherited disorder that presents with skin lesions such as small papules on the face, papillary changes in the oral mucosa, and keratotic papules at the ends of the extremities. This disease is characterized by the presence of hamartomatous polyposis throughout the gastrointestinal tract, including the esophagus, and is associated with an increased risk of several types of malignant tumors, including breast cancer and thyroid cancer.

### 6.5.2 Pathophysiology

Cowden's disease is caused by mutations in the tumor suppressor gene *PTEN* (phosphatase and tensin homolog deleted on chromosome 10) (80%) and is present in association with various malignancies, such as breast cancer and thyroid cancer, in >30% of cases.

### 6.5.3 Epidemiology

Cowden's disease is estimated to occur in 1/20,000 people.

### 6.5.4 Symptoms

The most common lesions are (1) multiple papules on the face, (2) keratotic papules at the ends of the extremities, (3) papillomas of the oral mucosa, (4) polyposis of the gastrointestinal tract, (5) hamartoma of multiple organs and various neoplastic lesions, and (6) familial or genetic development. Almost all patients present with skin lesions, and subjective symptoms are often observed depending on the development and progression of neoplastic lesions.

### 6.5.5 Clinical Examination

Multiple hamartomas occur throughout the gastrointestinal tract, and the disease is characterized by glycogenic acanthosis of the esophagus. Gastric lesions are observed from the gastric fundus to the pylorus, and in two-thirds of cases, multiple lesions are present in the small intestine, as well as many in the duodenum. In the colon, small elevated lesions tend to be observed in the descending colon, sigmoid colon, and rectum.

Skin lesions have multiple papules several millimeters in diameter, histologically presenting as trichilemmoma, multiple papillomas with small white elevations several millimeters in diameter in the oral mucosa, and verrucous keratotic papules at the ends of extremities. In addition, fibromatosis and cystic fibroma of the breast occur in 80% of female patients, and breast cancer is 2–5 times more common than in the general population. The incidence of thyroid cancer among patients with Cowden's disease is 3–10%, including follicular adenocarcinoma and papillary adenocarcinoma. Benign goiter develops in 70% of patients. In addition, complications such as ovarian cystoma, uterine myoma, renal cell carcinoma, meningioma, and schwannoma have been reported.

### 6.5.6 Treatment

While the polyps in individuals with Cowden's disease are not treatable, careful periodic examination for breast cancer and thyroid cancer should be performed.

### 6.5.7 Prognosis

The prognosis of individuals with Cowden's disease is influenced by the development of malignant tumors.

### 6.5.8 Recent Findings

Not all cases with inactivating germ cell mutations in the *PTEN* gene have a Cowden's disease phenotype; some have Bannayan-Riley-Ruvalcaba syndrome or Proteus syndrome phenotypes and are collectively referred to as *PTEN* hamartoma tumor syndrome.

## 6.6 Notes from Dentistry Perspective

Seiji Nakamura

Patients with gastrointestinal polyposis should be paid attention to the following possible oral symptoms.

### 6.6.1 Familial Adenomatosis of the Colon

Familial adenomatous colorectal disease may be associated with osteomas of the skull and jawbone; dental abnormalities such as unerupted teeth, supernumerary teeth, and odontomas; and soft tissue tumors such as fibromas. Gardner's syndrome, a subtype of the disease, is also well known, especially for the oral manifestations described above.

### 6.6.2 Peutz-Jeghers Syndrome

In Peutz-Jeghers syndrome, there may be multiple and punctate brown pigmentations on the lips and oral mucosa.

### 6.6.3 Cronkhite-Canada Syndrome

Cronkhite-Canada syndrome is also characterized by hyperpigmentation, mainly on the fingers with nail atrophy.

### 6.6.4 Cowden's Disease

Cowden's disease is characterized by the presence of papillomatosis of the oral mucosa and multiple small papules on the face and the distal of extremities.

Oral symptoms may lead to the diagnosis of polyposis of the gastrointestinal tract, and it is important to diagnose and treat the disease early, even though the frequency of canceration may vary. Dental treatment should be actively provided for the aforementioned dental abnormalities associated with familial adenomatous polyposis.

## References

1. Asaka M, Sugano K, Chiba T, editors. Gastroenterology (Shokakibyou-gaku). Tokyo: Nishimurashoten; 2013. p. 658–65. (in Japanese).
2. Yazaki Y, editor. Practice of internal medicine (Shin Rinsyo Naika-gaku). 10th ed. Tokyo: Igaku-shoin; 2020. p. 499–501. (in Japanese).
3. The Japanese Society of Gastroenterology, editor. Evidence-based clinical practice guidelines for peptic ulcer 2020. 3rd ed. Tokyo: Nanko-do; 2020.
4. Hammad TA, et al. Onset of acute myocardial infarction after use of non-steroidal anti-inflammatory drugs. Pharmacoepidemiol Drug Saf. 2008;17(4):315–21.
5. Sugano K, et al. Lansoprazole for secondary prevention of gastric or duodenal ulcers associated with long-term non-steroidal anti-inflammatory drug (NSAID) therapy: results of a prospective, multicenter, double-blind, randomized, double-dummy, active-controlled trial. J Gastroenterol. 2012;47(5):540–52.
6. Chan FK, et al. Management of patients on non-steroidal anti-inflammatory drugs: a clinical practice recommendation from the First International Working Party on Gastrointestinal and Cardiovascular Effects of Nonsteroidal Anti-inflammatory Drugs and Anti-platelet Agents. Am J Gastroenterol. 2008;103(11):2908–18.
7. Chaitanya B, et al. Rebamipide gargle in preventive management of chemo-radiotherapy induced oral mucositis. Oral Oncol. 2017;72:179–82.
8. Yatsuhashi H. Current trends in viral hepatitis - prevention of viral hepatitis. J Jpn Med Assoc. 2020;148(11):2185–9. (in Japanese).
9. Sasaki H. Recent advance in the treatment of chronic viral hepatitis. J Jpn Soc Intern Med. 2018;107(3):431–7. (in Japanese).
10. Garner JS, The Hospital Infection Control Practices Advisory Committee. Guidelines for isolation precautions in hospitals. Am J Infect Control. 1996;24:24–31.
11. CDC. Guidelines for infection control in dental health-care settings-2003. MMWR. 2003;52:1–61.
12. Japanese Association for Dental Science. Ministry of Health, Labour and Welfare Commissioned Project "Verification of nosocomial infection control in dental practice" guidelines for nosocomial infection control in general dental practice. 2nd ed. Tokyo: Japanese Association for Dental Science; 2019. (in Japanese). https://www.mhlw.go.jp/content/000510471.pdf. Accessed 30 Jan 2022.
13. Japan Dental Association, editor. Evidence-based practical manual for nosocomial infection control in general dentistry. (Evidence ni Motoduku Ippan Shika Shinryou niokeru Innai Kansen Taisaku Jissen Manual). Kyoto: Nagasueshoten; 2007. (in Japanese).
14. The Japan Society of Hepatology, Nishiguchi S, general editor. Cirrhosis of the liver by etiology 2018. (Kankouhen no Seiinbetsu Jittai 2018). Tokyo: Igakutosyo Shuppan; 2019. (in Japanese).
15. The Japan Society of Hepatology, editor. Medical guide for chronic hepatitis and cirrhosis 2019. (Mansei Kanen Kankouhen no Shinryo guide 2019). Tokyo: Bunko-do; 2019. (in Japanese).
16. The Japanese Society of Gastroenterology, editor. Guidelines for the treatment of liver cirrhosis 2015. (Kankouhen Shinryo Guideline 2015). Tokyo: Bunko-do; 2015. (in Japanese).
17. The Japanese Society of Gastroenterology, editor. Evidence-based Clinical Practice Guidelines for Gastroesophageal Reflux Disease (GERD) 2021. (Ishokudou Gyakuryu-shou (GERD) Shinryo Guideline 2021). 3rd edn. Tokyo: Nanko-do; 2015. (in Japanese).
18. Kinoshita Y. ed. New diagnosis and treatment ABC77/gastrointestinal 11 functional esophageal diseases - GERD and functional esophageal disorders - 2013 latest medical Supplement. (Atarashii Shindan to Chiryou no ABC77/Shoukaki 11, Kinousei Shokudou Shikkan – GERD to Kinousei Shokudou Shougai- 2013 nenn Saishin Igaku Bessatsu). Osakae: Saishin Igaku-sya; 2013. (in Japanese).
19. Kinoshita Y, et al. Future perspective of research and clinical practice in gastroesophageal reflux disease. (GERD no Kenkyuu to Shinryo niokeru Kongono Tenkai). J Jpn Soc Gastroenterol. 2017;114(10):1765–73. (in Japanese).
20. Kinoshita Y., et al., editors., Takigawa H, general editor. Practice of functional gastrointestinal care. (Kinousei Shoukakan Shinryou no Jissai). J Jpn Med Assoc. 2019;147(10). (in Japanese).
21. Miyawaki S, Lavigne GJ, et al. Association between sleep bruxism, swallowing-related laryngeal movement, and sleep positions. Sleep. 2003;26(4):461–5.
22. da Silveira MCM, Dalberto C, et al. Association between sleep bruxism and gastroesophageal reflux disease. J Prosthet Dent. 2013;110(5):349–55.
23. Ohmure H. Oikawa K et al.Influence of experimental esophageal acidification on sleep bruxism: a randomized trial J Dent Res. 90(5): 665–671. 2011.
24. Kanematsu K, Ohmure H, et al. Evaluation of therapeutic effects of proton pump inhibitor for sleep bruxism: a randomized, double-blind, placebo-controlled, crossover study. (Suiminji bruxism nitaisuru proton pump Sogaizai no Chiryoukoukano Kento: placebo Taisyou Nijyuouken crossover Hikakushiken). J

Jpn Soc Stomatognath Funct. 2014;21(1):38–9. (in Japanese).
25. The Japanese Society of Gastroenterology, editor. Evidence-based clinical practice guidelines for inflammatory bowel disease (IBD) 2020. 2nd edn. (Enshousei Cyoushikkann (IBD) Shindan Guideline 2020). Tokyo: Nanko-do; 2020. (in Japanese).
26. Health and Labor Sciences Research Grants, Intractable Disease Policy Research Project. Research on intractable inflammatory bowel disease (Suzuki group) in diagnostic criteria and treatment guidelines for ulcerative colitis and Crohn's disease, revised edn; 2020. (in Japanese). doc01.pdf (ibdjapan.org).
27. Omata M, Chiba T, editors. Gastroenterology for medical specialists. (Senmoni notameno Shoukakibyougaku). 3rd ed. Tokyo: Igakushoin; 2021. (in Japanese).
28. Ng SC, et al. Worldwide incidence and prevalence of inflammatory bowel disease in the 21st century: a systematic review of population-based studies. Lancet. 2017;390(10114):2769–78.
29. Thomas T, et al. Epidemiology, morbidity and mortality in Behçet's disease: a cohort study using The Health Improvement Network (THIN). Rheumatology. 2020;59:2785–95.
30. Skef W, et al. Gastrointestinal Bechet's disease: a review. World J Gastroenterol. 2015;21:3801–12.
31. Watanabe K, et al. The review of intestinal Behçet's disease: from epidemiology and diagnosis to future issue. Nihon Shokakibyo Gakkai Zasshi. 2022;119:217–26. (in Japanese).
32. Japanese Society for Cancer of the Colon and Rectum, editor. JSCCR guidelines 2020 for the clinical practice of hereditary colorectal cancer. (Idensei Daichougan Shinryo guideline). Tokyo: Kanehara Shuppan; 2020. (in Japanese).
33. Jenne DE, et al. Peutz-Jeghers syndrome is caused by mutations in a novel serine threonine kinase. Nat Genet. 1998;18:38–44.

# Malignant Diseases

# 11

Takeshi Terashima, Nobuaki Yagi, Shinya Maejima,
and Hiroyuki Harada

## 1 Lung Cancer/Bone Metastasis

Takeshi Terashima

### 1.1 Concept and Pathophysiology

Lung cancer is a malignant tumor arising from the epithelial tissue from the bronchi to the alveoli.

### 1.2 Epidemiology

Smoking and passive smoking are known to be reliable risk factors that increase the risk of developing lung cancer. In Japan, 112,000 people were diagnosed with lung cancer in 2014. The number of lung cancer-related deaths is the leading cause of death from malignancy, with approximately 74,000 death in 2017 in Japan.

T. Terashima
Department of Respiratory Medicine,
Tokyo Dental College, Ichikawa General Hospital,
Ichikawa, Chiba, Japan

N. Yagi
Department of Gastroenterology,
Asahi University Hospital, Gifu, Japan

S. Maejima (✉)
Department of Internal Medicine, Matsumoto Dental
University, Shiojiri, Nagano, Japan
e-mail: shinya.maejima@mdu.ac.jp

H. Harada
Graduate School of Medical and Dental Sciences,
Tokyo Medical and Dental University,
Bunkyo-ku, Tokyo, Japan

### 1.3 Classification

The major histologic types are adenocarcinoma, squamous cell carcinoma, neuroendocrine tumor, and large cell carcinoma. Neuroendocrine tumors include small cell carcinoma, large cell neuroendocrine carcinoma, and carcinoid tumor. The diagnosis is made based on not only morphological but also immunohistochemical characteristics (immunostaining patterns).

### 1.4 Symptoms

#### 1.4.1 Symptoms Caused by the Primary Tumor

Common symptoms include cough, sputum, wheezing, dyspnea, blood sputum, chest pain, anorexia, and general malaise. In some cases, the disease may be discovered by chance during a physical examination without any subjective symptoms.

#### 1.4.2 Symptoms Caused by Compression and Invasion of Adjacent Neighboring Organ

1. **Hoarse voice**: Lung cancer invasion or mediastinal lymph node metastasis causes recurrent


T. Chiba, H. Yamada (eds.), *Internal Medicine for Dental Treatments*,
https://doi.org/10.1007/978-981-99-3296-2_11

laryngeal nerve palsy, resulting in decreased vocal cord movement and hoarseness.
2. **Superior vena cava syndrome**: Edema of the face, neck, and upper limbs due to compression of the superior vena cava caused by tumor or lymph node metastasis.
3. **Pancoast tumor**: When a tumor in the apex of the lung invades the brachial plexus, it causes pain and dysesthesia from the shoulder to the upper limbs. If the tumor invades the cervical sympathetic nerves, it causes Horner's syndrome, which is characterized by unilateral pupil constriction, eyelid ptosis, enophthalmos, and hypohidrosis.
4. **Pleuritis carcinomatosa**: Exudative pleural effusion and sometimes bloody pleural effusion due to invasion or metastasis of cancer to the pleura. It causes thoracic back pain, respiratory failure, and dyspnea.

### 1.4.3 Symptoms Due to Distant Metastasis

The most frequent organs metastasized from lung cancer are the brain, bone, lung, liver, and adrenal gland, and symptoms of metastasis impair quality of life (QOL) and acitivities of dailiy living (ADL).

1. **Brain metastasis**: Lung cancer is the most common primary organ for metastatic brain tumors, accounting for more than 50%. It presents with symptoms of cranial nerve and intracranial hypertension. They include motor and sensory disturbances, headache, nausea, vomiting, convulsions, and disturbance of consciousness.
2. **Bone metastasis**: Bone metastasis occurs in 30–40% of patients with advanced lung cancer. The vertebrae are the most common site (42%), followed by the ribs (20%), pelvis (18%), and femur (6%). The prognosis for patients with bone metastases is approximately 8 months. Events that occur with the progression of bone metastases are called bone-related events. They include pathological fractures, spinal cord compression, worsening of bone lesions requiring radiation therapy or surgical treatment, and hypercalcemia. Bone-related events impair the QOL and ADL of cancer patients and affect their prognosis. The main symptom of bone metastasis is pain, and spinal cord compression caused by spinal metastasis can lead to hypoesthesia and muscle weakness. Simple X-ray (Fig. 11.1a), CT, and MRI (Fig. 11.1b) are useful for local diagnosis, while bone scintigraphy (Fig. 11.1c) and positron emission tomography (PET)/CT (Fig. 11.1d) are useful for systemic evaluation.

Radiotherapy is effective in relieving pain. Zoledronic acid, a bisphosphonate, and denosumab, an anti-receptor activator of NF-κB ligand (RANKL) antibody, are recommended to reduce the incidence of bone-related events. The most important adverse events associated with bisphosphonates and denosumab are osteonecrosis of the jaw and renal dysfunction. Denosumab may cause hypocalcemia, and it is recommended that calcium and vitamin D be supplemented and that serum calcium levels be measured regularly.

## 1.5 Clinical Examination and Diagnosis

When a tumor is suspected by chest X-ray (Fig. 11.2a), a chest CT scan (Fig. 11.2b) is useful to differentiate the tumor from other diseases and to determine the location, character, and range of the shadow.

For definitive diagnosis, pathological examination of specimens obtained by sputum, bronchoscopy, CT-guided lung biopsy, lymph node biopsy, pleurodesis, and thoracoscopic lung biopsy is performed.

The clinical stage is determined based on the TNM classification, where T indicates tumor: size and invasion of the primary tumor; N indicates lymph node: lymph node metastasis; and M indicates distant metastasis. For staging, contrast-enhanced CT of the chest and abdomen, contrast-enhanced MRI of the head, bone scintigraphy, and PET are performed. The treatment strategy is determined by histology, stage, and performance status. Tumor markers are useful as diagnostic aids and indicators of therapeutic efficacy. CEA is used for adenocarcinoma, SCC, and CYFRA for squamous cell carcinoma, and pro-GRP and NSE for small-cell lung cancer.

## 1.6 Treatment

### 1.6.1 Small-Cell Lung Cancer

Small-cell lung cancer is classified as limited disease (LD) and extensive disease (ED). LD is when the lesion is confined to the unilateral thorax, ipsilateral hilar lymph nodes, bilateral supraclavicular lymph nodes, or mediastinal lymph nodes, while ED is when malignant pleural effusion is present or when the lesion extends beyond LD. In LD, chemotherapy and radical thoracic radiotherapy are used simultaneously. Chemotherapy is the standard of care in ED.

### 1.6.2 Non-small Cell Lung Cancer

It includes adenocarcinoma and squamous cell carcinoma. Surgery is recommended as standard treatment for stage I, II, and IIIA tumors, in which the primary tumor has not invaded surrounding organs and lymph node metastasis is limited to the ipsilateral hilum.

Postoperative chemotherapy may also be used. Concurrent chemoradiotherapy is recommended for stage III patients with mediastinal lymph node metastasis. In recent years, maintenance therapy with immune checkpoint inhibi-

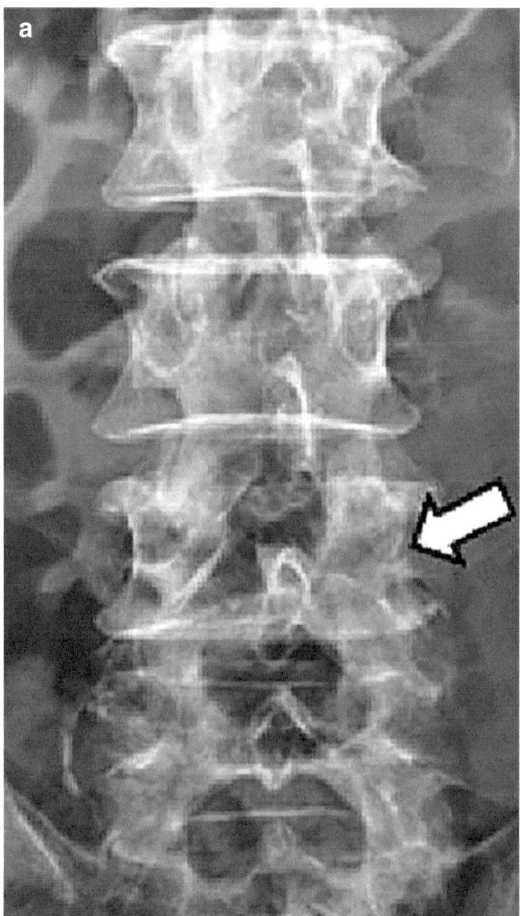


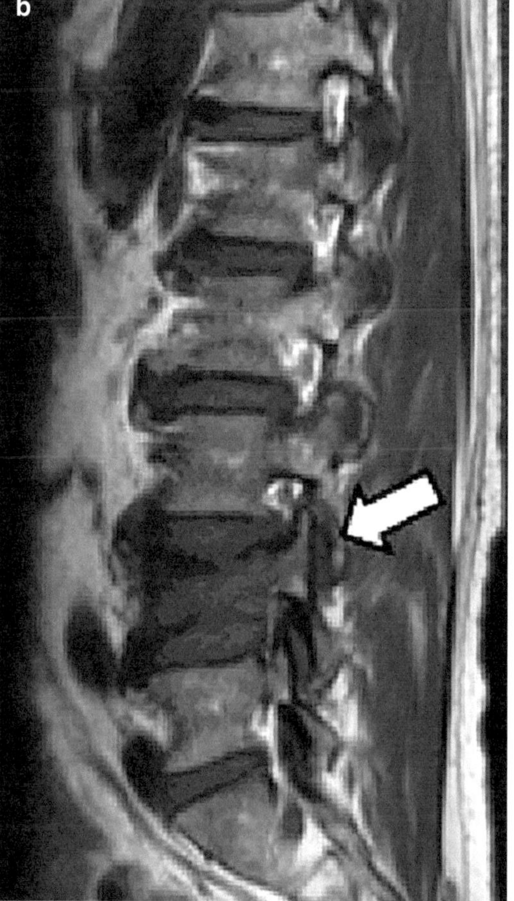


**Fig. 11.1** (**a**) Simple X-ray (frontal view) shows a winking owl sign (arrow) on the left side of the fourth lumbar vertebra. (**b**) MRI T1-weighted image shows a hypointense mass in the fourth lumbar vertebra with involvement of the vertebral arch (arrow). (**c**) Bone scintigraphy shows an increased uptake (arrow) in the fourth lumbar vertebra. (**d**) PET/CT showed an increased uptake (arrow) in the fourth lumbar vertebra in red color, extending to the vertebral arch

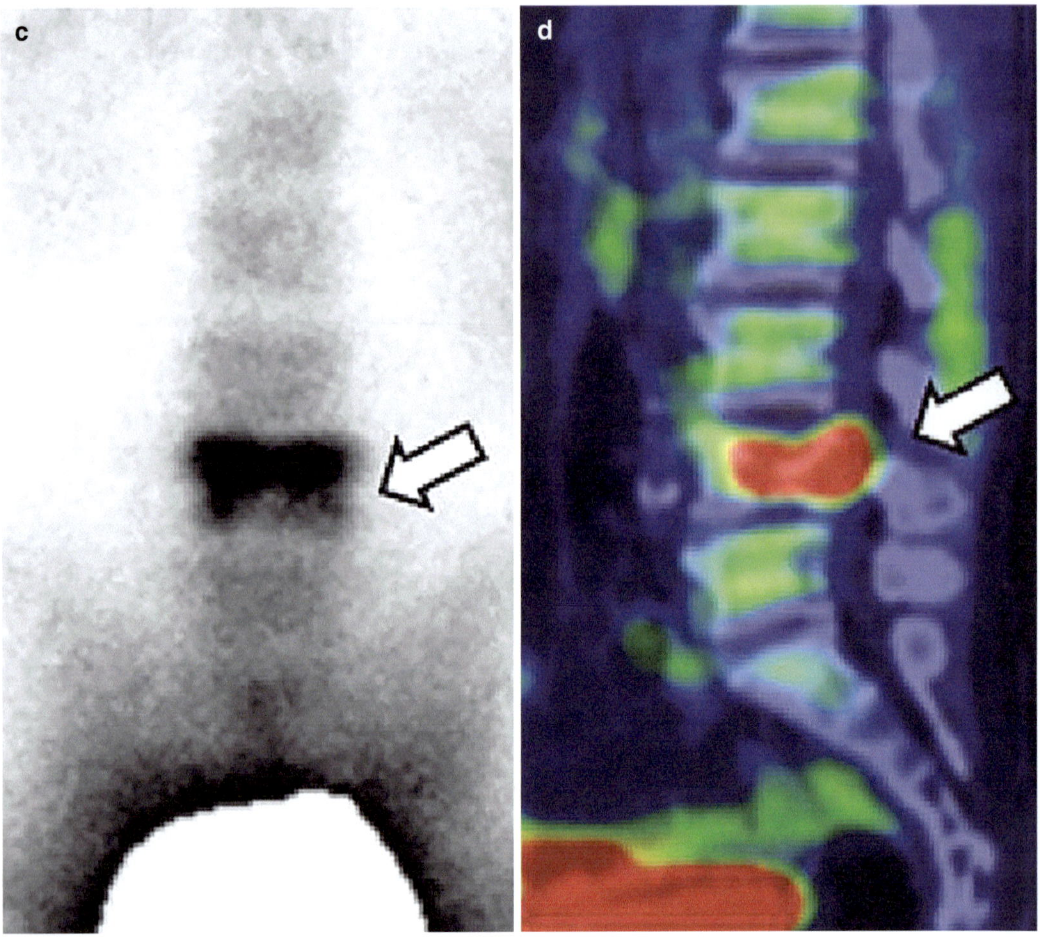

**Fig. 11.1** (continued)

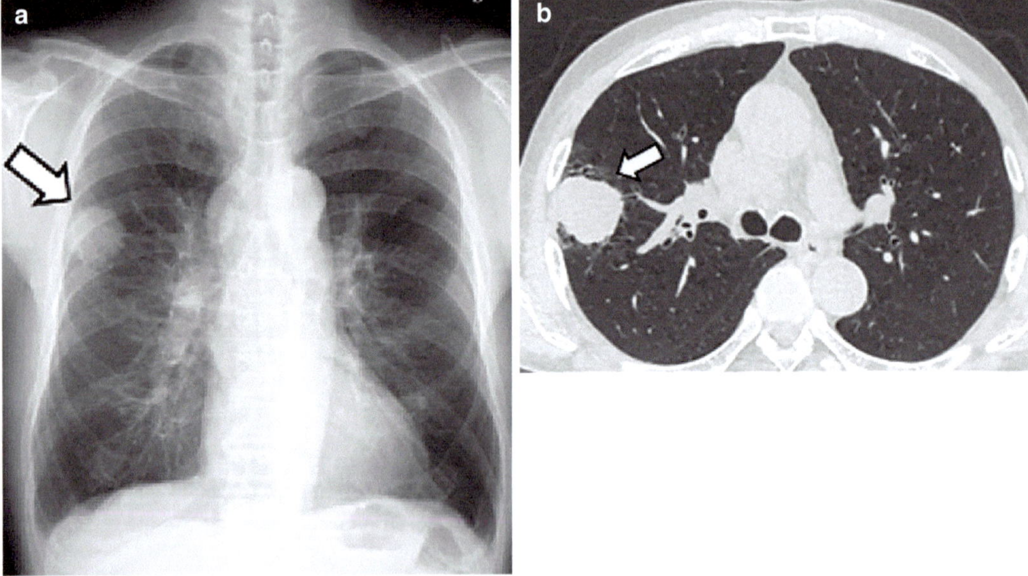


**Fig. 11.2** (**a**) Simple chest X-ray shows a mass lesion (arrow) in the peripheral right upper lung field. (**b**) Chest CT shows a mass lesion (arrow) with irregular margins in the right upper lobe

tors has been shown to be effective in patients who responded to concurrent chemoradiotherapy. Drug therapy is recommended for stage IV patients with malignant pleural effusion or distant metastasis. In the past, chemotherapy with cytotoxic drugs was the mainstay of treatment, but molecular-targeted therapy is now recommended for patients with positive driver gene mutations such as EGFR mutation, ALK gene translocation, ROS1 rearrangements, and BRAF gene mutation. In addition, immune checkpoint inhibitors are also used as immunotherapy.

### 1.7 Prognosis

The 5-year survival rates by clinical stage are approximately 80% for stages I and II, 25% for stage III, and 5% for stage IV.

### 1.8 Recent Findings

Personalized therapy using biomarkers is advancing. Biomarkers are laboratory findings that are useful for predicting the effect of treatment and selecting a treatment method. Cancer tissues and plasma are used as specimens.

One is a driver gene, which is defined as one whose mutations play a pivotal role in the development and progression of cancer. In lung cancer, EGFR gene mutation, K-ras, ALK gene translocation, MET amplification/overexpression, HER2 overexpression, ROS1 rearrangements, and BRAF gene mutation are known. In the past, each of these genes was tested individually, but multiplex genetic testing, which allows simultaneous testing of multiple genes, has become possible. In particular, cancer-related gene testing using next-generation sequencers is becoming possible.

The other is the emergence of immunotherapy. Surgery, irradiation, and chemotherapy were the mainstays of treatment in the past, but in recent years, immunotherapy has been added to them. Although cancer cells are originally recognized as non-self by the immune system and eliminated, the mechanism by which cancer cells escape from the surveillance of the immune system and proliferate and progress has been elucidated. The major immunosuppressive factors are PD-1, PD-L1, and CTLA-4, which are called immune checkpoints. Immune checkpoint inhibitors, such as anti-PD-1, anti-PD-L1, and anti-CTLA-4 antibodies, have been introduced to selectively inhibit these factors. The expression rate of PD-L1 in cancer tissues and the tumor mutation burden, which is an indicator of the number of gene mutations in cancer tissues, are expected to be biomarkers for predicting the response of immune checkpoint inhibitors.

## 2 Gastric Cancer

Nobuaki Yagi

### 2.1 Concept

Gastric cancer is defined as a malignant tumor of gastric mucosal epithelial origin. Gastric cancer accounts for more than 90% of all gastric malignancies and 15% of all cancers, and is the second most common carcinoma in men and the fourth most common in women (2017). It is classified into early gastric cancer and advanced gastric cancer according to the depth of the cancer lesion. In Japan, about 130,000 people (90,000 men and 40,000 women) are affected and about 45,000 people (30,000 men and 15,000 women) die annually. The age-adjusted mortality rate by sex is decreasing in both sexes, and the age-adjusted morbidity rate remains unchanged in males and is decreasing in females [1].

### 2.2 Pathophysiology

Early gastric cancer is characterized by a cancerous lesion localizing on the mucosa (m) or submucosa (sm), with or without lymph node metastasis. Advanced gastric cancer is characterized by invasion of the muscularis propria (mp), subserosa (ss), and serosa (se). The morphological type of gastric cancer is shown in Fig. 11.3 [2]. Histologically, gastric cancer can be divided into two types: differentiated gastric cancer with gland duct formation and undifferentiated gastric cancer with poor gland duct formation.

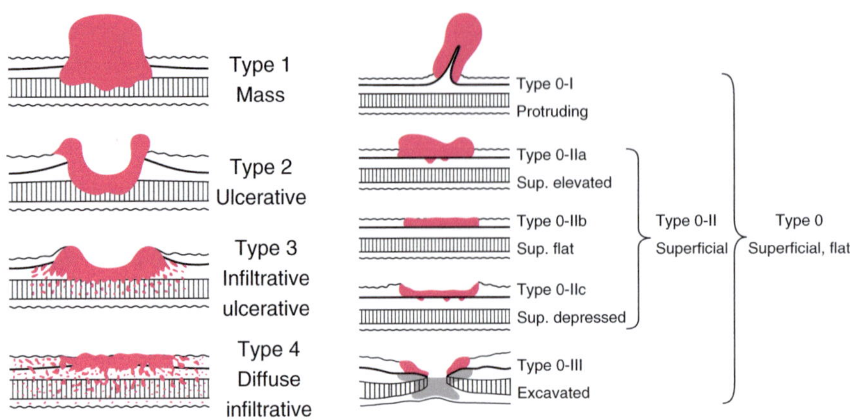


**Fig. 11.3** Macroscopic classification of gastric cancer. (Modified from [2])

Differentiated gastric cancer tends to occur in atrophic gastric mucosa with intestinal metaplasia, and is more common in elderly patients associated with *Helicobacter pylori* (*H. pylori*) infection. On the other hand, undifferentiated gastric cancer originates from the gastric mucosa with less atrophic changes and is more common in younger patients. *H. pylori* infection is considered to be a major cause of gastric cancer regardless of differentiated or undifferentiated type, and eradication therapy for chronic gastritis was covered by insurance in 2013 as a first step toward destruction of gastric cancer and is widely conducted. In a study of post-endoscopic resection of early gastric cancer, successful eradication was reported to reduce the risk of gastric cancer by about one-third.

## 2.3 Symptoms

Early stage gastric cancer without ulceration is often asymptomatic, while cases with ulceration and advanced cancer often present with symptoms such as epigastric pain, gastric discomfort, heartburn, nausea, anorexia, and weight loss. Anemia, hematemesis, and melena caused by bleeding from these lesions may be the trigger for detection. In addition, when advanced gastric cancer occurs in the cardia or pyloric region, patients often suffer from obstruction. Metastasis of advanced gastric cancer may cause enlargement of superficial lymph nodes (especially in the left supraclavicular node, called Virchow's node metastasis), Douglas' pouch metastasis, ovarian metastasis (Krukenberg tumor), and carcinomatous peritonitis.

## 2.4 Diagnosis

The presence of gastric cancer is diagnosed by X-ray examination, endoscopy, and biopsy specimens. Endoscopic images of early gastric cancer (Figs. 11.4 and 11.5) and advanced gastric cancer (Fig. 11.6) are shown. Next, endoscopic ultrasonography (EUS), computed tomography (CT), magnetic resonance imaging (MRI), and positron emission tomography (PET) are performed to investigate the depth of the cancer, invasion to organs adjacent to the stomach such as the pancreas, liver, and intestines, and metastasis to distant organs and lymph nodes in order to diagnose the degree of cancer progression (stage), which is important for determining the therapeutic strategy. Tumor markers may also be useful in detecting tumors and judgment of therapeutic effect.

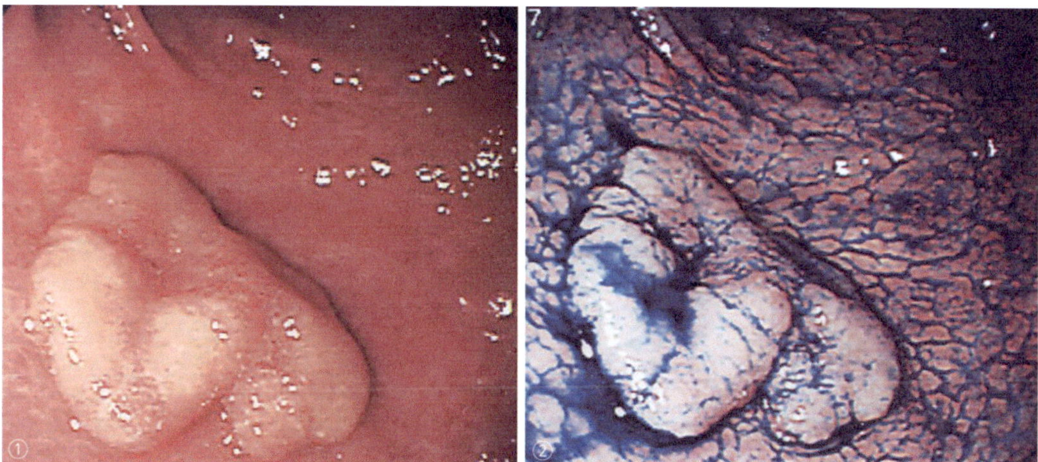

**Fig. 11.4** Early gastric cancer 0-IIa (slightly elevated), size in 30 mm, greater curvature of the antrum. ① White light observation. ② Chromoendoscopy with indigo carmine

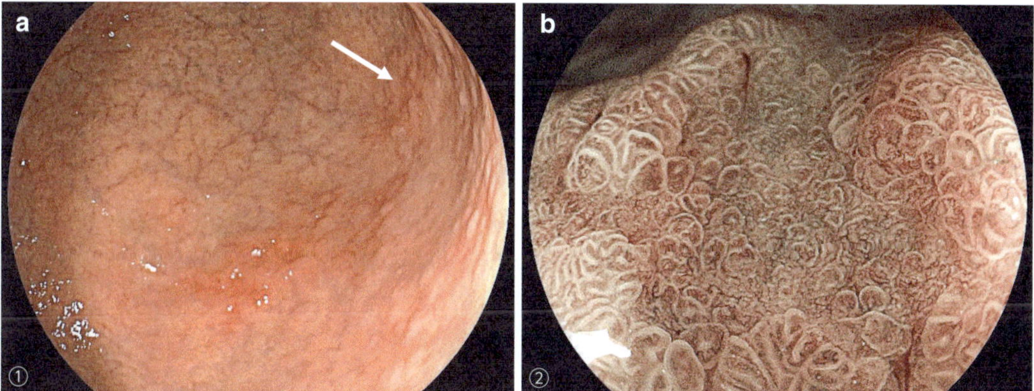

**Fig. 11.5** Early gastric cancer 0-IIc (slightly depressed), size in 45 mm, greater curvature of posterior wall in the lower body. (**a**) White light observation: A reddish depression was observed in the lower body. A biopsy specimen revealed carcinoma of the posterior wall (white arrow). (**b**) Magnified BLI observation. The reddish depression on the greater curvature of the posterior wall in the lower body shows irregular micro surface pattern and irregular micro vascular pattern with demarcation line

## 2.5 Prevention and Screening

In a gastric cancer epidemiological study targeting Japanese people, smoking cessation, moderate alcohol consumption, well-balanced diet, physical activity, proper body shape, and prevention of infection are effective in preventing cancer in general. The most common causes of gastric cancer are *H. pylori* infection and smoking. In addition, high-salt foods have also been reported to raise the risk of developing gastric cancer [3].

The purpose of cancer screening is to reduce deaths from cancer by early detection and appropriate treatment. In Japan, screening methods are defined in the "Guidelines for Priority Health

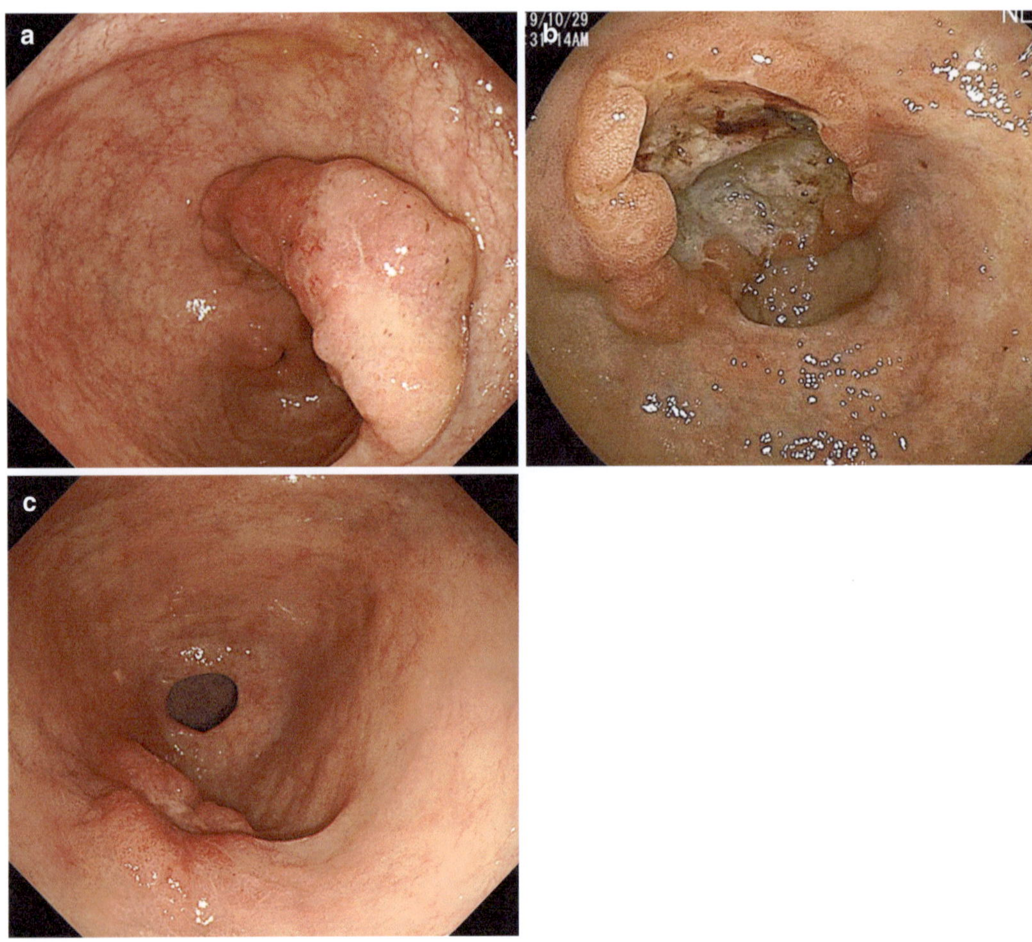

**Fig. 11.6** Advanced gastric cancer type 1, type 2, and type 3, surgical cases. (**a**) White light observation. Type 1 of the posterior wall of the antrum (Protruded type). (**b**) White light observation. Type 2 of the lesser curvature in the antrum (Ulcered carcinomas with sharp and raised margins type). (**c**) White light observation. Type 3 of the greater curvature in the antrum (Ulcered carcinomas without define limits type)

Education and Cancer Screening for Cancer Prevention (partially revised in 2016)" of the Ministry of Health, Labour and Welfare. The most effective screening methods for gastric cancer are "gastric X-ray examination" or "gastric endoscopy" in addition to "interview" for both men and women aged 50 years or older. The examinations should be carried out once every 2 years, but if there are symptoms of concern in between, it is important to visit a medical institution without waiting for the next screening [4].

## 2.6 Treatment

The treatment method is determined by discussing with the patients and their family based on the clinical stage of the cancer and the patient's general condition. Table 11.1 shows the clinical stage classification [2]. Treatment methods for gastric cancer include endoscopic therapy, surgery, and drug therapy.

Endoscopic resection is recommended for early-stage gastric cancer that is presumed to be

**Table 11** Clinical stage classification

| | MO | | M1 |
|---|---|---|---|
| | NO | N (+) | Any N |
| T1 (M, SM)/T2 (MP) | I | II A | IV B |
| T3 (SS)/T4a (SE) | II B | III | |
| T4b (S1) | IV A | | |

Clinical classification (cTNM, cStage: comprehensive diagnosis based on imaging, review laparoscopic or laparotomy findings)
(Reproduced with permission from [2])

free of lymph node metastasis. Endoscopic resection is performed by endoscopic mucosal resection (EMR) and endoscopic submucosal dissection (ESD). Recently, absolute indications for EMR/ESD have been defined as "UL0 intramucosal carcinoma (cT1a) ≤2 cm in length and differentiated carcinoma," and absolute indications for ESD have been defined as "(1) UL0 cT1a >2 cm in length and differentiated carcinoma; (2) UL1 cT1a ≤3 cm in length and differentiated carcinoma; and (3) UL0 cT1a ≤2 cm in length and undifferentiated carcinoma" [5]. Endoscopic resection is a minimally invasive and low-risk treatment method for the elderly and inoperable patients, and gastric cancer is a field in which early detection and early treatment have led to dramatic advances in treatment outcomes.

In advanced gastric cancer or the part of early gastric cancer that can be surgically resected, total gastrectomy, pyloric gastrectomy, pylorus-preserving gastrectomy, and ventrolateral gastrectomy are performed by laparotomy or laparoscopy. In the surgery, part or all of the lesion and the stomach are removed, and at the same time, lymph node dissection around the stomach and gastrointestinal reconstruction are performed. The major complications of surgery include dysraphia, pancreatic juice leakage, pulmonary embolization, etc.

When distant metastasis or local progression of gastric cancer makes curative resection difficult, anti-cancer drug therapy may be used. There are two main types of drug therapy: chemotherapy for advanced or recurrent gastric cancer that is difficult to remove by surgery and adjuvant chemotherapy for the prevention of recurrence. Gastric cancer can be treated with cytotoxic anticancer agents, molecular targeted agents, and immune checkpoint inhibitors. Because of the wide variety of side effects, patients should be treated by specialists with informed consent.

## 3 Colorectal Cancer [6–9]

Shinya Maejima

### 3.1 Concept

The colon is a gastrointestinal tract that reabsorbs water and electrolytes (minerals) and expels nondigestible food and wastes, and consists of the cecum, colon (ascending, transverse, descending, and sigmoid), and rectum. Malignant tumors occurring in the colon are called colorectal carcinomas, which are pathologically often highly differentiated adenocarcinomas.

### 3.2 Pathophysiology

It is associated with genetic and environmental factors. Many colorectal cancers develop from benign adenomas that undergo malignant transformation. Colorectal cancers are formed from the multistep accumulation of many genetic abnormalities, including activation of oncogenes and inactivation of tumor suppressor genes and mismatch repair genes. Inherited tumors include the APC gene in familial adenomatous polyposis and the mismatch repair gene in Lynch syndrome,[1] which causes microsatellite instability due to the accumulation of errors in repeated base sequences during DNA replication. Environmental factors such as diet, alcohol consumption, physical inactivity, obesity, and smoking are also considered to be important.

[1] Hereditary diseases that cause various malignant tumors such as colorectal cancer, uterine cancer, ovarian cancer, gastric cancer, renal pelvis and ureteral cancer, and brain tumor at a young age.

### 3.3 Epidemiology

The number of colorectal cancers in Japan continues to increase due to the aging of the population and changes in dietary habits. In terms of the number of cancer cases by site (2014), colorectal cancer is the third most common cancer in men after stomach and lung cancer, the second most common cancer in women after breast cancer, and the most common cancer in men and women combined. In terms of the number of cancer deaths (2017), it ranks first in women, third in men, and second in the total number of men and women after lung cancer.

### 3.4 Categories

In Japan, the colorectal cancer treatment rules are used [6]. Gross morphological classification is from type 0 to type 5 (Fig. 11.7, type 5 is unclassifiable). The superficial type (type 0), in which the depth of cancer invasion into the colon wall (depth) is limited to the mucosa and submucosa, is further divided into elevated and superficial types. Early-stage cancers are those whose depth is limited to the mucosa or submucosa, regardless of the presence or absence of lymph node metastasis. In advanced cancer, the ulcer-localized type (type 2) is common. The spread of cancer (degree of progression) is expressed by stage (staging) classification. The stage is determined by the depth of the colon wall and the presence or absence of lymph node metastasis or distant metastasis to other organs such as the liver or peritoneum. Accurate prediction of the stage before treatment is very important in determining the treatment strategy. There are two types of stage classification: the clinical stage, which is predicted by various imaging diagnoses before treatment, and the pathological stage, which is predicted after therapeutic resection. The final stage is the pathological stage, which determines whether additional adjuvant therapy is required.

### 3.5 Symptoms

There are no specific symptoms, and they vary according to the degree of cancer progression and the affected site. In particular, early stage cancers are often asymptomatic, regardless of the site. In right-sided colorectal carcinoma, symptoms do not appear until the disease progresses and worsens, because the intestinal contents are fluid and do not form a fecal mass. On the left side, transit disturbances such as bloody stool and constipation are more likely to occur. Chronic subclinical bleeding from the tumor may be detected during the examination for anemia.

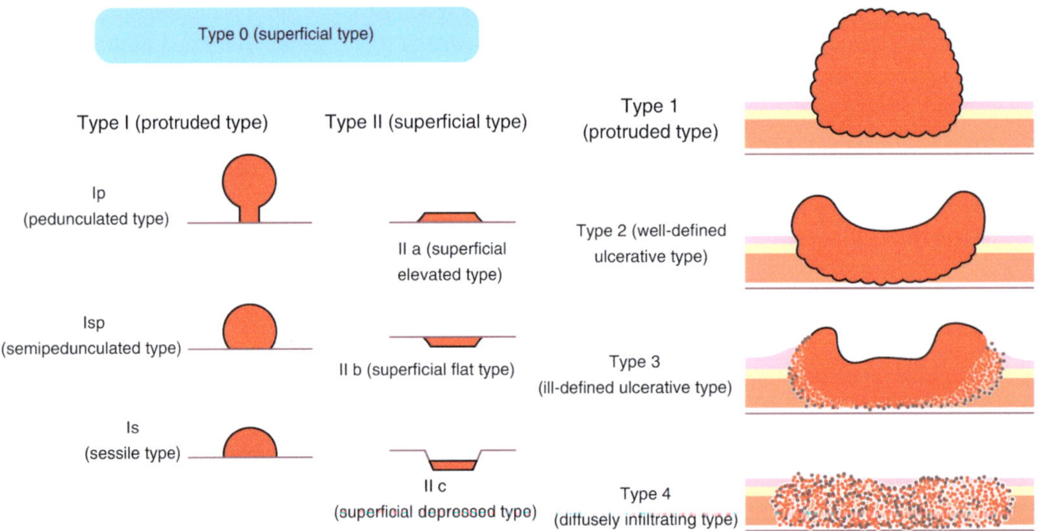


**Fig. 11.7** Macroscopic classification of colorectal cancer [6]

## 3.6 Clinical Examinations

### 3.6.1 Fecal Occult Blood Test

It is a screening test for the detection of colorectal cancer and is performed by collecting a small amount of stool during defecation. Early detection and treatment of colorectal cancer, as well as detection and resection of adenomas, is expected to reduce the incidence of colorectal cancer and has been demonstrated to reduce the risk of death.

### 3.6.2 Colonoscopy

An endoscope is inserted through the anus and observed from the inside. Although pretreatment with an intestinal cleaning is required, pathological diagnosis can be made not only by diagnosing the presence of the lesion but also by biopsy under direct vision. It is also excellent for qualitative diagnosis, such as the depth of the lesion, and the possibility of endoscopic treatment can be examined (Fig. 11.8).

IIa+Is

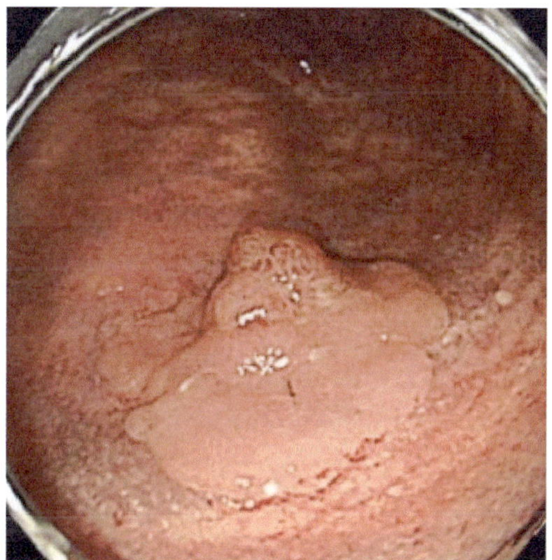

Small type 2 colorectal cancer

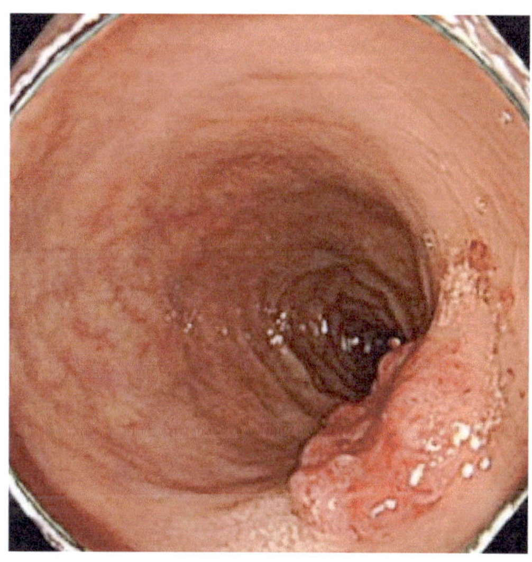

Type 2 colorectal cancer occupying 1/3 of the septa cavity

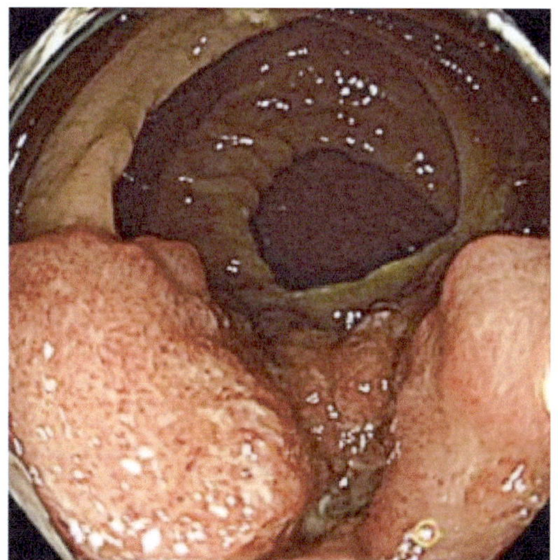

Type 2 colorectal cancer with stenosis of the duct cavity (Isp is also seen in the lower right)

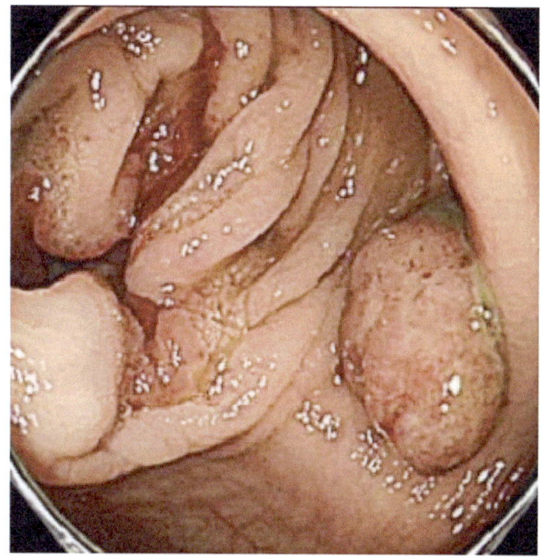

**Fig. 11.8** Endoscopic observation of colorectal cancer

### 3.6.3 Enterography

Contrast medium and air are injected through the anus, and the deformation of the colon is radiographed. With the development of endoscopy, the number of procedures is decreasing. The entire image and position of the colon can be confirmed (Fig. 11.9).

### 3.6.4 CT, MRI, PET Scan

Localized diagnosis, distant metastasis to other organs such as liver, and lymph node metastasis can be searched.

### 3.6.5 Capsule Endoscopy, CT Colonography

Capsule endoscopy and computed tomographic colonography have been developed as new examination methods.

In capsule endoscopy, a swallowed capsule is advanced to the anus by peristalsis, and the gastrointestinal tract is observed under physiological conditions during transit. The advantage of capsule endoscopy is that it is painless.

In addition, CT colonography, which is a virtual endoscope reconstructed from CT images, is said to have almost the same diagnostic ability as colonoscopy.

### 3.6.6 Blood Test

Carcinoembryonic antigen (CEA) is measured as a tumor marker. However, the positivity rate is not high and increases in proportion to the stage of the disease. It is recommended as an adjunct to postoperative monitoring.

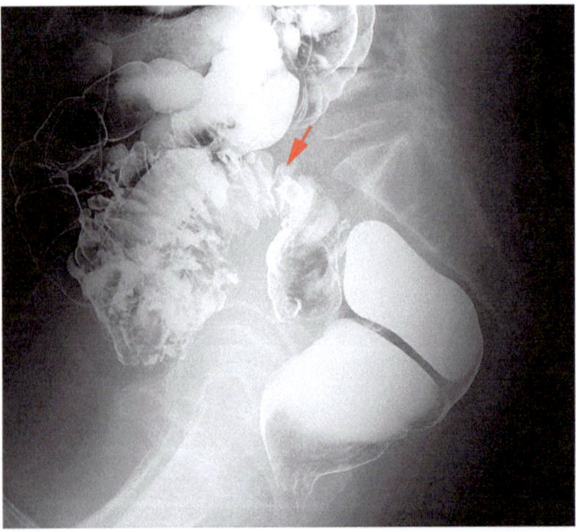

**Fig. 11.9** Stenosis due to colorectal cancer (apple core sign) at the transition of rectosigmoid colon

## 3.7 Treatment

The treatment includes endoscopic therapy, surgical treatment, chemotherapy, and radiotherapy. Based on the results of various examinations, the degree of progression (stage classification) is first determined, and then the treatment method is selected.

Endoscopic treatment is indicated for intramucosal carcinoma or mildly invasive carcinoma of the submucosa, which has little possibility of lymph node metastasis (Fig. 11.10). Technological advances have made it possible to remove lesions larger than 2 cm by endoscopic submucosal dissection (ESD).

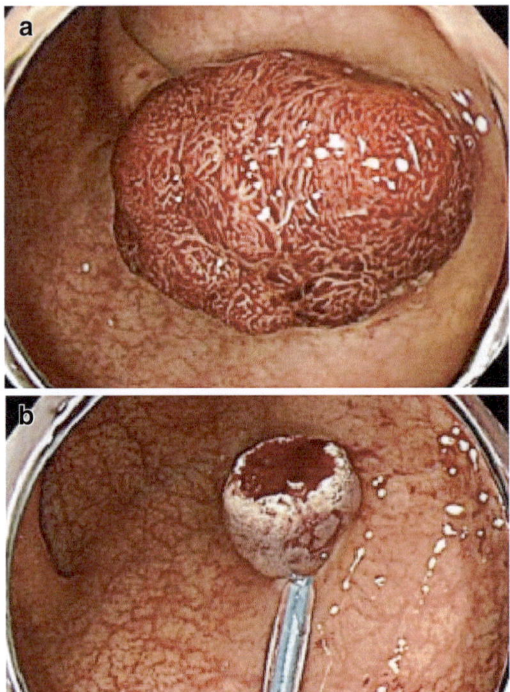


**Fig. 11.10** (**a**) 0-Ip, cancer in adenoma. (**b**) Resection with endoscopic ligation. The photograph shows the indwelling snare after resection

Surgical treatment consists of intestinal resection and lymph node dissection of those lymph nodes where the cancer may have spread. In principle, resection of the cancer lesion is performed, and even in stage IV patients with distant metastases, if resection of the primary lesion is possible, resection of the primary lesion and metastases should be considered.

Chemotherapy consists of postoperative adjuvant therapy to prevent recurrence in patients with resectable disease and systemic chemotherapy to prolong life and alleviate symptoms in patients with unresectable disease. In stage III, oral anticancer agents are administered for about 6 months as adjuvant therapy. In stage IV, molecular targeted agents are used according to the presence or absence of RAS mutation, and the patients are treated with other agents.

### 3.8 Prognosis

Colorectal cancer has a high curative ratio, and more than 90% of patients can be cured if detected early. The treatment of colorectal cancer in advanced, unresectable patients has been greatly improved by the development of various drugs and therapies. The survival time has been remarkably extended.

### 3.9 Recent Findings

Chemotherapy, in particular, has evolved in complexity with the development of novel anticancer agents, molecularly targeted therapies, and immune checkpoint inhibitors. Genetic testing has become inevitable not only for risk assessment of hereditary tumors but also for treatment decisions in chemotherapy using molecularly targeted agents and immune checkpoint inhibitors corresponding to the genetic mutations.

## 4 Perioperative Period

Hiroyuki Harada

### 4.1 Check the Stage of the Cancer

Malignant tumors are broadly classified into carcinomas (epithelial tumors), sarcomas (nonepithelial tumors), and others (hematologic neoplasm, myeloid tumors, malignant melanoma, etc). Staging is based on (T) the size of the local tumor, (N) the status of the involved lymph nodes, and (M) the presence or absence of distant metastases. Table 11.2 and Fig. 11.11 show the TNM classification (Union for International Cancer Control: UICC 8th edition, 2017) [10] and stage classification of lip and oral cancer. The TNM classification and the stage classification of

**Table 11.2** TNM classification of oral cancer and oral cavity cancer

| **T: Primary tumor** |
|---|
| TX: Primary tumor cannot be assessed |
| T0: No evidence of primary tumor |
| Tis: Epithelial carcinoma |
| T1: Tumor with a maximum diameter of 2 cm or less and a depth of 5 mm or less |
| T2: Tumors with a maximum diameter of 2 cm or less and a depth of more than 5 mm, or tumors with a maximum diameter of more than 2 cm but less than 4 cm and a depth of less than 10 mm |
| T3: Tumor with a maximum diameter greater than 2 cm but less than 4 cm and a depth greater than 10 mm, or a tumor with a maximum diameter greater than 4 cm and a depth less than 10 mm |
| T4a (lip): Tumor penetrating the cortical bone of the mandible, inferior alveolar nerve, floor of mouth, or skin (of the muzzle or external nose)[a] |
| T4a (oral cavity): Tumors with a maximum diameter greater than 4 cm and a depth greater than 10 mm, or tumors that penetrate the bony cortex of the mandible or maxilla or invade the maxillary sinus, or tumors that invade the facial skin[a] |
| T4b (lip and oral cavity): Tumor invading the masticatory muscle gap, pterygium, or skull base, or tumor encircling the internal carotid artery circumferentially |

(continued)

**Table 11.2** (continued)

| N: regional lymph node |
|---|
| NX: Unable to assess regional lymph node metastasis |
| N0: No regional lymph node metastasis |
| N1: Ipsilateral solitary lymph node metastasis with a maximum diameter of less than 3 cm and no extranodal invasion |
| N2: Transition described below: |
| N2a: Single ipsilateral lymph node metastasis with a maximum diameter greater than 3 cm but less than 6 cm and no extranodal invasion |
| N2b: Multiple ipsilateral lymph node metastases with a maximum diameter of 6 cm or less and no extranodal invasion |
| N2c: Bilateral or contralateral lymph node metastases with a maximum diameter of 6 cm or less and no extranodal invasion |
| N3a: Lymph node metastasis with a maximum diameter greater than 6 cm and no extranodal invasion |
| N3b: Single or multiple lymph node metastases with clinical extranodal involvement[b] |

| M: Distant metastasis |
|---|
| M0: No distant metastasis |
| M1: With distant metastasis |

(Reproduced with permission from [10])

[a] Cases in which the primary lesion is gingival and there is superficial erosion of bone and alveolus only are not considered T4a

[b] It is classified as a clinical extranodal invasion if there is skin involvement or soft tissue involvement with strong adherence or union to underlying muscle or adjacent structures, or if there are clinical signs of nerve involvement. The median lymph node is the ipsilateral lymph node

oral cancer are used to determine the treatment strategy and to predict the prognosis.

## 4.2 Confirmation of Treatment Plan

The treatment of malignant tumors can be broadly divided into surgical therapy, radiation therapy, and drug therapy. In advanced cases, multidisciplinary treatment is often performed by combining these methods.

## 4.3 Oral Environment

It is very important to maintain the oral environment during the perioperative period, not only for the performance of surgery but also for the prevention of postoperative complications.

During intubation for general anesthesia, preoperative oral treatment is necessary because severe carious teeth and periodontitis can cause tooth prolapse and fracture fragments to enter the airway. Postoperative periodontal cleaning and extraction of carious teeth and severe periodontitis are important because the patient often suffers from pneumonia and infection.

## 4.4 Radiation Therapy

Radiotherapy is classified into two types: interstitial irradiation, in which a small radiation source is inserted into the primary lesion (brachytherapy), and external irradiation. External irradiation includes electron beams, X-rays, gamma rays, proton beams, and heavy particle beams, and is used depending on the primary site, the condition of the patient, and the presence or absence of concomitant chemotherapy.

Because mucositis and dermatitis occur frequently as adverse events, management of these conditions is necessary (Figs. 11.12 and 11.13). For severe mucositis, patients should be advised to limit intake of irritants and avoid mechanical cleaning with toothpaste or a hard toothbrush. Relatively nonirritating gargles such as sodium azulene sulfonate hydrate are recommended. Ointments containing antibacterial or anti-inflammatory agents are effective against dermatitis. Other complications include osteonecrosis, xerostomia due to salivary gland damage, and radiation-induced cancer.

## 4.5 Drug Therapy

Drug therapy for cancer often includes cell-killing anticancer agents, molecularly targeted agents, and immunotherapy. The National Cancer Institute (NCI)-Common Terminology Criteria for Adverse Events (CTCAE) [11] is the standard method for evaluating adverse events, which are classified from grades 1 to 5, ranging from mild to fatal. The most common adverse events are gastrointestinal disorders, myelosuppression, pulmonary toxicity, nephrotoxicity, hepatotoxicity, cardiotoxicity, and mucositis. It is necessary to evaluate and control these adverse events.

| | N0 | N1 | N2 | N3 | M1 |
|---|---|---|---|---|---|
| Tis | 0 | | | | |
| T1 | I | III | IVA | IVB | IVC |
| T2 | II | III | IVA | IVB | IVC |
| T3 | III | III | IVA | IVB | IVC |
| T4a | IVA | IVA | IVA | IVB | IVC |
| T4b | IVB | IVB | IVB | IVB | IVC |

**Fig. 11.11** Chart for a disease stage

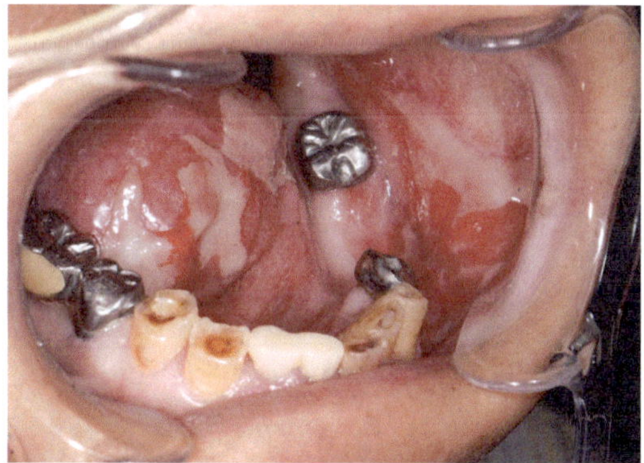

**Fig. 11.12** A patient underwent 50 Gy of radiotherapy after tongue cancer surgery. Mucositis with hemorrhage was observed on the left cheek mucosa and tongue

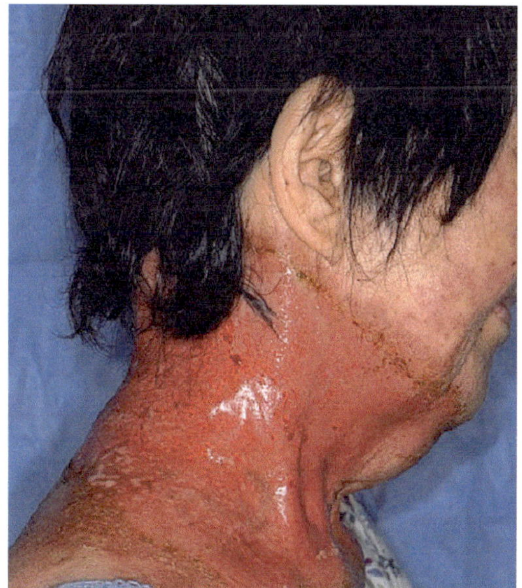

**Fig. 11.13** A patient underwent external beam radiation therapy of 50 Gy to the neck (with cetuximab). Severe erythema and hemorrhage were observed in the right side of the neck

## 4.6 Susceptibility to Infection

Patients with underlying diseases such as diabetes mellitus, liver cirrhosis, renal failure, malnutrition, malignancy, and hypogammaglobulinemia, and patients taking steroids, anticancer drugs, and immunosuppressive drugs are at high risk of infection, and care should be taken to avoid postoperative infection. Systemic findings include fever, leukocyte count and fraction, CRP, procalcitonin, and other results of blood test. Local findings include inflammatory symptoms

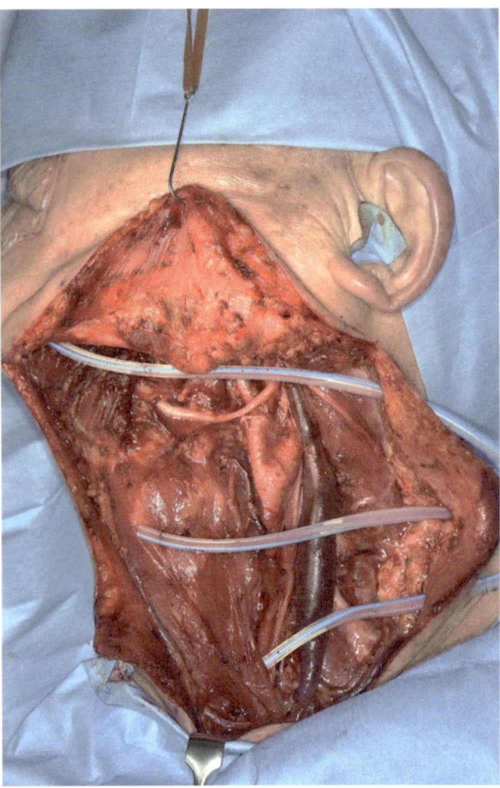

**Fig. 11.14** Neck dissection. A continuous suction drain should be placed before the wound is closed

such as redness and swelling, and drainage volume and characteristics. (Fig. 11.14).

## References


1. Katanoda K, Sobue T, Tanaka H, Miyashiro I, editors. JACR monograph supplement no. 2. Tokyo: Japanese Association of Cancer Registries 2016. (in Japanese). http://www.jacr.info/publicication/Pub/m_supp_02/m_supp2_all.pdf. Accessed 9 Feb 2022.
2. Japanese Gastric Cancer Association. Japanese classification of gastric carcinoma: 3rd English edition. Gastric Cancer. 2011;14:101–12.
3. Japanese Society of Medical Oncology, editor. Clinical oncology. (Shin Rinsho Shuyougaku). 5th ed. Tokyo: Nankodo; 2018 (in Japanese).
4. National Cancer Center Institute for Cancer Control. Guidelines for the screening for gastric cancer based on efficacy evaluation. (Yukousei Hyoukani Motozuku Igan Kenshin guideline). 2014 ed. Tokyo: National Cancer Center Institute for Cancer Control; 2015. (in Japanese). http://canscreen.ncc.go.jp/guideline/iganguide2014_150421.pdf.
5. Ono H, Yao K, Fujishiro M, et al. Guidelines for endoscopic submucosal dissection and endoscopic mucosal resection for early gastric cancer (second edition). Dig Endosc. 2021;33:4–20. https://doi.org/10.1111/den.13883.
6. Colorectal Cancer Research Society, editor. Guidelines for the treatment of colorectal cancer 2022. (Kanjyasanno Tameno Daichougan Chiryo guideline). Tokyo: Kanehara Shuppan; 2022. (in Japanese).
7. Committee of Accuracy Control for Colorectal Cancer Screening, Japanese Society of Gastrointestinal Cancer Screening. Manual of colorectal cancer screening (Daichogan Kenshin manual). Tokyo: Igakushoin; 2013. (in Japanese).
8. Quintero E. Colonoscopy versus fecal immunochemical testing in colorectal-cancer screening. N Engl J Med. 2012;366:697–706.
9. Japanese Society for Cancer of the Colon and Rectum, editor. Guidelines for the treatment of hereditary colorectal cancer 2022. (Idensei Daichougan Shinryo Guideline). Tokyo: Kanehara Shuppan; 2022. (in Japanese).
10. Brierley JD, et al., editors. TNM classification of malignant tumours. 8th ed. New York: Wiley; 2017.
11. National Cancer Institute. Cancer Therapy Evaluation Program, editor. Common terminology criteria for adverse events (CTCAE) version 5.0. https://ctep.cancer.gov/protocoldevelopment/electronic_applications/ctc.htm. Accessed 10 Feb 2022.

# 12 Metabolic Diseases

Kazutaka Aoki, Koichiro Ueki, Kunio Yoshizawa, Tadashi Toyama, Yasushi Ishigaki, Takayoshi Sakai, Masashi Watanabe, Ikuya Miyamoto, Fumiko Miyanaga, and Hiroyuki Yamada

## 1 Diabetes Mellitus

Kazutaka Aoki

### 1.1 An Overview of Diabetes Mellitus

Diabetes mellitus is a metabolic disease characterized by chronic hyperglycemia secondary to insufficient insulin action [1]. Complications of diabetes are associated with persistent chronic hyperglycemia.

### 1.2 Hormones Associated with Regulation of Blood Glucose Levels

#### 1.2.1 Insulin

Insulin, an important hormone secreted by the β-cells of the pancreatic islets of Langerhans lowers blood glucose levels. Hormones include basic secretion and additional secretion that is stimulated following food intake.

#### 1.2.2 Glucagon

Glucagon secreted by the α-cells of the pancreatic islets of Langerhans increases blood glucose levels.

K. Aoki
Department of Diabetes and Endocrinology, Kanagawa Dental University, Yokosuka, Kanagawa, Japan

K. Ueki · K. Yoshizawa
Department of Oral and Maxillofacial Surgery, Division of Medicine, Interdisciplinary Graduate School, University of Yamanashi, Chuo, Yamanashi, Japan

T. Toyama
Department of Nephrology and Rheumatology, Graduate School of Medical Sciences, Kanazawa University, Kanazawa, Ishikawa, Japan

Y. Ishigaki (✉)
Division of Diabetes, Metabolism and Endocrinology, Department of Internal Medicine, Iwate Medical University, Yahaba, Iwate, Japan
e-mail: ishigaki@iwate-med.ac.jp

T. Sakai
Department of Rehabilitation for Orofacial Disorders, Division of Growth and Development Dentistry, Osaka University Graduate School of Dentistry, Suita, Osaka, Japan

M. Watanabe
School of Life Dentistry at Tokyo, The Nippon Dental University, Chiyoda-ku, Tokyo, Japan

I. Miyamoto · H. Yamada
Division of Oral and Maxillofacial Surgery, Department of Oral and Maxillofacial Reconstructive Surgery, School of Dentistry, Iwate Medical University, Morioka, Iwate, Japan
e-mail: yamadah@iwate-med.ac.jp

F. Miyanaga
Osaka Dental University, Hirakata, Osaka, Japan


T. Chiba, H. Yamada (eds.), *Internal Medicine for Dental Treatments*,
https://doi.org/10.1007/978-981-99-3296-2_12

### 1.2.3 Incretins

Glucagon-like peptide-1 (GLP-1) is secreted by the L cells in the lower part of the small intestine, and glucose-dependent insulinotropic polypeptide (GIP) by K cells in the upper part of the small intestine. GLP-1 promotes insulin secretion in a glucose-dependent manner and inhibits glucagon secretion, whereas GIP promotes insulin secretion in a glucose-dependent manner.

## 1.3 Epidemiology

According to the National Health and Nutrition Survey performed by the Ministry of Health, Labour and Welfare in 2016, the number of individuals with “strongly suspected diabetes mellitus” and those in whom “the possibility of diabetes mellitus cannot be denied” is estimated to be approximately ten million each; therefore, this disease is known to affect a significantly large number of patients.

## 1.4 Classification

### 1.4.1 Etiological Classification (Table 12.1) [2, 3]

1. Type 1 diabetes mellitus: Type 1 diabetes mellitus is common in young individuals and is characterized by an absolute insulin deficiency, which necessitates insulin injections. This condition is classified into an autoimmune type, in which patients show positive islet-cell autoantibodies (the anti-glutamic acid decarboxylase [GAD] antibody and anti-insulinoma-associated protein-2 [IA-2] antibody, among others) and an idiopathic type. Based on the mode of onset, it may be classified into acute onset, fulminant, and slowly progressive disease.
2. Type 2 diabetes mellitus: Type 2 diabetes mellitus, the most common type of diabetes, is characterized by decreased insulin secretion or insulin resistance, with a consequent decrease in insulin action. It is more commonly observed in patients aged >40 years, although the incidence of type 2 diabetes mellitus is increasing in young patients in recent times. Patients with obesity or a family history of diabetes mellitus are predisposed to this metabolic disorder.
3. Diabetes associated with other specific mechanisms or diseases is categorized into the following groups:
   (a) Diabetes mellitus with identified genetic abnormalities: For example, maturity-onset diabetes of the young (MODY) and mitochondrial genetic abnormalities.
   (b) Certain types of diabetes are associated with other disorders and conditions: for example, blood glucose levels tend to increase with administration of glucocorticoids. Endocrine disorders such as Cushing’s syndrome and acromegaly are known to cause diabetes.
4. Gestational diabetes: This condition refers to abnormalities in glucose metabolism that are first detected or develop during pregnancy and do not lead to well-established diabetes mel-

**Table 12.1** Etiological classification of diabetes mellitus and glucose metabolism disorders [2]

| |
|---|
| I. Type 1 (Destruction of pancreatic β-cells, usually leading to absolute insulin deficiency)<br>A. Autoimmune<br>B. Idiopathic |
| II. Type 2 (Ranging from predominantly insulin secretory defect, to predominantly insulin resistance with varying degrees of insulin secretory defect) |
| III. Due to other specific mechanisms or diseases<br>A. Those in which specific mutations have been identified as a cause of genetic susceptibility<br>(1) Genetic abnormalities of pancreatic β-cell function<br>(2) Genetic abnormalities in the mechanism of transfer of insulin action<br>B. Those associated with other diseases and conditions<br>(1) Diseases of exocrine pancreas<br>(2) Endocrine diseases<br>(3) Liver disease<br>(4) Drug- or chemical-induced<br>(5) Infection<br>(6) Rare forms of immune-mediated diabetes<br>(7) Various genetic syndromes often associated with diabetes |
| IV. Gestational diabetes mellitus |

The occurrence of diabetes-specific complications has not been confirmed in some of these conditions. Those that cannot at present be classified as any of the above called unclassifiable

litus. The diagnostic criteria for gestational diabetes differ from those applicable for diabetes in non-pregnant women.

### 1.4.2 Pathophysiological Classification

1. Insulin-dependent state: this refers to a state of absolute insulin deficiency in which insulin injections are essential.
2. Insulin-independent state: this refers to a state of relative insulin deficiency.

## 1.5 Symptoms

Mild elevation in blood glucose levels is accompanied by few subjective symptoms; however, significant hyperglycemia manifests with thirst, polyuria, polyphagia, fatigue, and weight loss.

## 1.6 Blood Tests

1. Plasma glucose levels: The normal fasting blood glucose concentration is <110 mg/dL.
2. Hemoglobin A1c (HbA1c): HbA1c is an important indicator of blood glucose control over 1–2 months prior to blood sampling. The Guidebook for Diabetes Treatment published by the Japan Diabetes Society recommends a normal value of 4.6–6.2%; however, HbA1c around 6.2% may be associated with mixed normal, borderline, and diabetic types of glucose tolerance [4].
3. Glycoalbumin represents the mean blood glucose level measured over 2 weeks prior to blood sampling; normal values range between 11% and 16% [4].
4. 1,5-anhydroglucitol reflects rapid changes in glucose metabolism and is correlated with urinary glucose excretion. The normal value is >14.0 μg/mL [4].
5. The 75 g oral glucose tolerance test (75 g OGTT): Patients visit the hospital in a fasting state in the morning and are administered a drink containing 75 g glucose (TRAILAN G®), after which blood samples are drawn continuously. Figure 12.1 shows the classification and criteria [2, 5].

## 1.7 Diagnosis

"Diabetic type" is diagnosed based on fulfillment of one or two of the following criteria:

1. Fasting plasma glucose level of ≥126 mg/dL, a 2-h level of ≥200 mg/dL on the 75 g OGTT, or a random plasma glucose level of ≥200 mg/dL.
2. HbA1c ≥ 6.5%.

Definitive diagnosis of diabetes mellitus is established after the diabetic type is reconfirmed by tests performed on different days; however, at least one of the tests must meet the diagnosis of blood glucose levels. The patient is diagnosed with diabetes mellitus if both the blood glucose and HbA1c levels measured on the same day indicate diabetic type.

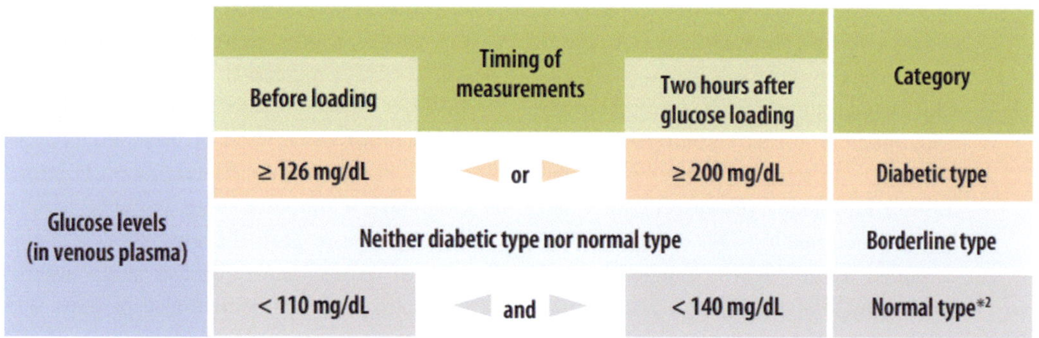


**Fig. 12.1** Categories of state of glycemia as indicated by fasting blood glucose levels and 75 g OGTT with reference value. (Excerpted with slight modification from [2, 5])

## 1.8 Complications

Complications of diabetes include acute complications secondary to severe deficiency of insulin action and chronic complications associated with persistent hyperglycemia.

### 1.8.1 Acute Complications

1. Hyperosmolar hyperglycemic state: This complication is commonly caused by extreme dehydration in elderly patients with type 2 diabetes.
2. Diabetic ketoacidosis: This is a serious metabolic disorder associated with severe deficiency of insulin action, which results in the accumulation of ketone bodies and metabolic acidosis, which often occur in patients with type 1 diabetes.

### 1.8.2 Chronic Complications

1. Microangiopathy: Microangiopathy, a specific complication of diabetes mellitus, represents the following three complications:
   (a) Diabetic retinopathy: This condition causes retinal hemorrhages, retinal white spots, and edema. Progressive retinopathy results in maculopathy, vitreous hemorrhage, and retinal detachment, which may lead to blindness. This condition is classified into the following three stages: (a) simple retinopathy; (b) pre-proliferative retinopathy; (c) proliferative retinopathy. Laser photocoagulation or surgery of the vitreous body is used to treat advanced retinopathy.
   (b) Diabetic nephropathy: Based on the 2014 classification, diabetic nephropathy is categorized into the following five stages. Stage 1 (pre-nephropathy); stage 2 (incipient nephropathy) with microalbuminuria; stage 3 (overt nephropathy) with persistent proteinuria; stage 4 (kidney failure); and stage 5 (dialysis therapy) [6].
   (c) Diabetic neuropathy: This complication is classified as polyneuropathy and mononeuropathy. Polyneuropathy is the most common type characterized by sensory nerve impairment in bilateral feet, which commonly manifests with numbness, pain, and dysesthesia in both lower extremities. Progression of hyposensitivity may lead to ulceration or gangrene of the feet. Autonomic nervous system impairment is associated with orthostatic hypotension, gastrointestinal motility disorders, such as diarrhea and constipation, neurogenic bladder, and erectile dysfunction.
2. Macroangiopathy: Macroangiopathy represents the following three complications:
   (a) Coronary artery disease: Patients with diabetes are at a high risk for angina pectoris and myocardial infarction. Some patients are asymptomatic.
   (b) Cerebrovascular disease: Patients with diabetes are also at a high risk of atherothrombotic cerebral infarction and show a high incidence of lacunar infarction secondary to concomitant hypertension [7].
   (c) Peripheral arterial disease (PAD): PAD is defined as arteriosclerosis of the peripheral arteries of the lower extremities; patients typically initially experience coldness of the affected extremity, and with intermittent claudication and lower extremity ulcers in advanced stages. Smoking, hypertension, and dyslipidemia are known to predispose patients to PAD.
3. Diabetic foot lesions such as ulcers and gangrene are likely to occur in patients with neuropathy-induced hypoesthesia concomitant with PAD, trauma, and infection. Appropriate foot care can prevent diabetic foot and should be recommended for high-risk patients.
4. Periodontal disease: Periodontal pathogens such as *Porphyromonas gingivalis* cause periodontal infection and subsequent chronic inflammation of periodontal tissues. Poor blood glucose control results in progressive periodontal disease; conversely, progressive periodontal disease worsens blood glucose control. Therefore, a bidirectional association is observed between periodontal disease and blood glucose control.
5. Dementia: Compared with patients without diabetes, those with diabetes show a higher risk of Alzheimer's disease and vascular dementia; onset of dementia in patients with diabetes is associated with worsening of glycemic control [8].
6. Cancer: Diabetes mellitus increases the risk of colonic, liver, pancreatic, breast, endometrial,

and bladder cancer [8]. A recent study that used Mendelian randomization to determine the risk of diabetes and cancer in the Japanese population did not provide strong evidence to support this association [9]. Insulin resistance and associated hyperinsulinemia, rather than diabetes mellitus itself, may be implicated in the increased risk of cancer.

## 1.9 Treatment

### 1.9.1 Objective

Antidiabetic therapy is aimed at prevention and progression of complications, maintenance of patients' quality of life as closely as possible to that of healthy individuals, and ensuring life expectancy similar to that of healthy individuals. Optimal blood glucose control and management of complications, such as hypertension and lipids are important to achieve these goals.

HbA1c < 7.0% is considered the target level to optimize glycemic control and prevent complications (Fig. 12.2) [10]. Figure 12.3 shows details regarding glycemic control in elderly patients with diabetes [11].

### 1.9.2 Actual Treatment

Diet, exercise, and medication represent the cornerstones of diabetic care.

1. Dietary therapy: Energy intake is calculated using the following formula: objective body weight × physical activity [12]. In patients aged <65 years, the objective body weight is calculated as (height [m])$^2$ × 22. In patients aged >65 years, objective body weight is calculated as (height [m])$^2$ × 22–25. Physical activity is considered as 25–30 kcal/kg objective body weight for light work, 30–35 kcal/kg objective body weight for normal work, and >35 kcal/kg objective body weight for heavy work. A food exchange list [13] is a user-friendly guide and forms an important element of actual dietary guidance. The amount of food-derived energy is set at 80 kcal/unit and is described based on the unit (e.g., 1 unit = 50 g of boiled rice). Patients with hyper-

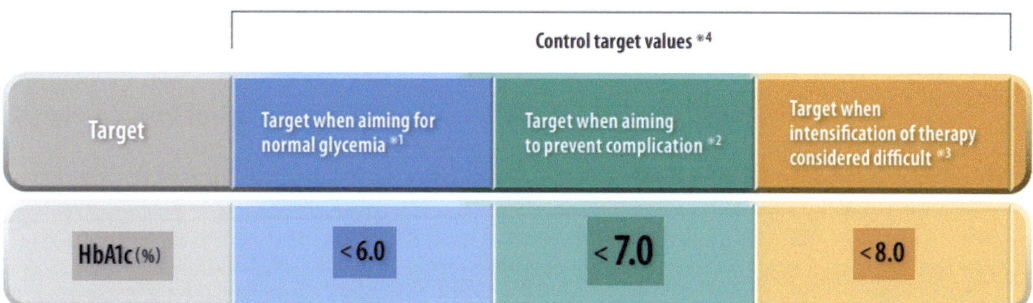


Control targets are established individually, in consideration of age, duration of disease, organ damage, risk of hypoglycemia, patient support, etc.

*1 In case, targets can be attained by appropriate dietary or exercise therapy, alone or by pharmacotherapy without the occurrence of side effects such as hypoglycemia.
*2 From the perspective of preventing complications, HbA1c target value is set below 7%. A fasting plasma glucose level <130 mg/dL and a 2-hour postprandial plasma glucose level < 180 mg/dL were used as an approximate estimate for the corresponding plasma glucose levels.
*3 Target in cases where intensification of treatment is considered difficult due to side effects such as hypoglycemia or for other reasons.
*4 All target values are for adults, not including pregnant women.

**Fig. 12.2** Glycemic control targets. (Reproduced from [10])

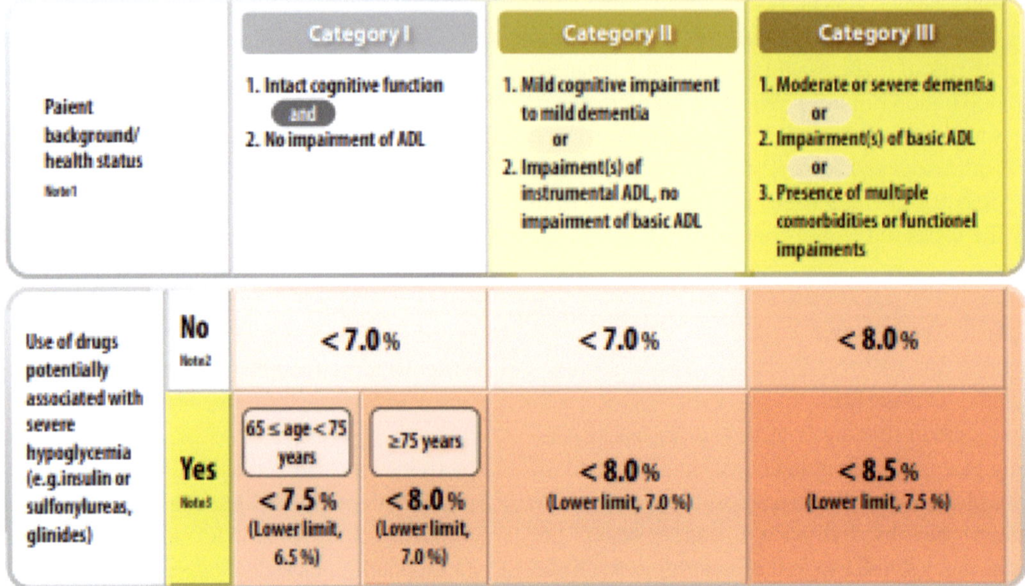

| | | Category I | | Category II | Category III |
|---|---|---|---|---|---|
| Paient background/ health status Note1 | | 1. Intact cognitive function and 2. No impairment of ADL | | 1. Mild cognitive impairment to mild dementia or 2. Impaiment(s) of instrumental ADL, no impairment of basic ADL | 1. Moderate or severe dementia or 2. Impairment(s) of basic ADL or 3. Presence of multiple comorbidities or functionel impaiments |
| Use of drugs potentially associated with severe hypoglycemia (e.g. insulin or sulfonylureas, glinides) | No Note2 | <7.0% | | <7.0% | <8.0% |
| | Yes Note3 | 65 ≤ age < 75 years<br><7.5% (Lower limit, 6.5%) | ≥75 years<br><8.0% (Lower limit, 7.0%) | <8.0% (Lower limit, 7.0%) | <8.5% (Lower limit, 7.5%) |

The glycemic target is to be determined for each patient by taking into account his/her age, duration of diabetes, risk for hypoglycemia, and any support available to the patient, as well as the patient's cognitive function, basic/instrumental ADL, and comorbidities/functional impairments. It should be noted that the potential risk of hypoglycemia increases with age in each patient.

*ADL* activities of daily living; *Note 1* Refer to the Japan Geriatrics Society website [http://www.jpn-geriat-soc.or.jp/tool/index.html], for the evaluation of the cognitive function, basic ADL (e.g. self-care abilities such as dressing, transferring, bathing, and toileting), and instrumental ADL (e.g. abilities to maintain an independent household such as shopping, meal preparation, taking medication, and handling finances,). In end-of-life care, priority is to be given to preventing significant hyperglycemia and subsequent dehydration and acute complications through appropriate therapeutic measures; *Note 2* As in other age groups, the glycemic target is set at <7.0% in the elderly for preventing diabetic complications. However, this could be set at <6.0% for those thought likely to achieve glycemic control through diet and exercise therapy alone or those likely to achieve glycemic control with drug therapy without adverse reactions, or 8.0% for those in whom intensifying therapy may prove difficult. In either case, no lower limit is specified for the glycemic target. A glycemic target of <8.5% may be allowed in patients thought to be in category III and therefore at risk of developing adverse reactions to multi-drug combination therapy or in those with serious comorbidities or poor social support; *Note 3* In patients in whom priority should be given to preventing the onset/progression of diabetic complications due to their duration of disease, the glycemic target or its lower limit may be set for each elderly patient with appropriate measures to prevent severe hypoglycemia. Current treatments are to be continued in those less than 65 years of age despite their HbA1c values falling below their glycemic target or lower limit while on therapy, but attention should be paid to potential severe hypoglycemia. Glinides may be classified as drugs unlikely to be associated with severe hypoglycemia, depending on the type and amount of glinide used in a particular patient relative to the patient's glucose level.

**Fig. 12.3** Glycemic targets (HbA1c values) for elderly patients with diabetes. (Reproduced from [11])

tension are recommended to consume <6 g of salt/day. A protein-restricted diet is required in patients with progressive nephropathy.

2. Exercise therapy: Exercise increases utilization of glucose and fatty acids and lowers blood glucose levels and improves insulin sensitivity. Exercise does not consume significant amounts of energy; therefore, increased exercise cannot utilize the extra energy associated with overeating.
3. Pharmacotherapy: This therapeutic strategy includes the administration of insulin secretagogues, non-insulin secretagogues, and insulin.
   (a) **Insulin secretagogues**
   - Sulfonylureas (SUs)
     These drugs bind with SU receptors on the pancreatic β-cell membrane and promote insulin secretion.
   - Glinides
     These agents dissociate from SU receptors within a short time; therefore, they stimulate insulin secretion during the early postprandial period and thereby improve postprandial hyperglycemia.
   - Dipeptidyl peptidase-4 (DPP-4) inhibitors
     GLP-1 and GIP are rapidly degraded by DPP-4; therefore, inhibition of DPP-4 activity increases endogenous GLP-1 and GIP production, promotes insulin secretion in a glucose-dependent manner, and suppresses glucagon secretion.
   - GLP-1 receptor agonists
     These agents bind to GLP-1 receptors on pancreatic β-cells and stimulate insulin secretion in a blood glucosedependent manner. Reductions in food intake and body weight are also expected. Oral and subcutaneous formulations are available for administration once or twice daily or once weekly. Mixed injections of GLP-1 receptor agonist and insulin are also available.
   - GIP and GLP-1 receptor agonist
     Tirzepatide is a dual GIP and GLP-1 receptor agonist. Reduction in food intake and body weight are also expected.
   - Imeglimin
     This novel orally administered drug was introduced in 2021 and is shown to have an effect on the mitochondria. It promotes insulin secretion in a blood glucose-dependent manner and improves insulin resistance in the liver and skeletal muscles.

   (b) **Non-Insulin secretagogues**
   - Biguanides
     These drugs suppress gluconeogenesis in the liver, improve insulin sensitivity in peripheral tissues, and inhibit glucose absorption in the gastrointestinal tract. They are contraindicated in patients with severe renal impairment and should be withdrawn prior to administration of contrast agents.
   - Thiazolidinediones
     These antidiabetic agents improve insulin resistance in adipose tissue and skeletal muscles. However, water retention is a known adverse effect of this drug.
   - Alpha-glucosidase inhibitors (α-GIs)
     These agents inhibit α-glucosidase activity and delay carbohydrate absorption by inhibiting the degradation of disaccharides to monosaccharides, which reduces postprandial hyperglycemia and insulin secretion. The most common adverse effects of α – GIs include gastrointestinal symptoms such as abdominal distention, flatus, constipation, and diarrhea.
   - Sodium-glucose co-transporter 2 (SGLT2) inhibitors
     These drugs inhibit glucose reabsorption by SGLT2 in the renal tubules and promote urinary excretion of glucose, thereby reducing hyperglycemia. The weight loss associated with these drugs is a benefit in patients with obesity. Some of the SGLT2 inhibitors are used in patients with heart failure and chronic kidney disease.

   (c) **Insulin therapy**
   Advances in genetic engineering have led to the emergence of novel insulin preparations. Furthermore, owing to the availability of innovative injection equipment and widespread use of self-monitoring blood glucose devices, insulin therapy is easier to administer.

## 1.10 Hypoglycemia

Hypoglycemia is a known adverse effect associated with the use of SUs, glinides, or insulin; patients should be instructed regarding prompt ingestion of glucose or supplemental food in such cases.

## 1.11 Metabolic Syndrome

Metabolic syndrome is characterized by insulin resistance. In Japan, patients who show accumulation of visceral fat and meet ≥two of the following criteria are diagnosed with metabolic syndrome: impaired glucose tolerance, impaired lipid metabolism, and hypertension (Fig. 12.4) [14].

## 1.12 Notes from Dentistry Perspective

Koichiro Ueki, Kunio Yoshizawa, Tadashi Toyama

### 1.12.1 Precautions on Dental Treatment

1. Removing psychological and painful stress

   Hormones such as adrenocorticotropic hormone, thyroid-stimulating hormone, and catecholamines secreted by stress have hyperglycemic effects, so it is important to engage in dental treatment to avoid psychological or painful stress as much as possible [15]. In addition, HbA1c level is generally emphasized as a major index of glycemic control (see Fig. 12.2), because it reflects the average blood glucose level over the past month or two, hyperglycemia may occur with treatment even if the HbA1c level is within the control target. Therefore, it is advisable to refer to fasting blood glucose and postprandial blood glucose to judge the patient's metabolic state comprehensively during treatment.
2. Be aware of periodontitis and other infections

   Diabetes mellitus treatment may significantly reduce bleeding on probing (BOP) in periodontal tissues and improve inflammation of periodontitis. It is rated as a recommended grade B for the CQ "Is diabetes treatment effective in ameliorating periodontal disease?" in Diabetes practice guidelines [16]. In addition, periodontitis is a risk factor for worsening glycemic control and progression of diabetes mellitus by increasing insulin resistance through inflammatory cytokines derived from bacterial infection [17]. On the other hand, it is known that periodontal disease tends to be more severe in diabetic patients, and the main reason is thought to be that macrophage function and bacterial phagocytosis of neutrophils, which are the infection defense functions of the body, are decreased by hyperglycemia and ischemia, and the growth of periodontal pathogens cannot be controlled [17]. Therefore, thorough prevention and treatment of periodontitis are indispensable in the dental treatment of diabetic patients.

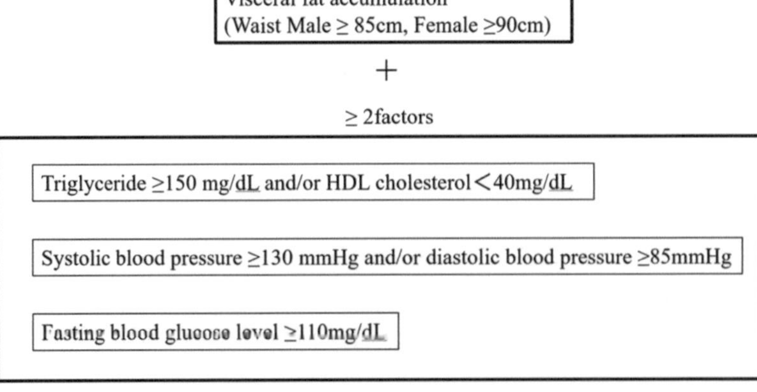


**Fig. 12.4** Diagnostic criteria of metabolic syndrome in Japan. (Modified from [14])

3. Sufficient attention should be paid to local bleeding

   Diabetic patients often suffer from complications of atherosclerotic diseases such as stroke and angina pectoris, and many of them take antiplatelet and anticoagulant drugs for their treatment. If the risk of thrombosis associated with the discontinuation of these antithrombotic agents is judged to be greater than the risk of bleeding, it is advisable to perform surgical treatment with careful attention to local hemostasis while continuing the medication.
4. Treatment time setting

   To prevent hypoglycemia associated with skipping meals, consideration should be given to the start time of the procedure. Outpatient dental procedures should be scheduled to begin around 1 h and 30 min after breakfast or lunch, and patients should be able to eat at their usual time before and after the procedure [15].
5. What to do in case of hypoglycemia

   Hypoglycemia is a common emergency during treatment of diabetes mellitus, especially in dental patients, who often suffer from hypoglycemia due to poor food intake caused by dental pain or restricted food intake after oral surgery. Hypoglycemia may also be caused by insulin injections or oral hypoglycemic agents in the management of diabetes mellitus. If hypoglycemic symptoms such as sweating, anxiety, palpitations, tremor, pallor, and drowsiness are observed, blood glucose should be measured and glucose should be administered. When disturbance of consciousness occurs, blood glucose monitoring is necessary to differentiate from hyperglycemic coma. If hypoglycemia occurs to the extent that the level of consciousness is decreased, even if the patient recovers temporarily with emergency treatment, there is a high possibility that the hypoglycemia will recur or prolong. If oral intake is possible, glucose (10 g) should be given. Sucrose requires at least double that amount (20 g), and other sugars delay the onset of effects. If oral intake is not possible or in an emergency, administer 20 mL of 50% glucose (40 mL of 20% glucose) intravenously. Hypoglycemia induced by sulfonylureas (SU) tends to be delayed, and hypoglycemic symptoms may recur after awakening. In addition, if the patient is taking an α-glucosidase inhibitor, glucose should always be chosen because sucrose delays the increase in blood glucose [18].

### 1.12.2 On the Use of Local Anesthetics and Epinephrine

A local anesthetic (lidocaine hydrochloride) containing epinephrine, a vasoconstrictor, is frequently used because of its high peripheral vasoconstrictor and anesthetic effects, but the stimulation of epinephrine is known to increase blood glucose by predominantly inhibiting insulin secretion [15]. Epinephrine-containing local anesthetics (lidocaine hydrochloride), which have high peripheral vasoconstrictor and anesthetic effects, can be used as usual in patients who receive only diet therapy or whose blood glucose is well controlled. However, if blood glucose control is poor or there are complications in the circulatory system or cerebrovascular disease, the use of 1–2 cartridges (1.8–3.6 mL) should be limited depending on the severity of the disease, or propitocaine hydrochloride containing felypressin should be used instead of lidocaine hydrochloride containing epinephrine. However, felypressin-containing local anesthetics are less vasoconstrictive and have a slightly lower anesthetic effect. Therefore, in some situations, it may cause painful stress to the patient, which may lead to adverse consequences such as increased blood pressure and blood glucose.

### 1.12.3 Oral Complications

There have been many reports of clostridial infection in the deep cervical region and severe dental infections in diabetic patients after tooth extraction. It should be noted that diabetic patients are more likely to have more serious dental infections than healthy people when their immunity is weakened. For example, if odontogenic infection arising from an untreated stump of tooth spreads to adjacent organs (Fig. 12.5), or if sepsis occurs, it may be fatal. For this reason, early treatment of dental infections in diabetic patients is recommended.

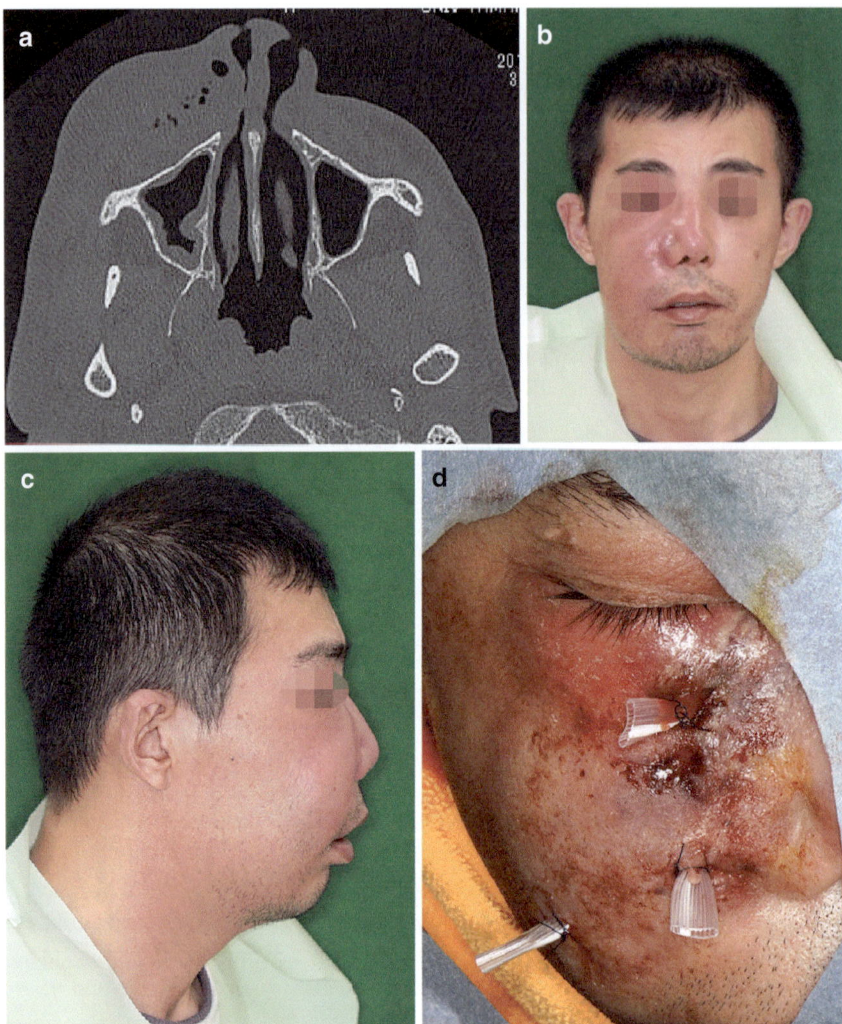


**Fig. 12.5** (**a**–**f**) Dental infections are more likely to be serious in diabetic patients than in normal subjects. Therefore, patients should pay attention to adequate oral cleaning and dental treatment of any oral infection foci before they worsen. (**a**) CT scan: swelling with gas production was observed from the lower orbit to the buccal area. (**b**, **c**) Patient with type 1 diabetes mellitus: The patient came to our hospital for cellulitis caused by periodontitis in the right maxillary molar. The blood glucose was in the 500 mg/dL range and CRP was 20.9 mg/dL. Gas-producing Bacteroides was detected. (**d**, **e**) The patient required antimicrobial therapy, incision and drainage, and tooth extraction. (**f**) Intraoral photograph (mirror image): after removal of the causative tooth. Poor intraoral cleanliness and numerous remaining roots were observed

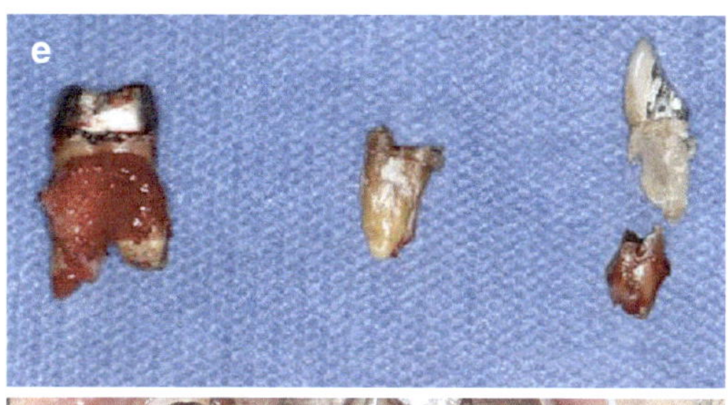


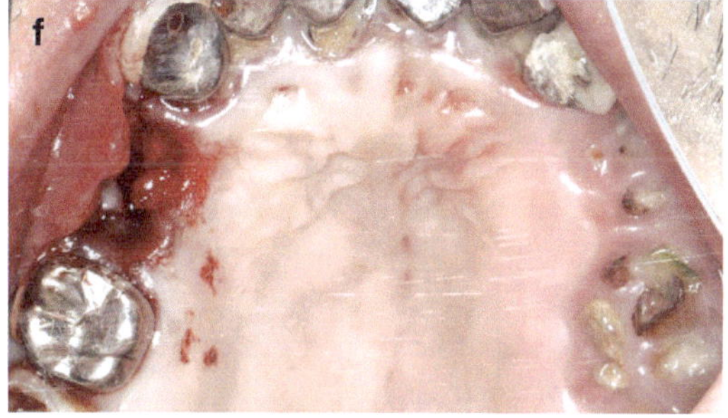


**Fig. 12.5** (continued)

### 1.12.4 What to Do in a Situation Where It Is Better to Extract a Tooth Even with a High HbA1c

According to the training guidebook for medical specialists of the Japanese Diabetes Association, preoperative glycemic control goals include fasting blood glucose <140 mg/dL, postprandial blood glucose <200 mg/dL, negative urine ketone bodies, and the amount of urinary glucose, but there is no clear indicator for HbA1c. Because high HbA1c levels are often associated with poor fasting and postprandial glucose control, it is advisable to improve glycemic control through inpatient management, continuation or introduction of insulin therapy, and improvement of diet and medication adherence before performing tooth extraction. If surgical stress is expected to be large, or if tooth extraction surgery under general anesthesia is indicated, the patient should be hospitalized 3–7 days before surgery to control the blood glucose level adequately.

If the HbA1c is high and there is a concern that postponing a surgical procedure such as tooth extraction will worsen the local condition and affect the general condition, it should be performed with adequate perioperative infection control and close coordination to the attending physician. Basically, the incidence of surgical site infection (SSI) in diabetic patients with appropriately controlled blood glucose, such as HbA1c (NGSP) less than 7.0%, is similar to that in healthy subjects, so there is no need to choose broad-spectrum antimicrobial therapy. However, because of the risk of perioperative infection in diabetic patients with poor glycemic control, more attention should be paid to the prevention of perioperative wound infection, such as administering antimicrobial agents from the day before tooth extraction [19].

## 2 Dyslipidemia

Yasushi Ishigaki

### 2.1 General Statement of Lipid Metabolism

Cholesterol and triglycerides (TG) are considered as the major lipids associated with dyslipidemia. Cholesterol is an essential component of cell membranes and is also used to produce bile acids, adrenocortical hormones, and sex hormones. On the other hand, TG is a combination of free fatty acids and glycerol, contributing to energy storage.

In general, lipids are insoluble in water. Since lipids cannot exist in the blood in their original form, cholesterol and TG are encapsulated in phospholipids and dissolved in the blood as the form of lipoproteins. Lipoproteins are roughly classified into five types according to the composition and content of lipids as well as the type of apoprotein (Fig. 12.6). Chylomicrons and VLDL, which have-low specific gravity, contain a large proportion of TG, while LDL and HDL, which have high specific gravity, contain a large proportion of cholesterol.

There are three pathways in lipid metabolism: the exogenous pathway, the endogenous pathway, and the reverse cholesterol transport pathway (Fig. 12.7). In the exogenous pathway, dietary lipids are absorbed from the small intestine, and flowing into the body circulation as chylomicrons, are finally to be hydrolyzed by lipoprotein lipase (LPL) before being taken up by the liver. In the liver, TG and cholesterol are synthesized independently of the lipids taken up from the blood, and both are combined and released into the blood as VLDL particle. VLDL

| Types of lipoproteins | CM | VLDL | IDL | LDL | HDL |
|---|---|---|---|---|---|
| | Chylomicron | Very low density lipoprotein | Intermediate density lipoprotein | Low density lipoprotein | High density lipoprotein |
| Role | Transporting lipids ingested through the diet to the liver | Released from the liver to provide free fatty acids | Intermediates between VLDL and LDL | Supply cholesterol to peripheral tissues | Draws excess cholesterol from peripheral tissues and redistributes it |
| Diameter(Å) | 800~10,000 | 300~800 | 250~300 | 200~250 | 75~200 |
| Structural component<br>Triglyceride<br>Cholesterol | | | | | |

Fig. 12.6 Types of lipoproteins

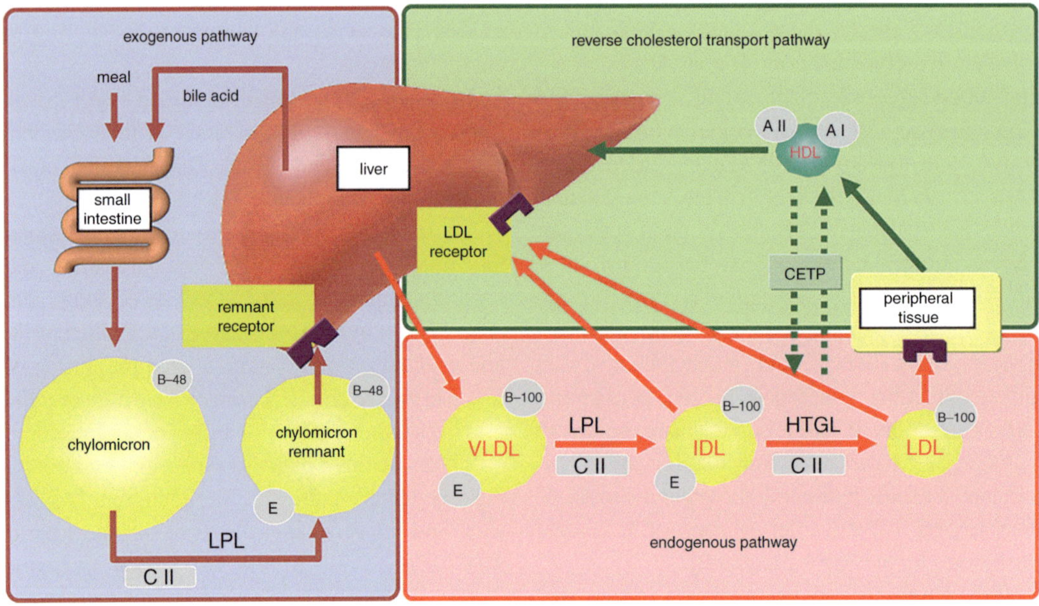


Fig. 12.7 Lipoprotein metabolic pathway

is metabolized to IDL and LDL by LPL, and supplies free fatty acids and cholesterol to peripheral tissues. This is called the endogenous pathway. The reverse cholesterol transport pathway plays a role of HDL in collecting excess cholesterol from peripheral tissues and returning it to the liver or redistributing it to VLDL and LDL.

## 2.2 Diagnosis of Dyslipidemia

In clinical practice, three or four lipid parameters are measured: total cholesterol (TC), TG, HDL cholesterol (HDL-C), and LDL cholesterol (LDL-C). Dyslipidemia is defined as hyper-LDL-C (high cholesterol in the LDL fraction), hyper-TG (high total TG of all lipoproteins combined), hypo-HDL-C (low cholesterol in the HDL fraction), and hyper-non-HDL-C (high total cholesterol minus HDL-C). The reference values for diagnosing abnormalities are LDL-C 140 mg/dL or more, TG 150 mg/dL or more, HDL-C less than 40 mg/dL, and non-HDL-C 170 mg/dL or more (Table 12.2), and early morning fasting blood sampling is recommended for diagnosis [20].

## 2.3 Pathogenesis of Dyslipidemia

Dyslipidemia is often caused by overeating, heavy alcohol consumption, lack of exercise, and obesity, as in other lifestyle-related diseases.

Some kinds of dyslipidemias associated with genetic abnormalities, referred to as primary dyslipidemias, show severe lipid abnormalities. Familial hypercholesterolemia (FH) is one of the most frequent and important genetic disorders of lipid metabolism. It is characterized by (1) high serum LDL-C (180 mg/dL or higher is suspicious, 250 mg/dL or higher is strongly suspicious), (2) xanthomas (e.g., Achilles tendon thickening), and (3) a family history of FH or coronary artery disease which developed in relatively young age (exhibit an autosomal dominant inheritance). Early intervention for FH is strongly recommended because of the high risk of developing coronary artery disease at a young age. In addition, family screening is also useful to find FH. There are some secondary lipid disorders associated with other diseases. Hypothyroidism and nephrotic syndrome are the most common disorders in which LDL-C is elevated. Diabetes mellitus often causes an increase in TG levels. Corticosteroid drugs may increase LDL-C and TG.

**Table 12.2** Serum lipid diagnostic reference values

| | |
|---|---|
| LDL cholesterol | 140 mg/dL or more |
| Triglyceride | More than 150 mg/dL |
| HDL cholesterol | Less than 40 mg/dL |
| Non-HDL cholesterol | 170 mg/dL or more |

## 2.4 Symptoms of Dyslipidemia

Most of patients with dyslipidemia are asymptomatic. However, dyslipidemia is generally recognized as a risk factor for atherosclerotic diseases such as coronary artery disease and cerebral infarction. In particular, hyper LDL-cholesterolemia has a strong impact on atherosclerosis, thereby, an important target for treatment. Since hypertriglyceridemia (increase in chylomicrons) is a risk factor for acute pancreatitis, drug therapy should be started as soon as possible if the blood concentration exceeds 1000 mg/dL.

## 2.5 Management Goals for Dyslipidemia

Even if serum lipid levels exceed the reference values shown in Table 12.2, not all patients are indicated for drug therapy. In accordance with the Japan Atherosclerosis Society Guidelines for Prevention of Atherosclerotic Cardiovascular Diseases [20], each patient is stratified according to their risk for establishing their LDL-C management target. At first, LDL-C management target for patients with the history of coronary artery disease, determined as secondary prevention, is established as less than 100 mg/dL, especially, less than 70 mg/dL for those with FH, acute coronary syndrome, or high-risk diabetes. For patients with primary prevention, if the patient has diabetes, chronic kidney disease, cerebrovascular disease, or peripheral arterial disease, LDL-C of less than 120 mg/dL should be established as the target. In the absence of any of the aforementioned concomitant diseases, the risk for predicting coronary artery disease is classified into high, intermediate, and low risk groups by calculating their itemized risks (age, gender, smoking status, blood pressure, HDL-C level, LDL-C level, presence of glucose intolerance, and presence of family history of coronary artery disease) in accordance with Japan Atherosclerosis Society Guidelines. The LDL-C management target values are less than 120 mg/dL, 140 mg/dL, and 160 mg/dL, respectively. The management targets for TG and HDL-C are <150 mg/dL and ≥40 mg/dL, respectively.

## 2.6 Treatment of Dyslipidemia

For all patients with dyslipidemia, lifestyle modification is required. It is recommended that total dietary energy intake should be optimized. In addition, it is also recommended that the maintenance for range of both fat/energy ratio 20–25%, and saturated fatty acids be 4.5–7%, restriction of cholesterol intake below 200 mg/day, increase for n-3 polyunsaturated fatty acids intake, and restriction of alcohol intake below 25 g/day as ethanol intake. Moreover, exercise therapy in combination with aerobic exercise, such as fast walking and swimming, and strength training is also recommended.

If lipid management is insufficient after 3–6 months of lifestyle modification, drug therapy should be considered. The most common drugs are HMG-CoA reductase inhibitors (statins), which act mainly by inhibiting cholesterol synthesis in the liver and increasing LDL uptake from the blood. They are the standard drugs for the treatment of dyslipidemia because of their strong LDL-C-lowering effect and many clinical results in reducing atherosclerotic diseases development. Muscle-related adverse effects, such as myalgia, weakness, and CK elevation, are characteristic, and in severe cases, rhabdomyolysis may occur. Ezetimibe, which inhibits cholesterol absorption from the small intestine, is also used as an LDL-C lowering agent. Recently, PCSK9 inhibitors, which have a very potent LDL-C-lowering effect, have been used in some high-risk patients. Fibrates, which inhibit TG synthesis in the liver and promote TG degradation in the blood, are used in patients with hypertriglyceridemia.

Because dyslipidemia is asymptomatic, patients often do not participate in medical care or discontinue treatment. Therefore, it is important to raise awareness for importance of disease treatment even if the serum lipid level is normalized by medication.

## 2.7 Notes from Dentistry Perspective

Takayoshi Sakai

### 2.7.1 Dyslipidemia and Oral Diseases

Dyslipidemia, also known as hyperlipidemia, is a condition in which the amount of cholesterol, neutral fat (triglycerides) and other lipids in the blood is higher than a certain standard. An excess of lipids in the blood tends to cause arteriosclerosis, which increases the risk of myocardial infarction and cerebrovascular disease. When patients with hypertension, which exerts strong pressure on blood vessels, develop dyslipidemia, their blood vessel walls are more easily damaged, increasing the risk of atherosclerosis. When insulin is insufficient due to diabetes mellitus, it becomes difficult for the body to utilize triglycerides. The increase in triglycerides in the blood tends to lead to dyslipidemia and the progression of arteriosclerosis. There are few subjective symptoms in patients themselves, and “sluggish blood” is generally applied to the condition. If the disease is discovered too late, it is not uncommon for patients to suffer a sudden attack such as a myocardial infarction. As a preventive measure, it is important to pay attention to lifestyle habits such as exercise and diet, and to take early action without delay if “suspicion of dyslipidemia” is pointed out in a medical checkup. It is clear that damage to blood vessels and blood flow caused by the progression of atherosclerosis can cause damage to the entire body, including the oral cavity. In this chapter, we will discuss the relationship between dyslipidemia and oral diseases.

#### Dyslipidemia and arteriosclerosis

According to the Vital Statistics of the Ministry of Health, Labour and Welfare in 2009, the leading causes of death in Japan is malignant neoplasm (cancer), followed by cardiovascular disease (excluding hypertension) and cerebrovascular disease. Heart disease and cerebrovascular disease together account for about 25% of all deaths. This is comparable to the total number of cancers, and approximately 310,000 Japanese die annually from cardiac and cerebrovascular diseases. It goes without saying that atherosclerosis is a major trigger of these cardiac and cerebrovascular diseases [21].

Atherosclerosis is a condition in which cholesterol is deposited on the arterial wall and blood vessels become stiffened due to tissue degeneration and loss of elasticity. When inflammatory cells accumulate in the area, an atherosclerotic mass (atherosclerotic plaque) is formed [22]. Plaque formation in coronary arteries reduces the supply of oxygen and nutrients to the myocardium by narrowing the vessel lumen, leading to angina pectoris with chest pain and feeling of thoracic compression as the main symptoms. Furthermore, thrombus formation due to plaque disruption can completely block blood flow, resulting in severe acute infarction. This phenomenon is called myocardial infarction in coronary arteries and cerebral infarction in cerebral vessels, and occurs not only locally in coronary arteries and cerebral arteries but also in distant organs through blood circulation by exfoliation of thrombi formed in other arteries throughout the body.

Age, gender, total cholesterol, LDL cholesterol, systolic blood pressure, and smoking have been identified as risk factors for the development of coronary artery disease. In addition to these classical risk factors, dyslipidemia, diabetes mellitus, and obesity have now been shown to be risk factors, and recently, high-sensitivity C-reactive protein (CRP) levels have been shown to be predictive of coronary artery disease [23]. It has been reported that high-sensitivity C-reactive protein (CRP) is elevated in the peripheral blood of patients with periodontal disease and is decreased by periodontal treatment [24], suggesting that an increased systemic inflammatory response due to periodontal disease is involved in the development and progression of vascular disorders.

### Relationship between periodontal disease and arteriosclerotic disease

C-reactive protein (CRP), a serum inflammatory marker, is useful not only as a marker of systemic inflammation but also as a risk marker for atherosclerosis and coronary artery disease. Atherosclerosis is characterized by thickening of the vascular endothelium, formation of atherosclerotic plaques covered with a thin fibrous film, and inflammatory infiltration. Risk markers for atherosclerotic disease include serum inflammatory markers hg.

Periodontal disease is a chronic inflammatory disease with destruction of periodontal tissues caused by infection of periodontal pockets by periodontopathogenic bacteria, *P. gingivalis* (invasion of vascular endothelial cells). Because periodontopathogenic bacteria are detected in atherosclerotic lesions, and because the pathogenesis of atherosclerotic disease cannot be explained by classical risk factors such as hypertension, dyslipidemia, and diabetes mellitus alone, the possibility of an association with periodontal disease has been suggested. It has been shown that serum CRP levels are significantly increased in patients with periodontal disease compared with healthy subjects [25]. It has also been reported that aggressive treatment of periodontal disease decreases IL-6, CRP, and other levels [26].

Dyslipidemia is an important risk factor for the development of atherosclerotic disease, and epidemiological studies have shown that an increase in serum LDL cholesterol or a decrease in HDL cholesterol increases the risk of developing the condition [27]. Recently, it has been reported that periodontal patients with high serum antibody titer against periodontopathogenic bacteria have significantly higher LDL cholesterol levels [28]. In addition, periodontal treatment has been shown to improve HDL levels. Furthermore, it has been reported that advanced periodontal therapy improves the condition of the arterial wall. However, it has been reported that there is no difference in serum lipid profiles between healthy individuals and those with periodontal disease [29], and a study by the American Heart Association (AHA) indicated that there is no evidence that periodontal disease is associated with the development or progression of ischemic heart disease [30]. Patients with periodontal disease often have obesity, diabetes mellitus, hypertension, and other lifestyle-related diseases due to their life background. Therefore, it is necessary to consider the co-occurrence of diseases in epidemiological studies, and further research is expected.

## 3 Osteoporosis [31–33]

Masashi Watanabe

### 3.1 Concept of the Disease

Osteoporosis occurs in the entire skeletal system and is a condition in which bone strength is reduced and the risk of fracture is increased as a result of decreased bone mass and disruption of the microstructure of bone tissue. Bone strength reflects both bone mineral density and bone quality, and bone quality is affected by the degree of calcification, collagen cross-linking components, and microfracture, in addition to bone microstructure. Fractures can occur at any site, but the major ones are vertebral fractures and femoral neck fractures.

### 3.2 Pathophysiology

In bone, old bone is always resorbed by osteoclasts, and then new bone is formed by osteoblasts. Bone remodeling occurs by repeating this process of bone resorption and bone formation. The amount and strength of bone are maintained by the equilibrium between bone resorption and bone formation. Therefore, when the equilibrium of bone metabolism is broken, bone mass decreases and osteoporosis occurs. Estrogen suppresses bone resorption by inhibiting the production of bone-resorbing cytokines (IL-1, IL-6, etc.) in bone. Therefore, when estrogen levels decline after menopause, osteoporosis mainly results from increased bone resorption and bone metabolic turnover. In men with osteoporosis, osteogenesis is reduced due to a decrease in bone formation-promoting factors, such as a decrease in Ca intake with aging and a decrease in sun exposure time and exercise, but bone resorption is not suppressed and bone resorption is relatively dominant, resulting in a breakdown of the bone metabolic equilibrium and osteoporosis. In immobilization osteoporosis, the mechanical load on bone is decreased, bone resorption is increased, and bone formation is decreased, resulting in a breakdown of the bone metabolic equilibrium and osteoporosis. In the elderly, patients with chronic liver disease, and patients with chronic kidney disease, vitamin D deficiency leads to secondary hyperparathyroidism, which is an important risk factor for osteoporosis. Long-term treatment with glucocorticoids suppresses bone formation and Ca absorption in the intestinal tract and renal tubules, resulting in increased bone resorption and osteoporosis.

### 3.3 Epidemiology

Osteoporosis is more common in postmenopausal women, but it also occurs in men and women who have diseases or major risk factors that cause bone decalcification. The exact frequency of osteoporosis in Japan is unknown, but the annual incidence is estimated to be about 50,000, with a sharp increase in both men and women over 70 years of age, and the rate is 2–2.5 times higher in women than in men.

### 3.4 Classification

Osteoporosis is classified into primary osteoporosis and secondary osteoporosis caused by other underlying diseases or drugs. Most of the primary osteoporosis are postmenopausal osteoporosis in postmenopausal women and male osteoporosis in elderly men. Other types of osteoporosis include juvenile osteoporosis, which occurs rarely in young people, and idiopathic osteoporosis, in which the cause is unknown.

## 3.5 Symptoms

Fracture is the most common subjective symptom, but vertebral fracture may occur without any symptoms. The vertebral fracture causes lumbar back pain and hump back due to spinal deformity, as well as nerve paralysis and pain in the lower limbs due to nerve compression caused by the vertebral fracture, resulting in a decrease in ADL and QOL.

## 3.6 Clinical Examination

Endocrine examination usually shows no abnormalities in serum Ca and parathyroid hormone. If abnormalities are found, secondary osteoporosis or osteomalacia due to abnormal Ca metabolism should be suspected. In bone metabolism, serum bone alkaline phosphatase (BALP) has been recognized as a marker of bone formation. As bone resorption markers, urinary and blood type I collagen cross-linked N-telopeptide (NTX), urinary type I collagen cross-linked C-telopeptide (CTX), and urinary deoxypyridinoline (DPD) are covered by insurance. Bone radiographs are performed to determine whether vertebral fractures have occurred. The bone density of the lumbar spine or proximal femur should be examined by dual-energy X-ray absorptiometry (DXA).

## 3.7 Diagnosis

Fracture is a frequent complication of osteoporosis, and it is necessary to proceed with the diagnosis with the indication of treatment in mind, with the prevention of fracture as the first priority. The diagnostic criteria for primary osteoporosis include the presence of fragility fractures and bone density less than 80% after differential diagnosis of secondary osteoporosis and after exclusion of osteoporosis-like diseases (osteomalacia, primary hyperparathyroidism, etc.). If bone mineral density is less than 70% of young adult mean (YAM), osteoporosis should be diagnosed even if there is no fragility fracture.

## 3.8 Treatment

Osteoporosis often becomes symptomatic only after a fracture occurs, but the primary goal of osteoporosis treatment is to prevent fragility fractures, so it is important to eliminate risk factors for osteoporosis and fractures. Since fractures can be caused by falls at home, it is necessary to improve the home environment and take measures to prevent falls. Moderate exercise is effective in maintaining bone strength and muscular power, and patients should be monitored and given appropriate exercise and rehabilitation. In daily life, vitamin D deficiency should be alleviated by sunbathing and Ca intake should be promoted by a Ca-rich diet such as dairy products. Nutritional intake of protein and other nutrients is also necessary. There are various types of drug therapy. Drug therapy should be initiated according to the criteria for initiation. Bisphosphonates, anti-RANKL antibodies (denosumab), and the osteogenic agent teriparatide (parathyroid hormone) are potent bone resorption inhibitors with high evidence of fracture prevention. In addition to bisphosphonates and selective estrogen receptor modulators (such as raloxifene hydrochloride), alfacalcidol, an active form of vitamin D, has been recommended for treatment and has been shown to prevent fractures, including vertebral bone and other bones. Vitamin K is approved only in Japan, but its mechanism of action on bone is unknown and its effect on fracture prevention has not been proven. Calcitonin acts directly on osteoclasts and inhibits bone resorption. In Japan, calcitonin is covered by insurance only for the relief of pain caused by osteoporosis.

## 3.9 Prognosis

Fracture of the neck of femur is the second most common cause of bedridden patients in Japan after stroke, accounting for about 13%. When patients become bedridden, they develop aspiration pneumonia, and the 5-year survival rate is about 50%. The mortality rate of patients with three or more vertebral fractures is four times higher than that of patients without vertebral fractures, and it is clear that vertebral fractures are a factor that worsens the prognosis of life.

## 3.10 Precautions in Dental Treatment: About RANKL

Bisphosphonates are potent inhibitors of bone resorption and are used in the treatment of osteoporosis, bone metastases of solid cancers, and multiple myeloma. Bisphosphonate-related osteonecrosis of the jaw (BRONJ) is a known side effect of bisphosphonates. Since it often occurs when a patient receiving this drug undergoes invasive dental treatment, such as tooth extraction. Since it often develops when patients receiving this drug receive invasive dental treatment that leads to bones such as tooth extraction, it is necessary to confirm whether or not they are taking this drug and consider for a treatment. Although the frequency of occurrence is unknown, injectable bisphosphonates are known to occur more frequently than oral bisphosphonates. The mechanism by which parathyroid hormone (PTH) matures bone precursor cells into osteoclasts through osteoblasts is the receptor activator of nuclear factor-kB (RANK) and the RANK ligand (RANKL) that binds to RANK. When PTH acts on osteoblasts, the osteoblasts secrete RANKL. Anti-RANKL antibodies are used for the treatment of osteoporosis and bone metastasis by inhibiting the action of RANKL and consequently suppressing bone resorption. However, osteonecrosis of the jaw has also been reported with denosumab, an anti-RANKL antibody, and is sometimes referred to as anti-resorptive agents-related osteonecrosis of the jaw (ARONJ) rather than BRONJ. If patients are receiving bisphosphonates or anti-RANKL antibodies in dental treatment, consult with the treating physician and allow an adequate withdrawal period.

## 3.11 Notes from Dentistry Perspective

Ikuya Miyamoto

### 3.11.1 Osteoporosis Is Increasing

It is estimated that there are 13 million patients with osteoporosis in Japan, and approximately one-third of the elderly population is affected. The number of patients is expected to increase further as the population ages.

### 3.11.2 Problems of Osteoporosis and Dental Treatment

Osteoporosis is not a direct risk for dental treatment. However, there are cases in which invasive procedures on bone require attention. For example, osteoporosis is a risk factor for implant treatment (Treatment Guidelines for Oral Implants 2020) [34].

### 3.11.3 Osteoporosis Medication and Osteonecrosis of the Jaw (ONJ)

Various treatment options are available for osteoporosis, and treatment with medication depends on the symptoms. Bisphosphonates (BPs) and other antiresorptive medications are used to treat osteoporosis. They can induce Osteonecrosis of the jaw (ONJ) following invasive bone treatment, such as tooth extraction or implant placement (Figs. 12.8, 12.9, 12.10, and 12.11). ONJ is closely associated with infected osteomyelitis; however, the detailed mechanisms are not clearly understood. Several terms are used to refer to this disease depending on the associated drug: bisphosphonate-related ONJ (BRONJ), anti-resorptive agent-related ONJ (ARONJ), and medication-related ONJ (MRONJ). There remains a lack of consensus regarding the management of ONJ. Based on the numerous published studies, the existing treatment strategies are based on regional associa-

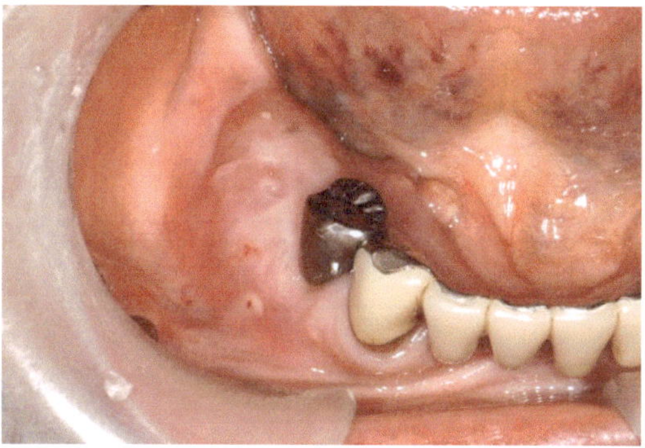

**Fig. 12.8** Osteonecrosis of the mandible on the right side. Multiple abscesses and pus discharge were observed in the alveolar region. The patient had been taking oral bisphosphonates for approximately 2 years for osteoporosis

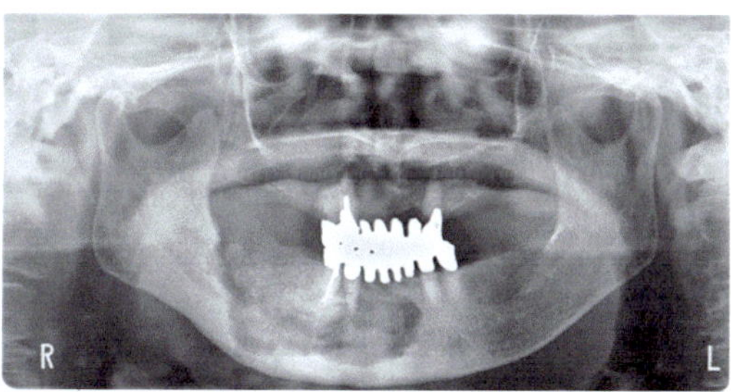


**Fig. 12.9** Panoramic radiograph of the same patient approximately 2 years after the photograph displayed in Fig. 12.8 was taken: separation of a large sequestrum separation is seen extending from the right premolar to right the molar region in the mandible

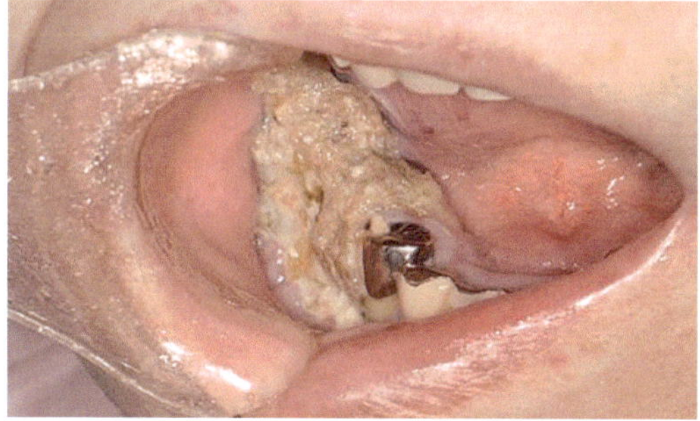

**Fig. 12.10** Approximately 2 years after the photograph presented in Fig. 12.8 was taken, bone exposure was observed in the same area, and sequestrectomy was performed

tions. A position paper on ONJ, "Management of osteonecrosis associated with antiresorptive medications," has been published in Japan. This

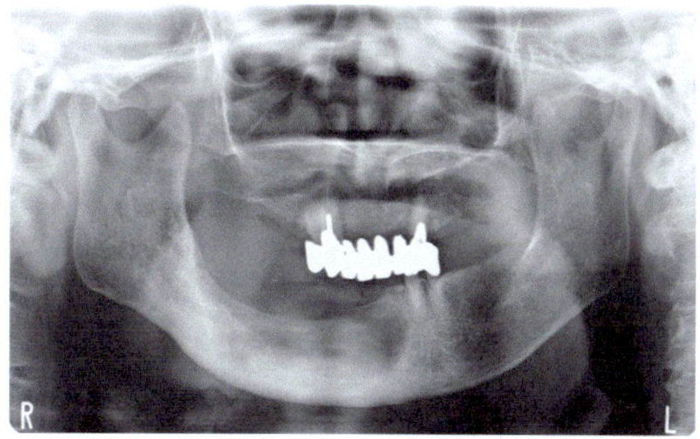


**Fig. 12.11** Panoramic radiograph of the patient taken after sequestrectomy: no sequestrum is seen

2016 position paper [35] classified ARONJ into stages and proposed treatment guidelines for each stage (Tables 12.3 and 12.4).

### 3.11.4 Common Sites and Risk Factors for ONJ

ONJ occurs predominantly in the mandible. The most common sites are the torus mandibularis, torus palatinus, and bony process in the mylohyoid of the mandibular molar lingual line, which is a sharp edge of bone with a thin oral membrane. In addition, periapical bone with chronic apical periodontitis or repeated periapical inflammation, decubitus ulcers with frequent bone exposure due to ill-fitting dentures, and bone protrusion prone to mucosal injury may increase risk of chronic damage to bone tissue. The main risk factors are listed in the position paper (Table 12.5).

### 3.11.5 Not All Osteoporosis Drugs Cause ONJ

BPs and anti-RANKL monoclonal antibody agents have the potential to cause ONJ. However, other drugs, such as hormones, active vitamins, selective estrogen receptor modulators, calcitonin, and parathyroid hormone, do not cause osteonecrosis.

### 3.11.6 Frequency of ONJ

According to the position paper, the incidence of ONJ in patients taking oral or intravenous nitrogen-containing BP medication for osteoporosis is estimated to be 0.001–0.01%. In contrast, the incidence of osteonecrosis in patients treated with denosumab ranges from 0 to 30.2 per 100,000 individuals.

**Table 12.3** Staging of ARONJ: clinical symptoms and imaging findings (Reproduced with permission from [35])

| | |
|---|---|
| Stage 0 | Clinical symptoms: no bone exposure/necrosis, deep periodontal pocket, loose tooth, oral mucosal ulcer, swelling, abscess formation, trismus, hypoesthesia/numbness of the lower lip (Vincent's symptom), non-odontogenic pain<br>Imaging findings: sclerotic alveolar bone, thickening and sclerosis of lamina dura, remaining tooth extraction socket |
| Stage 1 | Clinical symptoms: Asymptomatic bone exposure/necrosis without sign of infection, or fistula in which the bone is palpable with a probe<br>Imaging findings: Sclerotic alveolar bone, thickening and sclerosis of lamina dura, remaining tooth extraction socket |
| Stage 2 | Clinical symptoms: Bone exposure/necrosis associated with pain, infection, fistula in which bone is palpable with a probe or at least one of the following symptoms including bone exposure/necrosis over the alveolar bone (e.g., reaching the mandibular inferior edge or mandibular ramus, or reaching the maxillary sinus or mandibular ramus or the cheek bone), which result in pathologic fracture, extraoral fistula, nasal/maxillary sinus fistula formation, or advanced osteolydis extending to the mandibular inferior edge or maxillary sinus. |
| Stage 3 | Clinical symptoms: Bone exposure/necrosis associated with pain, infection, or at least one of the following symptoms, or fistula in which bone is palpable with a probe. Bone exposure/necrosis over the alveolar bone (e.g., reaching the mandibular inferior edge or mandibular ramus, or reaching the maxillary sinus or mandibular ramus or the cheek bone). As a result, pathologic fracture or extraoral fistula, nasal/maxillary sinus fistula formation, or advanced osteolysis extending to the mandibular inferior edge or maxillary sinus<br>Imaging findings: Osteosclerosis/osteolysis of the surrounding bone (cheek bone, palatine bone), pathologic mandibular fracture, and osteolysis extending to the maxillary sinus floor |

Note: Regardless of the stage of the disease, separated pieces of sequester should be removed without exposing the bone in the non-diseased area. Symptomatic teeth within the exposed necrotic bone should be considered for extraction, as the necrotic process is unlikely to be aggravated by extraction

**Table 12.4** Treatment of ARONJ (Reproduced with permission from [35])

| | |
|---|---|
| Stage 0/1 | Use of antimicrobial mouthwash, rinsing and cleaning of fistula and periodontal pocket, and topical application or injection of local antimicrobial agents |
| Stage 2 | Combination of antimicrobial mouthwash and agents; intractable case: Combination of multiple antimicrobial agents, long-term antimicrobial administration, continuous administration of intravenous antimicrobial agents, removal of sequestra, curettage of necrotic bones, and osteotomy |
| Stage 3 | Removal of sequestra, curettage of necrotic bones, osteotomy, extraction of tooth in exposed bone/necrotic bone as source of infection, maintenance of nutrition with supplements and infusions, and marginal or segmental resection of expanding necrotic bones |

Isolated sequestra are removed without exposing bones outside lesions, regardless of disease stage. A tooth with symptoms in exposed necrotic bones is extracted; extraction itself is unlikely to exacerbate necrosis

**Table 12.5** Risk factors for ARONJ (Reproduced with permission from [35])

| |
|---|
| 1. Local |
| Invasive dental treatments including bone (e.g., tooth extraction, dental implants, apical/periodontal surgery) |
| Ill-fitting dentures and excessive bite force |
| Poor sanitation in the oral cavity, periodontal disease, and gingival abscess inflammatory disease, including apical periodontitis |
| Common site: Mandible > maxilla, mandibular torus, palatal torus, and mylohyoid line torus |
| Root canal and orthodontic treatments are not considered to be risk factors |
| 2. Antiresorptive agents |
| Nitrogen-containing bisphosphonates (BPs) > non nitrogen-containing bisphosphonates (BPs) |
| Nitrogen-containing BPs: Zoledronate (Zometa), alendronate (Teiroc, Fosamac, Bonalon), risedronate sodium (Actonel, Benet), pamidronate (Aredia), incadronate (Bisphonal), minodronate (Bonoteo, Recalbon), ibandronate (Bonviva) |
| Non nitrogen-containing BPs: Etidronate (Didronel) |
| Denosumab (Ranmark, malignant tumor; Pralia, osteoporosis) |
| Drugs for malignant tumor > drugs for osteoporosis |
| Drugs for malignant tumor (Zometa, Aredia, Teiroc, Ranmark) |
| Drugs for osteoporosis (Didronel, Fosamac, Bonalon, Actonel, Benet, Bonoteo, Recalbon, Bonviva and Pralia) |

**Table 12.5** (continued)

| Dose and administration period |
|---|
| 3. Systemic |
| Cancer (breast, prostate, lung, renal and colon cancer, multiple myeloma, and other cancers) |
| Diabetes, rheumatoid arthritis, hypocalcemia, hypoparathyroidism, osteomalacia, vitamin D deficiency, renal dialysis, anemia, and Paget's disease of bone |
| 4. Congenital |
| Single-nucleotide polymorphisms (SNPs) in MMP-2 and cytochrome P450-2C genes |
| 5. Lifestyle |
| Smoking, drinking, and obesity |
| 6. Co-administered agents |
| Anticancer agents, corticosteroids, and erythropoietin |
| Angiogenic inhibitors (e.g., thalidomide, sunitinib, bevacizumab, and lenalidomide) |
| Tyrosine kinase inhibitors |

Note: These factors are proposed risk factors for ARONJ, but no evidence has been demonstrated

### 3.11.7 Drug Cessation

ONJ does not occur in all patients. Drug cessation at the time of tooth extraction has been suggested to avoid ARONJ; however, this hypothesis remains controversial. The position paper described a lack of clinical evidence to support drug cessation before invasive dental procedures. Osteoporosis medications are necessary for the treatment of osteoporosis, and drug cessation should not be recommended simply because of the risk of ONJ.

### 3.11.8 Dental Treatment of Patients Taking BP or the Other Anti-resorptive Agents

Generally, the dental treatment of patients taking this medication is not problematic. In cases of invasive dental treatment, such as tooth extraction, patients generally do not need drug cessation, and treatment, including tooth extraction, may be possible. However, patients at high risk of ONJ should be treated with caution. The risk factors include administration of injectable BP, chronic inflammation of the bone, poor oral hygiene, and concomitant intake of medications, such as corticosteroids, smoking, and alcohol consumption. In any case, to proceed with the treatment, a close relationship between the dentist and doctors acquainted with the patient's condition is necessary. In addition, if there is a risk of medication-related osteonecrosis of the Jaw (MRONJ), it is important to provide the patient an adequate explanation and obtain informed consent before treatment.

## 4 Amyloidosis [36–39]

Fumiko Miyanaga

### 4.1 Overview

Amyloidosis is a group of diseases in which fibrillar amyloid protein is deposited extracellularly in various organs of the body, causing organ damage.

### 4.2 Cause and Classification

Amyloid is structurally unique in that it has a beta-sheet structure, which makes it insoluble and resistant to the action of proteolytic enzymes, making it difficult to remove from the body, and various proteins aggregate to form a fibrous structure and deposit in tissues.

Amyloidosis can be classified into two types according to the mode of amyloid deposition: systemic amyloidosis, in which amyloid is deposited in various organs of the body, and localized amyloidosis, in which amyloid is deposited only in certain organs. Furthermore, there is a classification of clinical types corresponding to various amyloid proteins (precursor proteins) (Table 12.6). At least 36 types of amyloidosis have been identified, including AA derived from serum amyloid A, which is an acute phase protein, AL derived from immunoglobulin light chains (L chains), and AH derived from immunoglobulin H chains. There are still many unknown amyloidosis.

**Table 12.6** Classification of the main amyloidosis

| | Group of diseases | Amyloid protein | Precursor protein |
|---|---|---|---|
| Systemic amyloidosis | [Non-hereditary] | | |
| | Immunoglobulin-related amyloidosis | | |
| | AL amyloidosis | AL | Immunoglobulin L chain |
| | AH amyloidosis | AH | Immunoglobulin H chain |
| | Secondary/reactive amyloidosis | AA | Serum amyloid A |
| | Dialysis amyloidosis | $A\beta_2M$ | β2 microglobulin |
| | Senile systemic amyloidosis | ATTR | Transthyretin |
| | [Hereditary (familial)] | | |
| | FAP Type I, II | ATTR | Transthyretin |
| | FAP Type III | AApoA I | Apolipoprotein A-I |
| | FAP Type IV | Agel | Gelsolin |
| | Familial Mediterranean fever, muckle-Wells syndrome | AA | (Apo) SAA |
| Localized amyloidosis | Cerebral amyloidosis | | |
| | [Non-hereditary] | | |
| | Alzheimer's disease, cerebral amyloid angiopathy (CAA) | Aβ | AβPP |
| | Cretsfeldt-Jakob disease (CJD) (arcuate, acquired) | APrP | Prion protein (PrP) |
| | [Hereditary (familial)] | | |
| | Familial Alzheimer's disease, hereditary CAA (Dutch type) | Aβ | AβPP |
| | Hereditary prion disease | APrP | Prion protein (PrP) |
| | Endocrine amyloidosis | | |
| | Medullary thyroid cancer | ACal | Procalcitonin |
| | Type 2 diabetes mellitus | AIAPP | Amylin |
| | Localized atrial amyloidosis | AANF | ANP |
| | Prolactin-producing tumor | APro | Prolactin |
| | Localized nodular amyloidosis | AL | Immunoglobulin L chain |
| | Aortic tunica media amyloidosis | AMed | Lactoadherin |
| | Corneal amyloidosis | ALac | Lactoferrin |

*FAP*: familial amyloid polyneuropathy
(Created based on [34])

## 4.3 Clinical Image

Symptoms of systemic amyloidosis are latent and manifest in a variety of clinical manifestations due to the impairment of the function of the deposited amyloid organs. In many cases, amyloidosis is treated as a disease of unknown etiology because of the lack of symptoms specific to the disease, or it is diagnosed only after autopsy.

Symptoms of amyloidosis that should be noted are those of the kidneys, heart, gastrointestinal tract, and nerves.

1. Renal disorders: deposition on glomerular basement membrane, proteinuria, edema, nephrotic syndrome, renal failure, etc.
2. Cardiac disease: deposition in the endocardium, myocardium, and conduction system; heart failure symptoms such as palpitations, dyspnea, and edema; arrhythmia, etc.
3. Gastrointestinal symptoms: abdominal pain, macrognathia, hepatomegaly, gastrointestinal bleeding, anorexia, dysphagia, diarrhea, constipation, malabsorption/protein losing gastroenteropathy, etc.

4. Neurological symptoms: In amyloid polyneuropathy, autonomic neuropathy, and superficial sensory disturbance occur, and in localized amyloid neuropathy, median neuropathy is observed in carpal tunnel syndrome.

   Numbness in the lower limbs, muscle weakness, dizziness, dyshydrosis, urinary disturbance, impotency, etc.
5. Skin manifestations: It is mainly deposited on the walls of small blood vessels.

   Purpura, abnormal pigmentation, atrophy, etc.

## 4.4 Examination and Diagnosis

The diagnosis of amyloidosis should be suspected from the patient's symptoms. The definitive diagnosis is based on biopsy evidence of amyloid deposition in the affected organ. Amyloid is pathologically identified as an eosinophilic material by Congo-Red staining under light microscopy and an apple-green birefringence under polarized light microscopy (Figs. 12.12 and 12.13).

Once Congo-Red positive findings are obtained, immunostaining with specific antibodies against various amyloid proteins (AL, AA, A$\beta_2$MG, ATTR, etc.) is performed for the diagnosis of the disease type, assuming amyloid precursor protein. If the positive image of the specific antibody is consistent with the pattern of amyloid deposition, the type of the disease can be finally identified.

Functional tests of the affected organs include electrocardiography, echocardiography, blood tests, urinalysis, and bone marrow puncture.

## 4.5 Treatment and Prognosis

The treatment of amyloidosis consists of a combination of treatment of the deposited amyloid and symptomatic treatment of damage to the deposited amyloid organs. If myeloma or chronic inflammatory disease is the cause of the disease, the primary disease should be treated. In the past, amyloidosis was treated mainly through symptomatic treatment, but in recent years, therapies that strongly inhibit the production of amyloid precursor protein have been successful in clinical practice. These include liver transplantation for hereditary ATTR amyloidosis (FAP), autologous peripheral blood stem cell transplantation combined with high-dose melphalan chemotherapy as a fundamental treatment for AL amyloidosis, and biologics for AA amyloidosis. In addition, a large number of clinical trials are being conducted, and the development of new anti-amyloid therapies is progressing rapidly. On the other hand, there are some types of amyloidosis for

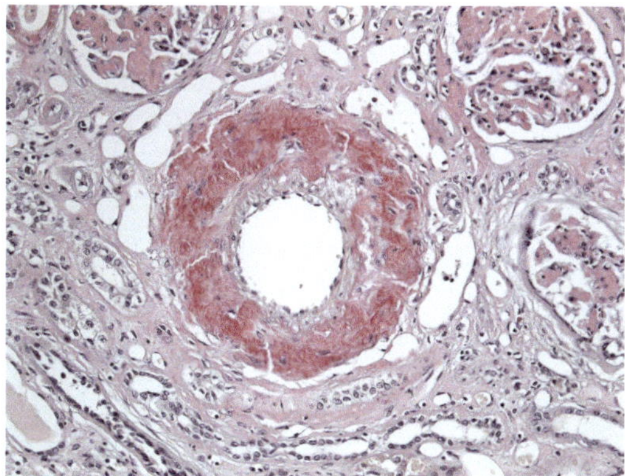

**Fig. 12.12** Congo-Red staining image of renal capillary blood vessels. The area of amyloid deposition is seen as a red-orange material. (Courtesy of Pathology Laboratory, Division of Clinical Laboratory, Osaka Dental University Hospital)

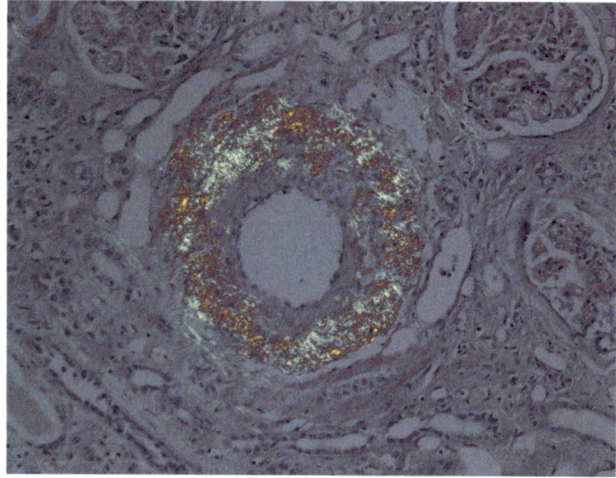

**Fig. 12.13** Polarized light microscopy image of renal capillary blood vessels. The amyloid deposition site shows an apple-green birefringence under polarized light. (Courtesy of Pathology Laboratory, Division of Clinical Laboratory, Osaka Dental University Hospital)

which no fundamental treatment has been established, and there are also many cases in which strong treatment is not possible because of advanced multiorgan damage or poor general condition. Therefore, we provide drug therapy for various symptoms and supportive therapy for poor general condition.

The prognosis of amyloidosis depends on the type of disease. Although there are individual differences, the course of the disease is basically progressive, and if not treated, the prognosis is poor.

## 4.6 Notes from Dentistry Perspective

Hiroyuki Yamada

In the oral and maxillofacial region, amyloid deposition has been reported in the tongue, lips, corners of the mouth, salivary glands, and buccal mucosa, with initial symptoms of swelling, presence of a mass, and hematoma [40–43]. Many cases feature deposition on the tongue, and as the disease progresses, dysphagia and dysphonia occur due to decreased mobility of the tongue. Ulceration and bleeding of the tongue may arise from mechanical stimulation of the teeth. In addition, dyspnea and upper airway stenosis caused by macroglossia, are also known to occur [44–46].

The treatment of systemic amyloidosis can be divided into two categories: causative therapy, for the process of amyloid deposition, and symptomatic therapy, for organ damage or symptoms resulting from amyloid deposition.

Oral amyloidosis has been treated with tracheotomy for dyspnea [44] and tongue reduction surgery for mouth closure problems due to macroglossia [47].

In the dental treatment of patients with amyloidosis, it is important to identify the type of amyloidosis the patient has and to treat the patient with the utmost care to avoid aggravating the condition. Therefore, the dentist should collaborate with the attending physician and share patient information prior to treatment to identify the type of amyloidosis. In particular, patients with cardiac or renal amyloidosis should be treated in the same way as patients with cardiac or renal disease by recognizing the possibility of impaired organ function. When highly invasive treatment is required for patients with cardiac deposits, adequate pain control should be provided and vital signs should be carefully monitored. When administering medication to a patient with renal deposits, special consideration should be given to selecting a drug with hepatic metabolism and adjusting the drug dose according to renal function, in line with chronic kidney disease guidelines [48].

It may be difficult to recognize amyloidosis when the presence of systemic disease is not known from the patient's history. However, it is important to include amyloidosis in the differential diagnosis of patients with macroglossia (Fig. 12.14) or multiple nodular lesions in the oral cavity (Figs. 12.15 and 12.16). Furthermore, if a biopsy from an oral lesion is histopathologically

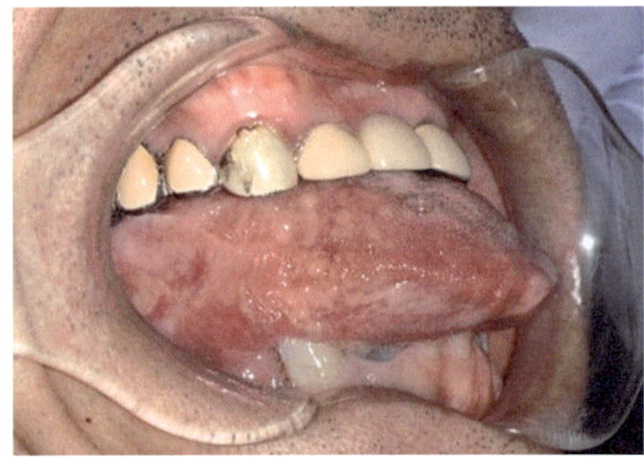

**Fig. 12.14** Pathological picture of macroglossia. Inability to close the mouth due to macroglossia

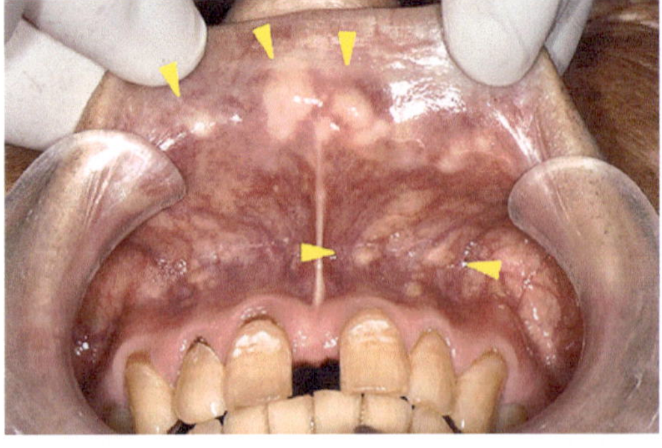

**Fig. 12.15** Multiple masses in the oral cavity. Multiple small masses (arrowhead) are seen in the upper lip mucosa

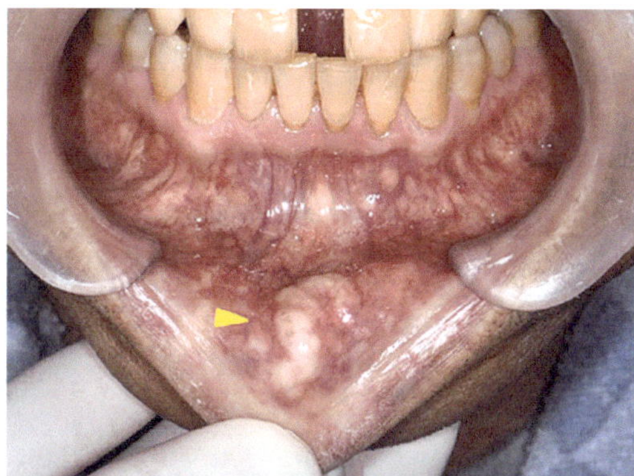

**Fig. 12.16** Mass of the lower lip. A mass (arrowhead) is seen in the mucosa of the lower lip

confirmed to be amyloidosis, the patient should be referred to a medical clinic even if the clinical symptoms related to the oral cavity are mild. This is because oral lesions may lead to the diagnosis of malignant diseases such as multiple myeloma. From this point of view, clinical knowledge of amyloidosis is essential for dentists.

## References


1. The Japan Diabetes Society, editor. Guidebook for diabetes treatment (Tonyobyo Chiryo Guide) 2022–2023 ed. Tokyo: Bunkodo; 2022. p. 14. (in Japanese).
2. Seino, Y., Nanjo, K., Tajima, N. et al. Report of the Committee on the classification and diagnostic criteria of diabetes mellitus. Diabetol Int 1, 2–20 (2010).
3. The Japan Diabetes Society, editor. Guidebook for diabetes treatment (Tonyobyo Chiryo guide). 2022–2023 ed. Tokyo: Bunkodo; 2022. p. 18. (in Japanese).
4. The Japan Diabetes Society, editor. Guidebook for diabetes treatment (Tonyobyo Chiryo Guide). 2022–2023 ed. Tokyo: Bunkodo; 2022. p. 15. (in Japanese).
5. The Japan Diabetes Society, editor. Guidebook for diabetes treatment (Tonyobyo Chiryo Guide). 2016-2017 ed. Tokyo: Bunkodo; 2020. p. 8.
6. The Japan Diabetes Society, editor. Guidebook for diabetes treatment (Tonyobyo Chiryo Guide). 2022–2023 ed. Tokyo: Bunkodo; 2022. p. 87. (in Japanese).
7. The Japan Diabetes Society, editor. Guidebook for diabetes treatment (Tonyobyo Chiryo Guide). 2022–2023 ed. Tokyo: Bunkodo; 2022. p. 92. (in Japanese).
8. The Japan Diabetes Society, editor. Guidebook for diabetes treatment (Tonyobyo Chiryo Guide). 2022–2023 ed. Tokyo: Bunkodo; 2022. p.94–95. (in Japanese).
9. Goto A, et al. Diabetes and cancer risk: a Mendelian randomization study. Int J Cancer. 2019;146(3):712–9.
10. The Japan Diabetes Society, editor. Guidebook for diabetes treatment 2016–2017. Tokyo: Bunkodo; 2016. p. 14.
11. The Japan Diabetes Society, editor. Guidebook for diabetes treatment 2016–2017. Tokyo: Bunkodo; 2016. p. 53.
12. The Japan Diabetes Society, editor. Guidebook for diabetes treatment (Tonyobyo Chiryo Guide). 2022–2023 ed. Tokyo: Bunkodo; 2022. p.49–50 (in Japanese).
13. The Japan Diabetes Society, editor. Food exchange lists-dietary guidance for persons with diabetes. 7th ed. Tokyo: Bunkodo; 2017.
14. Committee for the review of diagnostic criteria for metabolic syndrome. J Jpn Soc Intern Med. 2005;94:794–809. (in Japanese).
15. Furuya H ed. Shika Masuigaku (Dental Anesthesiology). 5th ed. Tokyo; Ishiyaku Syuppan. P. 189, 221. 1997. (in Japanese)
16. The Japan Diabetes Society, editor. Japanese clinical practice guideline for diabetes (Tonyobyo Shindan guideline). 2016 ed. Tokyo: Nanko-do; 2016. p. 293. (in Japanese).
17. Preshaw PM, et al. Periodontitis and diabetes: a two-way relationship. Diabetologia. 2012;55(1):21–31.
18. The Japan Diabetes Society, editor. Guidebook for diabetes treatment (Tonyobyo Chiryo Guide). 2020–2021 ed. Tokyo: Bunkodo; 2020. p. 95–6. (in Japanese).
19. Editorial Board for "Dental Treatment for Patients with Diseases", editor. Dental treatment for patients with diseases: advice to dentistry (Byoukiwo Motta Kanjyano Shikachiryou: Ika kara Shika heno advice). Revised ed. Nagasaki: Nagasaki Doctor & Dentist Association; 2017. p. 150–1. (in Japanese).
20. Japan Atherosclerosis Society. Clinical practice guidelines on dyslipidemia for prevention of arteriosclerotic disease (Doumyakukoukasei Shikkannyobou notameno Shishitsuijyousho Shinryo guide). 2018th ed. Tokyo: Japan Atherosclerosis Society; 2018. p. 4–10. (in Japanese).
21. Ministry of Health, Labour and Welfare Japan. Outline of Vital Statistics in Japan. Table 6: ranking of causes of death per sex and death rates (per 100,000 population). 2017. https://www.mhlw.go.jp/toukei/saikin/hw/jinkou/kakutei17/dl/10_h6.pdf (in Japanese). Accessed 22 Feb 2022.
22. Ross R. Atherosclerosis—an inflammatory disease. N Engl J Med. 1999;340(2):115–26.
23. Danesh J, et al. C-reactive protein and other circulating markers of inflammation in the prediction of coronary heart disease. N Engl J Med. 2004;350(14):1387–97.
24. Nakajima T, et al. Periodontitis-associated up-regulation of systemic inflammatory mediator level may increase the risk of coronary heart disease. J Periodontal Res. 2010;45(1):116–22.
25. Noack B, et al. Periodontal infections contribute to elevated systemic C-reactive. J Periodontol. 2001;72(9):1221–7.

26. Tonetti MS, et al. Treatment of periodontitis and endothelial function. N Engl J Med. 2007;356(9):911–20.
27. Gordon DJ, Rifkind BM. High-density lipoprotein—the clinical implications of recent studies. N Engl J Med. 1989;321(19):1311–6.
28. Kudo C, et al. Analysis of the relationship between periodontal disease and atherosclerosis within a local clinical system: a cross-sectional observational pilot study. Odontology. 2015;103(3):314–21.
29. D'Aiuto F, et al. Periodontal infections cause changes in traditional and novel cardiovascular risk factors: results from a randomized controlled clinical trial. Am Heart J. 2006;151(5):977–84.
30. Lockhart PB, et al. Periodontal disease and atherosclerotic vascular disease: does the evidence support an independent association? The evidence support an independent association? : A scientific statement from the American Heart Association. Circulation. 2012;125(20):2520–444.
31. The Committee for Developing Guidelines for Prevention and Treatment of Osteoporosis, editor. Guidelines for prevention and treatment of osteoporosis. Tokyo: Life Science Publishing; 2015. (in Japanese).
32. Sugimoto T, et al. ASAKURA internal medicine (Naikagaku). 9th ed. Tokyo: Asakura Shoten; 2007. (in Japanese).
33. Nishida J, et al. Internal medicine for the odontology (Shikanotameno Naikagaku). Revised 4th ed. Tokyo: Nankodo; 2018. (in Japanese).
34. Japanese Society of Oral Implantology, editor. Treatment guidelines for oral implants 2020 (Koukuu implant Chiryoushishin 2020 Kensahou Shindan kara risk management made). Tokyo: Ishiyaku Shuppan; 2020. (in Japanese).
35. Japanese Allied Committee on Osteonecrosis of the Jaw, Yoneda T, et al. Antiresorptive agent-related osteonecrosis of the jaw: position paper 2017 of the Japanese Allied Committee on Osteonecrosis of the Jaw. J Bone Miner Metab. 2017;35:6–19.
36. Amyloidosis Research Group, Health and Labor Sciences Research Grants, Research Project for Overcoming Intractable Diseases. Guidelines for the treatment of amyloidosis 2010. (in Japanese). http://amyloidosis-research-committee.jp/wp-content/uploads/2018/02/guideline2010.pdf. Accessed 22 Feb 2022.
37. Sanchorawala V, et al. Long-term outcome of patients with AL amyloidosis treated with high-dose melphalan and stem cell transplantation: a 20-year experience. Blood. 2015;126:2345–7.
38. Jaccard A, et al. High-dose melphalan versus melphalan plus dexamethasone for AL amyloidosis. N Engl J Med. 2007;357:1083–93.
39. Benson MD, et al. Amyloid nomenclature 2018: recommendations by the International Society of Amyloidosis (ISA) nomenclature committee. Amyloid. 2018;25(4):215–9.
40. Fijita T, Idou S, et al. A case of amyloidosis with multiple myeloma accompanied by rapidly growing macroglossia (Kyusokuni Zoudaishi Kyozetsuwo Teishita Tahatsusei Kotsuzuisyu nitomonau Amylodosis no Ichirei). Jpn J Oral Maxillofac Surg. 2014;61:25–30. (in Japanese).
41. Kawamata A, Yamada T, et al. A case report of localized nodular amyloidosis of the sublingual gland. (Zekkasenni Hasseishita Kyokugensei Kessetussei Amylodosis no Ichirei.). Jpn J Oral Maxillofac Surg. 2013;59:38–42. (in Japanese).
42. Shibata A, Shimizu T, et al. A case of bilateral primary localized amyloidosis of the angle of the mouth (Ryougawa Koukakuni Hassyoushita Genpatsusei Kyokugensei Amylodosis no Ichirei). Jpn J Oral Maxillofac Surg. 2012;58:252–6. (in Japanese).
43. Yamashiro T, Nakamatsu K, et al. A case of amyloidosis with massive hematoma of the lower lip and the buccal mucosa (Kashinto Hoonenmakuni Kouhanna Kessyuwo Keiseisita Amylodosis no Ichirei). Jpn J Oral Maxillofac Surg. 2010;56:705–9. (in Japanese).
44. Kimura Y, Shimahara M, et al. A case of systemic amyloidosis with swelling in the tongue and submandibular region as an initial symptom (Zetsu oyobi Gakukabu no Shucyou wokeikini Hakkennsareta Zenshinsei Amylodosis no Ichirei). Jpn J Oral Maxillofac Surg. 2009;55:71–5. (in Japanese).
45. Brenes-salazar JA, Grogan M, et al. A 66-year-old woman with an enlarged tongue. Cleve Clin J Med. 2013;80(11):696–7.
46. Liakou CI, Koh J, et al. A tongue lesion as a sign of a systemic disease. Case Rep Med. 2016;2016:6723575. https://doi.org/10.1155/2016/6723575.
47. Nakasone T, Matayoshi A, et al. A case of massive macroglossia caused by senile systemic amyloidosis (Roujinsei Zenshinsei amyloidosis niyori Shoujita Kyozetsusyou no ichirei). Jpn J Oral Maxillofac Surg. 2016;62:304–8. (in Japanese).
48. Japanese Society of Nephrology, editor. Evidence ni Motozuku CKD Shinryo guideline 2018 (Evidence-based clinical practice guideline for CKD 2018). Tokyo: Tokyo Igaku-sha; 2018. (in Japanese).

# Kidney Diseases

# 13

Masanori Tokumoto, Koichi Hayashi, Hiroshige Ohashi, and Akira Sasaki

## 1 Nephritis [1–3]

Masanori Tokumoto

Nephritis can be divided into glomerulonephritis and interstitial nephritis according to the site of inflammation in the kidney, and acute and chronic nephritis according to the degree of progression. In this section, acute glomerulonephritis, rapidly progressive glomerulonephritis, chronic glomerulonephritis, and acute interstitial nephritis, which are not partial diseases of systemic diseases but primary and relatively frequent diseases, are reviewed.

M. Tokumoto (✉)
Department of Nephrology, Japanese Red Cross Fukuoka Hospital, Fukuoka, Japan
e-mail: m-tokumoto@fukuoka-med.jrc.or.jp

K. Hayashi
Department of Emergency and Critical Care Medicine, St. Marianna University Yokohama Seibu Hospital, Yokohama, Kanagawa, Japan

H. Ohashi
Asahi University Hospital, Gifu, Japan

A. Sasaki
Okayama University, Okayama, Japan

Department of Dentistry (Oral Surgery), Kurashiki Central Hospital, Kurashiki, Okayama, Japan

### 1.1 Acute Glomerulonephritis

#### 1.1.1 Definition

It is a syndrome of acute onset of hematuria, proteinuria, decreased glomerular filtration rate (GFR), sodium (Na)/water retention, and hypertension.

#### 1.1.2 Pathophysiology

It develops after an incubation period of 1–2 weeks following upper respiratory tract infection. Some of the infectious pathogens become antigens, forming immune complexes and depositing them in the glomeruli, and inflammatory cells accumulate and endothelial cells and mesangial cells proliferate, resulting in obstruction of blood vessels in the glomeruli and impairment of glomerular blood flow. As a result, GFR and urine volume decreases, and sodium and water accumulate, causing hypertension and edema. Typically after hemolytic streptococcal (streptococcal) infection; conventionally, about 80–90% of cases were group A beta-hemolytic streptococcus, and streptococcus pneumoniae, staphylococcus aureus, fungi, and parvoviruses have been reported as causative pathogens in recent years.

#### 1.1.3 Epidemiology

It is common in children and adolescents, but also occurs in the elderly.



T. Chiba, H. Yamada (eds.), *Internal Medicine for Dental Treatments*,
https://doi.org/10.1007/978-981-99-3296-2_13

### 1.1.4 Symptoms

Hematuria, edema, and hypertension are the main symptoms. Gross hematuria (brown or cola color) is observed in about one third of cases, but it disappears in a few days to 2 weeks. Edema is present on the face and upper and lower extremities, and is more pronounced around the eyelids on waking. The patient may have oliguria with urine volume of less than 400 mL/day, and excessive circulating plasma volume may cause symptoms of heart failure.

### 1.1.5 Clinical Examination

Microscopic hematuria is always present, and most cases are accompanied by erythrocyte cast and proteinuria. Blood tests show a decrease in complements (CH50, C3) early in the course of the disease and an increase in serum antibody titers such as antistreptolysin O (ASO) and antistreptokinase (ASK) if after streptococcal infection. Bacteria may be detected in pharyngeal culture. GFR is decreased in about half of cases, and blood urea nitrogen (BUN) and serum creatinine (Cr) may be transiently elevated. Renal biopsy shows many inflammatory cells, including neutrophils filling the vascular lumen, such as endocapillary proliferation, and immunofluorescence microscopy shows granular deposition of C3 along the glomerular capillary wall and granular deposition of IgG in the early stages of the disease.

### 1.1.6 Treatment

Rest and diet therapy (high calorie intake, protein and salt restriction) are main, and rest in the early stages of illness is particularly important. If streptococcal infection is confirmed in the early stages of illness, antibacterial agents such as penicillin may be used, but not if the infection has been already cured. If hypertension and edema cannot be treated by salt restriction, diuretics should be administered. Antihypertensive agents may also be used to treat hypertension.

### 1.1.7 Prognosis

In children, more than 90% of cases are completely cured within 3–6 months, but the cure rate decreases with age, and the cure rate in adults is about 60–80% and the disease tends to become chronic.

## 1.2 Rapidly Progressive Glomerulonephritis

### 1.2.1 Definition

It is a syndrome of rapidly progressive renal failure over a period of weeks to months, accompanied by urinary abnormalities indicative of nephritis.

### 1.2.2 Pathophysiology

More than half of the cases have systemic vasculitis with positive of antineutrophil cytoplasmic antibodies (ANCA) in the blood, but acute glomerulonephritis, other primary glomerulonephritis, and infectious and collagen diseases may also be the cause.

### 1.2.3 Epidemiology

It is common in middle-aged and elderly people.

### 1.2.4 Symptoms

Most of the initial symptoms are non-specific, such as fever, arthralgia/myalgia, and loss of appetite. As renal dysfunction progresses, edema, hypertension, oliguria, and anuria are observed. Respiratory symptoms are also common.

### 1.2.5 Clinical Examination

Hematuria, proteinuria, and cylindruria are observed, and GFR is decreased and BUN and serum Cr are increased. Inflammatory findings such as elevated CRP and erythrocyte sedimentation rate, and severe anemia relative to the degree of renal dysfunction are often observed. ANCA and anti-glomerular basement membrane (GBM) antibodies are often positive, and reduced complements are not rare. The typical case is crescentic glomerulonephritis, in which more than 50% of glomeruli on renal biopsy show the formation of a crescent (increased epithelial cells of Bowman's capsule, monocytes, macrophages, and other cells that look like a crescent). There are various types in this disease. It can be divided into three types by immunofluorescence microscopy: (1) immunocomplex type, in which IgG is deposited in granular pattern on the glomerular capillary wall and mesangium; (2) anti-GBM antibody type, in which IgG is deposited in linear pattern on the glomerular capillary wall; and (3) pauci-immune type, in which immune complexes are less deposited. In Japan, pauci-immune type is the most common, and ANCA is found in many cases.

### 1.2.6 Treatment

Immunosuppressive therapy with corticosteroids and immunosuppressive drugs is the basic treatment. In the initial stage, oral corticosteroids are administered, and high-dose intravenous corticosteroids are used when there are severe inflammatory findings or multiple organ involvement. Immunosuppressive drugs are used in combination depending on the condition of the patient. In Europe and the United States, plasma exchange therapy is used for alveolar hemorrhage patients with ANCA-associated vasculitis or anti-GBM antibodies.

### 1.2.7 Prognosis

The renal prognosis and vital prognosis are both poor, and dialysis is often required, but there are cases of death during the course.

## 1.3 Chronic Glomerulonephritis

### 1.3.1 Definition

It is a primary glomerular disease in which abnormalities in urinalysis such as proteinuria, hematuria, and cylindruria persist for more than 1 year.

### 1.3.2 Pathophysiology

It is thought to be caused by an antigen-antibody reaction in the local glomeruli or by the deposition of immune complexes formed in the blood to the glomeruli, resulting in an immune reaction in the local glomeruli. With persistent inflammatory stimulation, glomerular component cells, infiltrating leukocytes, and platelets produce growth factors, proteolytic enzymes, and reactive oxygen species, resulting in inflammation not only in the glomeruli but also in the interstitium. Furthermore, hemodynamic changes in the glomerular region cause glomerular hypertension, which leads to glomerulosclerosis via glomerular hyperfiltration.

### 1.3.3 Epidemiology

It is the second most common primary cause of dialysis initiation and is more common in young patients than in the elderly.

### 1.3.4 Classification

Histopathologically, there are several types of nephropathy such as IgA nephropathy, mesangial proliferative glomerulonephritis, membranous nephropathy, membranoproliferative glomerulonephritis, minimal change nephrotic syndrome, focal glomerulosclerosis, etc. In Japan, the frequency of IgA nephropathy is the highest.

#### IgA Nephropathy

1. **Outline**: This is a mesangial proliferative glomerulonephritis with granular deposition of IgA in the mesangial region of the glomeruli.
2. **Epidemiology**: This is the most common primary chronic glomerulonephritis in Japan, accounting for more than 30% of chronic glomerulonephritis in adults. Because of the lack of symptoms, it is often detected by abnormal urine analysis.
3. **Symptoms**: In most cases, the symptoms are asymptomatic, but gross hematuria, edema, and hypertension may be observed with upper respiratory tract infection.
4. **Clinical Examination**: Microscopic hematuria is almost always observed, and deformed erythrocytes or erythrocytic cast may be seen in the urinary sediment. Proteinuria is also common. Serum IgA is elevated in more than half of patients, and renal function may be impaired at the time of diagnosis. Renal biopsy shows proliferation of mesangial cells and enlargement of the mesangial matrix, which may be accompanied by a crescent. Immunofluorescence microscopy shows granular IgA deposition mainly in the mesangial region, often accompanied by C3 deposition.
5. **Treatment**: Dietary therapy (high calorie intake, protein and salt restriction) and drug therapy are the basic treatments. In the group with low activity and low possibility of end-stage renal failure, the patient is observed without drug therapy. Patients with highly active acute lesion should be treated with

corticosteroids. Inhibitors of the renin-angiotensin system are often used to inhibit the increase in intraglomerular pressure and reduce proteinuria.

6. **Prognosis**: The prognosis had been thought to be good with a relatively gradual course, but it has become clear that approximately 20–40% of patients progress to end-stage renal failure and require hemodialysis more than 20 years after diagnosis. In general, the prognosis is poor in patients with hypertension and high levels of proteinuria in the early stage of the disease.

### 1.4 Acute Tubulointerstitial Nephritis

#### 1.4.1 Pathophysiology

Allergy to drugs such as antimicrobials, nonsteroidal anti-inflammatory agents, diuretics, uric acid synthesis inhibitors, and anti-ulcer agents is the main cause of the disease, which develops more than 2 weeks after initiation of the drug. All drugs are possible causes.

#### 1.4.2 Symptoms

Patients may be asymptomatic and may complain of anorexia, nausea and vomiting, and general malaise. They may also complain of back pain associated with renal enlargement, skin rash associated with drug allergy, fever, and arthralgia.

#### 1.4.3 Clinical Examination

Both proteinuria and hematuria are mild, but tubular injury results in increased urinary excretion of low-molecular-weight proteins (α1 and β2-microglobulin) that is absorbed from the tubular epithelium and N-acetylglucosaminidase (NAG) that is an enzyme in tubular epithelium. Sterile pyuria is characteristic, and eosinophils may be detected in the urine. In blood tests, both BUN and serum Cr are elevated, but the BUN/Cr ratio is characteristically less than 10. In drug allergy, there is an increase in peripheral blood eosinophils and serum IgE. In renal biopsy, glomeruli are almost normal, and there is marked inflammatory cell infiltration and edema in the interstitium surrounding the injured tubules.

#### 1.4.4 Treatment and Prognosis

In cases of drug-induced acute tubulointerstitial nephritis, renal function often recovers with discontinuation of the causative drug. The prognosis is good if the disease is detected early, and complete remission is usually achieved. If renal function does not improve after discontinuation of the causative drug, corticosteroids or immunosuppressive drugs may be administered. Oliguria and uremia may occur, and hemodialysis may be required.

## 2 Acute Renal Failure [4–7]

Koichi Hayashi

### 2.1 Disease Overview

Acute renal failure (ARF) is a life-threatening condition caused by a rapid decline in renal function, resulting in accumulation of metabolites, electrolyte abnormalities, disturbance of acid-base equilibrium, and dysregulation of fluid volume. Until now, there has been no definitive definition of the diagnosis of acute renal failure, but much attention has been mainly focused on the search for the cause and countermeasures against complications, rather than on early detection. In recent years, the concept of acute kidney injury (AKI) has been proposed to improve the prognosis by early diagnosis and intervention, and the definition of AKI has been established. The transition in perception from acute renal failure to AKI is now well established.

**Table 13.1** Diagnostic criteria for stage of acute kidney injury

| | sCr criteria | Urinary excretion criteria |
|---|---|---|
| Stage 1 | ΔCr ≥ 0.3 mg/dL or 1.5–1.9 times sCr elevated | 0.5 mL/kg/h or less for more than 6 h |
| Stage 2 | sCr elevated 2.0–2.9 times | 0.5 mL/kg/h or less for more than 12 h |
| Stage 3 | sCr elevated > 3.0 times or sCr > 4.0 mg/dL or start of renal replacement therapy | 0.5 mL/kg/h or less for more than 24 h or anuria for more than 12 h |

Definition

1. ΔCr ≥ 0.3 mg/dL (within 48 h)
2. 1.5 times higher than the reference value of sCr (within 7 days)
3. Urine output of 0.5 mL/kg/h or less for more than 6 h

Note: Diagnosis of AKI is made if one of definitions 1–3 is met; in severity classification by SCr and urine output, the higher severity is adopted

The RIFLE, AKIN, and KDIGO criteria have been proposed as definitions of AKI, and in 2016, Japanese guidelines for the treatment of AKI have been developed based on the KDIGO criteria. Thus, AKI is defined based on the degree of increases in serum creatinine levels and changes in urine volume (Table 13.1).

## 2.2 Pathophysiology

The rapid decline in renal function and urine output is central to the pathophysiology of the disease, but it does not matter whether the primary cause is renal or extrarenal. It includes not only direct renal damage such as acute tubular necrosis, nephritis, and vasculitis, but also functional renal damage such as heart failure, hypotension, hepatorenal syndrome, and sepsis. Consequently, decreased glomerular filtration and reduced urine volume and sodium excretion ensue.

Risk factors for AKI include age, male gender, pre-existing chronic kidney disease, diabetes mellitus, and heart failure, as well as sepsis, heart failure, and cardiac surgery (Table 13.2).

**Table 13.2** Risk factors for acute kidney injury

| Patient-specific AKI risk factors | AKI risk factors according to the disease state |
|---|---|
| Aging | Advanced disease |
| Male | Septicemia |
| Colored person | Cardiac surgery |
| Preexisting chronic kidney disease | Major non-cardiac surgeries |
| Albuminuria | Acute heart failure |
| Hypertension | Exposure to contrast media |
| Diabetes mellitus | Drug toxicity, nephrotoxic substances |
| Anemia | Injury |
| Complications of chronic liver disease and portal hypertension | |
| Heart failure, impairment of cardiac contractility | |
| Chronic obstructive pulmonary disease | |
| Peripheral vascular disease | |
| Malignant tumor | |

## 2.3 Epidemiology

The incidence of AKI has been increasing due to the aging of the population and the increase in lifestyle-related diseases. Although there are some issues such as the difference in data collection, there is a difference in the incidence of AKI between inpatients and outpatients. In hospitalized patients, the average incidence was 23%, and the incidence related to intensive care and cardiac surgery was particularly high, with the most common causes being renal ischemia, nephrotoxic substances, and sepsis. In contrast, the incidence of out-of-hospital AKI is higher in low- and middle-income countries, and the proportion of out-of-hospital AKI is higher in low-income countries. Factors associated with out-of-hospital AKI include dehydration, infection, and childbirth.

**Table 13.3** Classification of acute kidney injury

| | Prerenal | Renal | | Postrenal |
|---|---|---|---|---|
| Mechanism | Functional renal hypoperfusion | Renal parenchymal disorder | | Urinary tract excretion disorder |
| | | Glomerular and vascular disorders | Renal tubular impairment | |
| Cause | Shock<br>Dehydration<br>Bleeding<br>Burns<br>Postoperative period<br>Heart failure<br>Nephrotic syndrome | Malignant hypertension<br>Glomerulonephritis | Acute tubular necrosis<br>Interstitial nephritis | Prostatic hypertrophy<br>Bilateral ureteral obstruction<br>Neurogenic bladder |
| FENa | <1% | | >1% | |

FENa (fractional Na excretion) = 100 × (urine Na concentration × serum Cr concentration)/(serum Na concentration × urine Cr concentration). *Cr* creatinine

## 2.4 Categories

AKI is classified into prerenal, renal, and postrenal one according to the mechanism of renal involvement (Table 13.3). Fractional Na excretion (FENa) indicates sodium reabsorption in the renal tubules, and the response to AKI varies depending on the location of the lesion.

### 2.4.1 Prerenal

Prerenal AKI is defined as a condition in which glomerular filtration is reduced due to a decrease in renal blood flow. It is caused by dehydration, hemorrhage, burns, postoperation, heart failure, nephrotic syndrome, etc. FENa is low (<1%).

### 2.4.2 Renal

Renal parenchymal damage results in decreased glomerular filtration.

It is caused by glomerulonephritis with primary glomerular lesions, and acute tubular necrosis or acute tubulointerstitial nephritis presenting mainly tubular lesions.

FENa is low (<1%) in glomerular lesions and high (>1%) in tubular lesions.

### 2.4.3 Postrenal

Postrenal AKI is caused by an excretory disorder of the urinary tract, such as prostatic hypertrophy, bilateral ureteral obstruction, or neurogenic bladder. FENa is elevated (>1%).

## 2.5 Symptoms

Uremic symptoms such as oliguria, edema, hypertension, cardiac failure, pulmonary congestion due to fluid retention, anorexia, and nausea may occur. In acute and severe cases, disturbance of consciousness and convulsion may also occur.

Regarding hyperkalemia and hypocalcemia, as a result of electrolyte abnormalities, special attention should be paid to atrioventricular block and ventricular tachycardia (caused by hyperkalemia), and QT prolongation and ventricular tachycardia (caused by hypocalcemia).

## 2.6 Laboratory Examination

There is an increase in blood urea nitrogen level, serum levels of creatinine, potassium, and phosphorus due to acute renal dysfunction, a decrease in serum bicarbonate level due to metabolic acidosis, and an increase in serum chloride. On the other hand, serum sodium and calcium tend to decrease. In general, when renal function is totally impaired, serum creatinine is elevated by 0.5–1.0 mg/dL per day. Anemia may also be present.

### 2.7 Treatment

In prerenal cases, fluid correction or elimination of the cause of functional renal hypoperfusion should be done. In postrenal cases, the cause of urinary tract obstruction should be removed. In renal cases, drugs should be discontinued, steroid hormones may be administered, and immunosuppressive therapy should be used in rapidly progressive glomerulonephritis.

In all cases, dialysis therapy is indicated if no improvement is expected. In prerenal and postrenal cases, renal function may improve with elimination of the cause. In renal cases, there is relative improvement if the cause is drug-induced, but renal dysfunction often remains in other causes. In both prerenal and postrenal cases, the disease may progress to renal paremchymal AKI if appropriate treatment is not given.

Hemodialysis is often selected as dialysis therapy, but peritoneal dialysis may be used in cases of circulatory instability or cerebral hemorrhage. In hemodialysis, continuous or intermittent hemodialysis may be chosen depending on circulatory dynamics.

### 2.8 Prognosis

When comparing hospital-onset AKI with out-of-hospital-onset AKI, in-hospital-onset AKI is generally associated with a worse prognosis. Similarly, when septic AKI is compared with non-septic AKI, mortality is higher in septic AKI.

In AKI, renal dysfunction develops acutely but usually recovers, however, it may be irreversible depending on the pathogenesis of the primary disease. In recent years, a history of AKI has been recognized as a risk factor for chronic kidney disease and is considered to be a risk factor for future chronic kidney disease. Thus, it is important to prevent the development of AKI.

### 2.9 Recent Findings

Among urinary biomarkers, urine NGAL and urine L-FABP may be useful for early diagnosis of AKI.

The usefulness of low-dose atrial natriuretic peptide and low-dose dopamine in the prevention and treatment of AKI is not clear. Loop diuretics are not effective for prophylaxis or treatment, and their use is not recommended except for the correction of fluid overload.

## 3 Chronic Renal Failure [8–10]

Hiroshige Ohashi

### 3.1 Disease Overview

Chronic renal failure (CRF) is a syndrome in which the function of the kidneys declines to the point where they do not recover continuously for several months to several years or more, regardless of the primary disease, resulting in a variety of symptoms.

Decreased renal function means a decrease in the number of functioning nephrons in CRF. The remaining nephrons cannot withstand the excessive load and drop out, further reducing the number of nephrons and leading to end-stage renal failure.

In end-stage renal failure, systemic symptoms such as malaise, anorexia, and edema appear, resulting in uremia. In other words, uremia is an advanced state of chronic renal failure and is characterized by the appearance of systemic symptoms unrelated to the kidney.

### 3.2 Pathophysiology

Chronic renal failure differs significantly from acute renal failure in that it is irreversible with little chance of recovery.

Acute renal failure refers to the loss of renal function in a short period of time, hours or days. It may be caused by an abnormality in the kidney itself or by insufficient blood supply to the kidney due to shock, massive bleeding, severe diarrhea, or vomiting. However, acute renal failure is characterized by rapid healing.

Chronic renal failure (CRF) is a syndrome in which renal function declines over a chronic course, independent of the primary disease. It is important to understand the causes of chronic renal failure in order to determine treatment and prognosis.

When the number of nephrons decreases, the remaining nephrons are further overloaded, resulting in glomerular hyperfiltration, which further decreases the number of nephrons by hemodynamic mechanisms, decreases glomerular function, and increases creatinine:(Cr) in the blood.

Once chronic renal failure occurs, regardless of the primary disease, recovery is unusual and renal function declines further.

## 3.3 Epidemiology

It is estimated that there are 50,000–70,000 patients with chronic kidney disease stage 5 in Japan, and it is necessary to prevent the progression to dialysis and to suppress the development of complications such as cardiovascular disease during the course of the disease.

## 3.4 Symptoms

Symptoms of renal disease include abnormalities in urinalysis, such as proteinuria and hematuria, changes in urine volume, edema, and elevated blood pressure; further deterioration of renal function leads to uremia.

Symptoms of uremia include general malaise, anorexia, nausea with vomiting, uncontrollable blood pressure, dyspnea, and sleep disturbance.

1. Cardiovascular symptoms: The accumulation of sodium (Na) and water may cause heart failure, and hyperkalemia (K) may cause arrhythmia. Because the kidneys play an important role in sodium excretion and blood pressure control via the renin-angiotensin system, blood pressure often increases when renal function declines.
2. Gastrointestinal symptoms: The accumulation of uremic toxin causes anorexia and dysgeusia.
3. Renal anemia: Red blood cells are produced in the bone marrow, but when anemia occurs, erythropoietin is produced in the kidneys, and red blood cells are produced in the bone marrow to prevent anemia. Therefore, anemia appears and progresses when renal function declines.
4. Metabolic acidosis: Because the kidneys excrete acidic urine, when renal function is impaired, the body becomes acidic. The disease is asymptomatic, but hyperkalemia may occasionally occur.
5. Secondary hyperparathyroidism (osteitis fibrosa): Calcium (Ca) ingested orally is absorbed from the intestinal tract. In renal failure, hyperphosphatemia due to decreased phosphorus (P) excretion and hypocalcemia due to impaired vitamin D activation with reduction of Ca absorption from the intestinal tract are observed. In order to correct the hypocalcemia, the parathyroid gland increases its activity, producing more parathyroid hormone (PTH), mobilizing Ca from bone, and decreasing bone mineral density.

## 3.5 Clinical Examination

### 3.5.1 Urinalysis

This is the most important test, although it is simple. It is important to confirm whether there are any abnormalities in the urine sample, whether proteinuria is present alone or in combination with hematuria, and whether proteinuria is severe or not.

In diabetic nephropathy, hematuria is rare and proteinuria is predominant, and when proteinuria is accompanied by hematuria, chronic glomerulonephritis is more likely. In nephrosclerosis, there are often no abnormalities in urinalysis such as proteinuria or hematuria.

### 3.5.2 Blood Test

Depending on the degree of renal failure, elevated serum levels of Cr, urea nitrogen (UN), and uric acid (UA), decreased serum Na and Ca levels, and elevated serum K and P levels are often observed, and metabolic acidosis, renal anemia, and hyperparathyroidism develop.

Serum Cr level is widely used to evaluate renal function, but varies with gender and body size, because its production is proportional to muscle mass.

### 3.5.3 Diagnostic Imaging

With decrease in renal function, if the kidneys are atrophic, it is chronic renal failure; if they are enlarged, it may be acute renal failure.

### 3.5.4 Evaluation of Renal Function

1. Estimated glomerular filtration rate (eGFR): This test is widely used in recent years. eGFR is calculated by a formula based on serum Cr level, age, and gender, and is used to evaluate glomerular function.
2. Creatinine clearance (Ccr): Endogenous Ccr is measured using 24-h urine samples and is a commonly used method in clinical practice to evaluate glomerular function.

## 3.6 Treatment

Because the excretion of waste products, regulation of water and electrolytes, and erythropoietin production are dysfunctional, treatment is required for each condition. In particular, dietary therapy that restricts salt, water, protein, K, and P, and drug therapy for each condition are central of treatment.

### 3.6.1 Lifestyle Guidance and Diet Therapy

1. Salt and water: Excessive salt and water intake and extreme restriction are harmful. In conservative renal failure, fluid deficiency is likely to occur at the same time as fluid excess is easy to occur due to decreased accommodation ability. Basically, fluid intake should be equal to the volume of insensible perspiration plus the daily urine output, and salt intake should be 3–6 g/day.
2. Protein and energy intake**:** The basic principle of dietary therapy is to limit protein and salt intake with adequate energy intake. The recommended energy intake is 25–35 kcal/kg/day, depending on gender, age, and physical activity level. If serum Cr level is elevated and dialysis therapy may be required in the future, protein intake should be 0.6–0.8 g/kg/day.
3. Tasty thing**:** Smoking cessation is necessary to reduce the decline in renal function and to prevent cardiovascular disease. Appropriate alcohol consumption, in terms of ethanol, should be 20–30 mL/day or less for male and 10–20 mL/day or less for female.

### 3.6.2 Blood Pressure Control

The goal of antihypertensive therapy is to prevent the progression of chronic renal failure and to reduce the risk of cardiovascular disease and death, and the target of antihypertensive therapy is below 140/90 mmHg and, if possible, below 130/80 mmHg.

The first-line antihypertensive agents are angiotensin receptor blockade (ARB) and angiotensin converting enzyme (ACE) inhibitors, which inhibit the renin angiotensin system (RAS). If the target level is not reached, a Ca antagonist, an alpha blocker, a beta blocker, and a diuretic should be used in combination.

### 3.6.3 Anemia Management

Patients with chronic renal failure develop renal anemia due to decreased production of erythropoietin in the kidney. The erythrocyte stimulating agent (ESA) is administered, which should be started at a hemoglobin (Hb) concentration of 10 g/dL or less, and the therapeutic target Hb level should be 10–13 g/dL, not exceeding 13 g/dL.

### 3.6.4 Others

1. Dyslipidemia: The treatment of dyslipidemia is expected to decrease proteinuria and suppress renal function decline. The goal is to control low density lipoprotein (LDL) cholesterol below 120 mg/dL.

2. Mineral and bone disease (MBD): MBD develops and progresses with the progression of renal failure, and is collectively called chronic kidney disease (CKD) associated MBD (CKD–MBD). Because not only bone changes but also systemic abnormalities such as vascular calcification occur, CKD–MBD has an impact on life prognosis. In the latest studies, control of serum P is considered to be the most important factor.
3. Hyperuricemia: Hyperuricemia is defined as a serum uric acid level of 7 mg/dL or higher. As renal function declines, uric acid excretion function also declines, and the frequency of hyperuricemia increases. In order to lower the serum uric acid level, it is necessary to improve lifestyle and to administer appropriate drugs.
4. Avoidance of renal-impairing drugs: When renal function is impaired, renal excretory drugs may increase the frequency of side effects due to increased blood concentrations of the drugs. Since side effects can exacerbate renal impairment, when renal excretory drugs are used, renal function should be evaluated by eGFR and Ccr, and the dose of the drug should be reduced or the administration interval should be extended.

Antipyretic analgesic agents, contrast media, anticancer agents such as cisplatin, and antimicrobial agents such as aminoglycoside should be used with caution in patients with chronic renal failure.

## 3.7 Prognosis

As chronic renal failure progresses and uremic symptoms appear, patients are treated by hemodialysis (HD), peritoneal dialysis (PD), or renal transplantation. Hemodialysis is often chosen in Japan.

Renal transplantation is the only therapy that can restore renal functions and presents a good quality of life, more activated activities of daily living, and better vital prognosis. However, the low number of donated kidney transplants has become a social problem in Japan.

## 3.8 Notes from Dentistry Perspective

Akira Sasaki

The most common causes of chronic renal failure are diabetic nephropathy, chronic glomerulonephritis, and hypertensive nephrosclerosis, in that order. Especially, diabetic nephropathy is increasing year by year, and nephrosclerosis is also increasing. Therefore, when performing dental treatment for patients with chronic renal failure undergoing dialysis treatment (dialysis patients) or not, it is necessary to consider not only renal disease but also diabetes and hypertension, as well as associated anemia and bone metabolism disorder. In 2002, the concept of CKD was introduced, which broadly refers to the decline in renal function regardless of the causative disease, and prevention and treatment of CKD should be started from an early stage. The relationship between periodontal disease and systemic diseases such as diabetes mellitus has been pointed out, and it is necessary to understand CKD also from the standpoint of dentistry.

### 3.8.1 Oral Manifestations of Chronic Renal Failure

It is generally associated with multiple caries and parenchymal enamel defects due to the reduction of oral self-cleaning action and poor oral management. In particular, dialysis patients often present with xerostomia. The incidence of periodontal disease is also high. When bone metabolism is abnormal, the lamina dura disappears and the trabeculae are obscured, resulting in ground glass-like changes (Fig. 13.1). The oral mucosa is characterized by pallor of the gingival mucosa, stomatitis, and xerostomia due to anemia and peripheral circulatory disturbance caused by renal failure (Fig. 13.2). These symptoms are influenced not only by renal disease but also by concomitant diseases and their treatment.

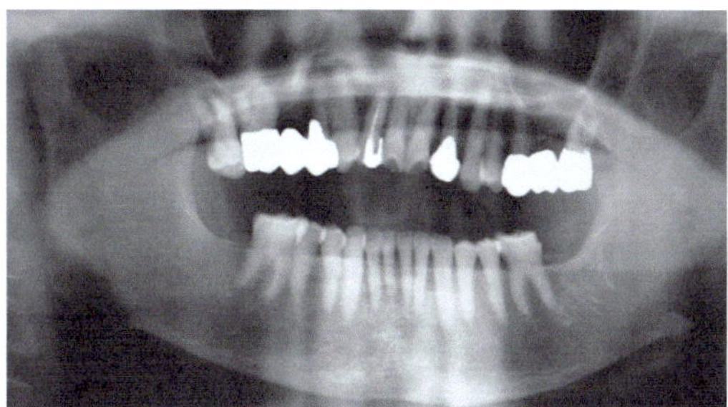

**Fig. 13.1** Panoramic radiograph of a dialysis patient

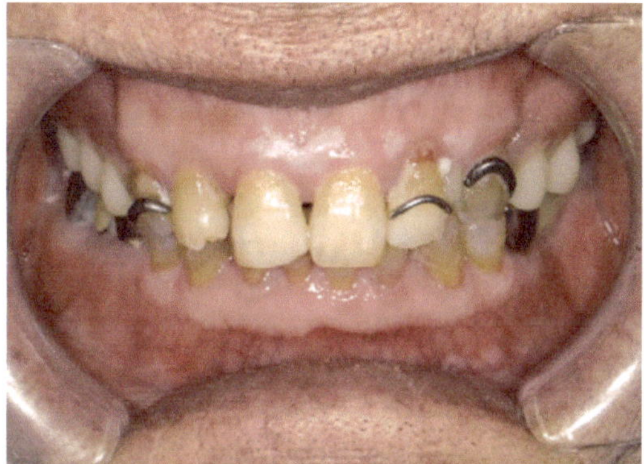

**Fig. 13.2** Oral photograph of a dialysis patient

### 3.8.2 Problems and Drug Metabolism During Dental Treatment

It is important to assess the patient's clinical symptoms and renal function with a thorough understanding of the patient's history and current medical condition. It is also necessary to understand the pathophysiology of concomitant diseases such as diabetes, hypertension, and bone metabolism disorders other than renal diseases, and the treatment status including medication. The severity of CKD is evaluated by the CGA classification, which consists of cause (C), renal function (GFR: G), and proteinuria (albuminuria: A). The correspondence to dental treatment depends on the severity of the CKD and the degree of invasiveness of the dental treatment. If the renal function is mildly impaired (G1A1, G2A1), usual dental treatment is possible, but it is important to consult with the attending physician to understand the condition of the patient and to confirm the precautions to be taken in dental treatment. In addition, oral implant treatment is contraindicated in patients with severe renal dysfunction or dialysis [11]. Because patients are often accompanied by cardiovascular disease, monitoring (blood pressure, pulse rate, and $SpO_2$) is necessary during dental treatment. The blood pressure manchette should be worn on the opposite upper arm to avoid the occlusion of arterio-venous fistula in hemodialysis patients.

The number of dialysis patients in the world is increasing, and the prevalence of oral diseases is high, so there are many opportunities for dental consultation. It is desirable to perform dental treatment on the day after hemodialysis when the patient is in good physical condition because of the time and physical burden on the day of hemodialysis. In performing surgical procedures such as tooth extraction, underlying diseases such as diabetes mellitus and cardiovascular disease should be noted, and bleeding tendency should be considered if they are receiving antithrombotic therapy, heparin during dialysis is not affected the day after dialysis. In general, surgical procedures should be performed under continuous antithrombotic therapy and local hemostasis should be used. In patients with renal disease, prophylactic administration of antibiotics is necessary because of decreased immunity and delayed wound healing. In dentistry, antibiotics and analgesics are frequently used, but their prescription should be based on (1) drug metabolism and excretion pathways and (2) renal function. The drugs, dosage, and administration schedule should be adjusted based on Ccr or the estimated GFR (glomerular filtration rate) calculated from serum Cr level based on age and gender. In dialysis patients, the dialyzability of the drug itself is also an important factor [12, 13]. In the guidelines, NSAIDs are recommended to be avoided as much as possible in the elderly and CKD patients because of the risk of acute renal failure due to renal ischemia caused by inhibition of prostaglandin synthesis, and acetaminophen is considered safer, but the safety of long-term administration is uncertain [14].

## References

1. Hishida A, et al., editors. Standard nephrology. Tokyo: Igaku Shoin; 2002. (in Japanese).
2. Schrier RW, et al. Schrier's diseases of the kidney. 8th ed. Philadelphia: Lippincott Williams & Wilkins; 2012.
3. Japanese Society of Nephrology, editor. Evidence-based clinical practice guideline for CKD 2018. Tokyo: Tokyo Igaku-sha; 2018. (in Japanese).
4. Horino T, Terada N. Clinical practice guideline for acute kidney injury 2016. Med Frontline. 2018;73(12):1582–7. (in Japanese).
5. Khwaja A. KDIGO clinical practice guideline for acute kidney injury. Kidney Int Suppl. 2012;2:1–138.
6. Yamamura Y, et al. Epidemiology and risk factors of AKI. Jpn Soc Dial Ther. 2018;51(2):123–8. (in Japanese).
7. Mori K, Mori N. Update and the prospect of prevention and treatment of AKI. J Jpn Soc Dial Ther. 2018;51(2):135–9. (in Japanese).
8. Uchiyama H, editor. Nephrology for specialists. 2nd ed. Tokyo: Igaku Shoin; 2009. p. 209–39. (in Japanese).
9. Fukagawa M, Yasuda T, editors. Manual of kidney diseases for residents. 3rd ed. Tokyo: Igaku Shoin; 2017. p. 281–307. (in Japanese).
10. Fukai T, Kurokawa K, Supervised. Harrison's principles of internal medicine. 5th ed. Tokyo: Medical Science International; 2015. p. 1861–71. (in Japanese).
11. Japanese Society of Oral Implantology, editor. Guidelines for oral implant treatment 2020. Tokyo: Ishiyaku Shuppan; 2020. (in Japanese).
12. KDIGO 2012 clinical practice guideline for the evaluation and management of chronic kidney disease. Kidney Int Suppl. 2013;3(1):1–150. https://kdigo.org/wp-content/uploads/2017/02/KDIGO_2012_CKD_GL.pdf.
13. Usui J, et al. Clinical practice guideline for drug-induced kidney injury in Japan 2016: digest version. Clin Exp Nephrol. 2016;20:827–31. https://doi.org/10.1007/s10157-016-1334-0.
14. Japanese Society of Nephrology, editor. Evidence-based CKD clinical practice guidelines 2018. Tokyo: Japanese Society of Nephrology; 2018. (in Japanese). https://cdn.jsn.or.jp/data/CKD2018.pdf.

# 14 Hematologic Diseases

Hirofumi Sawai, Masaatsu Yagi,
Kimihiro Matsumoto, Masahiro Ieko, Satoshi Goto,
Shigeki Ito, and Daishi Saito

## 1 Anemia [1–3]

Hirofumi Sawai

Anemia is a condition in which the hemoglobin concentration in the peripheral blood is decreased.

Anemia can be caused by bleeding (e.g., menstrual bleeding, gastrointestinal bleeding), hemolysis (e.g., spherocytosis, autoimmune hemolytic anemia), decreased red blood cell production in the bone marrow (e.g., aplastic anemia, leukemia, myelodysplastic syndrome), or abnormal blood distribution (e.g., idiopathic portal hypertension).

Common symptoms of anemia include those associated with decreased cerebral oxygenation due to impaired oxygen supply (lightheadedness, dizziness, headache, fainting, etc.) and those associated with cardiovascular overload due to compensatory increased blood flow (palpitations, shortness of breath, fatigue, general malaise, etc.).

According to red blood cell indices (mean corpuscular volume: MCV; mean corpuscular hemoglobin: MCH; and mean corpuscular hemoglobin concentration: MCHC) (Fig. 14.1), anemia is classified into three groups: (1) microcytic hypochromic anemia (Table 14.1); (2) macrocytic anemia (Table 14.2); and (3) normocytic normochromic anemia (Table 14.3).

### 1.1 Microcytic Hypochromic Anemia (Table 14.1)

Iron-deficiency anemia is the most common cause of microcytic hypochromic anemia.

#### 1.1.1 Iron-Deficiency Anemia

One hemoglobin molecule consists of four globin subunits (alpha chain, beta chain, etc.), and one heme is bound to each globin subunit. Heme is

H. Sawai
Kinki Health Care Center, Yodogawa-ku, Osaka, Japan

M. Yagi
Department of Dental and Oral Surgery, Iwate Prefectural Central Hospital, Morioka, Iwate, Japan

K. Matsumoto
Department of Internal Medicine, Tokyo Dental College, Ichikawa General Hospital, Ichikawa, Chiba, Japan

M. Ieko
Department of Nursing, Faculty of Health and Medical Sciences, Sapporo University of Health Sciences, Sapporo, Hokkaido, Japan

S. Goto
Department of Oral and Maxillofacial Surgery, National Hospital Organization Sendai Medical Center, Sendai, Miyagi, Japan

S. Ito (✉)
Division of Hematology & Oncology, Department of Internal Medicine, Iwate Medical University School of Medicine, Yahaba, Iwate, Japan
e-mail: shigei@iwate-med.ac.jp

D. Saito
School of Dentistry, Iwate Medical University, Yahaba, Iwate, Japan


T. Chiba, H. Yamada (eds.), *Internal Medicine for Dental Treatments*,
https://doi.org/10.1007/978-981-99-3296-2_14

**Fig. 14.1** Red blood cell index

1) Mean Corpuscular Volume (MCV)

$$\text{mean corpuscular volume (fl)} = \frac{\text{Ht (\%)}}{\text{RBC } (\times 10^4/\mu l)} \times 1000$$

(Reference value : 80 ~ 100 fl)

2) Mean Corpuscular Hemoglobin (MCH)

$$\text{mean corpuscular hemoglobin (pg)} = \frac{\text{Hb (g/dl)}}{\text{RBC } (\times 10^4/\mu l)} \times 1000$$

(Reference value : 27 ~ 34 pg)

3) Mean Corpuscular Hemoglobin Concentration (MCHC)

$$\text{mean corpuscular hemoglobin concentration (g/dl)} = \frac{\text{Hb (g/dl)}}{\text{Ht (\%)}} \times 100$$

(Reference value : 30 ~ 36 g/dL)

**Table 14.1** Microcytic hypochromic anemia

| Classification by erythrocyte index | Classification by etiology |
|---|---|
| Microcytic hypochromic anemia<br>MCV <80 (fL)<br>MCHC <30 (g/dL) | 1. Iron-deficiency anemia<br>2. Sideroblastic anemia<br>3. Thalassemia<br>4. Hemoglobinopathies |

**Table 14.2** Macrocytic anemia

| Classification by erythrocyte index | Classification by etiology |
|---|---|
| Macrocytic anemia<br>MCV >100 (fL)<br>MCHC >30 (g/dL) | 1. Megaloblastic anemia<br>(a) Vitamin $B_{12}$ deficiency: Pernicious anemia, post-gastrectomy, malabsorption syndrome, etc.<br>(b) Folic acid deficiency<br>2. Non-megaloblastic anemia<br>Secondary: Liver disease, etc. |

**Table 14.3** Normocytic normochromic anemia

| Classification by erythrocyte index | Classification by etiology |
|---|---|
| Normocytic normochromic anemia<br>MCV: 80–100 (fL)<br>MCHC: 30–36 (g/dL) | 1. Acute hemorrhage<br>2. Hemolytic anemia<br>3. Aplastic anemia<br>4. Leukemia, malignant lymphoma, myeloma, bone marrow metastasis of cancer<br>5. Secondary anemia |

synthesized in the mitochondria of erythroblasts, and has an iron atom in its center that binds reversibly to oxygen. When the body is deficient in iron, hemoglobin synthesis is reduced, leading to anemia. Causes of iron deficiency include bleeding (menstrual bleeding, gastrointestinal bleeding, etc.), inadequate iron intake, iron malabsorption, and increased iron requirements (pregnancy, etc.). Iron-deficiency anemia is the most common cause of anemia.

In addition to the common symptoms of anemia such as lightheadedness, palpitations, and shortness of breath, deformed nails (spoon nails), pica (eating dirt, paper, etc.), and Plummer-Vinson syndrome (atrophic glossitis, dysphagia) are also seen.

As examination findings, peripheral blood tests show microcytic hypochromic anemia, with no abnormalities in the leukocyte system, but an increased platelet count is common. Biochemical tests show a decrease in serum iron and ferritin (storage iron) and increased unsaturated iron binding capacity.

For treatment, iron is administered orally, but if gastrointestinal disturbances are observed as an adverse effect of iron or if the improvement of anemia is urgent, iron is administered intravenously. If bleeding is suspected as the cause of anemia, it is necessary to investigate and treat the causal disease of bleeding.

### 1.1.2 Sideroblastic Anemia

Due to impaired mitochondrial heme synthesis, erythroblasts accumulate iron in the absence of hemoglobin synthesis and collapse. Sideroblastic anemia includes hereditary sideroblastic anemia, myelodysplastic syndromes, and secondary sideroblastic anemia due to vitamin $B_6$ deficiency or drugs.

Examination findings include microcytic hypochromic anemia, increased serum iron and ferritin, and decreased unsaturated iron-binding capacity. In the bone marrow, iron staining shows ringed sideroblasts.

Vitamin $B_6$ may be effective as a treatment. Drug-induced sideroblastic anemia can be improved by the discontinuation of the causative drug.

### 1.1.3 Thalassemia

Thalassemia is an inherited disorder in which globin synthesis is decreased due to abnormalities in the globin genes, resulting in microcytic hypochromic anemia. Thalassemia includes alpha-thalassemia in which alpha-globin decreases and beta-thalassemia in which beta-globin decreases.

## 1.2 Macrocytic Anemia (Table 14.2)

Macrocytic anemia is classified into two categories: megaloblastic and non-megaloblastic.

### 1.2.1 Megaloblastic Anemia

1. **Pernicious anemia**: Vitamin $B_{12}$ is absorbed in the ileum by binding to (gastric) intrinsic factor produced by gastric parietal cells. Since vitamin $B_{12}$ acts as a cofactor for enzymes involved in DNA synthesis, vitamin $B_{12}$ deficiency causes maturation disorders not only in red blood cells (megaloblastic anemia) but also in all blood cells.

   Pernicious anemia is induced by impaired absorption of vitamin $B_{12}$ due to decreased secretion of intrinsic factor associated with the loss of gastric parietal cells caused by atrophic gastritis, or due to the production of anti-intrinsic factor antibody (a type of autoantibody).

   In addition to the common symptoms of anemia, Hunter glossitis (associated with redness and pain of the tongue) may be observed. As neurological symptoms, subacute combined degeneration of spinal cord (numbness of the limbs, loss of deep sensation, ataxia, etc.) may occur.

   As examination findings, peripheral blood tests show macrocytic anemia as well as leukopenia, thrombocytopenia (pancytopenia), and neutrophil hypersegmentation (five or more lobes). In the bone marrow, proliferation of megaloblasts is observed. Anti-intrinsic factor antibody can be detected in the serum of about 60% of patients.

   For treatment, vitamin $B_{12}$ should be administered by intramuscular injection (because orally-administered vitamin $B_{12}$ is not absorbed).

   In addition to pernicious anemia, postgastrectomy (due to lack of secretion of intrinsic factor) and small intestinal lesions (e.g., Crohn's disease) may reduce vitamin $B_{12}$ absorption, resulting in macrocytic anemia.
2. **Folic acid deficiency anemia**: Since folic acid acts as a cofactor in various enzymatic reactions, DNA synthesis is impaired by folic acid deficiency, resulting in megaloblastic anemia. Folic acid deficiency is mainly caused by inadequate folic acid intake due to nutritional disorders or alcoholism. Folic acid deficiency also occurs in folic acid metabolism disorders caused by folic acid antagonists (methotrexate).

   The symptoms are similar to pernicious anemia, but neurological symptoms are absent.

   Examination findings include low levels of serum folic acid.

   For treatment, oral administration of folic acid and improvement of dietary habits are recommended.

### 1.2.2 Non-megaloblastic Macrocytic Anemia

In secondary anemia associated with chronic hepatitis and liver cirrhosis, macrocytic anemia without megaloblasts in the bone marrow is observed.

## 1.3 Normocytic Normochromic Anemia (Table 14.3)

The causes of normocytic normochromic anemia include acute hemorrhage, hemolytic anemia, aplastic anemia, leukemia, secondary anemia, etc.

### 1.3.1 Aplastic Anemia

A disorder of bone marrow hematopoietic stem cells results in decreased production of all blood cells. It may be idiopathic, hereditary, or secondary to the effects of drugs or radiation.

As symptoms, not only the common symptoms of anemia but also susceptibility to infection associated with leukopenia, and bleeding tendency associated with thrombocytopenia are observed.

Examination findings include pancytopenia in peripheral blood tests and decreased all hematopoietic cells without abnormal cells in bone marrow tests. An increase in serum iron and ferritin, a decrease in unsaturated iron-binding capacity, and a marked increase in erythropoietin are observed.

For treatment, blood transfusions (red blood cells, platelets) are administered as supportive care. Drugs include anabolic hormones, erythropoietin, granulocyte colony-stimulating factor (G-CSF), immunosuppressive agents, etc. Bone marrow transplantation is performed as a radical treatment.

### 1.3.2 Hemolytic Anemia

Hemolytic anemia is either hereditary (abnormalities in red blood cells) or non-hereditary (causes other than red blood cells). Common symptoms of hemolytic anemia include splenomegaly, jaundice, and gallstones, in addition to the symptoms of anemia. Compensatory erythroblast hyperplasia in the bone marrow is associated with increased reticulocytes (immature red blood cells) in the peripheral blood. Biochemical findings include an increase in indirect bilirubin and a decrease in haptoglobin.

1. **Hereditary spherocytosis**: Hereditary spherocytosis is caused mainly by autosomal dominant inheritance, in which red blood cells are spherical in shape and cannot pass through the endothelial cell space in the spleen and are phagocytosed by macrophages, resulting in hemolytic anemia.

   As examination findings, peripheral blood smears show spherocytes.

   For treatment, splenectomy is performed, which results in clinical cure, including improvement of anemia and disappearance of jaundice.
2. **Sickle cell anemia**: Mutations in the beta-globin gene cause hemoglobin S, which lead to sickle-shaped (crescent-shaped) red blood cells, resulting in hemolysis in the spleen and vascular occlusion. Sickle cell anemia is common in malaria-prone areas such as Central Africa owing to its malaria resistance.
3. **Hereditary hemolytic anemia due to enzyme abnormalities**: Genetic abnormalities of enzymes in red blood cells cause hemolytic anemia.

   Glucose-6-phosphate dehydrogenase (G6PD) deficiency is inherited as an X-linked recessive trait and occurs almost exclusively in males. It is common in Africa and the Mediterranean, and is rare in Japan. Acute hemolytic attacks are induced by infections, drugs, surgery, or ingestion of fava beans, although anemia is usually absent.

   Pyruvate kinase (PK) deficiency is inherited as an autosomal recessive trait and causes hemolysis in the spleen, resulting in splenomegaly, jaundice, and gallstones.
4. **Paroxysmal nocturnal hemoglobinuria**: A deficiency of GPI-anchored membrane protein due to an abnormality in the PIGA gene causes increased complement sensitivity, resulting in intravascular hemolysis during nighttime sleep and reddish-brown hemoglobinuria in the early morning. Since abnormalities exist in hematopoietic stem cells, pancytopenia occurs, and the disease may progress to acute leukemia. Bone marrow transplantation is performed as a radical treatment.
5. **Autoimmune hemolytic anemia**: The production of anti-erythrocyte antibodies (autoantibodies against red blood cells) causes hemolytic anemia. It is usually caused by warm autoantibodies (autoantibodies that are active at 37 °C), but can be caused by cold autoantibodies (autoantibodies that are active at low temperatures).

(a) **Autoimmune hemolytic anemia caused by warm autoantibodies (IgG)**: It may be idiopathic (of unknown cause) or secondary (associated with systemic lupus erythematosus, lymphocytic leukemia, etc.). Hemolytic anemia is sometimes complicated by thrombocytopenia and is called Evans syndrome.

As examination findings, the direct Coombs test (detection of anti-erythrocyte antibodies bound to the surface of red blood cells) and the indirect Coombs test (detection of anti-erythrocyte antibodies in serum) are positive. Corticosteroids and immunosuppressants are used for treatment.

(b) **Cold agglutinin disease**: Cold agglutinin (IgM), which is active at low temperatures, causes hemolytic anemia, resulting in its aggravation in winter and relief in summer. The acute form, secondary to mycoplasma or viral infections, is more common in the young, while the chronic form, associated with idiopathic type or malignant lymphoma, is more common in the elderly. Raynaud's phenomenon may be observed in cold weather. To prevent hemolysis, it is recommended to avoid exposure to cold.

(c) **Paroxysmal cold hemoglobinuria**: Donath-Landsteiner antibodies (IgG), which bind to red blood cells at low temperatures and activate complement at 37 °C, causes hemolysis, resulting in chills, shivering, headache, abdominal pain, and hemoglobinuria after exposure to cold. It is often secondary to syphilis or viral infections.

6. **Drug-induced immune hemolytic anemia**: Hemolytic anemia may occur as adverse effects of drugs (penicillin, quinidine, methyldopa, etc.). Recovery from anemia is observed within 1–2 weeks after discontinuation of the drugs.

### 1.3.3 Secondary Anemia

Anemia caused by diseases other than hematologic disorders is called secondary anemia, and it occurs not infrequently.

1. **Anemia of chronic disease**: Anemia caused by chronic infections (e.g., tuberculosis), collagen diseases, malignant tumors, etc. usually presents as normocytic normochromic anemia. As examination findings, serum iron and total iron-binding capacity are low, and ferritin is high (ferritin is low in iron-deficiency anemia). However, when iron deficiency (hemorrhage) is associated, microcytic hypochromic anemia is observed.
2. **Renal anemia**: In chronic renal failure, erythropoietin production in the kidney is decreased, resulting in normocytic normochromic anemia. For the treatment of renal anemia, erythropoietin preparation is administered.
3. **Anemia associated with liver disease**: In chronic hepatitis and liver cirrhosis, macrocytic anemia is observed.

## 1.4 Notes from Dentistry Perspective

Masaatsu Yagi

### 1.4.1 Types of Anemia

There are several types of anemia, but iron-deficiency anemia, megaloblastic anemia, and aplastic anemia, which are most frequently associated with oral manifestations, are reviewed.

#### Iron-Deficiency Anemia

Iron-deficiency anemia (IDA) is a common form of hypochromic microcytic anemia that accounts for more than 80% of all anemias. It is more common in women than in men. It is caused by iron deficiency due to impaired heme synthesis or inadequate iron absorption, and is common in patients who have undergone gastrectomy.

Systemic symptoms include fatigue, tachycardia, palpitations, and spoon nails.

Oral symptoms include a smooth tongue (red, flat tongue) due to atrophy of tongue papillae, angular cheilitis, atrophy of the pharyngeal and cervical esophageal mucosa, and dysphagia, known as Plummer-Vinson syndrome (Figs. 14.2 and 14.3).

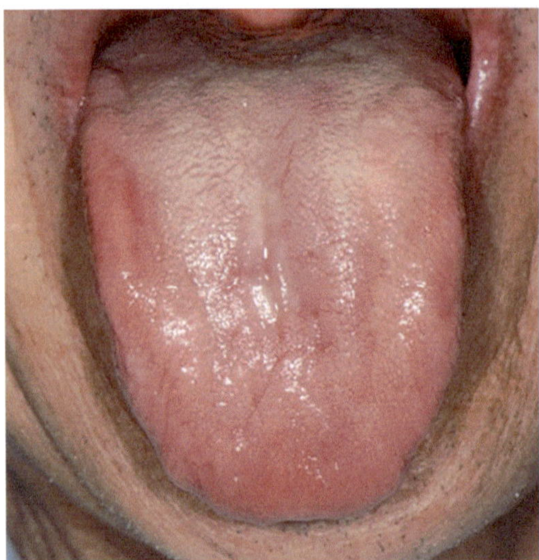

**Fig. 14.2** Smoothing of the tongue is seen

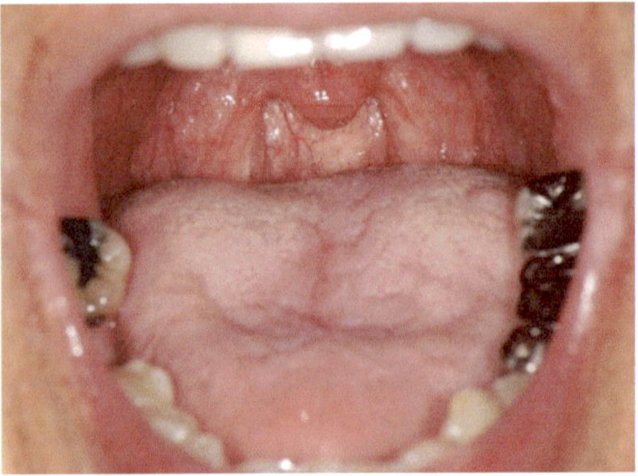

**Fig. 14.3** Atrophy of the pharyngeal mucosa is seen

As for dental treatment, if Hb is 9.0 g/dL or higher, there is no problem with surgical procedures such as tooth extraction. For tongue pain caused by atrophic glossitis, the treatment of the primary disease should be prioritized, and iron supplements should be administered.

#### Megaloblastic Anemia

Macrocytic megaloblastic anemia is caused by deficiency of vitamin $B_{12}$ or folic acid, and vitamin $B_{12}$ deficiency is more common. Vitamin $B_{12}$ is often found in patients who have undergone gastrectomy because it is not absorbed into the body when the intrinsic factor secreted by the gastric mucosa is deficient. Even without gastrectomy, megaloblastic anemia caused by decreased secretion of intrinsic factor or anti-intrinsic antibodies is called pernicious anemia.

The oral manifestations include a smooth tongue with atrophy of tongue papillae, dysgeusia, and dysphagia, which is called Hunter's glossitis.

As in iron-deficiency anemia, there is no problem in dental treatment if Hb is 9.0 g/dL or higher. Vitamin $B_{12}$ or folic acid may be effective in the treatment of tongue pain, but only injectable vitamin $B_{12}$ is effective.

#### Aplastic Anemia

Aplastic anemia is normocytic normochromic anemia caused by damage to hematopoietic stem cells due to abnormal bone marrow function. It is said to be caused by anticancer agents or radiation exposure, but the cause is often unknown in Japan. Because not only red blood cells but also white blood cells and platelets are reduced, oral symptoms include worsening of inflammatory symptoms such as periodontitis and gingival bleeding. The problem in dental treatment is that platelets should be kept above 50,000/mm$^3$ when performing surgical procedures such as tooth extraction. Because the white blood cell count is also low, antimicrobial agents (in normal doses) should be administered from the day before tooth extraction. In any case, when performing surgical procedures, it is necessary to consult with the attending hematologist and to make adequate preparations.

## 2 Leukemia

Kimihiro Matsumoto

### 2.1 Disease Overview, Pathogenesis, and Symptoms

In the bone marrow, the site of hematopoiesis in adults, normal hematopoiesis is impaired by the space-occupying proliferation of leukemic cells derived from mutated hematopoietic stem cells and progenitor cells. Leukemia is a life-threatening disease that progresses into blood flow (peripheral blood) due to an increase in leukemia cells (leukocyte formation and blood cell increase) and is complicated by multiple organ involvement, impaired blood flow, thrombosis, DIC, infection, and anemia. Since acute myelogenous leukemia (AML) and acute lymphoblastic leukemia (ALL) progress on a daily basis, urgent treatments should be taken compared to chronic myelogenous leukemia (CML) and chronic lymphocytic leukemia (CLL), which progress on a monthly to yearly basis.

## 2.2 Causes of Leukemia

Leukemia is a cancerous state of hematopoietic stem cell (HSC) or hematopoietic progenitor cell due to abnormalities or disruptions in genes, growth factors, transcription factors, and epigenetics related to hematopoietic differentiation, proliferation, and the surrounding microenvironment. Radiation exposure and chemotherapy are risk factors.

## 2.3 Epidemiology

The incidence rate is a few per 100,000 age-adjusted persons, and the incidence rate increases in older age groups.

ALL is more common in children, and AML is more common in adults. In the elderly, the proportion of secondary AML from myelodysplastic syndrome (MDS) etc. increases, and in ALL, the proportion of Philadelphia chromosome-positive of ALL increases.

## 2.4 Classification

### 2.4.1 Classification of Acute Leukemia

Of the French–American–British (FAB) classification of blood cell morphology (M0–7 for AML and L1–3 for ALL) published in 1976, M0–7 is the most important conventional morphological classification and is still used in clinical practice. The WHO classification [4], which is based on histology and genotyping, is also included.

Other than de novo acute leukemia, MDS and/or myeloproliferative neoplasm (MPN)-based AML is occasionally generated. Acute leukemia is defined as the ratio of myeloblasts greater than 20% by bone marrow puncture (30% in the FAB classification), except in the presence of specific chromosomal abnormalities characteristic of acute leukemia (e.g., 8;21 translocation, inversion 16, 9;22 translocation). Acute promyelocytic leukemia (APL), which is more likely to be associated with DIC and is more likely to benefit from vitamin A derivatives, and Ph+ ALL, which is more likely to benefit from tyrosine kinase inhibitors (TKIs) in ALL are especially subclassified from each leukemia. The term "Ph leukemia" refers to Ph+ ALL and CML. In addition, the elderly and the AYA generation (16–24 years old) are classified according to different treatment guidelines (intensity), such as chemotherapy and bone marrow transplantation.

### 2.4.2 Classification of Chronic Leukemia

1. **CML**: It is defined by a single mutation in a hematopoietic stem cell (HSC) that results in acquisition of the BCR/ABL chimeric gene, and has myeloproliferative tumor characteristics. It progresses from the chronic phase (CP) to the accelerated phase (AP) and blastic phase (BP) in the natural course of 4–5 years, and is usually found in the CP phase. The prognostic risk classification by Sokal score (low, intermediate, high) is still useful in the era of tyrosine kinase inhibitors (TKIs).
2. **CLL**: It is a mature lymphoma identical to low-grade B-cell lymphoma and is defined as a peripheral blood lymphocyte count of 5000/μL or higher. The presence of TP53 mutation is an important adverse prognostic factor.

## 2.5 Symptoms

Compromised hosting is caused by varying degrees of depression of defense mechanisms such as the cutaneous mucosal barrier, neutrophil count, humoral immunity, and cellular immunity. Sepsis and febrile neutropenia occur frequently due to neutropenia caused by disease or treatment, resulting in severe infection of bacteria, candida, or aspergillus, etc. In lymphoid leukemia (ALL, CLL), cellular immunity is also impaired because systemic steroid-containing regimens are often used in addition to decreased humoral immunity.

Symptoms other than those of infection are described below.

### 2.5.1 Acute Leukemia

Specific symptoms during the course of the disease include leukostasis due to marked leukocytosis, hypoglycemia, hyperfibrinolytic DIC, and tumor lysis syndrome after chemotherapy either before or after treatment. Initial symptoms include fatigue (due to anemia), bleeding tendency (sometimes due to DIC, but mainly due to thrombocytopenia), fever (due to pneumonia, bacterial infections such as anal or dental infections, or deep mycosis such as pulmonary aspergillosis), bone pain (due to myeloproliferation), night sweats, masses, and local pain (in patients with extramedullary masses).

### 2.5.2 Chronic Leukemia

Abdominal distention due to hepatosplenomegaly, left hypochondrial pain due to splenomegaly or splenic infarction, or abnormalities in regular medical checkup (leukocytosis, thrombocytosis).

## 2.6 Clinical Examination

### 2.6.1 Blood Test

Leukopenia (neutropenia), leukocytosis (increase from the beginning in CML, but decrease followed by increase in acute leukemia), anemia, thrombocytopenia (increase in CML), increased LDH, increased FDP (in patients with DIC), and increased CRP (in patients with infectious diseases or non-infectious inflammation such as MDS) are observed. In CML, immature granulocytes, eosinophils, and basophils are increased, and leukemic hiatus are not formed; in APL, promyelocytes and blasts are increased, and in CLL, mature lymphocytes are increased.

### 2.6.2 Bone Marrow Examination

The ilium is mainly punctured. As with peripheral blood, the cells are stained with Giemsa stain and examined to determine their morphology (Fig. 14.4). Special stains such as peroxidase stain (POX), esterase stain, and PAS stain are applied as necessary, and myeloid (M0–7) and lymphoid are determined on the day of examination. At the time of bone marrow specimen collection, cell surface antigen test, chromosome test, and genetic test should be submitted at the same time to assist in morphological diagnosis.

### 2.6.3 Imaging Tests (X-Ray, CT, Etc.)

It detects hepatosplenomegaly, pneumonia, deep mycosis, and enlarged lymph nodes.

## 2.7 Treatment

After achievement of improved hematopoiesis by remission induction therapy, three to four courses of the same treatment are performed as consolidation therapy. For high-risk or relapse-refractory patients, hematopoietic stem cell transplantation is performed except in elderly patients [5]. A certain period of time is required for appropriate donor selection and preparation.

### 2.7.1 Chemotherapy

Patients with AML should receive anthracycline plus cytarabine (AraC), and patients with APL should receive ATRA (all-trans-retinoic acid) plus anthracycline or arsenite; patients with ALL should receive systemic steroids plus combination chemotherapy, and patients with Ph+ ALL should receive TKIs (tyrosine kinase inhibitors). TKI monotherapy is the first choice for CML, and anti-CD20 antibody chemotherapy, BTK (Breton-type kinase) inhibitors, and BCL2 inhibitors are useful for CLL.

### 2.7.2 Irradiation Therapy

Local irradiation of extramedullary tumors or total body irradiation (TBI) during hematopoietic stem cell transplantation are performed before or after chemotherapy.

### 2.7.3 Intrathecal Therapy

MTX and AraC are administered intrathecally to patients with or at high risk for central nervous system involvement (ALL, some forms of AML). Systemic side effects often occur. MTX or AraC should be administered two to three times a week for treatment and once a month for prophylaxis, but this has not been standardized.

### 2.7.4 Transplantation Therapy

Hematopoietic stem cell transplantation. Except for APL, which can be treated with autologous transplantation, allogeneic transplantation is often indicated for leukemia in the absence of favorable prognostic factors and in patients younger than 60 years of age. It is important to strengthen oral hygiene before transplantation and to deal with oral problems caused by graft-

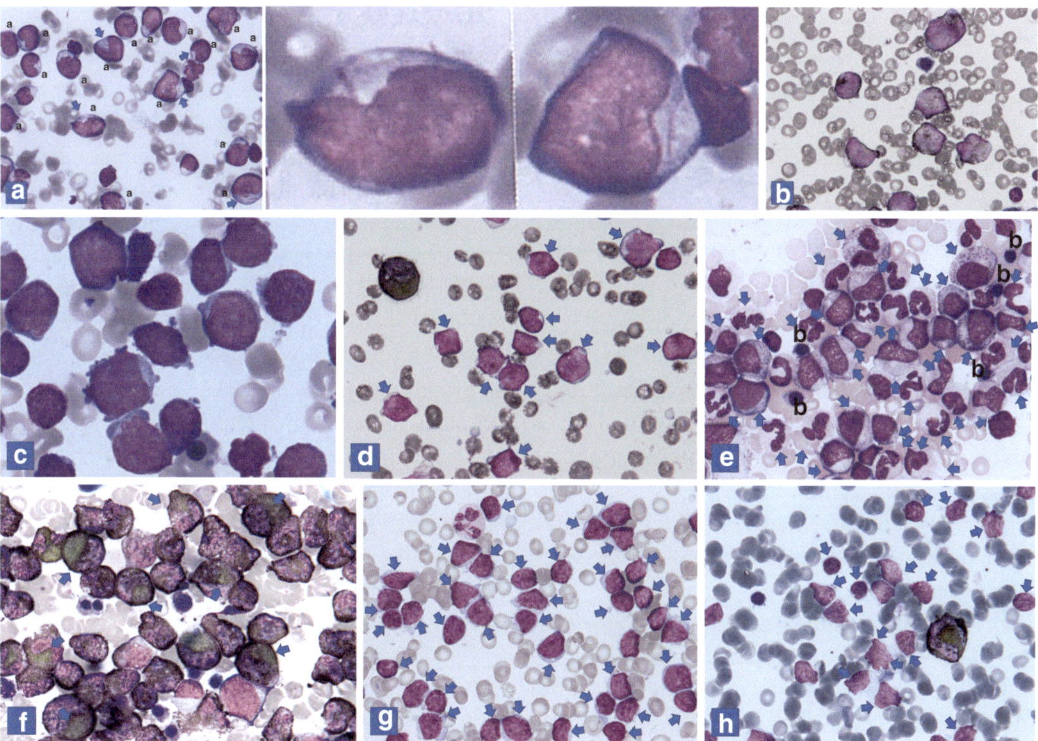

**Fig. 14.4** (**a**–**h**) Bone marrow findings of leukemia. *AML* acute myelogenous leukemia (**a**, **b**), *ALL* acute lymphocytic leukemia (**c**, **d**), *CML* chronic myelogenous leukemia (**e**, **f**), *CLL* chronic lymphocytic leukemia (**g**, **h**). May-Giemsa (**m**–**g**) staining (**a**, **e**, **c**, **g**) and peroxidase (POX) staining (**b**, **d**, **f**, **h**). (**a**, **left picture**) Increased of medium to large myeloblasts (a) are found, and some of them have auer rods (arrows: red club-shaped lines) with granules characteristic of AML. (**a**, **right picture**) Enlarged view of myeloblasts possessing Auer rods (arrows in (**a**) left picture). (**b**) Many blasts are POX positive (brown cytoplasm). (**c**) Medium- to large-sized blasts with a high nuclear cytoplasmic (N/C) ratio without cytoplasmic granules are uniformly produced, and some nucleoli are prominent. (**d**) POX negative blasts (arrows) are increasing uniformly. (**e**) Compared to the background erythroblasts, the number of granulocytic cells (arrows) (= having cytoplasmic granules) at each differentiation stage is overwhelmingly increased. Granulocytes predominate over erythroblasts, but myeloblasts are inconspicuous, corresponding to the chronic stage. (**f**) Granulocytes (arrows) of each maturation stage cell size are POX positive. (**g**) There is a marked increase in the number of small- to medium-sized mature lymphocytes (arrows) with a high N/C ratio that lack cytoplasmic granules. (**h**) Proliferating lymphocytes (arrows) are POX negative

versus-host disease (GVHD) after transplantation.

## 2.8 Prognosis

Various new drugs and advances in allogeneic hematopoietic stem cell transplantation, including bone marrow transplantation, have improved the prognosis. When a long-term prognosis is achieved, it is important to consider the deterioration of QOL due to chronic GVHD.

## 2.9 Recent Findings

The International Scale (IS%) of peripheral blood BCR/ABL chimera gene (RT-PCR) is now covered by insurance in Japan. In terms of treatment, the development of drug therapy has been remarkable along with the progress of hematopoietic stem cell transplantation methods. In recent years, FLT3 inhibitors for relapsed and refractory AML, cytotoxin-conjugated anti-CD22 antibody, anti-CD19 antibody and CD3 double antibody (blinatumomab) as antibody therapy for ALL, and T cells (CAR-T) modified to recognize and attack specific cancer antigens by chimeric antigen receptor (CAR) have been developed.

In addition, ponatinib, a third-generation TKI for T315I-resistant mutations in Ph leukemia, and BCL2 inhibitors for relapsed and refractory CLL were launched.

## 2.10 Notes from Dentistry Perspective [3]

Masaatsu Yagi

Leukemia, also known as cancer of the blood, is one of the most common hematologic neoplasms. It is a disease in which the number of leukocytes increases abnormally in general, although there is a period of temporary decrease in the number of leukocytes. The bone marrow function is abnormal and thrombocytopenia occurs, causing gingival bleeding (Fig. 14.5). Although the number of leukocytes increases, the abnormal function of the leukocytes results in decreased immunity and increased gingivitis and periodontitis, and gingival swelling is a characteristic symptom. In addition, hematologic neoplasms are more likely to develop DIC than solid tumors, and the bleeding tendency is stronger and the general condition is more likely to deteriorate.

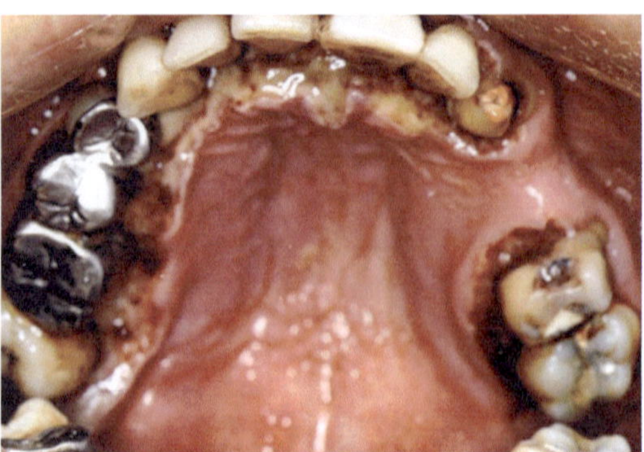

**Fig. 14.5** Gingival bleeding due to leukemia

Since gingival swelling and bleeding are characteristic symptoms of leukemia, it is common for leukemia to be detected during a dental examination. If you notice any abnormalities in the oral cavity, you should take measures such as referring the patient to a hematologist or having a blood test performed, and avoid performing surgical procedures such as tooth extraction. Systemic symptoms include palpitations, shortness of breath, malaise, and fever. Easy bleeding, such as bruising of the hands and feet, petechiae, and epistaxis, and swelling of the liver and spleen may also be seen. Lumbago, arthralgia, and headache may also be seen.

### 2.10.1 Types of Leukemia

There are two types of leukemia, acute and chronic, myeloid and lymphoid, and the oral and systemic manifestations are similar, although lymphadenopathy is added in the lymphoid form. In addition, the white blood cell count is usually higher in chronic than in acute cases. Acute promyelocytic leukemia has been difficult to treat because it is more likely to be associated with

DIC and progresses more rapidly than other leukemias. Still, the introduction of all-trans retinoic acid (ATRA) has improved treatment outcomes.

Adult T-cell leukemia is caused by infection with the HTLV-1 virus. It is transmitted from mother to child through breast milk, blood transfusion, or sexual intercourse. The incubation period is very long (30–50 years), and it was once thought to be a hereditary disease.

Chemotherapy with anticancer agents or molecular targeted drugs and hematopoietic stem cell transplantation are used for treatment. Chemotherapy further lowers the immune system, making the patient more susceptible to fungal infections such as candida and viruses such as herpes. Oral candidiasis, herpes labialis, and herpes zoster are common complications of chemotherapy, and antifungal and antiviral agents may be necessary.

#### 2.10.2 GVHD

Although hematopoietic stem cell transplantation (HSCT) has improved treatment outcomes, the incidence of graft-versus-host disease (GVHD) has also increased. In contrast to peripheral blood stem cell transplantation, bone marrow transplantation involves HLA compatibility testing, but because the transplant is from another person, GVHD often develops even after immunosuppressive drugs are administered after transplantation. There are two types of GVHD: acute GVHD and chronic GVHD, and it is chronic GVHD that generally causes oral symptoms. Lichen planus-like mucosal symptoms and xerostomia are known as oral symptoms. It is difficult to distinguish GVHD from oral lichen planus even by histopathological examination, so it is important to confirm a history of hematopoietic stem cell transplantation by interview for diagnosis.

Immunosuppressive drugs such as cyclosporine and steroids are the mainstay of treatment for GVHD, while azulene mouthwash and steroid ointments are applied for lichen planus-like symptoms and symptomatic treatment for xerostomia.

## 3 Hemophilia

Masahiro Ieko

### 3.1 Disease Overview

Due to X-chromosome-linked recessive inheritance, hemophilia A is an inherited deficiency in coagulation factor VIII (F VIII), and hemophilia B is an inherited deficiency in F IX, which is a typical hereditary hemorrhagic predisposition that causes bleeding tendency. The disease usually affects boys, with heterozygous females being carriers (Fig. 14.6). The disease is characterized by recurrent deep hemorrhage in joints and muscles that occurs from childhood. Treatment basically replaces the deficient coagulation factor preparation.

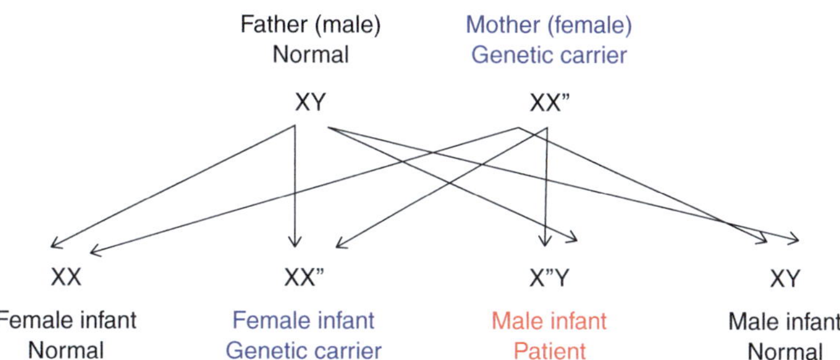


**Fig. 14.6** X-chromosome-linked recessive inheritance (hemophilia). Children born to healthy fathers and a mother of a hemophilia gene carrier have a 1/2 chance of developing hemophilia in boys and being a carrier in girls, respectively

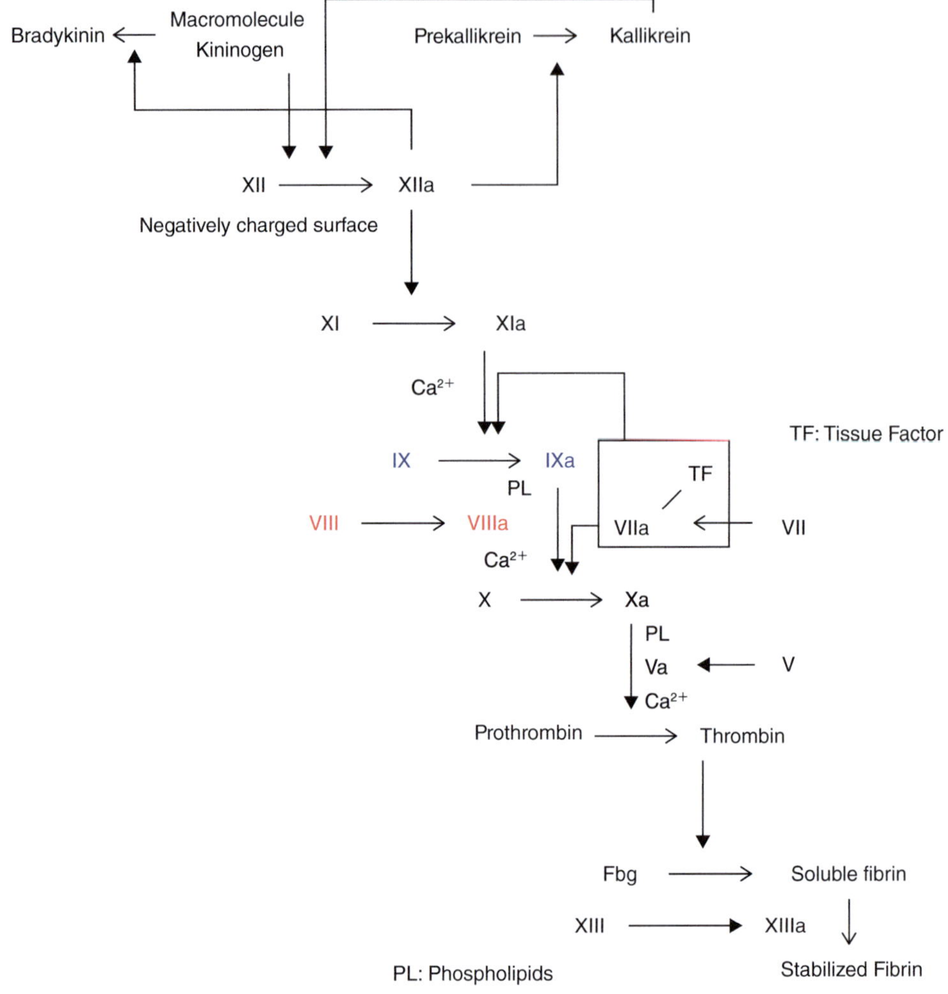


**Fig. 14.7** Cascade of coagulation reaction. F VIIIa amplifies FX activation of F IXa by 20,000-fold

## 3.2 Pathophysiology

F VII is a large gene located on Xq28 at the end of the long arm of the X chromosome and is composed of 26 exons and an intervening intron. Hemophilia A is caused by a genetic abnormality (point mutation, inversion, deletion, etc.) such as an intron 22 inversion. The F IX gene is located at Xq27.1 and consists of eight exons and seven introns. In hemophilia B, more than 90% of the genetic abnormalities are point mutations [6].

F VIII and F IX are essential factors for the FX activation reaction (Xase) in the coagulation reaction system, activated factor VIIIa (F VIIIa) amplifies FX activation by F IXa about 20,000-fold. (Fig. 14.7). Therefore, a decrease in F VIII and F IX leads to a significant bleeding tendency.

## 3.3 Epidemiology

Hemophilia A is the most common congenital blood coagulation disorders in Japan, with an incidence of 1 per 5,000–10,000 boys. The ratio of hemophilia A to hemophilia B is 5:1. About 30% of cases are solitary with no family history. Female hemophiliacs also occur, although they are extremely rare.

### 3.4 Classification

Severity is categorized according to the activity value of the applicable coagulation factor. F VIII or F IX activity of <1% is classified as severe, 1–5% as moderate, and >5% (to <40%) as mild.

### 3.5 Symptoms [6, 7]

In hemophilia, bleeding that exudes (Oozing) is common, subcutaneous, intra-articular, intramuscular, and oral bleeding and hematuria are common clinical manifestations of hemophilia.

1. **Subcutaneous bleeding**: This is the most common type of hemorrhage. Mottled subcutaneous bleeding occurs from infancy, sometimes forming a subcutaneous hematoma. Occasionally, bruising is palpable.
2. **Intra-articular bleeding**: This is a characteristic clinical manifestation of the disease, most commonly in the foot, knee, and elbow joints. It generally appears after the age of 1 year, when the child begins to walk. In the acute stage, intra-articular bleeding causes discomfort in the joints, severe pain and swelling, as well as movement disorders that greatly limit the range of motion of the joints. Repeated intra-articular bleeding leads to progressive degeneration and inflammation of the synovial membrane of the joint, and chronicity leads to irreversible bone deformation and destruction, resulting in hemophilic arthropathy.
3. **Intramuscular bleeding**: The hemorrhage tends to occur in the gastrocnemius muscle, soleus muscle, lower limb muscles such as muscle of thigh, causing swelling, pain, and motor impairment. In iliopsoas bleeding, the characteristic hip flexion position is called the psoas position.
4. **Intraoral hemorrhage**: Bleeding from the gingiva and tongue due to small cuts and bites is common. Periapical inflammation, deciduous teeth, and the eruption period of permanent teeth are also common causes of oral bleeding. The fibrinolytic activity of the oral mucosa makes it difficult to stop bleeding and prone to rebleeding, requiring appropriate treatment and replacement therapy.
5. **Other bleeding symptoms**: Hematuria occurs in adults with hemophilia and recurs frequently. Intracranial hemorrhage is the most frequent central nervous system hemorrhage and the most common cause of death in hemophilia. It is most often caused by trauma, but spontaneous hemorrhage also occurs. Hemoperitoneum may cause significant anemia. Hemorrhage within the intestinal wall causes severe abdominal pain and may lead to ileus.

### 3.6 Clinical Examination

The screening test shows a prolonged APTT with a normal PT and platelet count. A definitive diagnosis confirms a decrease in F VIII or F IX activity. The von Willebrand factor (vWF) activity is normal and this is an essential test for differentiating von Willebrand disease. To exclude acquired hemophilia A, anti-F VIII antibody activity and APTT cross-mixing test should also be performed.

### 3.7 Treatment

In principle, the main treatment is to replace the deficient coagulation factors. Currently, heat-treated plasma-derived products and genetically modified products are used. Recently, bispecific antibodies that bind to both F IXa and F X have been developed to replace the cofactor function of F VIII, and are used in the treatment of hemophilia A.

1. **Blood preparation replacement therapy**: F VIII preparation is administered for hemophilia A and F IX preparation for hemophilia B. Plasma-derived products and genetically modified products are available. There are bleeding replacement therapy, regular replacement therapy, and preliminary replacement therapy, depending on the timing of replacement. Regular replacement therapy is widely

used for the prevention of hemophilic arthropathy, which is performed once to three times a week using a formulation with a long half-life. On the other hand, preliminary replacement therapy involves infusion prior to events with a high risk of bleeding (such as athletic events).

For oral bleeding, replacement therapy should be given at a target level of F VIII activity of 20–40%, but should be limited to a single dose. If hemostasis is difficult, supplementation should be given every 12–24 h to maintain the peak factor level above 20% (until hemostasis). In patients with bleeding of the tongue or laceration of the palate, the target level of F VIII activity should be 40–60%.

2. **Desmopressin acetate (DDAVP)**: DDAVP, a treatment for central diabetes insipidus, causes the release of vWF from vascular endothelial cells and simultaneously increases F VIII blood levels. DDAVP is often used in mild to moderate hemophilia A patients during procedures such as tooth extraction. The effect is attenuated by continuous administration.
3. **Emicizumab (IgG-type recombinant humanized bispecific monoclonal antibody: bispecific antibody)**: Subcutaneously administered at a dose of 3 mg/kg four times at weekly intervals for the purpose of regular replacement therapy, followed by 1.5 mg/kg once every week, 3 mg/kg once every 2 weeks, or 6 mg/kg once every 4 weeks.

## 3.8 Inhibitor-Possessing Hemophilia and Its Treatment

Coagulation factor replacement therapy may result in the development of allogeneic antibodies (inhibitors) to F VIII and F IX in coagulation factor preparations, which invalidates the administered preparation. Inhibitors occur in about 30% of patients with hemophilia A and 3% of patients with hemophilia B. Inhibitor titers are measured by the Bethesda method (1 BU/mL is defined as the inhibitor activity that reduces 100% of the factor activity to 50%), with 5 BU/mL or more defined as a high-titer inhibitor and less than 5 BU/mL as a low-titer inhibitor. The risk of developing inhibitors is thought to be influenced by the severity of hemophilia, the type of genetic mutation, genetic background such as family history, and the amount of drug administered at the time of initial treatment.

In patients with low inhibitor titers, high-dose coagulation factor preparations are repeatedly administered to eliminate inhibitors (referred to as immune tolerance induction (ITI) therapy). In hemostatic therapy, a coagulation reaction that avoids the deficient coagulation factor (exogenous coagulation reaction) is used to stop bleeding, and activated prothrombin complex preparation (APCC), recombinant activated factor VII preparation (rF VIIa), and dried concentrated human coagulation factor X plus activated factor VII are administered. This is called bypass therapy.

## 3.9 Physical Treatment

When hemophilia bleeds, in addition to hemostatic treatment, the bleeding site should be rested, elevated with a cold compress, and immobilized. Intra-articular puncture should be considered for acute severe intra-articular bleeding.

## 3.10 Prognosis

The two leading causes of death in hemophilia are hemorrhagic death and liver disease caused by hepatitis C virus (HCV) transmitted by previously administered blood products. Death from AIDS-related complications due to human immunodeficiency virus (HIV) infection is also common.

In recent years, the prognosis of hemophilia is good due to the improvement of therapeutic agents such as the safety of blood coagulation factor preparations. As a result, the number of adult to elderly patients with hemophilia has increased, and the disease is now associated with atherosclerosis, such as hypertension. Coagulation control has become more complicated in patients with ischemic heart disease who also take antithrombotic drugs.

## 3.11 Notes from Dentistry Perspective

Satoshi Goto

### 3.11.1 Clinical Examination

In hemophilia, which is generally a blood coagulation disorder, PT is normal and APTT is prolonged.

### 3.11.2 Precautions for Dental Treatment

Dental treatment of patients with hemophilia begins with knowing the severity of the disease (Table 14.4). Since most hemophilic patients know that they have hemophilia, it is important to obtain information from their physician. However, some patients with mild hemophilia do not have bleeding episodes and do not know that they have hemophilia.

The first step in risk assessment is a medical interview. Most patients with severe or moderate disease have had episodes of bleeding in the past and have taken measures in their daily lives. First, write a letter of introduction to the patient's primary care physician and ask about the patient's current condition and the precautions and measures to be taken in case of surgical treatment. The patient should be able to undergo normal dental treatment without any problems, and if a surgical procedure is to be performed, it should be performed after replacement therapy of coagulation factors according to the instructions and local hemostatic treatment such as sutures should be taken [8]. Since platelet function is normal, there is no problem with temporary hemostasis. Therefore, it is important to monitor the postoperative course because bleeding, extensive swelling, and subcutaneous hemorrhage may occur several days after the patient returns home, even if hemostasis appears to have been achieved in the clinic, such as after tooth extraction (Fig. 14.8).

In the case of patients with mild hemophilia who do not know that they have hemophilia, dental treatment can be performed normally because bleeding stops spontaneously even if the patient falls and bleeds in daily life. In general, surgical procedures such as tooth extraction are no problem. However, hemostasis may be difficult to achieve during relatively invasive dental surgery that requires bone drilling. There have been cases in which hemophilia has been identified due to difficulty in stopping bleeding after dental surgery. If it is judged that hemostasis is difficult to achieve with normal hemostatic treatments after surgery, the patient should consult with the oral surgery department of a general hospital while trying to achieve local hemostasis by applying gauze to the area.

Bleeding from advanced marginal periodontitis is difficult to stop even in healthy individuals. Therefore, it is recommended that periodontal management and oral hygiene guidance be given to patients with hemophilia, and a management plan should be developed to maintain healthy gingival conditions.

**Table 14.4** Severity classification of hemophilia

| |
|---|
| Severe: Coagulation factor activity <1% |
| Moderate: Coagulation factor activity 1–5% |
| Mild disease: Coagulation factor activity >5% |

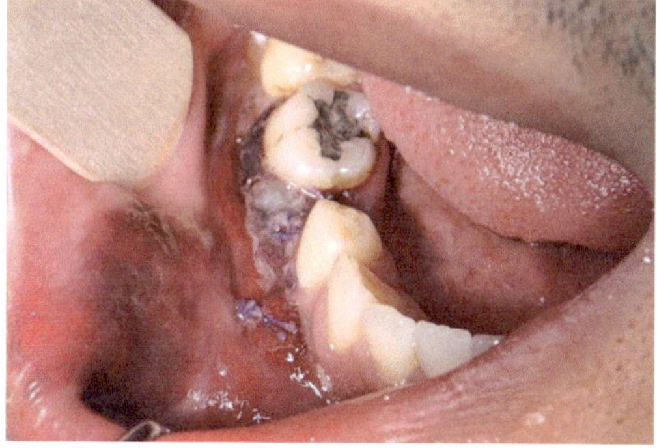

**Fig. 14.8** Swelling and ecchymosis after extraction of mandibular right second premolar

## 4 Malignant Lymphoma (ML)

Shigeki Ito

### 4.1 Disease Concept

Malignant lymphoma is a neoplastic disease of lymphocytes that develops from various stages of lymphocyte differentiation. Malignant lymphoma occurs mainly in lymphoid tissues such as lymph nodes, spleen, and tonsils, but it also occurs in many other tissues. It can occur in any organ, including the gastrointestinal tract, thyroid gland, lungs, liver, skin, bone marrow, and central nervous system, and presents a variety of symptoms depending on the site of development.

### 4.2 Pathophysiology

Genetic abnormalities are mainly involved in the pathogenesis of malignant lymphoma. It is thought that the accumulation of chromosomal translocations and genetic abnormalities leads to tumorigenesis through a multistep process. Diffuse large B-cell lymphoma (DLBCL), a typical malignant lymphoma, is classified into two types based on its cellular origin: germinal center type and non-germinal center type. In the germinal center type, epigenetic mutations and activation of the PI3K/AKT pathway are involved in the pathogenesis. On the other hand, in the non-germinal center type, mutations in the nuclear factor-κB (NF-κB) signaling pathway gene cluster, which is involved in cell survival and proliferation, are linked to the pathogenesis of the disease. In particular, mutations in cell surface molecules such as B-cell receptors and Toll-like receptors, and their downstream genes such as *TNFAIP3*, *CARD11*, *MYD88*, and *CD79B* are observed and are involved in pathogenesis. Double expression lymphoma, which co-expresses the anti-apoptotic molecule BCL2 and the transcription factor MYC protein, is a subgroup with poor prognosis [9]. Follicular lymphoma is characterized by translocation of *BCL2* gene and immunoglobulin heavy chain gene. Lymphoma progression requires secondary genetic mutations such as *p53* mutations. Mucosa-associated lymphoid tissue lymphoma has a high incidence in extralymphatic sites such as the stomach, lung, orbit, thyroid gland, and salivary gland, which often develops on the basis of autoimmune diseases such as chronic thyroiditis and Sjögren's syndrome.

### 4.3 Epidemiology

The crude morbidity rate of malignant lymphoma is estimated to be 29.6 males and 24.5 females per 100,000 population (2016), and the number of cases is increasing worldwide [10]. In Europe and the United States, the proportion of Hodgkin's lymphoma and B-cell lymphoma is high, while in Asia, the proportion of Hodgkin's lymphoma is lower and the proportion of T-cell lymphoma is higher than in Europe and the United States. On the other hand, the crude morbidity rate is estimated to be 11.9 for males and 8.9 for females per 100,000 population (2018) [10]. There are various types of malignant lymphoma, and the incidence varies depending on geographical conditions and race. In Japan, adult T-cell leukemia–lymphoma caused by human T-cell leukemia virus type 1 is the most common type of T-cell lymphoma, but the incidence varies greatly depending on the invasive status of the virus. The incidence of extranodal NK/T-cell lymphoma, nasal type, caused by Epstein–Barr virus is more common in East Asia. Hepatitis C virus, HIV virus, infections such as *Helicobacter pylori*, immunodeficiency and autoimmune diseases, and the use of methotrexate have been reported as risk factors for the development of the disease [11, 12].

### 4.4 Classification

According to the World Health Organization (WHO) classification, the disease is broadly classified into B-cell, T and NK cell, and Hodgkin lymphoma according to cellular origin [13]. Furthermore, each disease unit is formed by the postulated normal cellular counterparts/cell of origin, chromosomal/genetic abnormality, and

**Table 14.5** Classification of lymphoid neoplasms

| |
|---|
| 1. Precursor lymphoid tumor |
| 2. Mature B-cell neoplasms<br>• Diffuse large B-cell lymphoma<br>• Follicular lymphoma<br>• Mucosa-associated lymphoid tissue lymphoma<br>• Mantle cell lymphoma<br>• Burkitt lymphoma<br>• Intravascular large B-cell lymphoma, etc. |
| 3. Mature T- and NK-cell neoplasms<br>• Adult T-cell leukemia/lymphoma<br>• Extranodal NK/T-cell lymphoma, nasal type<br>• Peripheral T-cell lymphoma<br>• Undifferentiated large cell lymphoma, etc. |
| 4. Hodgkin lymphoma<br>• Nodular lymphocyte-predominant Hodgkin lymphoma<br>• Classical Hodgkin lymphoma |
| 5. Post-transplant lymphoproliferative disorders |
| 6. Histiocytic and dendritic cell neoplasms |

clinical picture. In the fourth edition (WHO-2017), revised in 2017, the number of classification items for lymphoid tumors is 112 [14]. Since it is not possible to show all of them in this paper, a rough classification is given (Table 14.5).

## 4.5 Symptoms

Malignant lymphoma can involve any part of the body. Lymphadenopathy is the main symptom, but organ-specific symptoms (abdominal distention due to hepatosplenomegaly, dyspnea due to pleural effusion, diarrhea and intestinal obstruction due to gastrointestinal tract involvement) may occur if extralymphatic organs are involved. Fever, sweating, and weight loss (symptom B) may be observed as systemic symptoms.

## 4.6 Clinical Examination

The examination of malignant lymphoma can be divided into two main categories: definitive diagnosis and staging. Definitive diagnosis is based on histopathological diagnosis using tumors obtained by surgical resection or biopsy of lymph nodes. Once a definitive diagnosis is made, staging is performed to determine the treatment strategy. Imaging tests such as CT scan and PET-CT scan, bone marrow examination, and cerebrospinal fluid examination are used for staging.

## 4.7 Treatment

Chemotherapy and radiation therapy are the mainstay of treatment for malignant lymphoma. The treatment strategy is determined based on the patient's general condition, histopathological diagnosis, grade, and clinical stage. Stages are classified as stages I–IV, as shown in Table 14.6, with stages I and II being the localized stages and stages III and IV being the advanced stages.

In the localized stage, radiation therapy may be added after chemotherapy. In the advanced stage, chemotherapy is the mainstay. Since chemotherapy depends on the type and grade of the disease, this article discusses representative lymphomas.

### 4.7.1 Hodgkin's Lymphoma

Doxorubicin, bleomycin, vinblastine, and dacarbazine combination therapy (ABVD therapy) is the initial standard of care. Recently, the combination of brentuximab vedotin (BV), an anti-CD30 monoclonal antibody conjugated with the anticancer agent monomethyl auristatin E, and doxorubicin, vinblastine, and dacarbazine has been covered by insurance in Japan and has been positioned the standard of care. The combination of BV, high-dose chemotherapy with autologous transplantation, and immune check-

**Table 14.6** Stages of lymphoma

| | |
|---|---|
| Stage I | One lymph node region or one extranodal lesion |
| Stage II | Lesions in two or more lymph node areas that are confined to either the upper or lower part of the diaphragm, or one extranodal lesion and a lesion in the lymph node region on the ipsilateral side of the diaphragm |
| Stage III | Multiple lymph node areas on both sides of the diaphragm or extranodal lesions |
| Stage IV | Diffuse and disseminated lesions of extranodal tissue |

point inhibitors such as nivolumab and pembrolizumab is used for patients with refractory disease.

### 4.7.2 Diffuse Large B-Cell Lymphoma

For DLBCL, the most common form of the disease, the standard of care is R-CHOP therapy, a combination of rituximab, an anti-CD20 monoclonal antibody, and cyclophosphamide, doxorubicin, vincristine, and prednisolone.

### 4.7.3 Follicular Lymphoma

Follicular lymphoma, the second most common type of lymphoma, is a low-grade lymphoma that progresses on a yearly basis. It progresses slowly and often without subjective symptoms, but is difficult to cure. After evaluating the stage, tumor volume, and course of the disease, the following options should be selected for each patient: (1) careful observation, (2) rituximab monotherapy, or (3) rituximab combination chemotherapy.

### 4.7.4 Extranodal NK/T-Cell Lymphoma, Nasal Type

Most of them are rare lymphomas derived from NK cells. About 70% of patients have localized stage disease, mainly in the nasal cavity or surrounding tissues. Because of the low efficacy of CHOP therapy even in the localized stage, chemoradiation with concurrent radiotherapy and chemotherapy (2/3 dose of DeVIC; dexamethasone, etoposide, ifosfamide, and carboplatin) is recommended [15].

## 4.8 Prognosis

Prognosis varies according to clinical stage and disease type; in DLBCL, age (≥61 years), LDH (>normal), performance status (≥2), stage (stage III–IV), and extranodal disease (≥2 sites) are prognostic factors, and the 4-year survival rate is 94% for 0 factors, 79% for 1 or 2 factors, and 55% for 3 or more factors [16].

## 4.9 Recent Findings

As the molecular pathogenesis has been clarified, classification of diseases based on genetic abnormalities has progressed; in DLBCL, the classification of germinal center B-cell type and activated B-cell type was proposed using DNA microarray [17]. For follicular lymphoma, a prognostic index (m7-FLIPI) incorporating the seven gene mutation states of *EZH2*, *ARID1A*, *MEF2B*, *EP300*, *FOXO1*, *CREBBP*, and *CARD11* has been proposed, and prognostic stratification has been performed [18]. It is expected that novel therapies for the poor prognosis group will be developed in the future.

## 4.10 Notes from Dentistry Perspective [5, 19, 20]

Daishi Saito

### 4.10.1 Malignant Lymphoma Arising in the Oral Cavity

Between 2001 and 2014, diffuse large B-cell lymphoma accounted for about 40% of reported cases of ML in the oral cavity in Japan, followed by MALT lymphoma (about 30%), extranodal NK/T-cell lymphoma, and Burkitt lymphoma. The palate, maxillary gingiva (Fig. 14.9), and mandibular

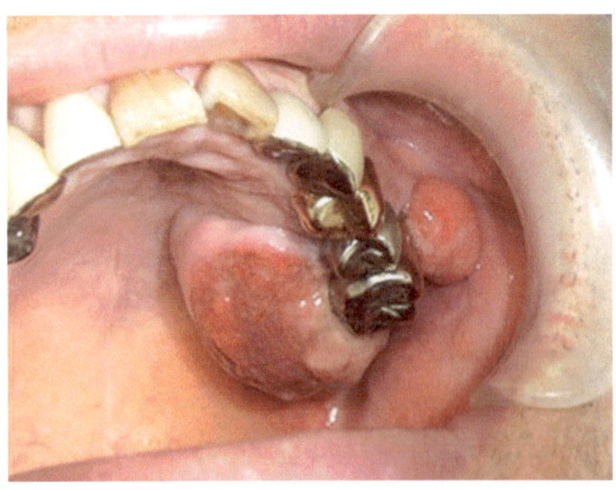

**Fig. 14.9** Malignant lymphoma of maxillary gingiva

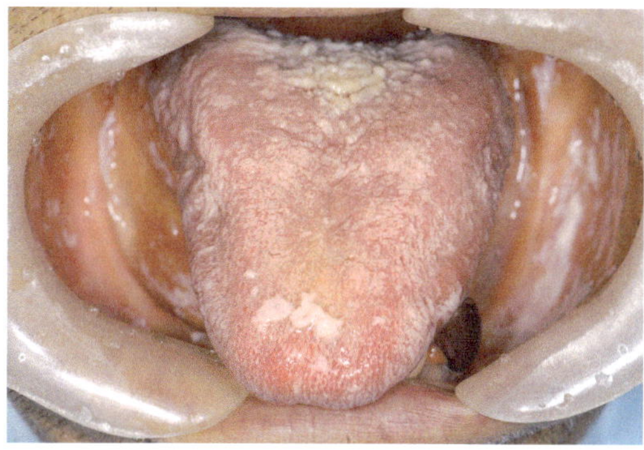

**Fig. 14.10** Oral candidiasis. White pseudomembranes are seen on the tongue and buccal mucosa

gingiva are the most common initial sites in the oral cavity (20% each), followed by the mandible and buccal mucosa. Intraoral findings included masses or swellings in about 70% of cases and ulcers or necrosis in about 20% of cases [20].

### 4.10.2 Treatment

Histopathological examination by biopsy is essential for the definitive diagnosis of ML, and ML may be detected by biopsy of intraoral lesions. When ML is suspected by histopathological findings, immediate consultation with a specialist is necessary. Drug therapy (chemotherapy, molecular targeted therapy), radiotherapy, and hematopoietic stem cell transplantation are available for the treatment of ML, and side effects such as stomatitis and other oral mucosal problems are common during any of these treatments. In addition, since the source of infection in the oral cavity may lead to serious infections such as bacteremia and sepsis due to immunosuppression during treatment, it is necessary to collaborate with the attending physician and to conduct thorough oral screening before treatment and oral care during treatment (Fig. 14.10).

## References


1. Yazaki Y, editor. ASAKURA internal medicine. (Naikagaku). 11th ed. Tokyo, Asakura Shoten; 2019. (in Japanese).
2. Nishida J, et al., editors. Internal medicine for the odontology. (Shika no tame no Naikagaku). Revised 4th ed. Tokyo: Nankodo; 2018. (in Japanese).
3. Shirasuna K, Kogo M, editors. Oral surgery. (Kouku Gekagaku). 3rd ed. Tokyo: Ishiyaku Shuppan; 2010. (in Japanese).
4. Kizaki M, Tamaru J, editors. Pathogenesis of leukemia and lymphoid tumors according to the revised fourth edition of the WHO classification. (WHO Bunrui Kaitei Dai 4 han niyoru Hakketsubyo Lympakei Shuyou no Byoutaigaku). Tokyo: Chugai Igaku-sha; 2019. (in Japanese).
5. The Japanese Society of Hematology, editor. Practical guidelines for hematological malignances, 2018, revised version (Zouketsuki Shuyou Shinryou guideline). 2018 ed. Tokyo: Kanehara Shuppan; 2018. (in Japanese).
6. Shima M. Chapter XI: thrombotic and hemostatic diseases, 8. Hemophilia. (Dai XI Shou: Kessen Shiketsu Shikkan, 8. Ketsuyubyo). In: Japanese Society of Hematology, editor. Textbook of hematology (Ketsueki Senmon-I text). Revised 2nd ed. Tokyo: Nanko-do; 2015. p. 396–400. (in Japanese).
7. Ieko M. 13. Symptoms of lymphatic and vascular disease, 2. Petechiae, purpura. Internal medicine diseases diagnosed from symptoms. (13. Lympa Kekkan no Shoujyou, 2. Tenjyou Shukketsu, Shihan). In: Watanabe J, Sawada K, editors. Internal medicine diseases diagnosed from symptoms. (Shoujyoukara miru Naika Shikkan). Tokyo: Medical View; 2005. p. 404–8. (in Japanese).
8. The Japanese Society on Thrombosis and Hemostasis. Guideline for the treatment of haemostasis in patients with haemophilia without inhibitors (Inhibitor nonai Ketsuyubyo Kanjya nitaisuru Shiketsu Chiryo guideline). In: Hemostatic therapy guideline for patients with hemophilia without inhibitors: 2013 Revised ed. Tokyo: The Japanese Society on Thrombosis and Hemostasis; 2013. p. 1–24. (in Japanese). https://www.jsth.org/wordpress/wpcontent/uploads/2015/04/03_inhibitor_H1_B.pdf.
9. Horn H, et al. MYC status in concert with BCL2 and BCL6 expression predicts outcome in diffuse large B-cell lymphoma. Blood. 2013;121:2253–63.
10. National Cancer Center Japan Information Service. Latest cancer statistics. (in Japanese). https://ganjoho.jp/reg_stat/statistics/stat/summary.html.
11. Morton LM, et al. Rationale and design of the International Lymphoma Epidemiology Consortium (InterLymph) non-Hodgkin lymphoma subtypes project. J Natl Cancer Inst Monogr. 2014;48:1–14.
12. Morton LM, et al. Etiologic heterogeneity among non-Hodgkin lymphoma subtypes: the InterLymph non-Hodgkin lymphoma subtypes project. J Natl Cancer Inst Monogr. 2014;48:130–44.
13. Swerdlow SH, et al. WHO classification of tumours of haematopoietic and lymphoid tissues. 4th ed. Lyon: IARC Press; 2008.
14. Swerdlow SH, et al. WHO classification of tumours of haematopoietic and lymphoid tissues. Revised 4th ed. Lyon: IARC Press; 2017.
15. Yamaguchi M, et al. Phase I/II study of concurrent chemoradiotherapy for localized nasal natural killer/

T-cell lymphoma: Japan Clinical Oncology Group Study JCOG0211. J Clin Oncol. 2009;27:5594–600.
16. Sehn LH, et al. The revised International Prognostic Index (R-IPI) is a better predictor of outcome than the standard IPI for patients with diffuse large B-cell lymphoma treated with R-CHOP. Blood. 2007;109:1857–61.
17. Alizadeh AA, et al. Distinct type of diffuse large B-cell lymphoma identified by gene expression profiling. Nature. 2010;403:503–11.
18. Pastore A, et al. Integration of gene mutations in risk prognostication for patients receiving first-line immunochemotherapy for follicular lymphoma: a retrospective analysis of a prospective clinical trial and validation in a population-based registry. Lancet Oncol. 2015;16:1111–22.
19. National Cancer Center Japan. Cancer information service. (in Japanese). https://ganjoho.jp/reg_stat/index.html.
20. Kawamata A, et al. A clinical study of malignant lymphomas arising in the oral and maxillofacial region with a review of case reports in Japan. Oral Oncol. 2015;27:119–25. (in Japanese).

# Immune System Diseases 15

Yoshihiro Matsukawa, Natsumi Ikumi,
Yoshiki Hamada, Noriyuki Seta, Keiko Aota,
Masayuki Azuma, Yuh Baba, and Satoshi Takada

## 1 Rheumatoid Arthritis [1–4]

Yoshihiro Matsukawa, Natsumi Ikumi

### 1.1 What Is Rheumatoid Arthritis (RA)?

Rheumatoid arthritis (RA) is a chronic inflammatory disease caused by an autoimmune mechanism in which joints become the target of immune responses. It is a chronic inflammatory disease involving mainly in the synovium and other joint components repeatedly featuring remissions and relapse. It can affect every joint in the body, and the inflammation causes arthralgia (tenderness and spontaneous pain), swelling, heat sensation, and dysfunction of joints, leading to loss of joint cartilage and bone, and eventually to joint destruction with deformity. Finally, RA patients could result in locomotive syndrome that tends toward "bedridden" status, in which motor ability is significantly reduced due to joint destruction and deformation.

It is also characterized by the presence of a variety of extra-articular symptoms, and should be regarded as a systemic disease rather than an osteoarticular disease. Among them, those with vasculitis are designated as malignant RA (MRA) (this is a diagnosis unique to Japan).

### 1.2 Pathoetiology

Although pathoetiology of RA is still to be resolved, it is accepted to be caused or induced by a complex combination of factors, including viral and bacterial infections[1], hormones, drugs, physi-

[1]Viruses such as Human parvovirus B19, EB virus, and Retrovirus, as well as Mycoplasma, *Porphyromonas gingivalis,* etc.

Y. Matsukawa
Department of Internal Medicine, Tsurumi University Dental Hospital, Yokohama, Kanagawa, Japan

N. Ikumi
Division of Cutaneous Science, Department of Dermatology, Nihon University School of Medicine, Itabashi-ku, Tokyo, Japan

Y. Hamada
Department of Oral & Maxillofacial Surgery, School of Dental Medicine, Tsurumi University, Kanagawa, Yokohama, Japan

N. Seta (✉)
Department of Internal Medicine, Tokyo Dental College, Ichikawa General Hospital, Ichikawa, Chiba, Japan
e-mail: nseta@tdc.ac.jp

K. Aota · M. Azuma
Graduate School of Biomedical Sciences, Tokushima University, Tokushima, Japan

Y. Baba · S. Takada
Department of General Clinical Medicine, Ohu University School of Dentistry, Koriyama, Fukushima, Japan


T. Chiba, H. Yamada (eds.), *Internal Medicine for Dental Treatments*,
https://doi.org/10.1007/978-981-99-3296-2_15

cal stress, smoking, and periodontal disease, against a background of genetic abnormalities[2].

## 1.3 Epidemiology

It is estimated that 0.5% to 1% of the world population is affected, although there are racial differences. The ratio of males to females is reported to be 1:3 to 1:4, with a little difference among races or regions. The incidence is lower in Asians and Hispanic than in Caucasians. According to patients' survey conducted by the Japanese Ministry of Health, Labour and Welfare (MHLW) in its FY 2018 report (first Committee on Rheumatism and Other Related Diseases), the estimated number of patients in FY 2014 was 33.6/1,000, which would be about 4.3 million if the total population is just under 130 million[3]. The total number of patients is on the rise and has increased 1.2 times in the last 20 years.

## 1.4 Pathophysiology

It is accepted that the inflammation is induced by various cytokines such as TNF-α produced by the abnormally proliferated synovium, as well as by inflammation-inducing substances such as prostaglandins and leukotrienes.

## 1.5 Symptoms of RA

The initial symptoms are morning stiffness and symmetrical, multiple, and migratory arthralgia. In addition, it should be noted that patients with temporomandibular arthritis tend to visit a dentist. RA should be considered when polyarthralgia persists for more than 1 month and cannot be explained by other diseases[4]. Initial changes are limited to articular malfunction due to swelling, redness, warmth, and pain, but when RA is insufficiently controlled, articular destruction progresses and finally leads to functionless deformity. We therefore have to establish the most suitable anti-rheumatic strategy as soon as possible. The frequently affected joints are the proximal interphalangeal joints, metacarpophalangeal joints, hand/shoulder/knee joints, and metatarsophalangeal joints. As the lesion progresses, deformities unique to RA such as swan-neck deformity, button hole deformity, and ulnar deviation, are completed.

Extra-articular manifestations include (1) subcutaneous nodules (rheumatic nodules): they appear on the extensor side of the joint where pressure is applied, but can occur anywhere in the body; (2) interstitial pneumonia, pleurisy, and intrapulmonary rheumatic nodules (which must be differentiated from lung cancer); (3) eye manifestations: uveitis and episcleritis; (4) neurologic manifestations: carpal tunnel stenosis, paresthesia, motor paralysis, and vertigo due to neck deformity; (5) vasculitis: skin ulcer; and (6) renal failure(mainly due to ADE).

## 1.6 Diagnosis

The diagnosis should be established by referring to the ACR/EULAR classification criteria after confirming arthritis and various symptoms, and taking into account blood tests and imaging studies (Table 15.1) [3].

## 1.7 Clinical Examination

Anti-cyclic citrullinated peptide (Anti-CCP) antibody, rheumatoid factor (RF), CRP, and erythrocyte sedimentation rate (ESR), are required for diagnosis (Table 15.1), and in addition, the destruction of articular cartilage should be evaluated by matrix metalloproteinase-3 (MMP-3). Serum complement titer (CH50) is also useful in assessing RA activity.

## 1.8 Imaging Findings of RA

Although plain radiography is the basic method, it is insufficient for early diagnosis because it only confirms the established anatomical

[2]It has been suggested that class II MHC, especially HLA-DR antigens, are involved.

[3]This number is higher than the previous estimates of 700,000 to 1,000,000, but it is close to the actual number because it is based on patients who visited medical institutions.

[4]RA cannot be ruled out only because it is monoarthritis.

**Table 15.1** Rheumatoid arthritis classification criteria. The 2010 ACR/EULAR classification criteria (American College of Rheumatology/European College of Rheumatology classification criteria). Clinically observed synovitis (joint swelling) in one or more joints that cannot be explained by any other disease is graded A–D

| | |
|---|---|
| A: Joint involvement | |
| 1 large joint[a] | (0) |
| 2–10 large joints | (1) |
| 1–3 small joints (with or without involvement of large joints)[b] | (2) |
| 4–10 small joints (with or without involvement of large joints) | (3) |
| >10 joints (at least 1 small joint) | (5) |
| B: Serology[c] | |
| Negative RF and negative ACPA | (0) |
| Low-positive RF or low-positive ACPA | (2) |
| High-positive RF or high-positive ACPA | (3) |
| C: Acute-phase reactants | |
| Normal CRP and normal ESR | (0) |
| Abnormal CRP or abnormal ESR | (1) |
| D: Duration of symptoms | |
| <6 weeks | (0) |
| ≥6 weeks | (1) |

A score of 6 or more classifies it as rheumatoid arthritis. *ACPA* anti-cyclic citrullinated peptide antibody

[a] Large joints refers to shoulders, elbows, hips, knees, and ankles

[b] Small joints refers to the metacarpophalangeal joints, proximal interphalangeal joints, second through fifth metatarsophalangeal joints, thumb interphalangeal joints and wrists

[c] Low-positive refers to IU values that are higher than the upper limit of normal (ULN) but ≤3 times the ULN for the laboratory and assay; high-positive refers to IU values that are >3 times the ULN for the laboratory and assay

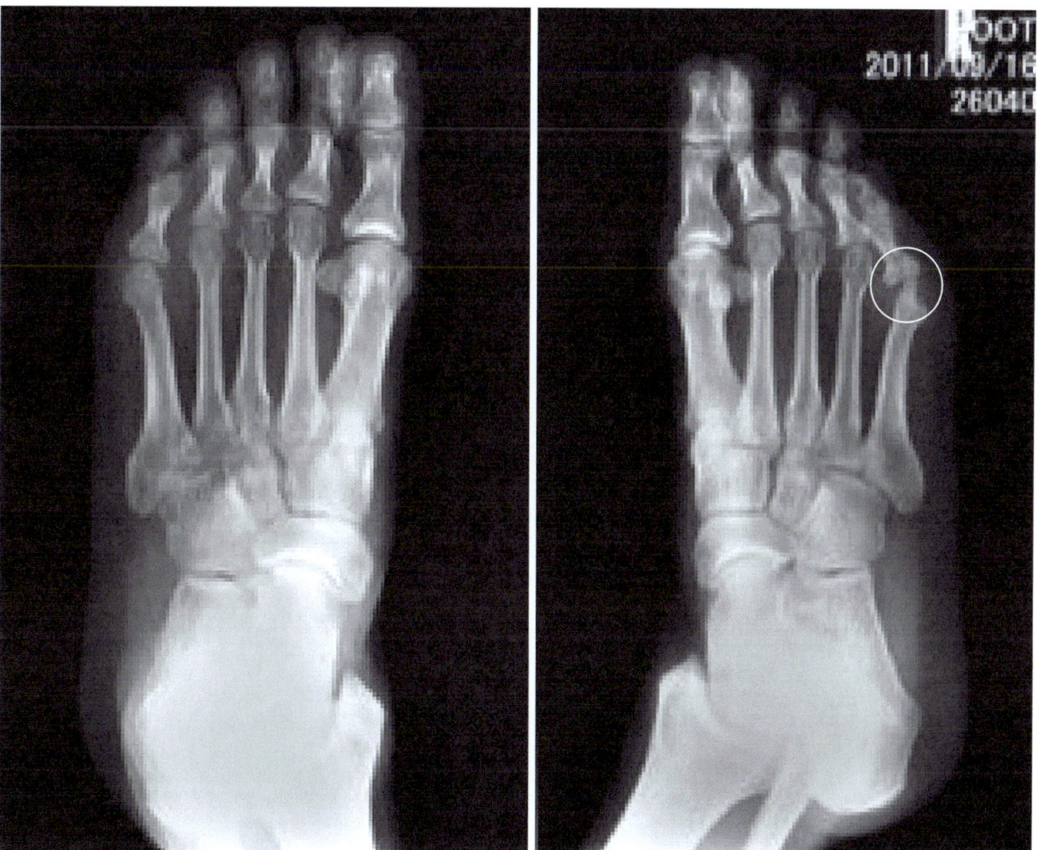


**Fig. 15.1** Plain radiographs of both toes at the time of the first visit to RA: bone erosion limited to the head of proximal phalanx of the right fifth toe

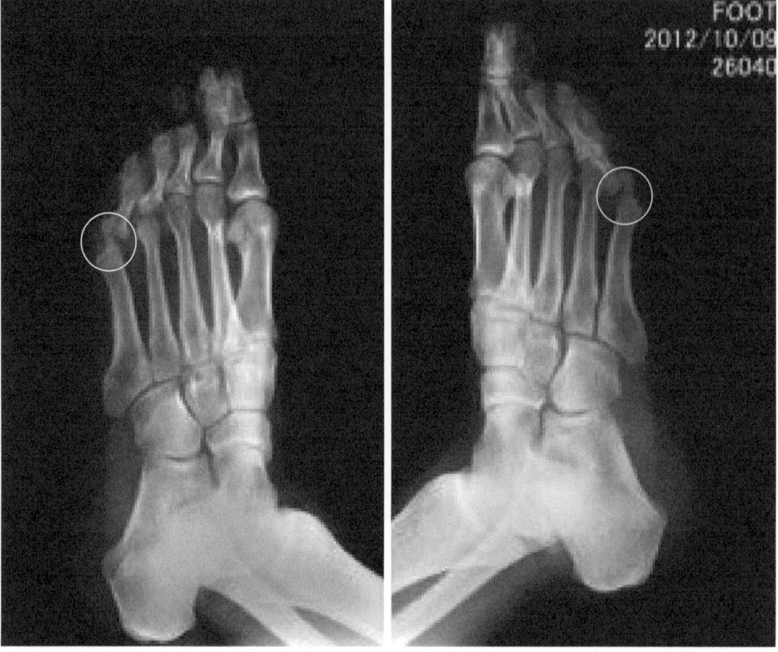


**Fig. 15.2** One year after the start of MTX, bone erosion extends to the left 4/5 toes

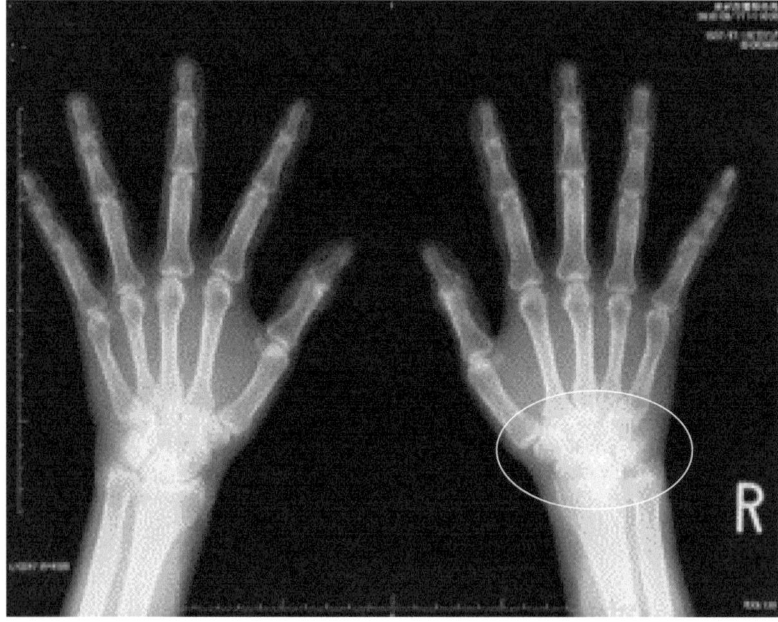


**Fig. 15.3** Right carpal bone lumping is observed

changes. Narrowing of the joint space indicates destruction of articular cartilage, and bone erosion indicates destruction of bone (Figs. 15.1 and 15.2). In the terminal stage of RA, the constituent bones of the joint would be fused into a mass and no longer could maintain the articular function (ankylosis) (Fig. 15.3). Recently, articular echography and contrast-enhanced MR have been used to visualize ongoing inflammation.

## 1.9 Treatment

Drug therapy is the basic treatment, but rehabilitation and surgery are also essential to improve patients' quality of life.

Non-steroidal anti-inflammatory drugs (NSAIDs) and corticosteroids are used for symptomatic relief, and disease-modifying anti-rheumatic drugs (DMARDs) have been developed to control RA. Currently, methotrexate (MTX) is accepted as the key drug of first choice, and the dose can usually be increased to 16 mg/week in Japan.

Biologics should be considered for patients with insufficient response to MTX or with contraindications to MTX such as interstitial pneumonia or renal dysfunction. Biologics are injectable drugs that effectively control RA by inhibiting the action of cytokines such as TNF-α, IL-1/IL-6/IL-8, and CTLA4. Oral Janus kinase (JAK) inhibitors, which are as effective as biologics, can also be used. However, due to their potent immunosuppressive effects, consideration for tuberculosis and viral infections is essential[5]. Both biologics and JAK inhibitors are expensive and are not recommended for patients who cannot afford them. Tacrolimus is another kind of immunosuppressive agent commonly used. Adrenocorticosteroids have a potent anti-inflammatory effect and are used during remission induction, but long-term administration should be avoided because of side effects. Other classical DMARDs are applied in mild cases (salazopyrin, gold formulations, penicillamine, etc). All of RA treatments suppress the immune response, we therefore should always pay attention to compromised infection.

## 1.10 Notes from Dentistry Perspective

Yoshiki Hamada

### 1.10.1 Rheumatoid Arthritis of the Temporomandibular Joint [5–9]

Rheumatoid arthritis (RA) also affects the temporomandibular joint (TMJ), and the frequency of RA in the TMJ varies from 5 to 86%, depending on each report, that is probably because there are no clear diagnostic criteria for rheumatoid arthritis of the TMJ (TMJ RA). Symptoms of TMJ RA correlate with the duration and severity of RA, but are less severe and progress more slowly than in other joints. Incidentally, in rare cases, RA symptoms can first occur in the TMJ. In the early stage of the disease, however, it is difficult to distinguish RA symptoms from those of temporomandibular joint disorder (TMD), especially TMJ osteoarthritis (OA), because there are no characteristic imaging findings. Therefore, in the cases of RA which symptoms first occur in the TMJ, the definitive diagnosis of RA may be established after the development of systemic symptoms and/or polyarthritis.

On the other hand, it is important to establish the definitive and start treatment as early as possible because RA can lead to serious conditions such as progressive condylar resorption and ankylosis of the TMJ (Figs. 15.4 and 15.5). The viewpoints for clinical differential diagnosis

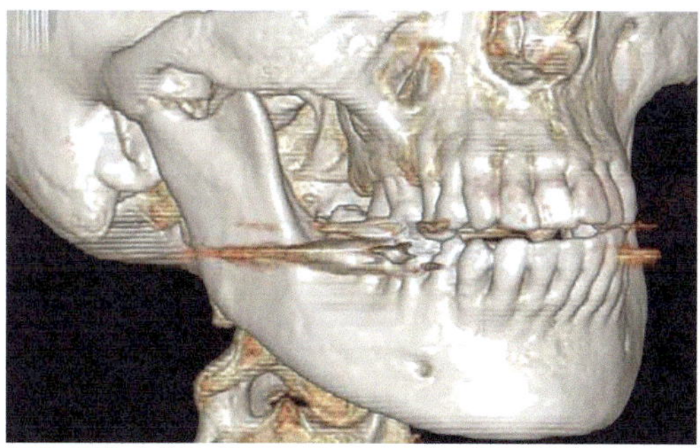

**Fig. 15.4** Bony ankylosis of the TMJ due to RA

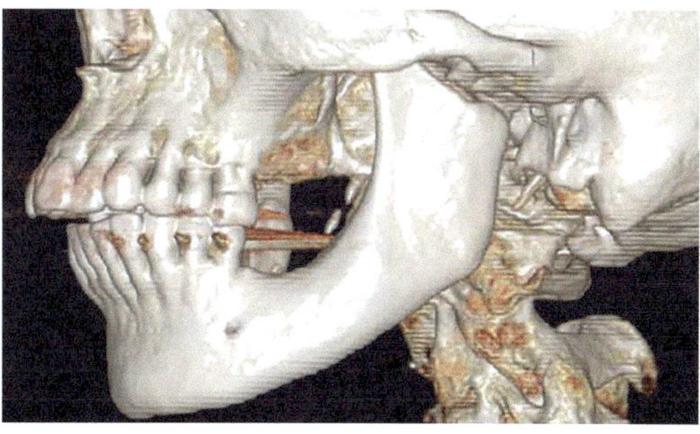

**Fig. 15.5** Condylar resorption due to RA

[5]Hepatitis B reactivation (de novo hepatitis) during and after quitting of biologics or MTX has become a serious problem because of the high mortality. It is essential to check for hepatitis B before initiation of biologics and MTX.

between RA and TMJ OA are: (1) worsening of symptoms over time without response to the standard treatment for TMD; (2) spontaneous pain and tenderness in the TMJ area; and (3) unilateral onset of symptoms on the opposite side. If symptoms develop in other joints, the patient should be immediately referred to a rheumatologist.

The symptoms of TMJ RA depend on the severity of RA, but the basic treatment is same as that for TMD. In the advanced case with ankylosis of the TMJ or open bite with retrotrusive mandible due to severe condylar resorption, surgical mobilization of TMJ, orthognathic surgery, reconstruction of the condylar process, or artificial TMJ replacement is indicated to recover jaw function and occlusion.

#### 1.10.2 Methotrexate-Associated Lymphoproliferative Disease (MTX-LPD) and RA Drug-Induced Stomatitis

Currently, the basic concept of treatment for RA is to suppress or delay the onset of dysfunction due to joint destruction as much as possible, and methotrexate (MTX), an immunosuppressive agent, is recommended as a standard drug for this purpose. On the other hand, serious side effects include acute interstitial pneumonia, myelosuppression and associated infections, and MTX-associated lymphoproliferative disorders (MTX-LPD).

In the oral cavity, in addition to stomatitis caused by RA drugs such as MTX, there are several reports of ulceration caused by MTX-LPD (Fig. 15.6), which may be accompanied by bone exposure, and commonly diagnosed as histopathological diffuse large B-cell malignant lymphoma. Clinically, local pain and contact pain at the ulcer site are observed, and systemic symptoms, including fever and weight loss, are recognized. In addition, elevated IL-2R level is often observed, and if its level is abnormally high of exceeding 1000 U/mL, it is necessary to consider the possibility of existence of other undetected lesions in the areas outside of oral cavity.

As a general rule, MTX-LPD is treated with MTX withdrawal, and if no remission is observed, chemotherapy is generally considered after consultation with a hematologist or other physician, but radiotherapy may be applied depending on the histological type. Regarding the prognosis, it has been reported that remission rate of 21 to 60% can be achieved with drug suspension alone, but recurrence occurs in 33 to 67%. On the other hand, a review of 24 Japanese cases of MTX-LPD in the oral cavity reported a remission rate of 92%.

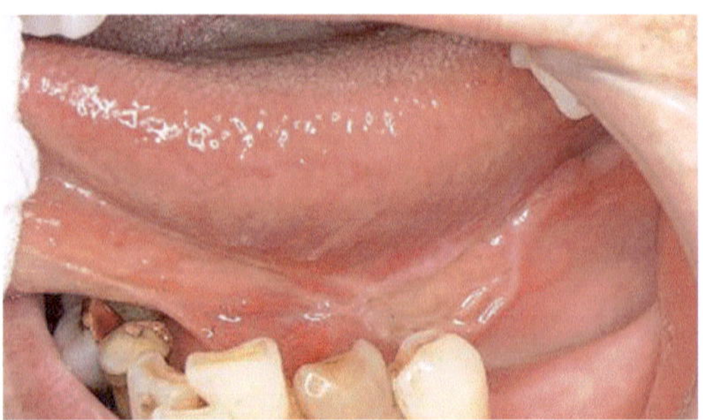

**Fig. 15.6** Ulceration of the left floor of mouth due to MTX-LPD. (Courtesy of Dr. Toshikatsu Horiuchi, Department of Oral and Maxillofacial Surgery, Saiseikai Yokohamashi Tobu Hospital)

Although the pathogenesis of MTX-LPD is unclear, EBV-positive patients account for more than half of the cases, and it has been suggested that EBV, which has the ability to proliferate and transform B cells, causes lymphoma under the condition of MTX-induced immunosuppression. It has also been reported that RA-related biologics may be a cause of MTX-LPD, and that RA itself increases the risk of developing LPD. On the other hand, no significant findings have been found in relation to the duration and dosage of MTX and concomitant medications such as prednisolone and bisphosphonates.

## 2 Collagen Disease [10–13]

Noriyuki Seta

### 2.1 Systemic Lupus Erythematosus: SLE

#### 2.1.1 Disease Overview

It is one of the most common collagen diseases and causes damage to multiple organs due to the production of a variety of autoantibodies. The pathogenesis is extremely variable, ranging from cases that do not require treatment to severe, life-threatening cases. Anti-double-stranded DNA antibodies and anti-Sm antibodies are disease-specific antibodies, and complications of renal lesions affect the prognosis.

### 2.1.2 Pathophysiology

The basis of the pathogenesis of SLE is an autoimmune phenomenon centered on B cell hyperactivation. Inflammation and tissue damage are caused by the persistent activation of lymphocytes due to the acquisition of tolerance of T cells and B cells that recognize self-antigens and the dysfunction of regulatory T cells. Activated B cells produce an excessive amount of autoantibodies, such as anti-DNA antibodies, and the immune complexes formed by binding with self-antigens are deposited in tissues, activating the complement system and causing persistent inflammation.

### 2.1.3 Epidemiology

The age of onset is 20 to 40 years, with those in their 20 s accounting for 40% of all cases. The male to female ratio is approximately 1:20, with females being overwhelmingly affected. The prevalence in Japan is estimated to be about 100 per 100,000 people.

### 2.1.4 Symptoms

1. **Mucocutaneous manifestations:** The most characteristic eruption in SLE is erythema of the cheeks, which is also called butterfly rush because of the shape of the eruption. This edematous erythema often appears as the first symptom of SLE and is found almost symmetrically on both cheeks, centered on the dorsum of nose, with healthy skin remaining inside the nasolabial sulcus (Fig. 15.7). The other specific eruption is erythema with keratotic scales, which is called discoid erythema, and is found on the exposed areas of the head, face, auricles, and dorsum of the fingers. Raynaud's phenomenon, in which the fingers and toes show a triphasic color change of white, purple, and red, and alopecia may also occur. Oral ulcers are also frequently seen, but they are characterized by being painless and located on the hard palate (Fig. 15.8).

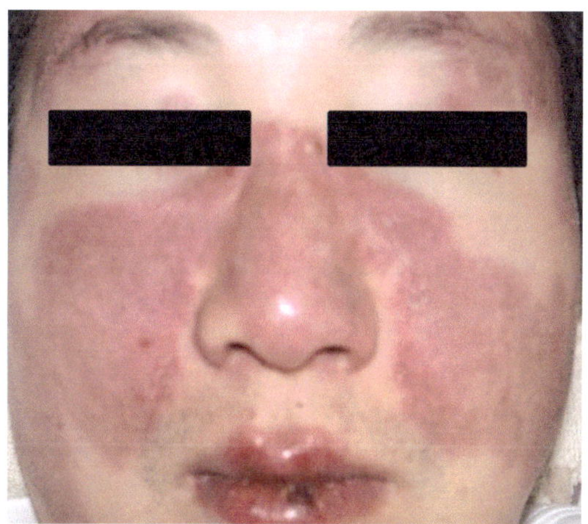

**Fig. 15.7** Butterfly rash of systemic lupus erythematosus

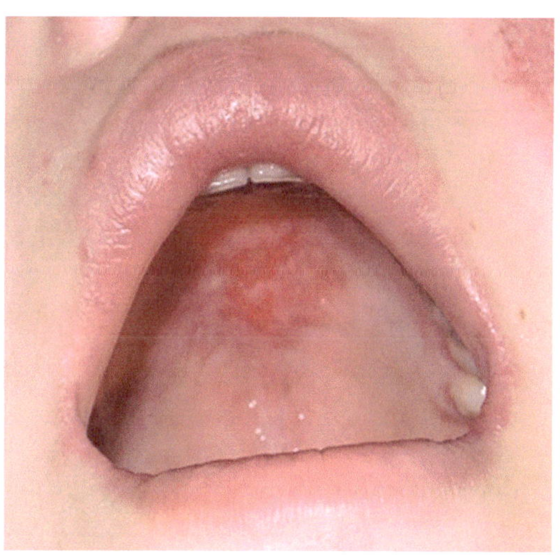

**Fig. 15.8** Oral ulceration in systemic lupus erythematosus

2. **Bone and joint symptoms:** Arthritis with joint swelling, heat sensation, and pain may occur. Joint deformity may occur with laxity of periarticular tissues, but unlike arthritis of rheumatoid arthritis (RA), it is nondestructive and can generally be temporarily corrected by passive reposition (Jaccoud's arthropathy). Aseptic necrosis of bone may occur in patients with SLE treated with corticosteroids, and the femur head is the most common site of necrosis.
3. **Respiratory and cardiovascular symptoms:** Aseptic pleurisy and pericarditis may occur,

accompanied by chest pain, dyspnea, and fever. When myocarditis occurs, nonspecific ST-T changes and arrhythmias appear on the electrocardiogram. In the pulmonary parenchyma, interstitial pneumonia and alveolar hemorrhage may appear during the active phase of the disease. Pulmonary arterial hypertension (PAH) may also occur, and is an important factor in determining the prognosis.
4. **Renal manifestations:** The nephropathy associated with SLE is known as lupus nephritis and is present in about half of all patients with SLE. Proteinuria, erythrocyturia, leukocyturia, and cylindruria occur early in the course of the disease, leading to nephrotic syndrome and renal failure as the disease progresses. In some cases, dialysis may eventually be required.
5. **Neuropsychiatric symptoms:** Neuropsychiatric lupus (NPSLE) is a disorder of the nervous and mental systems associated with SLE. Neuropathy is diverse and can manifest as central, peripheral, or autonomic symptoms.
6. **Gastrointestinal symptoms:** Peritonitis may occur, resulting in abdominal pain and ascites. Vasculitis of the mesenteric artery causes intestinal ischemia, which may lead to infarction, ulceration, and hemorrhage of the intestine. It may also cause intestinal obstruction (lupus enteritis).

### 2.1.5 Clinical Examination

1. **Inflammation reaction:** In the active stage of SLE, the erythrocyte sedimentation rate and serum gammaglobulin are increased, but there is usually no significant increase in CRP. If CRP is strongly positive, the presence of arthritis, serositis, vasculitis, or infection should be suspected.
2. **Hematologic test:** In the active phase of SLE, all three blood cell systems (white blood cells, red blood cells, and platelets) may be decreased. Among the white blood cells, lymphocytes are mainly decreased. Autoimmune hemolytic anemia associated with the production of autoantibodies against red blood cells results in a marked decrease in red blood cells, a decrease in haptoglobin levels, an increase in indirect bilirubin, and a positive Coombs test. The decrease in platelets is often due to decreased platelet production or platelet destruction in the periphery by antiplatelet antibodies, and thrombocytopenia may also occur in patients with anti-phospholipid antibody syndrome.
3. **Immunological test:** Anti-nuclear antibodies (ANA) are positive in almost 100% of patients with SLE. Anti-double-stranded DNA antibodies and anti-Sm antibodies are known as disease-specific antibodies, and anti-double-stranded DNA antibodies are also used as an indicator of disease activity. In some cases, serum immune complexes increase and serum complement titers decrease during the active phase of SLE. Antibodies against cardiolipin and lupus anticoagulant are also positive in SLE, which tends to cause (1) arteriovenous thrombosis, (2) habitual abortion, and (3) thrombocytopenia, which is called anti-phospholipid antibody syndrome.
4. **Renal function tests and urinalysis:** In patients with lupus nephritis, urine protein is persistently positive, and erythrocyte and leukocyte columns are seen in the active stage of nephritis. As renal damage progresses, serum creatinine and BUN increase, leading to renal failure.

### 2.1.6 Treatment

The mainstay of treatment for SLE is corticosteroid therapy. The dosage of corticosteroids is determined based on the following factors: (1) disease activity, type and severity of the affected organ, and (2) complications. Small doses of corticosteroids (<20 mg/day of prednisolone equivalent) are used for mild cases such as arthritis and rash, moderate doses (30–40 mg/day of prednisolone equivalent) are used for moderate cases such as pleurisy, pericarditis, and some thrombocytopenia, and high doses (about 60 mg/day of prednisolone equivalent) are used for severe cases such as refractory lupus nephritis, alveolar hemorrhage, and marked hemolytic anemia. In cases where it is difficult to reduce the dose of adrenal corticosteroids, immunosuppressive drugs should be used in combination. The effectiveness of immunosuppressive drugs has been established in the treatment of refractory lupus nephritis, and active concomitant use of corticosteroids and immunosuppressive drugs is considered.

### 2.1.7 Prognosis

The short-term prognosis of SLE is good except in some patients with refractory disease such as alveolar hemorrhage, but the long-term prognosis is still poor. In order to improve the long-term prognosis, it is necessary to establish treatment aimed at remission of lupus nephritis and to avoid deaths due to infectious diseases such as sepsis resulting from immunosuppressive therapy.

## 2.2 Systemic Sclerosis (SSc)

### 2.2.1 Disease Overview

It is a connective tissue disease characterized by fibrotic lesions of the skin and visceral organs such as the esophagus, intestines, and lungs, and peripheral circulatory disturbances such as Raynaud's phenomenon and digital ulcers.

### 2.2.2 Pathophysiology

The etiology is unknown, whereas it is considered to be an autoimmune disease because specific antibodies are detected. In patients with SSc, activation of immunocompetent cells such as fibroblasts and T cells, vascular endothelial cell damage, and subsequent repair mechanisms are observed in the lesions. These cells are closely related to each other to form pathological conditions such as skin sclerosis and peripheral circulatory disorders.

### 2.2.3 Epidemiology

The number of patients in Japan is estimated to be more than 20,000, and the male-to-female ratio is 1:12, with the overwhelming majority being women, and the preferred age group is 30 to 50 years old.

### 2.2.4 Classification

SSc is classified into two types based on the extent of cutaneous sclerosis. Limited cutaneous SSc (lcSSc), in which the cutaneous sclerosis is distal to the knee and elbow, and diffuse cutaneous SSc (dcSSc), in which the cutaneous sclerosis extends proximally to the knee and elbow. The prognosis of lcSSc is generally better than that of dcSSc, but attention should be paid to complications of pulmonary arterial hypertension (PAH).

### 2.2.5 Symptoms

1. **Peripheral vascular lesions:** Raynaud's phenomenon is the most common initial symptom of SSc. This phenomenon is caused by transient constriction of arteries induced by cold exposure or mental tension, resulting in pallor (ischemia), followed by purple (cyanosis), and flushing (recanalization) during recovery (Fig. 15.9). In cases of severe peripheral circulatory disturbance, intractable skin ulceration or necrosis of the tips of the fingers or toes may occur.
2. **Skin lesions:** In the early edematous stage, the fingers become swollen rather than sclerotic (sausage-like fingers). The skin becomes hard and shiny as the disease progresses, and telangiectasia and pigmentation may also occur. In dcSSc, skin sclerosis extends to the entire body (sclerosis phase). After reaching its peak, skin sclerosis slowly improves (atrophy phase), and in some cases it disappears completely.
3. **Joint and muscle lesions:** Complications of arthritis are observed in approximately 20%

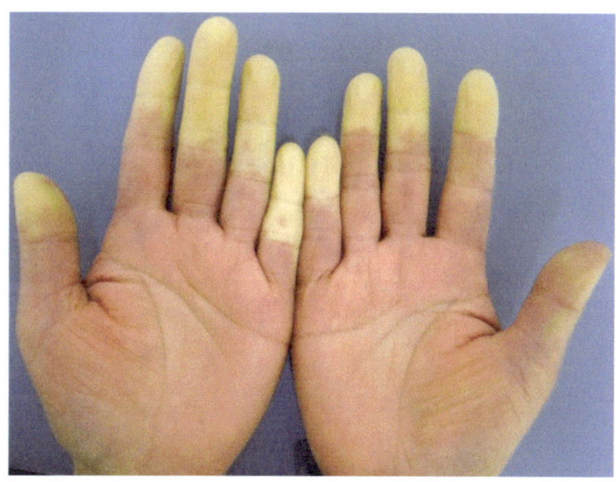

**Fig. 15.9** Raynaud's phenomenon

of patients. Inflammation and fibrosis of the neighboring tissue to the tendon cause impaired tendon mobility, and joint contracture and muscle atrophy occur with the progression of skin sclerosis.

4. **Oral lesions:** In patients with significant facial skin sclerosis, sclerosis of the skin around the mouth and impaired range of motion of the temporomandibular joint cause opening difficulties. In addition, tongue movement is restricted due to shortening and thickening of the lingual frenum. Atrophy of the oral mucosa and telangiectasia are also observed.
5. **Gastrointestinal lesions:** Dysphagia, heartburn, and nausea may occur due to decreased peristalsis associated with sclerosis of the lower esophagus. Similar lesions may also be seen in the small and large intestines, and in some cases, abnormal overgrowth of intestinal bacterium due to decreased peristalsis in the small intestine may result in malabsorption syndrome. In rare cases, intestinal gas may flow into the wall of the thinning colon or into the abdominal cavity, causing pneumatosis cystoides intestinalis.
6. **Respiratory lesions:** Interstitial pulmonary lesions are seen in about 60% of patients with SSc, and when they progress to pulmonary fibrosis, they are an important prognostic complication. The initial symptoms are dry cough and dyspnea on exertion, and progressive fibrosis leads to respiratory failure. About 10% of patients with SSc have PAH, which is also an important prognostic complication.
7. **Cardiac lesions:** Not only complications of secondary heart failure associated with pulmonary fibrosis and PAH, but also conduction defect and myocardial damage may occur due to peripheral angiostenosis of coronary arteries and fibrosis of myocardium itself.
8. **Renal lesions:** Sudden constriction of the renal arteries causes a marked decrease in renal blood flow and progressive renal dysfunction, called scleroderma renal crisis, which often occurs in patients who are positive for anti-RNA polymerase III antibodies.

### 2.2.6 Clinical Examination

1. **Blood tests:** ANA is detected by immunoserological tests in 50% to 90% of cases. Disease-specific antibodies such as Scl-70, anti-centromere and anti-U1-RNP antibodies may be found. Scl-70 antibodies are associated with dcSSc, anti-centromere and anti-U1-RNP antibodies with lcSSc.
2. **X-ray examination:** In SSc, bone X-ray findings may include resorption of the distal phalanges of the fingers and subcutaneous calcification. Gastrointestinal contrast radiography shows decreased peristalsis and dilatation of the lower esophagus, and plain chest radiography shows linear and reticular shadows suggestive of interstitial lung disease.

### 2.2.7 Treatment

Although there is no radical treatment, symptomatic therapy is the basic treatment, and it is important to protect the fingertips from cold and to encourage smoking cessation. For Raynaud's phenomenon and skin ulcers, peripheral vasodilators (calcium channel blockers, prostanoids) are used, and for gastroesophageal reflux disease due to decreased esophageal peristalsis, antacids (proton pump inhibitors) and prokinetic agents (mosapride) are used. For PAH, pulmonary artery dilators (veraprost, phosphodiesterase 5 inhibitors, endothelin receptor inhibitors) are used, and angiotensin-converting enzyme inhibitors are used for scleroderma renal crisis. Bosentan, an endothelin receptor inhibitor, is used to prevent the development of hand ulcers.

### 2.2.8 Prognosis

In dcSSc, skin sclerosis progresses rapidly during the first 3 to 5 years after the onset of the disease, but improves slowly after the peak in most cases. In contrast, in lcSS, skin sclerosis is mild and unchanging over a long period of time. The most common cause of death is the progression of interstitial lung lesions, followed by PAH, and these lung lesions account for about half of all deaths.

## 2.3 Polymyositis/ Dermatomyositis: PM/DM

### 2.3.1 Disease Overview

PM is a chronic inflammatory muscle disease that causes widespread damage to striated muscle. The symptoms are muscle weakness of the trunk, proximal muscles of the extremities, cervical muscles, and pharyngeal muscles. It is called DM when it is accompanied by characteristic cutaneous symptoms, such as heliotrope eruption and Gottron's sign, in addition to myositis symptoms. Patients with dermatomyositis, especially the elderly, should be monitored for malignancy.

### 2.3.2 Pathophysiology

Although the etiology is unknown, myopathology shows infiltration of mononuclear cells, such as T cells, B cells, and macrophages, around unnecrotic myofibers, and degeneration, necrosis, and regeneration of myofibers in cases with myositis. Clinically, there are two types of DM: myositis-only PM and dermatitis-only DM. It is considered to be an autoimmune inflammatory myopathy that develops myositis and dermatitis at the severity of each case.

### 2.3.3 Epidemiology

The estimated total number of patients with PM/DM in Japan is about 17,000, and the number of patients with PM and DM is about the same. The ratio of males to females is 1:3, and the onset of PM/DM peaks in the age groups of 5 to 9 years and 50 years.

### 2.3.4 Symptoms

1. **Muscular symptoms:** The muscle weakness of the trunk, proximal muscles of the extremities, neck muscles, and pharyngeal muscles progresses slowly and symmetrically, and the patient has difficulty climbing stairs, squatting, lifting heavy objects, and raise the head in the supine position. When the pharyngolaryngeal muscles are severely damaged, dysphagia and dysarthria appear.
2. **Cutaneous manifestations:** Erythema with purplish-red edema on the eyelids is called heliotrope eruption, and erythema with purplish-red edema or papules with hyperkeratosis and skin atrophy on the dorsal of finger joints is called Gottron's sign. A skin rash resembling Gottron's sign appearing on the extensor surfaces of the elbows and knees is also a characteristic skin finding of DM.
3. **Respiratory symptoms:** Interstitial lung lesions are a common complication in patients with PM/DM. The subjective symptoms are dry cough and dyspnea on exertion, but respiratory failure occurs in some patients. Particularly in patients with DM who have few myositis symptoms, interstitial pneumonia progresses rapidly and can be fatal.
4. **Joint symptoms:** Although polyarthritis may occur, unlike in RA, bone erosion does not occur and, in principle, joint deformity due to bone destruction does not occur.
5. **Others:** Although subjective symptoms are rare, arrhythmias, conduction disturbances, and abnormalities in cardiac wall motion associated with myocarditis may be observed. Carcinoma of the digestive organs, lungs, mammary glands, or reproductive organs may develop within 2 years before or after the diagnosis of PM/DM.

### 2.3.5 Clinical Examination

1. **Blood tests:** The myogenic enzymes CK, aldolase, AST, ALT, LDH, and myoglobin are elevated in myositis. In addition, CK-MB and cardiac troponin are elevated in the presence of myocardial damage. Leukocytosis and elevation of C-reactive protein (CRP) may also be observed, reflecting inflammation. ANA is detected by immunoserological tests in about 80% of cases. Anti-aminoacyl-tRNA synthetase antibodies, such as anti-Jo-1 antibody, are known as disease-specific antibodies, but their detection rate is low (10–20%). Anti-MDA-5 antibodies are also disease-specific antibodies, and are positive in 20 to 30% of cases, and are closely associated with rapidly progressive interstitial pneumonia, which is fatal due to rapid progression of respiratory failure.
2. **Electromyography:** The appearance of resting activity such as fiber-spontaneous potentials and positive sharp waves with a regular

cycle is characteristic of muscles affected by myositis. During contraction at any time, so-called myogenic changes, which are low-amplitude, short-duration motor unit potentials, can be seen and are useful for diagnosis.
3. **Magnetic resonance imaging (MRI):** It can be used for qualitative diagnosis of muscle tissue, such as edema caused by inflammatory changes in muscle tissue, fibrosis and steatosis. MRI, which is a non-invasive examination, is useful for diagnosis and evaluation of therapeutic effect.
4. **Muscle biopsy:** In muscle affected by myositis, inflammatory cell infiltration, degeneration and necrosis of myofibers, and uneven size of myofibers can be seen, which is important for definitive diagnosis.

### 2.3.6 Treatment

If the symptoms are only the skin, the main treatment is to avoid skin exposure and topical corticosteroids should be used. For muscle symptoms, rest is necessary during the acute phase of the disease, but after the disease has stabilized, rehabilitation should be performed aggressively to restore muscle strength. For drug therapy, high-dose corticosteroids (60 mg/day of prednisolone equivalent) are initially administered, and the dose is gradually decreased as the disease progresses. In cases in which corticosteroids alone are ineffective or in which it is difficult to reduce the dose of corticosteroids, immunosuppressive drugs should be used in combination. High-dose gamma globulin therapy may be used for refractory myositis. Patients with rapidly progressive interstitial pneumonia are also treated initially with high-dose corticosteroids and, in some cases, with steroid pulse therapy using higher doses of corticosteroids administered intravenously. Anti-MDA-5 antibody-positive patients are especially susceptible to fatal interstitial pneumonia, and should be treated with immunosuppressive drugs.

### 2.3.7 Prognosis

Patients with rapidly progressive interstitial pneumonia or malignancy have a poor prognosis. The 5-year survival rate for all patients is about 80%, but treatment methods are improving, and further improvement is expected in the future.

## 2.4 Sjögren's Syndrome (SS)

### 2.4.1 Disease Overview

Chronic inflammation and destruction of glandular tissue occur mainly in the lacrimal and salivary glands due to inflammatory cell infiltration, and the main symptoms are dry eye due to decreased lacrimal fluid secretion and xerostomia due to decreased salivary secretion.

### 2.4.2 Pathophysiology

Although the etiology is still unknown, it is thought to be an autoimmune disease because of the appearance of various autoantibodies, such as anti-SS-A, anti-SS-B, and rheumatoid factor, and hypergammaglobulinemia. Pathologically, there is a marked mononuclear cell infiltration, mainly lymphocytes, around the conduits of salivary glands and lacrimal gland, atrophy and disappearance of acinar tissues, and stenosis of the lumen of the duct. This causes decreased lacrimal and salivary secretion.

### 2.4.3 Epidemiology

The estimated total number of patients with SS in Japan is about 70,000. The male to female ratio is 1:17.4, and the peak age of onset is in the 50 s and 60 s.

### 2.4.4 Classification

SS can be divided into primary, uncomplicated by other autoimmune diseases, and secondary, complicated by autoimmune diseases such as RA and SLE. Primary SS can be divided into glandular type, in which the lesions are confined to the lacrimal and salivary glands, and extraglandular type, in which the active lesions extend to other organs.

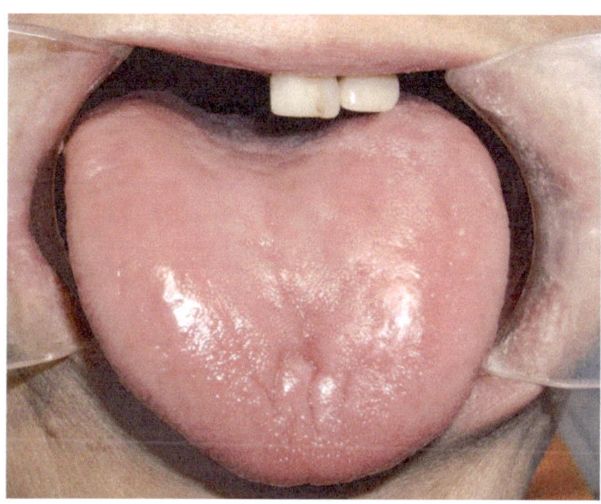

**Fig. 15.10** Flat tongue

### 2.4.5 Symptoms

1. **Xerostomia:** The oral cavity becomes dry due to decreased salivary secretion, and the tongue becomes smooth due to atrophy of the tongue papillae (Fig. 15.10). In addition, since oral cleansing effect of saliva is reduced, tooth caries frequently occurs.
2. **Ocular dryness:** Decreased lacrimal fluid secretion causes dry keratoconjunctivitis, which leads to foreign body sensation, burning sensation, and redness of the eyes.
3. **Extraglandular symptoms.**
   (a) Arthritis: Primary SS may be complicated by polyarthritis. However, it is rarely accompanied by joint destruction as in RA.
   (b) Lymphatic malignancies: The frequency of malignant lymphoma is clearly higher in SS than in normal subjects. The frequency of mucosa-associated lymphoid tissue extranodal follicular marginal zone lymphoma (MALT lymphoma) is also high, especially in the salivary glands.
   (c) Skin lesions: Erythema annulare, Raynaud's phenomenon, and purpura associated with hypergammaglobulinemia and cryoglobulinemia may be seen.
   (d) Organ lesions: SS is often associated with autoimmune thyroid diseases such as chronic thyroiditis (Hashimoto's disease) and Graves' disease. Although infrequent, interstitial pneumonia may complicate the disease, and symptoms such as cough and dyspnea may be observed. As a renal lesion, tubular acidosis due to interstitial nephritis may be a complication of renal disease. Primary biliary cholangitis may also occur, although it is rare. Peripheral neuropathy is associated with sensory disturbance and numbness.

### 2.4.6 Clinical Examination

1. **Blood tests:** High incidence of hypergammaglobulinemia, mainly IgG, accompanied by increased blood sedimentation, but elevated CRP is rare. Antinuclear antibodies are detected in 80% to 90% of patients, and anti-SS-A and anti-SS-B antibodies are also often positive, although anti-SS-B antibodies are more specific for SS than anti-SS-A antibodies.
2. **Ophthalmologic examination:** Decreased lacrimal secretion is assessed by Schirmer's test (positive when tears wet the filter paper less than 5 mm in 5 min), and dry keratoconjunctivitis is assessed by Rose Bengal or fluorescein staining.
3. **Salivary gland function tests:** Decreased salivary secretion is determined by the gum test (chewing gum for 10 min and measuring saliva volume: positive when the volume is less than 10 mL) or the Saxon test (chewing gauze for 2 min and measuring weight gain: positive when the weight is less than 2 g). In the past, salivary gland contrast was used to observe structural changes in salivary glands, but this has been discontinued recently because of problems such as pain and infection. Salivary gland scintigram using $^{99m}TcO_4$ is useful for objective evaluation of salivary gland function. The accumulation in the parotid and submandibular glands decreases reflecting a decrease in salivary gland function, and in severe salivary gland disorders, accumulation is rarely seen.
4. **Minor salivary gland biopsy and lacrimal gland biopsy:** Biopsy of the lower lip where minor salivary glands are distributed and lacrimal gland shows lymphocytic infiltration and disruption of glandular structures around

the conduits of salivary glands and lacrimal gland.

### 2.4.7 Treatment

In the absence of serious extraglandular lesions, symptomatic treatment is the mainstay of therapy. Although M3-type muscarinic acetylcholine receptor stimulants are often effective in stimulating salivary secretion, they are associated with a high incidence of hyperhidrosis and should be started in small doses. Steroids may be used for organ lesions such as interstitial pneumonia and interstitial nephritis.

### 2.4.8 Prognosis

The prognosis is good, with few life-threatening complications except for severe extraglandular lesions such as severe interstitial pneumonia or malignant lymphoma.

**Table 15.2** Organ/tissue lesions included in IgG4-related diseases

| Organ and tissue | Diseases |
|---|---|
| Pancreas | Autoimmune pancreatitis |
| Lacrimal gland/ ophthalmology | Dacryoadenitis (Mikulicz' disease), orbital inflammation (IgG4-related eye disease) |
| Salivary gland | Sialadenitis (Mikulicz' disease), Küttner tumor |
| Arteries | Inflammatory aortic aneurysm, periaortitis, arteritis |
| Renal/ retroperitoneal | Tubulointerstitial nephritis, retroperitoneal fibrosis |
| Prostate | Prostatitis |
| Dural/pituitary/ thyroid | Hypertrophic Pachymeningitis, autoimmune hypophysitis, Riedel's thyroiditis |
| Lung/mediastinum | IgG4-related lung disease, inflammatory pseudotumor, mediastinal fibrosis |
| Liver and biliary system | Sclerosing cholangitis, IgG4-related liver disease |
| Lymph nodes | IgG4-related lymphadenopathy |

## 2.5 Mikulicz' Disease

Mikulicz' disease is a persistent swelling associated with inflammation of the salivary and lacrimal glands. The swollen glandular tissue is markedly infiltrated with mononuclear cells, and it was previously thought to be a subtype of SS. However, while typical SS is more common in women, Mikulicz disease is more common in men. Furthermore, Mikulicz' disease differs from SS in that the dryness is milder and the response to corticosteroid therapy is better, despite the marked adenopathy. Since serum IgG4 is often elevated, and IgG4-producing plasma cells are found in the lacrimal gland and salivary gland, Mikulicz' disease is now included in IgG4-related disease. The organs and tissues affected by IgG4-related diseases are shown in Table 15.2.

## 2.6 Behçet's Disease (BD)

### 2.6.1 Disease Overview

BD is an intractable multiorgan invasive disease proposed by Behçet in Turkey. The main symptoms are recurrent oral aphthous ulcers, cutaneous manifestations, uveitis, recurrent genital ulcers, and repeated acute inflammatory attacks. Among the main symptoms, visual disorder caused by uveitis is the most problematic, but special lesions such as gastrointestinal, vascular, and neurological lesions can cause organ derangement.

### 2.6.2 Pathophysiology

Although the etiology of the disease is still unknown, the strong correlation with HLA-B51 suggests that some environmental factors may be added to the genetic predisposition, leading to the onset of the disease. It is assumed that trace chemical substances and indigenous oral bacteria are involved as environmental factors. The basic pathogenesis of this disease is thought to be an increase in neutrophil function based on a hypersensitivity reaction of T cells.

### 2.6.3 Epidemiology

Patients are accumulating along the former Silk Road, the estimated number of patients in Japan is 20,000, and the peak age of onset is in the 30 s, with a male to female ratio of 1:1.

### 2.6.4 Symptoms

1. **Recurrent aphthous ulcers of the oral mucosa:** Almost always present and often the first symptom. The buccal mucosa, malar mucosa, gingival mucosa, and tongue are covered with shallow, painful, round ulcers with well-defined margins. They heal without scarring in about a week, but recurrence is common.
2. **Skin manifestations:** Erythema nodosum-like rash, a painful subcutaneous nodule, and superficial thrombophlebitis, a painful funicular, are most common on the lower legs. Acneiform eruption and folliculitis-like eruptions are found on the face, neck, and back. Severe redness of the skin at the site of shaving in men, blood sampling, or injection reflects the increased irritability of the skin and is detected on examination as a needle reaction.
3. **Ocular lesions:** Paroxysmal iridocyclitis (anterior segment ocular type) and retinal uveitis (ocular fundus type) are repeated. During the anterior segment ocular type attacks, photophobia, conjunctival injection, and eye pain are seen, and in typical cases, hypopyon iritis occurs. During ocular fundus type attacks, patients have blurred vision and decreased visual acuity, which may affect the prognosis of vision.
4. **Genital ulceration:** Painful, well-demarcated, punched ulcers, most commonly on the scrotum and penis in males and on the labia majora and minora in females, which may leave scars after healing.
5. **Arthritis:** Redness, pain, and swelling appear transiently in large joints of the extremities such as the knee, elbow, and shoulder, and disappear within a few weeks.
6. **Epididymitis:** Transient and recurrent swelling and pain in the testicles. The frequency of occurrence is low, but it is highly specific to BD.
7. **Gastrointestinal lesions:** In intestinal Behçet's disease, punched-out ulcerations are seen in the gastrointestinal tract. The lesions can occur anywhere from the esophagus to the rectubem, and the ileocecal region is the most common site; abdominal pain, bloody stool, and diarrhea are the main symptoms.
8. **Vascular lesions:** Angio-Behçet disease can cause vasculitis in both arteries and veins regardless of the size of the vessel, but venous lesions such as deep vein thrombosis of the lower extremities are more common. Depending on the location of the lesion, aortic aneurysm, brain circulatory disturbances, superior vena cava syndrome, Budd-Chiari syndrome, and many other conditions may occur.
9. **Central nervous system disorders:** Neuro-Behçet disease can be divided into acute and chronic progressive forms. The acute form develops as meningitis or brainstem encephalitis. The chronic progressive type is more intractable, and in addition to neurological symptoms such as leukomalacia, necrosis of white matter, hemiplegia due to demyelination, cerebellar symptoms, dysarthria, and dysphagia, gradually progressive personality changes and dementia are problems.

### 2.6.5 Clinical Examination

1. **Blood tests:** In the active stage, elevated erythrocyte sedimentation rate, elevated CRP value, and leukocytosis are observed. No disease-specific antibodies have been found to confirm the diagnosis, but HLA-B51 and A26 may be helpful.
2. **Other examinations:** Intestinal and skin lesions are often biopsied for pathologic evaluation. CT and MRI are also useful to examine vascular lesions and central nervous system lesions.

### 2.6.6 Treatment

For oral aphthous ulcers, genital ulcers, and skin lesions, local treatment centered on external corticosteroids is used. Nonsteroidal anti-inflammatory drugs are used to treat arthritis and epididymitis. On the other hand, ocular lesions that can cause severe visual disorder and specific types (intestinal, vascular, and neuro-Behçet's disease) that affect the prognosis of life require aggressive treatment, including systemic administration of steroids and immunosuppressive drugs. In recent years, anti-TNF-α antibody biologics have been used to treat refractory uveitis and intestinal, vascular, and neuro-Behçet's disease, and are expected to improve the prognosis.

### 2.6.7 Prognosis

Although symptoms appear chronically and repeatedly, the prognosis is not bad except for ocular lesions and specific lesions such as intestinal, vascular, and neuro-Behçet's disease. As mentioned above, the use of anti-TNF-α antibody biologics is expected to improve the prognosis of ocular lesions and specific lesions.

## 2.7 Notes from Dentistry Perspective

Masayuki Azuma, Keiko Aota

The problems in dental treatment of patients with collagen disease can be roughly divided into two categories: problems caused by the oral symptoms of collagen disease itself and problems caused by the drugs used to treat collagen disease.

### 2.7.1 Dental Treatment Problems Caused by Collagen Disease Itself

#### Systemic Lupus Erythematosus (SLE)

Erythema and ulcers of the oral mucosa are among the many organ lesions that may occur. It is generally painless, appears in the acute phase, and disappears in response to treatment. In SLE, the incidence of secondary Sjögren's syndrome has been reported to be 13%, and xerostomia should also be noted [14].

#### Systemic Scleroderma

Oral manifestations include ankyloglossia (44%) due to fibrosis of the lingual frenum and trismus (26%) due to sclerosis of the skin around the lips [15].

#### Sjögren's Syndrome

Oral symptoms include significant xerostomia. With decreased salivary secretion, various oral symptoms such as oral candidiasis, dental caries, taste disorder, dysphagia, halitosis, glossalgia, and denture incompatibility may occur.

### 2.7.2 Dental Treatment Problems Caused by Collagen Disease Drugs

Adrenocortical steroids are frequently used in the treatment of collagen diseases to control chronic inflammation and immune abnormalities. Because steroids have a wide range of physiological effects, attention should be paid to various side effects. When steroids are used, drugs for osteoporosis are also used to prevent secondary osteoporosis. In addition, immunosuppressive agents, biological agents, and antithrombotic agents are used in the treatment of collagen diseases (Table 15.3).

**Table 15.3** Drugs most commonly used by patients with collagen diseases

| Type | Main effect | Side effects to be especially careful about |
|---|---|---|
| Adrenocorticosteroid | Anti-inflammatory action, immunosuppressive action | 1. Inducement of infectious diseases and serious illness<br>2. Osteoporosis<br>3. Atherosclerotic lesions (myocardial infarction, cerebral infarction, aneurysm, thrombosis)<br>4. Induction and exacerbation of diabetes mellitus<br>5. Gastrointestinal disorders<br>6. Adrenal insufficiency, steroid withdrawal syndrome<br>7. Mental disorder |
| Immunosuppressant (drug) | Immunosuppressive action | Induction of infections, severe disease |
| Biological drug | Regulatory action of molecular targeted therapy target molecules | Induction of infections, severe disease |
| Antithrombotic agents (anticoagulants, antiplatelet agents) | Antithrombotic | Bleeding |
| Osteoporosis drugs (bisphosphonates) | Decreased bone formation | Osteomyelitis, osteonecrosis of the jaw |

#### Infectious Disease Problems

According to the Practical Guidelines for the Appropriate Use of Antimicrobial Agents in the Prevention of Postoperative Infections (2016), the use of steroids and immunosuppressive drugs is a high-risk factor for surgical site infection. Therefore, in patients using this drug, a single dose of amoxicillin to 48 h postoperatively is recommended for invasive dental treatment such as tooth extraction (clindamycin for patients allergic to β-lactam antibiotics).

#### The Problem of Steroid Coverage

When the hypothalamic–pituitary–adrenal system is suppressed by steroids, secondary adrenal insufficiency occurs due to insufficient cortisol production under stress conditions such as surgical invasion. In general, steroid coverage is not necessary for local anesthesia surgery of about 1 h in duration with a dose of less than 5 mg/day of prednisone equivalent. However, steroid coverage may be necessary in cases of high doses of prednisone or depending on the degree of surgical invasion and operative time.

#### Problems with Osteoporosis Drugs

The first recommended drug for steroid-induced osteoporosis is a bisphosphonate (BP). The Japanese Osteonecrosis of the Jaw Review Committee position paper (2016) does not recommend withdrawal of BP before invasive dental procedures in osteoporotic patients receiving BP. On the other hand, the American Association of Oral and Maxillofacial Surgeons position paper (2014) advocates that patients who have received BP for more than 4 years or who have osteoporosis with risk factors for osteonecrosis of the jaw undergo invasive dental treatment, if their general condition permits, should discuss and consider withdrawal of BP for approximately 2 months with their attending physician. Invasive dental treatment should be performed in accordance with the latest guidelines.

#### Problems in Antithrombotic Therapy

For minor surgery such as tooth extraction, antiplatelet agents and anticoagulants should be continued, and local hemostasis should be maintained. For surgery with a high risk of bleeding, consult your family physician and consider suspending antiplatelet and anticoagulant medications. Patients taking warfarin have been treated with heparin as an alternative therapy during the perioperative period, but the Japanese Circulation Society (JCS)/Japanese Heart Rhythm Society (JHRS) 2020 Guideline on Pharmacotherapy of Cardiac Arrhythmias do not recommend preoperative replacement therapy with heparin, based on the results of the BRIDGE study, however, it is classified as IIb in the recommended classification, and its efficacy and usefulness have not been established based on evidence and opinions.

### 2.7.3 Precautions for Implant Treatment in Patients with Xerostomia

Although xerostomia is a risk factor for implant treatment, it is not an absolute contraindication. Denture treatment is recommended for patients with xerostomia, but in many cases, dentures cannot be used because of pain during denture placement due to mucosal atrophy. Implant treatment should be carried out after thorough evaluation and informed consent, and strict maintenance is necessary.

The use of steroids, immunosuppressive drugs, and osteoporosis drugs in patients with collagen diseases should be carefully considered, bearing in mind that there is a significant risk in acquiring and maintaining osseointegration, as well as a risk of drug-related osteomyelitis and osteonecrosis of the jaw.

## 3 Allergic Disease

Satoshi Takada, Yuh Baba

### 3.1 General Discussion

Allergic disease is defined as a condition in which an excessive immune response to a specific antigen (allergen) is induced to the detriment of the host. In the past, allergic reactions were classified into four types [16], but recently, the concept of type V allergy has been proposed. However, considering the underlying immune response, type V allergy can be classified as subtype of type II allergy (Table 15.4).

**Table 15.4** Classification of allergic reactions

| | Type I reaction | Type II reaction | Type III reaction | Type IV reaction | Type V reaction |
|---|---|---|---|---|---|
| Synonym | Immediate type<br>Anaphylactic type | Cytotoxic type<br>Cytolysis type | Immune complex type<br>Arthus type | Late reaction type<br>Cell-mediated immunity type<br>Tuberculin type | Cell function control type |
| Action factor | IgE (reagin) | IgG, IgM | IgG, IgM (immune complex) | Sensitized T-cell | IgG, IgM |
| Mechanism of occurrence | When the antigen binds again to the IgE bound to the mast cell, the mast cell releases chemical mediators and symptoms appear | Antibodies bind to surface antigens of autologous cells and damage the cells | Immune complexes, which are a combination of multiple antigens and antibodies, are deposited in tissues, activating complement and causing tissue damage | Sensitized T-cell and cytotoxic T-cell react with antigens, resulting in cellular immune responses that damage cells | Anti-receptor antibodies bind to the receptors of target cells and enhance or reduce the function of the target cells |
| Major related diseases | Anaphylactic shock<br>Allergic rhinitis<br>Bronchial asthma<br>**Oral allergy syndrome**<br>**Allergy to local anesthetics (type I + type IV)** | Autoimmune hemolytic anemia<br>Immunologic (idiopathic) thrombocytopenic purpura<br>ABO incompatible blood transfusion | Serum sickness<br>**Systemic lupus erythematosus (SLE)**<br>Acute glomerulonephritis | Granuloma formation due to tuberculosis infection<br>Tuberculin test<br>**Graft-versus-host disease (GVHD)**<br>**Metal allergy** | Hyperthyroidism (graves' disease)<br>Myasthenia gravis |
| Examination | Specific IgE measurement<br>Histamine release test<br>Challenge test | Coombs test<br>Antibody measurement | Complement and immune complex assay<br>Antibody measurement | Patch test<br>Lymphocyte stimulation test<br>Cytokine measurement | Antibody measurement |

#### 3.1.1 Type I Allergy

It is also called the immediate type or anaphylactic type because symptoms appear immediately after the reaction between the causative antigen (allergen) and IgE antibody. Antigens are taken up by antigen-presenting cells, which are recognized by Th2 cells, and Th2 cells produce cytokines related to allergic inflammation. The cytokines induce the production of IgE by B cells, and the IgE antibodies produced adhere to mast cells, resulting in a sensitized state that is susceptible to repeated stimulation by the same antigen. When the antigen binds again to the IgE bound to the mast cell, various chemical mediators are released from the mast cell, resulting in increased vascular permeability, smooth muscle contraction, and increased glandular secretion, causing symptoms such as angioedema, hypotension, wheezing, dyspnea, and nasal discharge. Typical diseases include anaphylactic shock, allergic rhinitis, bronchial asthma, urticaria, atopic dermatitis, and Latex allergy.

Anaphylactic shock is a condition in which allergens cause anaphylactic reactions due to type I allergy, resulting in symptoms such as hypotension, dyspnea, and loss of consciousness. It is caused by administration of drugs such as antimicrobial agents, taking of eggs, wheat, dairy products, bee venom, contrast media, and analgesic-antipyretic. In severe cases, loss of consciousness and death may occur within a few minutes. In the treatment of anaphylactic shock, prompt treatment determines the prognosis, and adrenaline injection should be given at the same time as assessment of the airway, respiration, circulation, and consciousness. One type of anaphylaxis caused by occupational allergy is Latex allergy. This is an immediate allergic reaction to proteins contained in natural rubber products. High-risk groups include healthcare workers, people with a predisposition to atopic dermatitis, patients who repeatedly undergo medical procedures due to congenital diseases such as spina bifida or chronic diseases, and people with occupations that require frequent use of natural rubber gloves. Type I allergic diseases related to dentistry include oral allergy syndrome and allergy to local anesthetics (type I and type IV allergy to local anesthetics are seen).

### 3.1.2 Type II Allergy

Type II allergy is caused by the binding of autoantibodies (IgG, IgM) to surface antigens of autologous cells, resulting in cellular and tissue damage. The mechanisms include phagocytosis, cytolysis, and antibody-dependent cell-mediated cytotoxicity (ADCC). Typical diseases include autoimmune hemolytic anemia, immunologic (idiopathic) thrombocytopenic purpura, Goodpasture's syndrome (anti-glomerular basement membrane disease), and ABO-incompatible blood transfusion.

### 3.1.3 Type III Allergy

Type III allergy is also called immune complex type or Arthus type. It is a reaction in which multiple antigens and antibodies are bound together, and immune complexes are deposited in tissues, activating complement, resulting in tissue destruction. Typical diseases include serum sickness, systemic lupus erythematosus (SLE), hypersensitivity pneumonitis, acute glomerulonephritis, and cryoglobulinemic vasculitis.

### 3.1.4 Type IV Allergy

Unlike type I–III allergies, allergies caused by T-cell rather than antibodies are called type IV allergies. Helper T-cell activated by antigens release a variety of cytokines that activate macrophages and cytotoxic T-cell, resulting in tissue damage. The formation of granuloma due to tuberculosis infection, tuberculin reaction, graft versus host disease (GVHD), allergic contact dermatitis, and metal allergy are involved in type IV allergic reactions.

### 3.1.5 Type V Allergy

Type V allergy is a subtype of type II allergy in which anti-receptor antibodies bind to the receptors of target cells, and unlike type II allergy, the target cells are not destroyed and the anti-receptor antibodies exhibit ligand-like effects or inhibit the effects of the ligands. In Graves' disease (hyperthyroidism), anti-TSH receptor antibodies increase thyroid function, while in myasthenia gravis, anti-acetylcholine receptor antibodies cause muscle weakness.

## 3.2 Notes from Dentistry Perspective

### 3.2.1 Allergies Related to Dentistry

#### Oral Allergy Syndrome [17]

It is an immediate type allergy in which swelling and itch sensation appear in the mucosa of the oral cavity and pharynx immediately after ingestion of specific foods such as fruits and vegetables. It develops as a cross-reaction to sensitizing antigens and is often associated with pollinosis. Symptoms appear within 15 min, but the antigenicity of apples, peaches, and pears, which are easy to become antigens, is easily lost by heating or digestive enzymes, symptoms are localized to the oral cavity and pharynx unless taken in large quantities (Fig. 15.11). The radioallergosorbent test (RAST), prick test, and scratch test are useful for diagnosis. The most important treatment is to avoid antigen without ingesting the causative food.

#### Allergy to Local Anesthetics

The incidence of anaphylaxis due to lidocaine is extremely low, with an incidence of 0.00007%. It is considered to the immediate allergy if it developed within 1 h, and to the delayed allergy within 72 h. In most cases,

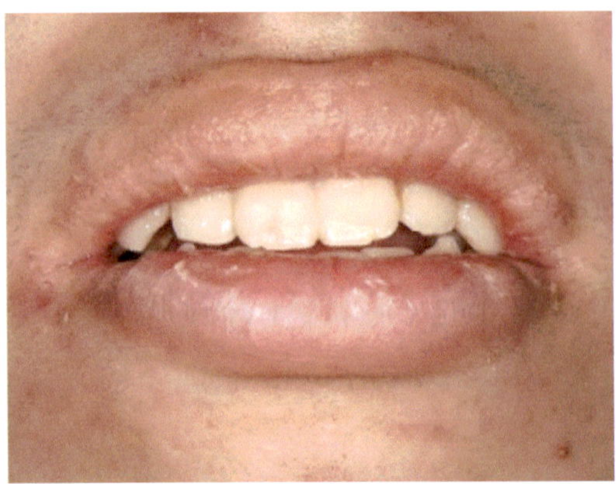

**Fig. 15.11** Oral allergy syndrome. Pruritus and swelling of the lips are seen after ingestion of melon

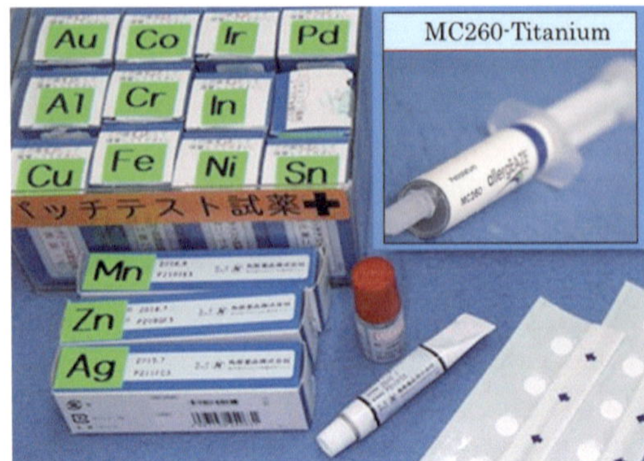


**Fig. 15.12** Patch test reagent for metal allergy

however, it causes allergy not to the local anesthetic itself but to the preservative paraben (paraoxybenzoate) on the antioxidant sodium sulfite. Also other allergic reactions might be caused by gloves (latex) and disinfectant used during local anesthesia, and antibacterial, analgesic agents used before and after local anesthesia which must be differentiated. In addition, vasovagal reflexes before local anesthesia, anomaly of sensation, motor paralysis, discomfort are often thought to be allergic reactions to local anesthesia. Furthermore, it is necessary to differentiate from odontophobia, aichmophobia, local anemia due to excessive injection volume, necrosis of the tissue at the insertion point, and peripheral nerve injury.

#### Allergy to Dental Materials (Metal)

It is delayed type allergy to metals used in dental treatment. About 15 types of metals are used for it. Titanium (Ti) and vanadium (V) have also been used due to the spread of dental implant treatment (Fig. 15.12) in recent years. Symptoms range from systemic to local, including pruritus, dysgeusia, discomfort in the mouth, and contact dermatitis. These are rarely diagnosed as allergy to dental metals at the initial examination, and are often treated symptomatically with unknown cause, or as climacteric disturbance or xerostomia in some cases. Metal allergies can be diagnosed by testing for metals, and also cements and resins which are included in dental materials should be tested as well. In addition to the patch test, a metal lymphocyte stimulation test (MLST) is also used for diagnosis. The test should be performed on the back, arms, legs, or other skin with little hair, and the results are basically checked at 48 h with checking after 24 h, 72 h and 1 week as well. Because of the strong contact, dermatitis or immediate allergic reaction may rarely occur, symptoms should be immediately monitored after the test. Treatment is to change the causative material to the appropriate therapeutic material.

Stomatitis, oral lichen planus (Fig. 15.13), palmoplantar pustulosis (Fig. 15.14), dermatitis, erythema, and urticaria are related to dental materials, and they are in some cases relieved by metal removal. On the other hand, as in contact dermatitis, it may cause redness, erosions, papules and bullae within 24 h with contact of dental materials with the oral mucosa (Fig. 15.15).

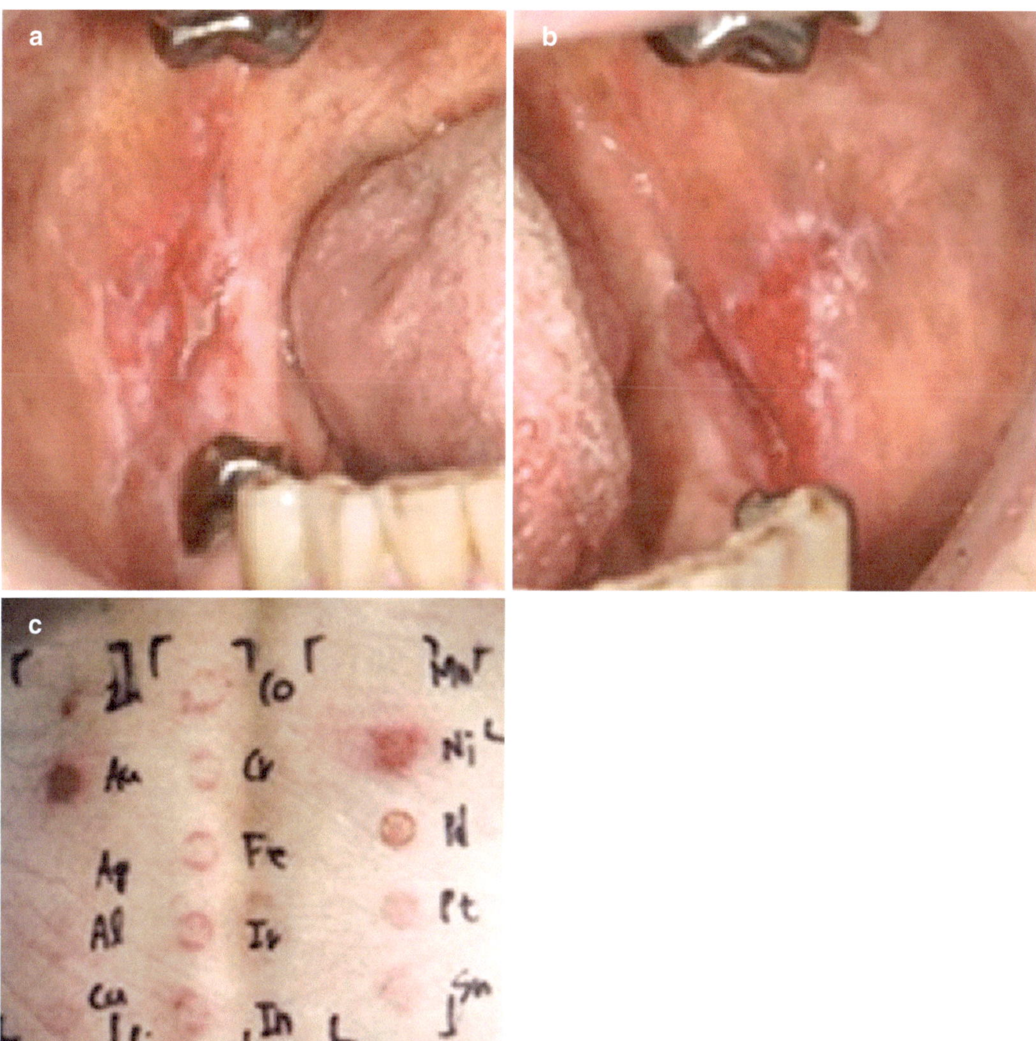


**Fig. 15.13** Lichen planus of the oral cavity. (**a**, **b**) White lacy erosions and erythema are seen on both buccal mucosae. (**c**) Patch tests showed positive reactions to Au, Ni and Pd

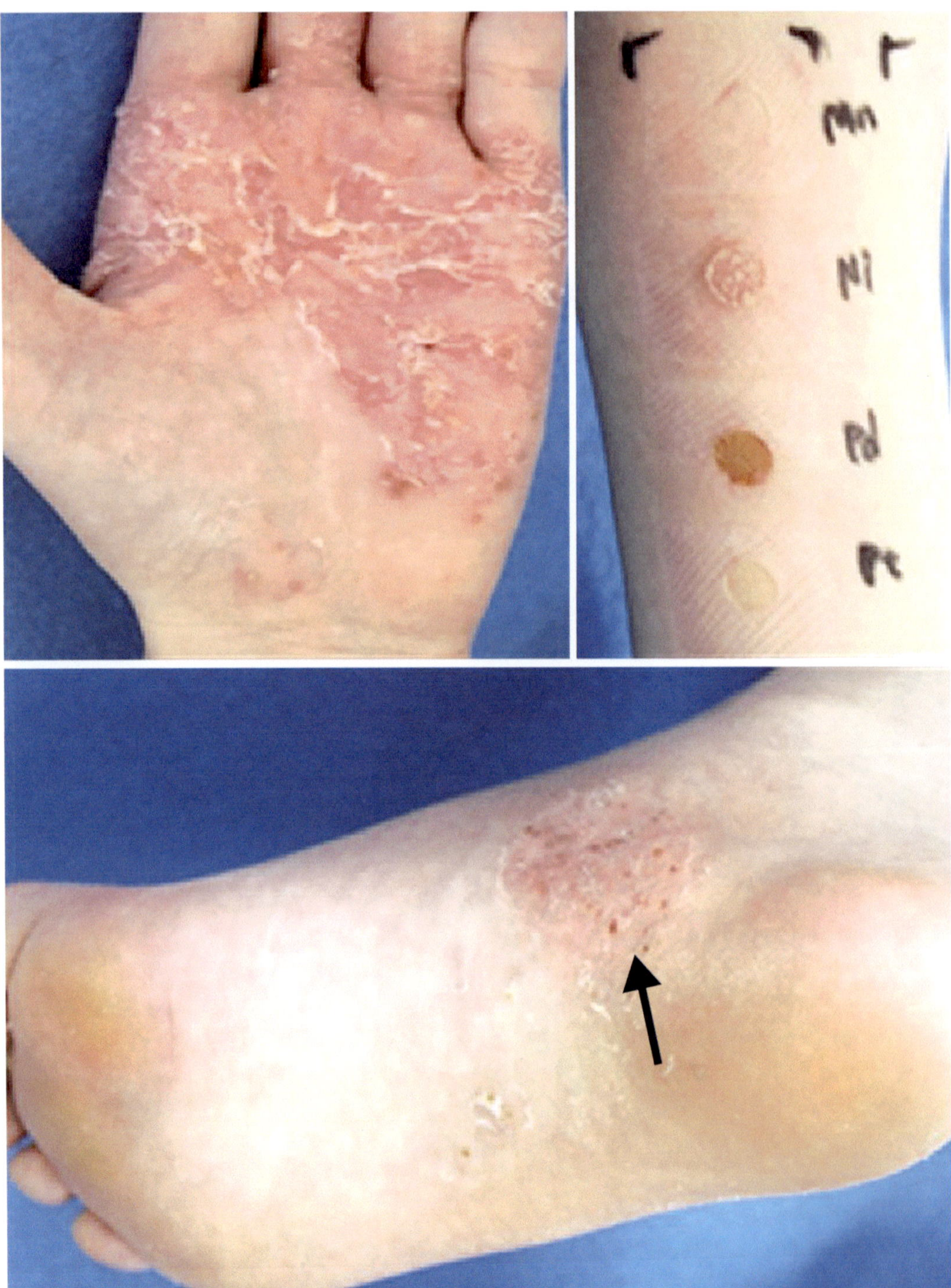


**Fig. 15.14** Palmoplantaris pustulosis. Patch test showed positive reaction to Ni and Pd, and formation of vesicles in the Ni area

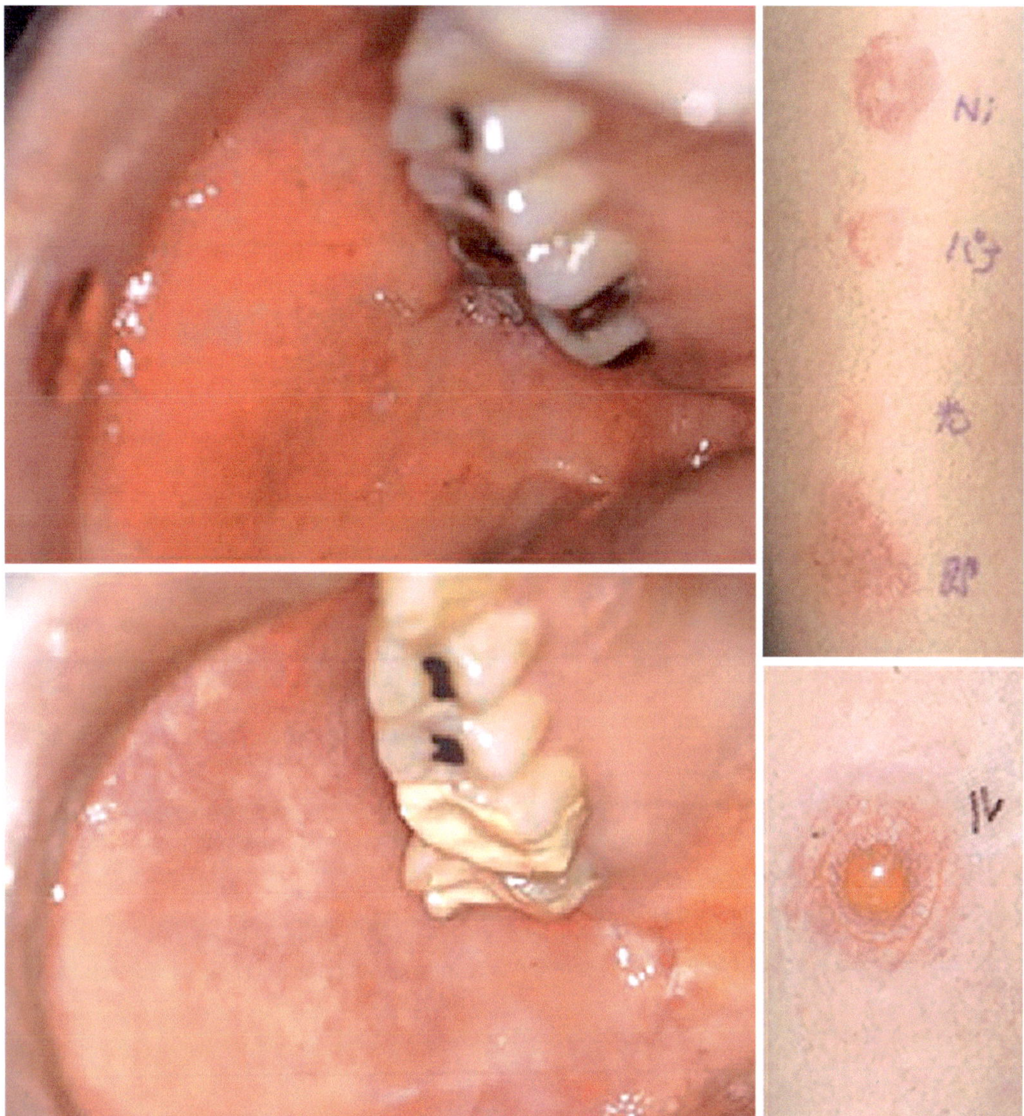


**Fig. 15.15** Allergy to luting cement. Erythema appeared on the buccal mucosa immediately after luting the restoration, which resolved after removal. A patch test showed large blisters reacting to the luting cement

## References


1. Japan College of Rheumatology. 2020 Japan College of Rheumatology Clinical Practice Guidelines for the Management of Rheumatoid Arthrits (Kansetsu Ryumachi shinryo guideline 2020). Tokyo: Shindan to Chiryousya; 2020; (in Japanese).
2. Ministry of Health, Labour and Welfare. Committee on Rheumatism and Other Diseases, Disease Control Committee, Health Sciences Council. Tokyo; Ministry of Health, Labour and Welfare. 2018. (in Japanese). https://www.mhlw.go.jp/stf/shingi2/0000199527.html (in Japanese).
3. Aletaha D, et al. American College of Rheumatology/European league against rheumatism:2010 rheumatoid arthritis classification criteria. Arthrit Rheum. 2010;62:2569–81.
4. Klippel JH, et al., editors. Primer on the rheumatic diseases. New York, NY: Springer; 2008.
5. The Japanese Society for Temporomandibular Joint (ed.) New edition: Temporomandibular joint disorders, Revised Ed. Kyoto; Nagasueshoten. 2013 (in Japanese).
6. Gaulard P, et al. Other iatrogenic immunodeficiency-associated lymphoproliferative disorders. In: Swerdlow SH, Campo E, et al., editors. WHO classification of tumors of haematopoietic and lymphoid tissues. Lyon: IARC Press; 2008.
7. Fukushima M, et al. Primary central nervous system malignant lymphoma in a patient with rheumatoid arthritis receiving low-dose methotrexate treatment. Br J Neurosurg. 2013;27:824–6.
8. Obata K, et al. A case of methotrexate-associated lymphoproliferative disorders arising in the maxillary gingiva: a review of the literature of cases arising in the oral region in Japan. Jpn J Oral Maxillofac Surg. 2015;61:20–4; (in Japanese).
9. Ichiki T, et al. A case of methotrexate-associated lymphoproliferative disorder diagnosed on detection of ulceration of the gingiva. Jpn J Oral Diag/Oral Med. 2017;30:187–92; (in Japanese).
10. Japan Rheumatism Foundation Educational Training Committee. Japan College of Rheumatology. Life Education Committee (ed.) Textbook of rheumatology 2nd. Tokyo; Shindan to Chiryousha. 2016; (in Japanese).
11. Hashimoto H. Clinical manual of systemic lupus erythematosus (Zenshinsei Erythematousus rinsho manual). Nihon ijishinpousha: Tokyo; 2012; (in Japanese).
12. Domic RT, et al. Disease subsets in clinical practice. In: Varga J, et al., editors. Scleroderma. From pathogenesis to comprehensive management. New York, NY: Springer; 2017.
13. Research Group on Autoimmune Diseases. Polymyositis dermatomyositis subcommittee polymyositis, dermatomyositis treatment guidelines. (Tahatsusei Kinen Hifukinen Bunkakai Tahatsusei Kinen · Hifukinen Chiryou Guideline). Tokyo: Shindan to Chiryosha; 2015; (in Japanese).
14. McDonagh JE, Isenberg DA. Development of additional autoimmune diseases in a population of patients with systemic lupus erythematosus.Ann Rheum Dis 59: 230–232, 2000.
15. Kondo H. Recent advances in pathogenesis and treatment of systemic sclerosis (SSc, scleroderma) Kitasatoigaku (Kyouhishou no byoutaito saishinno chiryou). 2007;37(2): 95–104. (in Japanese).
16. Gell PGH and Coombs RRA.The classification of allergic reactions underlying disease. In Clinical aspects of immunology, RRA Coombs, PGH Gell (eds) 1st.Oxford; Blackwell Science. 1963, 317–337.
17. Amlot PL, Kemeny DM, Zachary C, Parkes P and Lessof MH.Oral allergy syndrome (OAS):symptoms of IgE-mediated hypersensitivity to foods Clin Exp Allergy 17:33–42 1987.

# Neurological Diseases 16

Makiko Nishina, Tomoaki Shintani, Tetsuji Okamoto, Kazuhiro Muramatsu, Tadashi Kawai, Kanako Yamahara, Tetsuya Maeda, Yasuo Terayama, Satoshi Okada, and Takaaki Kamatani

## 1 Dementia and Alzheimer's Disease

Makiko Nishina

### 1.1 Definition

Dementia is diagnosed when there is a significant decline from the previous level of behavior in one or more of the following cognitive domains: complex attention, executive function, learning and memory, language, perceptual-motor function, and social cognition, which interferes with daily life [1].

### 1.2 Pathophysiology

It is caused by the loss of neurons and networks in the central nervous system, which are involved in cognitive functions. In pathological changes, degenerative diseases are common and each causative disease has characteristic findings [2, 3].

### 1.3 Epidemiology

The prevalence of dementia is on the rise, with a prevalence of approximately 15% in a 2012 survey. With the aging of the population, it is esti-

M. Nishina
Department of Internal Medicine, Tokyo Dental College, Ichikawa General Hospital, Ichikawa, Chiba, Japan

T. Shintani
Center for Oral Clinical Examination, Hiroshima University Hospital, Hiroshima, Japan

T. Okamoto
School of Medical Sciences, University of East Asia, Shimonoseki, Yamaguchi, Japan

K. Muramatsu
Yokohama Tsurumi Rehabilitation Hospital, Yokohama, Kanagawa, Japan

T. Kawai
Division of Oral and Maxillofacial Surgery, Department of Reconstructive Oral and Maxillofacial Surgery, School of Dentistry, Iwate Medical University, Morioka, Iwate, Japan

K. Yamahara · T. Maeda (✉)
Division of Neurology and Gerontology, Department of Internal Medicine, School of Medicine, Iwate Medical University, Yahaba, Iwate, Japan
e-mail: maeda@iwate-med.ac.jp

Y. Terayama
Neurological institute, Shonan Keiiku Hospital, Fujisawa, Kanagawa, Japan

S. Okada
Department of Neurology, Tokyo Dental College, Ichikawa General Hospital, Ichikawa, Chiba, Japan

T. Kamatani
Department of Oral and Maxillofacial Surgery, School of Dentistry, Showa University, Ota-ku, Tokyo, Japan



T. Chiba, H. Yamada (eds.), *Internal Medicine for Dental Treatments*,
https://doi.org/10.1007/978-981-99-3296-2_16

mated that the number of dementia patients will reach 7.3 million by 2025 [4].

## 1.4 Classification

There is a wide range of diseases that cause dementia as shown in Table 16.1 [5]. Some neurosurgical diseases such as normal pressure hydrocephalus and chronic subdural hematoma, and some medical diseases such as hypothyroidism and vitamin $B_{12}$ deficiency are treatable dementia, should be diagnosed and treated as early as possible.

The most common cause of dementia is Alzheimer's disease, which accounts for about 68% of cases, followed by vascular dementia (19%) and dementia with Lewy body (4.5%) [6].

**Table 16.1** Diseases and conditions that cause major cognitive impairment (created based on [5])

| 1. Central neurodegenerative diseases | 6. Associated with systemic diseases |
|---|---|
| Alzheimer's disease<br>Frontotemporal dementia<br>Lewy body dementia<br>Huntington's disease, etc. | Hypothyroidism<br>Vitamin $B_1$ deficiency<br>Vitamin $B_{12}$ deficiency<br>folic acid deficiency<br>Liver failure<br>Neurosyphilis, etc. |
| 2. Vascular dementia | 7. Drug-induced |
| Multi infarct dementia<br>Chronic subdural hematoma<br>Cerebral hemorrhagic dementia, etc. | Psychotropic drug<br>Sedative drug<br>Hypnotic<br>Antidepressant<br>Analgesics opioids, NSAIDs, etc. |
| 3. Normal pressure hydrocephalus | |
| 4. Brain tumor | |
| 5. Neurological infections | 8. Others |

## 1.5 Symptoms

We focus on the symptoms of Alzheimer's disease, which accounts for the majority of cases.

### 1.5.1 Cognitive Dysfunction

Forgetfulness and memory impairment are characteristic and often the first symptoms. They forget appointments, misplace objects, and repeat the same story. The patient is unable to remember new things, recall them, and use them. A slow and progressive disorientation, executive function disorder, and visual-spatial impairments occur as the disease progresses. Many constructive apraxia are also observed, the patient loses the ability to use daily tools and to imitate by verbal and visual commands, and there is a decrease in the ability to perform work and housekeeping (Table 16.2) [7]. In daily life, the ability to per-

**Table 16.2** Examples of major cognitive dysfunction in dementia (created based on [7])

| Cognitive function | Symptoms | Examples |
|---|---|---|
| Generalized disorder | Generalized attention disorder | More mistakes in various tasks<br>Blurred and slow to react |
| Executive functioning | Executive functioning disorder | Cannot get things done in a timely manner |
| Memory | Forgetfulness | Inability to remember new things (anterograde amnesia)<br>Inability to remember what happened before (retrograde amnesia) |
| Language | Aphasia<br>Agraphia | Disorders of speech, comprehension, calling, recitation, reading, and writing<br>Dysgraphia |
| Count | Acalculia | Trouble handling money and paying bills |
| Visual-spatial cognition | Constructive apraxia geographic disorientation<br>Visual hallucination/optical illusion | Inability to imitate figures and finger shapes<br>Get lost in familiar places<br>Seeing things that are not there |
| Conduct | Apraxia (inability to purposely perform some actions) | Difficulty completing familiar tasks |
| Social cognitive | Disinhibition | Inability to recognize the surrounding situation and take appropriate action |

form activities, such as paying bills and managing medication become impaired from an early stage.

### 1.5.2 Behavioral and Psychological Symptoms of Dementia: BPSD

Behavioral and psychological symptoms such as impaired motivation and emotion, delusion, hallucination, wandering behavior, agitation, and aggression occur. Indifference, decreased spontaneity, and depression are also common. In Alzheimer's disease, delusions of robbery and delusion of persecution are common, and characteristic interpersonal behaviors such as lack of disease awareness and mending reactions are observed. On the other hand, visual hallucination is common in Lewy body dementia.

### 1.5.3 Others

Depending on the cause of cognitive impairment, there are characteristic symptoms other than cognitive dysfunction, such as parkinsonism in Lewy body dementia.

## 1.6 Clinical Examination

### 1.6.1 Psychological Test

Patients with cognitive complaints should undergo a careful mental states examination. The Mini-Mental State Examination (MMSE) is the most widely used screening scale for cognitive dysfunction in dementia, and a score of 23 or lower is considered suspicious for dementia.

### 1.6.2 Blood Test

To differentiate cognitive dysfunction associated with medical diseases, blood count, blood biochemistry, thyroid function, electrolytes, fasting blood glucose, vitamin $B_{12}$, folic acid, and serum syphilis tests should be performed.

### 1.6.3 Neuroimaging

1. **Brain MRI and CT:** The first step is to exclude treatable dementia. The pattern of atrophy and signal changes in the cerebral atrophy are useful for distinguishing the cause of dementia.
2. **Single-photon emission tomography (SPECT):** Alzheimer's disease is characterized by hypoperfusion in the posterior cingulate gyrus, precuneus, and parietal association areas.

## 1.7 Diagnosis

The diagnosis of dementia is based on history, physical and neurological examination, and laboratory and neuroimaging findings. Many drugs that cause cognitive impairments, and it is necessary to confirm the contents of medication. In particular, anticholinergic agents and benzodiazepines are at risk of causing dementia.

## 1.8 Treatment

Treatment of dementia aims to improve cognitive function and quality of life (QOL), which are the core symptoms. For behavioral and psychological symptoms of dementia (BPSD) such as paranoia and irritability, environmental adjustment and non-pharmacotherapy may provide maximal benefits.

### 1.8.1 Drug Therapy

Three cholinesterase inhibitors, donepezil, galantamine, and rivastigmine, and an *N*-methyl-D-aspartate (NMDA) receptor antagonist, memantine, are available symptomatic medications for cognitive function in Alzheimer's disease.

### 1.8.2 Non-Drug Therapy

These include cognitive function training, cognitive stimulation, exercise therapy, music therapy, and training in activities of daily living. Dental treatment and oral care are also vital, and preventive and continuous oral hygiene management is necessary.

## 1.9 Prognosis

As the disease progresses, almost all memory is impaired, and the patient eventually loses the ability to perform self-care tasks such as dressing, eating, toileting, bathing, and understanding and speaking. Basic motor skills are also lost, and the patient eventually becomes bedridden. In the terminal stage, the patient dies from complications such as malnutrition, dehydration, and infections such as aspiration pneumonia [8].

## 1.10 Recent Findings

Many patients with dementia show eating behavior change, low nutrition, and weight loss due to eating disorders and dysphagia. Therefore, it is important to evaluate nutrition, prevent aspiration, and review drugs, depending on the progress. However, percutaneous endoscopic gastrostomy (PEG) does not prolong long-term survival in patients with severe dementia [9].

Diabetes mellitus, obesity in middle age, hypertension, depression, hearing impairment, and smoking are risk factors for the development of dementia, and intervention in these areas is expected to prevent the onset of dementia. In addition, regular exercise and social participation have been shown to have preventive effects [10]. Recently aducanumab, recombinant monoclonal antibody directed against amyloid beta, is approved by the US Food Drug Administration (FDA) for the treatment of mild Alzheimer's disease. At present, there is uncertainty about whether patients benefit clinically from aducanumab [11].

## 1.11 Notes from Dentistry Perspective

Tetsuji Okamoto, Tomoaki Shintani

### 1.11.1 Periodontitis and Alzheimer's Disease

The etiology of Alzheimer type dementia (hereafter referred to as Alzheimer's disease) remains unclear, and effective prevention and treatment have not yet been established. There have been many reports on the relationship between Alzheimer's disease and the oral cavity, and it has been shown that "tooth loss" and "periodontitis" are risk factors, each of which induces Alzheimer's disease by its own mechanism [12, 13]. Regarding the relationship between tooth loss and Alzheimer's disease, it has been suggested that tooth loss reduces chewing efficiency and decreases blood flow to the brain, causing cognitive dysfunction [13]. Oue et al. found that the maxillary bilateral molar extraction group showed a decrease in cognitive function and a significant decrease in the number of neurons in the hippocampus compared with the non-extraction group, but there was no difference in the deposition of amyloid β protein (Aβ) in the brains of the two groups using the Alzheimer's disease transgenic mice [14].

On the other hand, periodontitis is a chronic infection caused by periodontopathic bacteria, and it has been reported that periodontitis is a risk factor for systemic diseases such as diabetes mellitus, myocardial infarction, atherosclerosis, preterm and low birth weight, endocarditis, aspiration pneumonia, and rheumatoid arthritis [15]. DNA of *Porphyromonas gingivalis* (*P.g*), a periodontopathic bacterium, has been detected in the placenta of mothers who delivered preterm or low birth weight babies and in atherosclerotic plaques in the aortic wall of patients with atherosclerosis (Fig. 16.1) [16]. Furthermore, bacterial components of *P.g* have been detected in the liver parenchyma of patients with nonalcoholic steatohepatitis (NASH), suggesting that they may be involved in the progression of NASH. Since microglia, a type of macrophage, are activated in the brains of patients with Alzheimer's disease, Alzheimer's disease is considered a chronic inflammation of the brain [17], and many studies have investigated its relationship with periodontitis.

Serum antibody titers against *Fusobacterium nucleatum* and *Prevotella intermedia* were increased in Alzheimer's disease patients [18], and the presence of lipopolysaccharide (LPS) from *P.g* in the brain was confirmed [19, 20]. In the Alzheimer's disease transgenic mice infected with *P.g*, cognitive function is further reduced

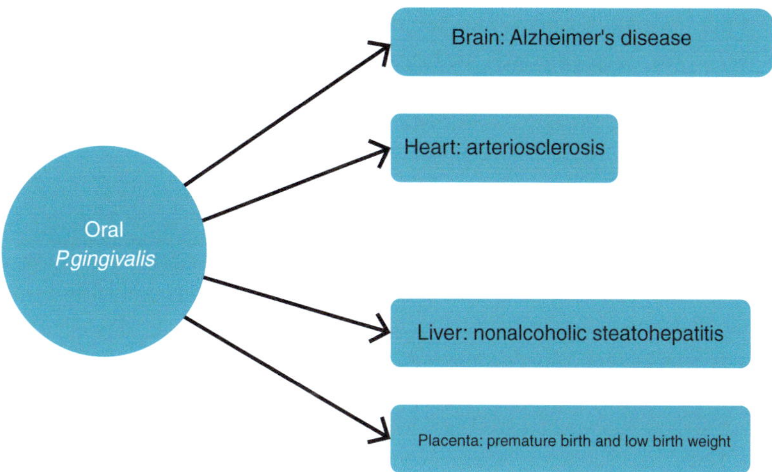


**Fig. 16.1** Organs and diseases in which *P.g* bacteria were detected

and the deposition of Aβ in the brain is increased [21]. In addition, periodontopathic bacteria and bacterial-derived LPS activate macrophages, and inflammatory mediators such as TNF-α, IL-1, IL-6, and CRP produced by macrophages in the periodontal region are transported to the brain via the bloodstream and induce inflammatory reactions in neurons, which may exacerbate the pathogenesis of Alzheimer's disease [22]. Although periodontopathic bacteria cannot invade the brain parenchyma because of the blood-brain barrier (BBB) in the brain, it is thought that periodontopathic bacteria may reach the brain by increasing the permeability of the BBB due to inflammatory cytokines in the blood and aging of cerebral blood vessels [23]. After inflammatory cytokines and periodontopathic bacteria reach the brain parenchyma, abnormal aggregation and deposition of Aβ induces neuronal apoptosis, resulting in the appearance of symptoms of Alzheimer's disease [17]. It has been reported that *P.g* exist in the brains of Alzheimer's disease patients and that DNA of *P.g* exists in spinal cord secretions, and gingipains, proteolytic enzymes produced by *P.g*, have been detected in the brains of Alzheimer's disease patients [24]. In the brains of patients with Alzheimer's disease, tau and ubiquitin, proteins strongly associated with Alzheimer's disease, were found to be present in large amounts [24], and clinical studies of the molecular target therapy targeting gingipains for the disease have already been initiated [24]. On the other hand, it was found that the number of bacteria of the genus *Bacteroides* was significantly lower in the intestinal microflora of elderly patients with dementia than that of non-demented elderly patients [25].

Thus, periodontitis is considered to be a risk factor for Alzheimer's disease, and treatment of periodontitis may prevent Alzheimer's disease or delay the progression of the disease.

### 1.11.2 Dysphagia in Patients with Alzheimer's Disease

With the progression of Alzheimer's disease, memory impairment, impaired judgment, and disorientation, which are the main symptoms of the disease, progress, and it is difficult to recognize how to eat food and what food is offered. As dementia progresses and ADL (Activities of Daily Living) decline significantly, swallowing function declines and nutritional status deteriorates. A characteristic feature of Alzheimer's disease is that the onset of eating and deglutition disorders is different. In addition, as Alzheimer's disease becomes more severe, patients may require assistance to wear dentures, or they may refuse to wear or use dentures. Denture refusal not only makes it difficult to consume food, but also leads to deterioration of masticatory function and aspiration, which in many cases leads to deterioration of nutritional status and dehydration.

#### 1.11.3 Dental Treatment and Oral Care for Patients with Alzheimer's Disease

Dental treatment in patients with Alzheimer's disease should be planned in accordance with the progression of dementia [26]. In the early stage, patients with Alzheimer's disease can be treated with conventional dentistry, including tooth extraction, endodontic treatment, and prosthetic treatment. In the middle stage of the disease, the patient has difficulty in following detailed instructions and in taking long dental treatments. In addition, masticatory dysfunction is observed, and assistance during meals and changes in eating patterns become necessary. In the latter stage, communication becomes difficult, and not only normal dental treatment but also denture cleaning and oral self-care cannot be performed, and oral hygiene deteriorates, so the intervention of oral care is essential.

In addition, to prevent aspiration pneumonia, oral care is necessary to reduce the number of oral bacteria as much as possible. Furthermore, nutritional management is also important because dentures become difficult to wear. In order to make oral care as smooth as possible, it is important to perform it in a familiar environment and with dental staffs, and to talk to the patient in a way that gives a sense of security. Patients with impaired swallowing function should receive oral care while taking care to avoid aspiration. Patients who cannot control their body movements should not be forced to perform oral care.

Although there are individual differences in Alzheimer's disease, it is a progressive disease and oral care is essential for many patients. Therefore, when planning treatment, it is important to intervene to create an oral environment that facilitates better oral care, such as preserving residual root teeth as much as possible and avoiding the fabrication of dentures that are difficult to put on and take off.

## 2 Epilepsy [27–29]

Kazuhiro Muramatsu

### 2.1 What Is Epilepsy?

Epilepsy is a chronic brain disease that causes repetitive seizures of the brain due to the overexcitement of nerve cells in the cerebrum. The seizures are sudden and cause unusual physical symptoms and changes in consciousness, movement, and sensation. If there are obvious convulsions, epilepsy is the most likely cause. In addition to convulsions, epilepsy can cause a variety of other symptoms, such as lightheadedness, body twitching, and moving around while unconscious. Epilepsy is characterized by recurrent episodes. Various tests, mainly electroencephalography, are necessary to confirm the diagnosis.

### 2.2 Epidemiology

Epilepsy is one of the most common central nervous system diseases, along with Alzheimer's disease and cerebrovascular disease. The prevalence of epilepsy is 4 to 8 per 1,000 of the general population in developed countries. In Japan, the number of patients is estimated to be 650,000 to 900,000. The incidence of epilepsy is about 45 cases per 100,000 people per year in developed countries. The incidence of epilepsy has been shown to be higher in infants and the elderly. It is estimated that there are about 300,000 people with epilepsy in the elderly in Japan.

### 2.3 Classification

Classification of epileptic seizures is essential for subsequent patient handling, testing, and selection of antiepileptic drugs, and the International League Against Epilepsy (ILAE) classification is used. Until now, the 1981 classification for epileptic seizure types and the 1989 classification for epilepsy, epilepsy syndromes, and related seizure disorders have been widely used, but in 2017, the ILAE proposed a new epileptic seizure and classification (Figs. 16.2 and 16.3). The ILAE proposed that epileptic focal epilepsy should be referred to as focal epilepsy when the epileptic focus is in neural circuits in one hemisphere and generalized epilepsy when the epileptic focus is in neural circuits spanning both hemispheres.

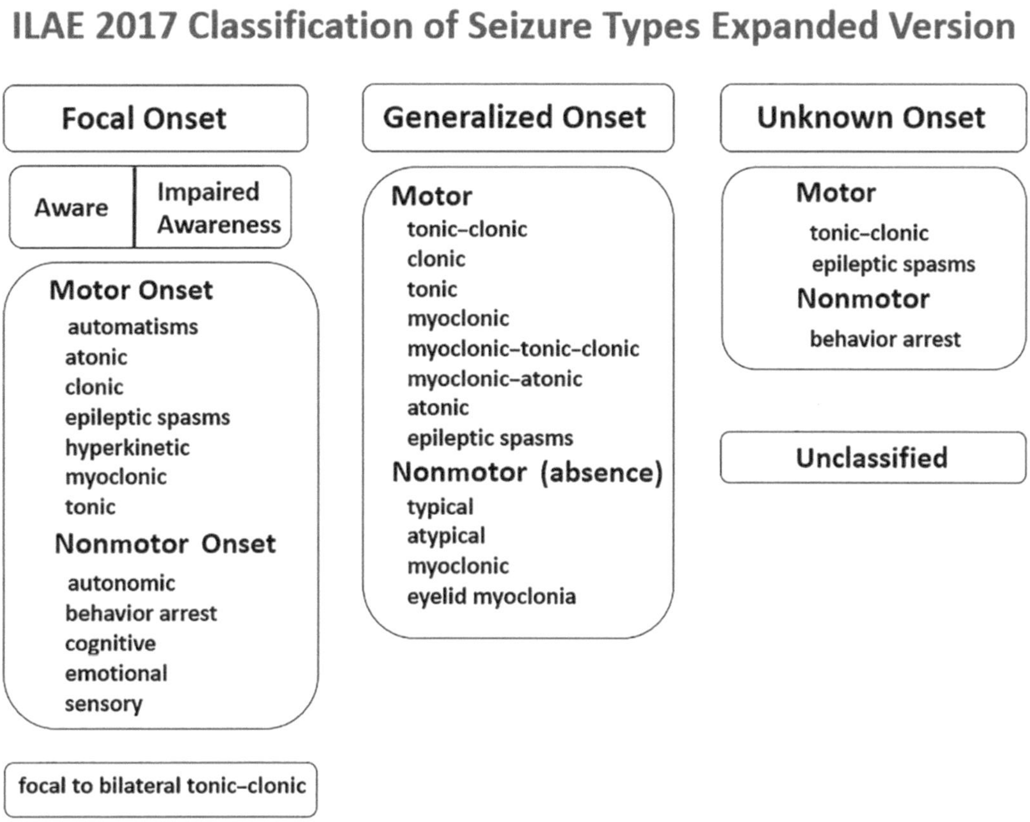

**ILAE 2017 Classification of Seizure Types Expanded Version**

**Focal Onset**

Aware | Impaired Awareness

**Motor Onset**
automatisms
atonic
clonic
epileptic spasms
hyperkinetic
myoclonic
tonic

**Nonmotor Onset**
autonomic
behavior arrest
cognitive
emotional
sensory

focal to bilateral tonic-clonic

**Generalized Onset**

**Motor**
tonic-clonic
clonic
tonic
myoclonic
myoclonic-tonic-clonic
myoclonic-atonic
atonic
epileptic spasms

**Nonmotor (absence)**
typical
atypical
myoclonic
eyelid myoclonia

**Unknown Onset**

**Motor**
tonic-clonic
epileptic spasms

**Nonmotor**
behavior arrest

**Unclassified**

**Fig. 16.2** ILAE 2017 Classification of seizure types (reproduced with permission from [27])

## 2.4 Interview for Epilepsy Diagnosis

Gathering sufficient information and witnessing the seizures are most helpful in diagnosing epilepsy. Although the chief complaint is often a convulsive seizure (and sometimes a nonconvulsive seizure), more than one seizure is usually necessary to diagnose epilepsy. Patients and seizure witnesses may provide information on seizure frequency, seizure circumstances and triggers (e.g., photosensitivity), symptoms before and during seizures (physical and mental symptoms and disturbance of consciousness), persistence of symptoms, symptoms following seizures, presence of trauma, bite tongue, urinary incontinence, headache and muscle pain after seizures, age of first attack in patients with multiple seizures, seizure and changes/transitions in seizure type, last seizure, relationship between seizures and wakefulness/sleep, etc.

## 2.5 Diseases that Need to be Differentiated from Epilepsy (Table 16.3)

Neurally mediated syncope/psychogenic nonepileptic seizures account for 40% of patients presenting to the emergency department with sudden-onset loss of consciousness, followed by epilepsy in 29% and cardiogenic seizures in 8%. To diagnose epilepsy, it is important to investigate the cardiovascular cause. The characteristic feature of syncopal seizures is that they are not accompanied by altered consciousness, fatigue, or malaise. The overall risk of developing epilepsy in patients who have an acute seizure within

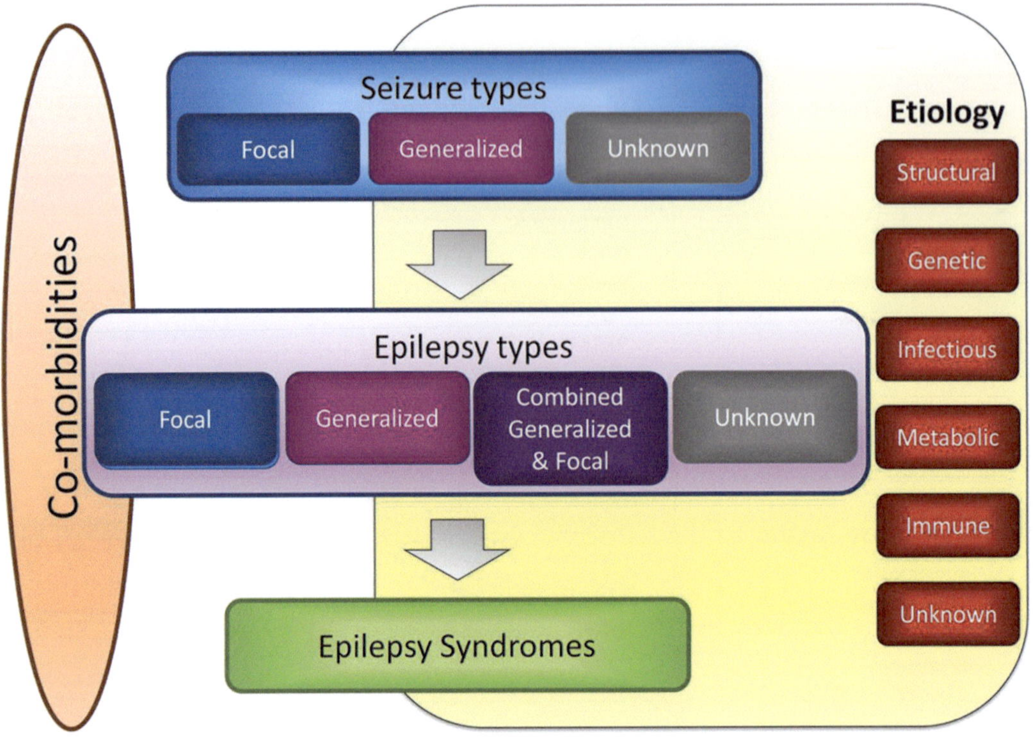


**Fig. 16.3** ILAE 2017 Framework for classification of the epilepsies (three levels of epilepsy diagnosis) (reproduced with permission from [28])

**Table 16.3** Diseases that should be differentiated from epilepsy

| |
|---|
| Fainting (neuromodulatory, cardiogenic, etc.) |
| Psychogenic non-epileptic seizure |
| Hyperventilation and panic attacks |
| Stroke (cerebral infarction, cerebral hemorrhage), transient ischemic attack |
| Sleep-related disorders (abnormal REM sleep behavior, non-REM parasomnias) |
| Acute poisoning (drugs, alcohol), drug withdrawal, alcohol withdrawal |
| Acute metabolic disorder (hypoglycemia, tetany) |
| Acute renal failure |
| Head trauma (within 1 week) |
| Involuntary movements (tics, tremors, myoclonus, paroxysmal dyskinesia, etc.) |
| Paroxysmal ataxia |

1 week of head injury is about 25%. Alcohol withdrawal may cause convulsive seizures.

## 2.6 Procedure for the Diagnosis of Epilepsy [29]

Electroencephalography (EEG) (including photic stimulation, hyperventilation, and sleep) should be recorded for the first unprovoked epileptic seizure. Sleep-activated EEG can increase the frequency of epileptic discharge recordings. If necessary, neuroimaging and simultaneous video-EEG recording should be performed.

In the diagnosis of epilepsy, EEG is the most useful test, but it may not be possible to make a diagnosis with only one conventional EEG, and multiple EEGs, including sleep activation, are necessary. Prolonged video-EEG monitoring is useful in the definitive diagnosis, typing, and localization of epilepsy.

Neuroimaging studies (MRI or CT) should be performed to diagnose epilepsy. MRI is particularly useful when focal-onset epilepsy is suspected. When an MRI or CT scan of a patient with a first unprovoked seizure shows organic lesions suggestive of stroke, central nervous system infection, or traumatic brain injury, the patient should be diagnosed as epilepsy even if it was the first seizure, because of the high risk of recurrence.

## 2.7 What to Do During an Epileptic Seizure

First, it is important to ensure safety and observe seizure symptoms. It is necessary to confirm that the place where the seizure occurred is not dangerous and that there are no dangerous things around, and depending on the situation, it may be necessary to assist the patient or keep away from dangerous things. Observation of seizure symptoms is the basis for the "symptomatic diagnosis" of epilepsy.

For cases of vomiting during or after seizure, there is also impaired consciousness and the vomit tends to get stuck in the throat, the patient should be placed on their side so that vomit can go out. After a seizure, the patient becomes sleepy, so let him sleep for a while. Patients with normal seizures recover after 30 min to 1 h of sleep, or 2 h at most.

Seizures that last more than a certain length of time or are repeated even if they are short and without recovery of consciousness are called status epilepticus, and treatment should be started immediately.

## 2.8 Drug Treatment of Epilepsy

As a rule, antiepileptic drug therapy should not be initiated for the first unprovoked seizure. Patients with neurological abnormalities, electroencephalographic abnormalities, brain imaging lesions, or a family history of epilepsy are more likely to have recurrent seizures and should be considered for treatment.

Antiepileptic drug therapy is usually initiated as a single agent. The choice of drug should be based on the seizure type and the diagnosis of epilepsy, taking into account the patient's individual condition. Carbamazepine, lamotrigine, and levetiracetam are recommended as first-line agents in patients with focal-onset epilepsy, while valproate is recommended as first-line therapy in patients with generalized-onset epilepsy.

If the patient is well controlled with medication, all dental procedures can be performed almost normally. Epinephrine-containing cannabis is not a problem. Problems arise in patients who are off medication or who have complications such as infection or fatigue.

## 2.9 Notes from Dentistry Perspective [30–34]

Tadashi Kawai

### 2.9.1 Oral Cavity of Epileptic Patients

Patients with epilepsy are often treated with single or multiple medications, and patients taking phenytoin may develop drug-induced gingival hyperplasia, with an incidence of about 50%. It is thought that phenytoin increases the proliferation of gingival fibroblasts, increases the synthesis of extracellular matrix by gingival fibroblasts, and decreases their resolving power. Gingival hyperplasia can be improved by oral cleaning. Still, if symptoms are marked, the dentist should ask the patient's physician to change the medication, and if this is difficult, a gingivectomy may be performed.

### 2.9.2 Confirmations Before Dental Treatment

Before dental treatment, the dentist should consult with the patient's physician for details of the patient's condition, history, current condition, medications, and precautions for dental treatment. Information on the severity of the epileptic seizures is also necessary, such as whether they are minor seizures with a brief loss of consciousness or major seizures leading to convulsions (seizures). The presence or absence of other comorbidities should also be confirmed. Even if the patient claims that his or her symptoms have calmed down, dental treatment involves a variety of invasive procedures, and if we believe the patient's words and proceed with treatment without paying attention to the patient's condition, the invasive procedures may trigger an epileptic seizure and cause serious problems. Therefore, dental treatment should be performed with care to prevent epileptic seizures. The presence or absence of epileptic aura and how to respond to seizures at home should also be confirmed.

#### 2.9.3 Precautions for Dental Treatment

A variety of invasive procedures can be expected at the beginning of dental treatment. Even if the treatment has not started, a long waiting time in the waiting room may induce epileptic seizures due to nervousness about dental treatment. Therefore, it is advisable to avoid a long waiting time after the patient arrives at the clinic. The patient's physical condition should be checked before the treatment begins. Check that the patient is tired or not, and that they have not forgotten to take the medicine. If there are any problems, it is advisable to postpone the treatment. Attention should also be paid to the environment during dental treatment. Loud noises, such as dropping objects on the floor and light stimulation can be very stressful. Proceeding with treatment without talking to the patient can also cause anxiety and distress, and should be treated appropriately. With regard to local anesthetics, there are no contraindications to epinephrine or concomitant use of antiepileptic drugs, but it is advisable to check other drugs, such as psychotropic drugs, that are prescribed concomitantly. Concerning prescription drugs from dentists, concomitant use of acetaminophen in patients taking phenytoin is cautioned because of the increased risk of liver dysfunction.

#### 2.9.4 What to Do During an Epileptic Seizure

Even if the above information is considered during treatment, seizures may still occur because dental treatment itself is invasive for the patient. If the patient is unresponsive or has a seizure, stop treatment and observe the patient until they regain consciousness in a few seconds. After that, give only first aid and postpone treatment. If a grand mal occurs, as many people as possible should assemble to prevent the patient from falling off the dental unit. Administer diazepam, if available. Intravenous injection is preferable, but intramuscular injection is also acceptable if convulsions make it difficult. Convulsions often subside in a few minutes, and the patient should be kept under control until then. Because the patient is not breathing spontaneously, the oxygen saturation level ($SpO_2$) drops to about 80%. Oxygen may be administered during convulsions, but it may not be effective because spontaneous breathing is not stable. In fact, it is better to administer oxygen after the patient regains consciousness because of the fatigue caused by the convulsions. After the seizure subsides, the patient should rest for a while, and when consciousness is clearly restored, treatment should be terminated and the planned treatment should be postponed.

For subsequent treatment, the reasons for the seizures should be reviewed and analyzed. If there is an obvious cause, it should be noted in the next treatment. It is also advisable to report the seizure to the patient's doctor. The doctor may consider changing the medication to control the seizures.

## 3 Parkinson's Disease

Kanako Yamahara, Tetsuya Maeda, and Yasuo Terayama

### 3.1 Introduction

Parkinson's disease (PD) is the second most common neurodegenerative disease next to Alzheimer's disease (AD). A neurodegenerative disease is a disorder in which a specific group of neurons in the brain and spinal cord are damaged and lost. In AD, cortical neurons in the cerebrum are affected, whereas in PD, dopaminergic neurons in the substantia nigra of the midbrain are selectively degenerated and lost. As a result, the striatal level of dopamine decreased, resulting in dysfunction of the basal ganglia circuits and the emergence of various movement disorders. The cause of PD remains unknown, but the involvement of genetic and environmental factors is known to be important. The prevalence of PD in Japan is 100 to 180 per 100,000 people, but increases with age and is estimated to be 1 in 100 for people aged 70 years or older. The number of patients with PD continues to increase with the aging of society, and it is predicted that the global PD population will exceed 13 million by 2040 at the lowest estimate [35].

## 3.2 Pathogenic Factors

PD is a sporadic disease in general and usually develops in the 60 s. Those with onset age at 40 or younger are associated with genetic abnormalities, and hereditary PD accounts for about 10% of all. Pathologically, PD is characterized by the presence of intracellular inclusions called Lewy body in the residual dopaminergic neurons in the substantia nigra pars compacta. The main component of Lewy body is α-synuclein, which is formed by abnormal aggregation in the presence of genetic and environmental risks. α-synuclein has been shown to propagate between neurons and is thought to be a key molecule involved in the onset, progression, and treatment of PD.

## 3.3 Parkinson's Disease Clinical Syndrome

PD is a movement disorder characterized by motor symptoms. However, it is clinically considered a systemic neurological syndrome that also presents with non-motor symptoms. Cardinal motor symptoms include (1) tremor at rest: 4–6 Hz constant involuntary movements of fingers, hands, arms, and legs; (2) rigidity: an abnormal increase of muscle tone evoked by passive movement of limb joints; (3) akinesia and bradykinesia: small voice, poor facial expression, and decrease of body spontaneous movements which takes time to perform daily activities; and (4) postural instability: leading poor postural balance and frequent fall. Due to these symptoms, the patient has a lack of facial expression, leans forward, and walks in a small, unsteady manner. The tremor tends to disappear during movement and to increase with tension and anxiety. These symptoms respond well to anti-parkinsonian agents and can be maintained with activities of daily living if appropriate treatment is initiated. However, as the disease progresses and becomes more severe, patients may require assistance in turning and rising from bed, and dysarthria and decreased swallowing function may be observed. Since risks of aspiration pneumonia and bone fracture due to falls increases, prevention through oral care and rehabilitation is important.

On the other hand, PD has a variety of non-motor symptoms as shown in Table 16.4 [36], which are difficult to treat in clinical practice. The most common symptoms in the early stages of the disease are constipation, sleep disturbance, depressive mood

**Table 16.4** Indications of nonmotor symptoms (cited from [36])

| |
|---|
| • Neuropsychiatric symptoms |
| Depression and depressive symptoms |
| Anxiety and anxiety symptoms |
| Apathy |
| Psychosis |
| Impulse control and related disorders |
| Dementia |
| Cognitive impairment (other than dementia; mainly mild cognitive impairment) |
| • Autonomic dysfunction |
| Drooling |
| Orthostatic hypotension |
| Urinary dysfunction |
| Erectile dysfunction |
| Gastrointestinal dysfunction |
| Excessive sweating |
| Disorders of sleep and wakefulness |
| Sleep fragmentation and insomnia |
| Rapid eye movement sleep behavior disorder |
| Excessive daytime sleepiness |
| • Others |
| Pain |
| Fatigue |
| Olfactory dysfunction |
| Ophthalmologic dysfunction |

disorders, fatigue, hyposmia, and pain. About 10 years after the onset of PD, orthostatic hypotension appears as a symptom of autonomic failure and the frequency of dizziness and falls increases. Even if there are no subjective symptoms, systolic blood pressure may drop 30 to 50 mmHg after repositioning or urinating. Sudden repositioning should be avoided, especially in dehydration cases. Cognitive decline is also a common symptom of PD. In the early stage, cognitive processing speed is mainly affected and making plans and recalling words become difficult. Gradually, cortical symptoms such as memory disorder, decreased attentiveness, and executive function impairment become apparent. After dementia becomes apparent, clear visual hallucinations of people and small animals are often experienced. These non-motor symptoms are known to deteriorate the quality of life (QOL) in PD patients. Therefore, management of non-motor symptoms are clinically important as well as motor symptoms.

## 3.4 Diagnosis

In PD, clinical examinations including blood tests and brain MRI are not abnormal. These are performed to exclude other diseases with similar symptoms to PD. Multiple system atrophy, progressive supranuclear palsy, and corticobasal degeneration are well known as important differential diagnoses of PD. In contrast to PD, these diseases often have a short period of time until gait disturbance and easy falling appear. Clinical course is important for diagnosis, and neuroimagings used with nuclear medicine, such as MIBG cardiomyography and dopamine transporter scintigraphy, are also employed (Fig. 16.4a–d). The most important practical difference between PD and other movement disorders with parkinsonism is the response to dopaminergic agents. Clear and dramatic beneficial response to the initial therapy using with

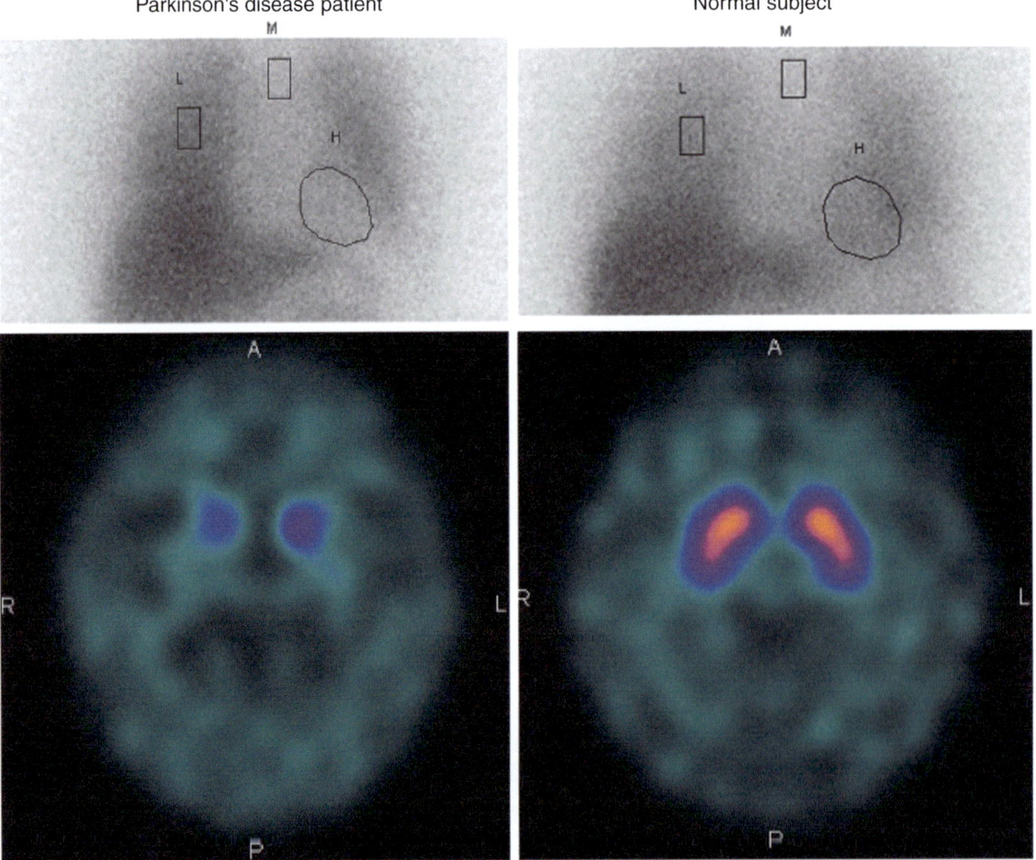


**Fig. 16.4** MIBG myocardial scintigraphy (upper panel) and dopamine transporter SPECT (lower panel): Parkinson's disease patient on the left and normal subject on the right. Decreased accumulation in the patient with Parkinson's disease, respectively

**Table 16.5** Classification of severity of Parkinson's disease and impairment of life

| Hoehn & Yahr's severity classification | | Ministry of Health, Labour and Welfare's classification of functional disability in daily life (Research Group for Abnormal Motor Diseases) |
|---|---|---|
| I | Unilateral disorder with unilateral tremor and muscle stiffness. It is a mild case | The patient needs little assistance in daily life and hospital visits |
| II | It is a bilateral disorder with postural changes but without postural instability. There is some disability in daily life and employment due to the bilateral presence of muscle rigidity and bradykinesia to akinesia | Partial assistance is required for daily life and hospital visits |
| III | The patients have obvious gait disorder. They have postural instability, and fall easily when changing direction but can walk. They are able to live without assistance and can work depending on their occupation, although their activities are limited | The patient needs full assistance in daily life and is unable to walk or stand up by himself |
| IV | There is a marked decrease in activities of daily living, such as standing and walking, and the ability to work is lost. It is difficult to live only by oneself | |
| V | The patient becomes unable to stand and is wheelchair-bound or bedridden with assistance | |

L-dopa is supportive to diagnose PD. Clinical severity of PD is usually evaluated by Hoehn & Yahr staging (Table 16.5), which is a simple and standard assessment method in the world.

## 3.5 Treatment

Treatment of PD is classified into medical, surgical, and exercise therapy. There is no curative treatment for PD, and the most common treatment is dopamine replacement therapy.

The mainstay of medical therapy is L-dopa and dopamine agonists. L-dopa is the most effective agent, but its duration of action is short, and long-term administration is associated with motor complications (wearing-off phenomenon, dyskinesia). Therefore, concomitant therapy with dopamine agonists is common, which have variable formulations, including oral pills, subcutaneous self-injection, and transdermal patch. All of them can be selected according to the patient's lifestyle. Since sleep attacks and psychiatric symptoms have been reported as major side effects, it is recommended that patients with cognitive decline or suspected impulse control disorders refrain from using the drug. Selective monoamine oxidase B (MAO-B) inhibitors, catechol-o-methyl transferase (COMT) inhibitors, adenosine $A_{2A}$ receptor antagonists, and zonisamide as activator of dopamine system are also used as adjunctive agents with L-dopa. The motor symptoms respond well to dopamine replacement therapy in the early stage, and honeymoon period follows in which the primary symptoms become less prominent. However, as the disease progresses, the effectiveness of the anti-parkinsonian drugs are ameliorated and symptomatic fluctuation (wearing-off phenomenon) and hyperkinetic abnormal involuntary movements (dyskinesia) may emerge. These are defined as motor complications and the clinical phase with them is defined as the advanced stage. In the advanced stage, therapeutic strategies such as increasing the frequency of medication or usage of a longer-lasting effect are necessary to maintain the motor complications.

Malignant syndrome is the most important issue in patients using anti-parkinsonian drugs. PD patients usually take multiple drugs in combination. Abruptly discontinuation of their drugs due to poor physical condition or fasting periods associated with surgery or examination may result in the development of serious symptoms such as high fever, disturbance of consciousness, rigidity of extremities, and rhabdomyolysis. When a fasting period is required for examination, treatment, or surgery, supplementation with L-dopa by intravenous infusion or concomitant use of transdermal patch should be considered to prevent this malignant syndrome.

Functional surgery should be considered for patients with advanced PD who have uncontrollable motor complications with anti-parkinsonian medications. Practically, eligible conditions for surgical treatment are patients who do not respond to anti-parkinsonian medication even for a short period, who are independent during on state but cannot get up and walk without assistance when off state. In Japan, deep brain stimulation and intraduodenal L-dopa carbidopa intestinal gel therapy are the two options, called device-assisted therapy in terms of treatment using medical equipment.

In recent years, dopaminergic neuronal cell transplantation derived from induced pluripotent stem (iPS) cells and nucleic acid therapy targeting the *SNCA* gene encoding an α-synuclein are noticed as attracting treatments, which also involves surgical procedures. In the former treatment, iPS-derived dopaminergic progenitor cells are stereotactically injected into the putamen to replace lost dopaminergic neurons. The latter is a treatment using a nucleic acid drug called AmNA-modified antisense nucleic acid, which has been reported to suppress the accumulation of α-synuclein in brain cells by inhibiting the expression of the *SNCA* gene. Treatment development is constantly underway, and these studies are also highly promising areas.

Finally, exercise therapy is essential for the maintenance of motor function, because it can be performed at any stage of the disease, from early onset to advanced stages, in parallel with pharmacotherapy and surgical treatment. In recent years, clinical studies have been conducted and scientific evidence for the efficacy of exercise therapy has been accumulated. However, motivation is often low in PD patients, and it is important to inspire patients to continue exercise therapy.

## 3.6 Notes from Dentistry Perspective [37–39]

Tadashi Kawai

### 3.6.1 Oral Cavity of Patients with Parkinson's Disease

Patients with Parkinson's disease have difficulty moving their bodies smoothly, and various symptoms such as decreased chewing and swallowing functions and sialorrhea appear in the oral cavity. The oral environment is also affected by oral medications. When anticholinergic drugs, which are parasympathomimetic drugs, are prescribed, their effects suppress saliva secretion at rest, resulting in xerostomia. This may increase the risk of dental caries and periodontal disease, and may be accompanied by other oral mucosal diseases and mucosal damage due to denture incompatibility. In patients with advanced disease, involuntary movements (oral dyskinesia) such as lip gagging and tongue twisting may occur in the mouth.

### 3.6.2 Confirmations Before Dental Treatment

Prior to dental treatment, the patient's physician should be consulted about the details of the disease, the patient's history, current condition, medications, and precautions for dental treatment. Depending on the severity of Parkinson's disease, there is a limit to the content of dental treatment that can be performed. Even patients with Parkinson's disease who have relatively little difficulty in daily life or who require only minor assistance may have diurnal variation in symptoms. The presence of other complications such as cerebrovascular disease, malignant tumors, and infections should also be checked.

### 3.6.3 Precautions for Dental Treatment

#### In the Treatment Room

Patients with Parkinson's disease may have difficulty moving due to movement disorder, and it is necessary to pay attention to their feet when moving around in the clinic room and transferring to the unit. Patients with Parkinson's disease may also have difficulty in conversation, so it is necessary to communicate with them in a relaxed manner to avoid stress.

#### Clinic Hours

Because of the lack of efficacy of oral medications for Parkinson's disease (wearing-off phenomenon), once diurnal variation in symptoms has been identified, treatment should be performed to the time of day when the medication is most effective.

The morning hours are often chosen. It is not advisable to carry out treatment for too long, so treatment should be completed promptly.

**Local Anesthetics**

In patients taking levodopa-containing drugs, epinephrine may induce marked increases in blood pressure and tachycardia because the metabolism of epinephrine with a catechol group is inhibited. Monoamine oxidase inhibitors and catechol-*O*-methyltransferase inhibitors also induce elevated blood pressure and tachycardia with epinephrine. Patients taking dopamine receptor stimulators should be cautioned against concomitant use of epinephrine because of its vasoconstrictive effects and blood pressure increasing effects, although the mechanism of action is not clear. Since many Parkinson's patients are taking these drugs, it is advisable to avoid epinephrine-containing local anesthetics.

**During Dental Treatment**

Orthostatic hypotension may occur in 20 to 30% of patients with Parkinson's disease who are taking medication. Therefore, patients with Parkinson's disease should move slowly when raising the dental unit during treatment. The patient should be careful about aspiration because of dysphagia. Be careful about vacuuming during treatment with water. In patients with significant dysphagia, it is advisable to set the angle of the dental unit at 45° to prevent aspiration of saliva or water stored in the mouth. Since the patient's facial expression may be poor, check their condition by talking to them as appropriate. During treatment, blood pressure and arterial oxygen saturation ($SpO_2$) should be monitored because of fluctuations in blood pressure and the effect of aspiration on respiration.

### 3.6.4 Oral Management

Although dental treatment is not easy due to the nature of the disease, regular oral management every 3 to 4 months is necessary. If oral management is inadequate, occlusion may collapse due to the high risk of dental caries and periodontal disease, and oral nutritional intake may become difficult due to pain caused by oral mucosal disease. This may lead to weight loss. In addition, in patients with advanced symptoms and marked akinesia, aspiration pneumonia may occur repeatedly.

The pathogenesis of Parkinson's disease should be understood, and dental treatment should proceed with consideration to changes in the oral environment and the resulting effects on the whole body.

## 4 Amyotrophic Lateral Sclerosis [40, 41]

Satoshi Okada

### 4.1 Concepts and Definitions

Motor neurons include lower neurons from the brain stem motor neurons and anterior horn cells of the spinal cord to skeletal muscles, and upper neurons that travel through the pyramidal tract from the motor area of the cerebral cortex and connect to the lower neurons. Amyotrophic lateral sclerosis (ALS) is a neurodegenerative disease in which both higher and lower motor neurons are progressively impaired. The skeletal muscles of the whole body are damaged, resulting in marked muscle weakness and atrophy. The disease is often solitary, but it may occur familial.

### 4.2 Pathophysiology

Although the etiology of sporadic ALS is still unclear, it has been postulated that TDP-43 protein accumulates in the cytoplasm of motor neurons and is involved in RNA dysfunction. In addition, glutamate-induced excitotoxicity, mitochondrial abnormalities, axonal transport disorders, and oxidative stress have been proposed to be involved.

In familial cases, causative genes such as SOD1, FUS, TARDBP, C9ORF72, optineurin, UBQLN2, and ERBB4 have been identified. Among these, SOD1 is the most common, accounting for about 20%. It is not unusual for phenotypic differences to occur even within the same family.

## 4.3 Epidemiology

The prevalence is 7 to 11 per 100,000 population, and the incidence is 1.1 to 2.5 per 100,000 population. The male to female ratio is 3:2, with a slightly higher incidence in males. The age of onset is usually in the 60 s to 70 s. Familial ALS accounts for 5% to 10% of cases.

## 4.4 Symptoms

### 4.4.1 Subjective Symptoms

Muscle weakness in all four limbs, dysarthria, and dysphagia appear and progress. In the initial stage, it is commonly observed muscle weakness on one side of the hand or upper limb. It becomes difficult to use chopsticks and writing becomes poor. In many cases, the inability to open the lid of a plastic bottle is noticed. Dysarthria and dysphagia may be the first symptoms. The onset of lower extremity disease is often noticed by difficulty in walking or climbing of stairs. Muscle atrophy and weakness extend to the extremities, trunk, and globe, and the patient becomes bedridden. In addition, respiratory muscle dysfunction leads to respiratory failure and death, or the need for a ventilator.

### 4.4.2 Objective Symptoms

The presence of both upper and lower neuron signs is essential for a definitive diagnosis. The upper neuron signs include increased tendon reflexes in the extremities, spasticity, and pathological reflexes such as clonus and Babinski's sign (Table 16.6). Lower neuron signs include muscle atrophy and weakness, often asymmetrical in appearance. Fasciculation is a characteristic sign and is often observed at rest in muscle groups with progressive atrophy, such as the quadriceps muscle, shoulder girdle muscles, intrinsic muscles, and tongue. In addition, dysarthria, dysphagia, and atrophy of the tongue are observed due to bulbar palsy. Decreased cognitive function is another symptom that should be noted. About half of the patients have cognitive decline detectable by neuropsychological examination. Some patients are diagnosed as having frontotemporal dementia due to significant cognitive decline. Negative symptoms include ocular motility disorder, sensory disturbance, and rectovesical disturbance; however, even in the late stage, the extraocular muscles, anal sphincter, urinary muscles, cardiac muscles, and smooth muscles are usually unaffected, and bedsores do not occur.

**Table 16.6** Upper and lower neuron signs

| | Upper neuron sign | Lower neuron sign |
|---|---|---|
| Muscle weakness | Advanced | Slight degree |
| Muscle atrophy | Advanced | Without |
| Clumsiness | Advanced | Slight degree |
| Fasciculation | Existence (at the present moment) | Without |
| Muscle tension | Decreased | Accelerated |
| Tendon reflex | Decreased or absent | Accelerated |
| Pathologic reflexes of the lower extremities | Without | Occasionally appears |

## 4.5 Clinical Examination

### 4.5.1 Needle Electromyogram

It is an important test to identify disorders of the lower motor neurons. Acute denervation findings include fibrillation potentials, fasciculation potentials, and positive sharp waves. Chronic denervation findings include increased amplitude, polyphasic motor units, and prolonged duration.

### 4.5.2 Peripheral Nerve Conduction Test

A decrease in the amplitude of compound muscle action potentials and a decrease in the frequency of F waves may be observed. This is important to rule out demyelinating neuropathy.

### 4.5.3 MRI

T2-weighted images of the head may show high signal in the pyramidal tract and low signal in the motor cortex. However, the positive rate is not high. MRI of the spinal cord is useful in differentiating cervical spondylosis.

## 4.6 Classification

As mentioned above, the onset type is sporadic and hereditary. It can be divided into the following three groups according to the degree of impairment of the upper motor neurons and lower motor neurons. (1) Classical type: the upper and lower motor neurons are damaged to the same degree. (2) Progressive muscular atrophy type: almost only lower motor neurons are affected, and muscle atrophy and weakness are observed, but no increased tendon reflexes or pathological reflexes as signs of upper motor neurons are observed. The differentiation from the adult form of spinal muscular atrophy can be difficult. (3) Primary lateral sclerosis type: almost all upper motor neurons are affected, and there is no muscle atrophy or weakness.

## 4.7 Treatment

There is still no fundamental treatment for the disease. The effectiveness of currently available drugs is limited, and symptomatic treatment and nursing care are the mainstays of treatment. Riluzole and edaravone have been used to slow the progression of the disease. Riluzole is thought to have a protective effect on neurons mainly by inhibiting glutamate-induced excitotoxicity. Riluzole has a limited effect, prolonging survival by only 2 to 3 months. In addition, edaravone, a free radical scavenger, was covered by insurance in 2015 in Japan, which has been shown to have an inhibitory effect on the progression of the early stages of the disease. Many ALS patients experience pain. The causes include painful muscle spasms, spasticity, contractures, pressure from immobility, and psychological factors. Antiepileptic drugs, muscle relaxants, and nonsteroidal anti-inflammatory drugs are used, and morphine is used when these drugs are not effective. Dysphagia may cause sialorrhea. Tricyclic antidepressants may be effective. The use of a low-pressure continuous aspirator dedicated to saliva is also recommended. As ALS progresses, respiratory failure may occur due to respiratory muscle damage. Noninvasive positive pressure ventilation (NPPV) and tracheostomy positive pressure ventilation (TPPV) are available as ventilatory therapies, and the survival time of TPPV patients (mean 49.1 months) is significantly longer than that of non-TPPV patients (mean 35.8 months).

## 4.8 Recent Findings

Research is being actively conducted to develop more effective therapies; as of June 2019, clinical trials of several drugs are underway, including a new ALS treatment candidate found by a drug screening approach using patient-derived iPS cells.

## 4.9 Notes from Dentistry Perspective

Takaaki Kamatani

Amyotrophic lateral sclerosis (ALS) is a neurodegenerative disease first described by Charcot in France in 1869, characterized by rapid symptom progression and an average survival of 2 to 5 years. It is designated as an intractable neurological disease in Japan [42].

About one quarter of ALS patients are said to have bulbar palsy type, in which the initial symptoms are dysarthria and eating disorder caused by the dysfunction of the IX to XII cerebral nerves. Patients may not be diagnosed even if they visit multiple medical institutions with the main complaints of difficulty in speaking and swallowing. The diagnosis of ALS requires a differential diagnosis based on many professional examinations in the field of neurology, including motor neuron disorders, peripheral neuropathies, neuromuscular junction diseases, and cerebrospinal diseases. When findings such as atrophy of the tongue and fasciculation, which is a small spasm of the muscle surface, are observed, the dentist should exclude temporomandibular joint disease and dental disease and then refer the patient to a neurologist [43].

In advanced cases of bulbar palsy, muscle atrophy causes tongue movement disorder, so tongue massage is recommended. In cases of severe spasticity, the patient may have difficulty in opening the mouth due to increased muscle tone; instruct rehabilitation that opens the mouth wide consciously several times daily. If the patient bites down hard on the teeth, the cheek or tongue may be bitten. In such cases, a mouthpiece can be made to protect the cheek and tongue [44].

As the symptoms of bulbar palsy progress, it becomes difficult to bolus formation in the oral cavity and feed them into the pharynx, resulting in increased residual bolus of food in the pharynx and a higher risk of aspiration. In patients with advanced ALS, abnormalities in the neuromodulation of saliva secretion can lead to increased saliva production at rest, resulting in severe sialorrhea and aspiration of saliva. In such cases, the use of a low-pressure continuous aspirator for saliva that mechanically aspirates saliva is effective [45].

Anticholinergics can decrease salivary secretion in patients with increased salivation, but are contraindicated in patients with glaucoma or prostatic hypertrophy. Application of scopolamine ointment to the parotid gland equivalent and tricyclic antidepressants can decrease salivation in patients with depression or emotional dysregulation [45, 46]. Since these drugs are prescribed by physicians, dentists need to work closely with them in providing oral care. Although botulinum toxin is reported to be effective for sialorrhea [45, 46], it is not covered by health insurance in Japan and is contraindicated in ALS. Patients with ALS severity I or II may receive intravenous edaravone [47]. When renal excretion antimicrobial agents are administered from the dentist to such patients, caution should be exercised because concomitant use may exacerbate renal dysfunction.

In addition, impaired respiratory function increases the risk of aspiration by reducing the ability to cough adequately. Peak cough flow (PCF) is a simple test to estimate the risk of aspiration, and cough assistance is required when the PCF is below 270 L/min, and noninvasive positive pressure ventilation (NPPV) is required when the PCF is below 160 L/min [45].

Thus, the degree of dependence on medical care increases as ALS progresses. While sharing information with specialists, occupational therapists, speech therapists, home visit nursing care stations, and nursing care workers, visiting dentists, together with dental hygienists, need to support patients' recuperation by providing dental treatment focusing on oral care [45]. The dentist plays a major role in preventing aspiration pneumonia by maintaining oral hygiene, giving instructions on the form of meals, and providing swallowing training [44].

## References


1. American Psychiatric Association. Diagnostic and statistical manual of mental disorders. Fifth Ed. DSM-5. Arlington, TX: VA: American Psychiatric Association; 2013.
2. Braak H, Braak E. Neuropathological staging of Alzheimer-related changes. Acta Neuropathol. 1991;82(4):239–59.
3. Braak H, Del Tredici K, Rub U, et al. Staging of brain pathology related to sporadic Parkinson's disease. Neurobiol Aging. 2003;24(2):197–211.
4. Research group on future projections of the elderly population with dementia in Japan. Health and labor science research Grant-in-aid for special research on health, labour and welfare sciences. Research on the future estimation of the elderly population with dementia in Japan. 2015. (in Japanese).
5. The Japanese Society of Neurology (Supervised). Guidelines for the Treatment of Dementia Diseases Committee. Dementia Disease Diagnosis Guidelines for Dementia Care 2017 (Ninchishou shikkan shinryou guideline). Tokyo; Igakushoin. 2017. p 6–7; (in Japanese).
6. MHLW Science research Grant Comprehensive research project for dementia control: prevalence of dementia in urban areas and response to functional impairment of life in dementia: a comprehensive research report for 2011–2012 (Toshibu niokeru ninchishou yuubyouritsu to ninchishou no seikatsukinoushougai heno taiou H23–24). 2013; (in Japanese).
7. The Japanese Society of Neurology. Committee for "Guidelines for the Diagnosis and Treatment of Dementia" Guidelines for the Diagnosis and Treatment of Dementia 2017. (Ninchishou shikkan shinryou guideline 2017). Tokyo; Igakushoin. 2017. p 19–22; (in Japanese).
8. The Japanese Society of Neurology Committee for "Guidelines for the Diagnosis and Treatment

of Dementia" Guidelines for the Diagnosis and Treatment of Dementia 2017. (Ninchishou shikkan shinryou guideline 2017). Tokyo; Igaku Shoin. 2017. p 204–205; (in Japanese).
9. Goldberg LS, Altman KW. The role of gastrostomy tube placement in advanced dementia with dysphagia: a critical review. Clin Interv Aging. 2014;9:1733–9.
10. The Japanese Society of Neurology. Committee for "Guidelines for the Diagnosis and Treatment of Dementia" Guidelines for the Diagnosis and Treatment of Dementia 2017. (Ninchishou shikkan shinryou guideline 2017). Tokyo; Igaku Shoin. 2017. p 118–138; (in Japanese).
11. FDA Grants Accelerated Approval for Alzheimer's Drug. US Food and Drug Administration. https://www.fda.gov/news-events/press-announcements/fda-grants-accelerated-approval-alzheimers-drug. Accessed 7 Jun 2021.
12. Aragón F, et al. Oral health in Alzheimer's disease: a multicenter case-control study. Clin Oral Investig. 2018;22:3061–70.
13. Tonsker PP, et al. Periodontal disease, tooth loss and dementia: Is there a link? A systemic review. Gerodontology. 2017;34:151–63.
14. Oue H, et al. Tooth loss induces memory impairment and neuronal cell loss in APP transgenic mice. Behav Brain Res. 2013;252:318–25.
15. The Japanese Academy of Clinical Periodontology. HP: http://www.jacp.net/perio/effect/ (in Japanese).
16. Shintani T, et al. Serum antibody titer test against Porphyromonas gingivalis infection (Kansenshou nitaisuru kesseikoutaika kensa). Nichikokukenkaishi. 2018;10(1):39–43; (in Japanese).
17. Shankar GM, et al. Amyloid-beta protein dimers isolated directly from Alzheimer's brains impair synaptic plasticity and memory. Nat Med. 2008;14(8):837–42.
18. Engelhart MJ, et al. Inflammatory proteins in plasma and the risk of dementia: the Rotterdam study. Arch Neurol. 2004;61(5):668–72.
19. Sparks SP, et al. Serum antibodies to periodontal pathogens are a risk factor for Alzheimer's disease. Alzheimers Dement. 2013;8(3):196–203.
20. Poole S, et al. Determining the presence of periodontopathic virulence factors in short-term postmortem Alzheimer's disease brain tissue. J Alzheimers Dis. 2013;36(4):665–77.
21. Ishida N, et al. Periodontitis induced by bacterial infection exacerbates features of Alzheimer's disease in transgenic mice. NPJ Aging Mech Dis. 2017;3(5):15. https://doi.org/10.1038/s41514-017-0015-x.
22. Kamer AR, et al. TNF-alpha and antibodies to periodontal bacteria discriminate between Alzheimer's disease patients and normal subjects. J Neuroimmunol. 2009;219:92–7.
23. Holmes C, et al. Systemic inflammation and disease progression in Alzheimer disease. Neurology. 2009;73(10):768–74.
24. Dominy SS, et al. Porphyromonas gingivalis in Alzheimer's disease brains: evidence for disease causation and treatment with small-molecule inhibitors. Sci Adv. 2019;5(1):eaau3333. https://doi.org/10.1126/sciadv.aau3333.
25. Saji N, et al. Analysis of the relationship between the gut microbiome and dementia:a cross-sectional study conducted in Japan. Sci Rep. 2019;9(1):1008.
26. Michikawa S, et al. Dentistry and dementia (Shika to ninchishou). Tokyo: Media; 2015; (in Japanese).
27. Fisher RS, et al. Operational classification of seizure types by the international league against epilepsy: position paper of the ILAE commission and terminology. Epilepsia. 2017;58(4):522–30.
28. Sheffer IE, et al. ILAE classification of the epilepsies: position paper of the ILAE commission for classification and terminology. Epilepsia. 2017;58(4):512–21.
29. Japanese Society of Neurology, Committee for Epilepsy Treatment Guidelines. Guidelines for the treatment of epilepsy 2018, 1st Ed. Tokyo; Igakushoin; 2018, p 15–16; (in Japanese).
30. Shirasu K, Furusato K. Oral surgery (kouku gekagaku). 3rd ed. Tokyo: Ishiyakushuppan; 2011. p. 229–30; (in Japanese).
31. Casetta I, et al. Phenytoin-induced gingival overgrowth: a community-based cross-sectional study in Ferrara, Italy. Neuroepidemiology. 1997;16(6):296–303.
32. Kato T. Study on the mechanism of collagen metabolism in phenytoin-induced gingival overgrowth. (Fenitoin yuuhatsusei shiniku zoushokushou ni kansuru koragen taishakikou no kaiseki). Shiyakuryohou. 2008;27:86–91; (in Japanese).
33. Shinotsuka O. Epilepsy and dentistry for the disabled (Tenkan to shougaisha shika). Epilepsy. 2013;7(2):107–11; (in Japanese).
34. Sugiyama K. Hiyari-hatto: what to do in such a situation? First aid techniques during dental treatment (Hiyari-hatto: Konnatoki Dousuru? Shikachiryou no Kyukyu Technique). Tokyo: Nagamatsu shoten; 2005. p. 74–9; (in Japanese).
35. Seppi K, et al. Update on treatments for nonmotor symptoms of parkinson's disease—an evidence-based medicine review. Mov Disord. 2019;34(2):180–98.
36. Seppi K, Ray Chaudhuri K, Coelho M, Fox SH, Katzenschlager R, Perez Lloret S, Weintraub D, Sampaio C. The collaborators of the Parkinson's disease update on non-motor symptoms study group on behalf of the movement disorders society evidence-based medicine committee. Update on treatments for nonmotor symptoms of Parkinson's disease-an evidence-based medicine review. Mov Disord. 2019;34:180–98.
37. DeBowes SL, et al. Parkinson's disease:considerations for dental hygienists. Int J Dent Hyg. 2013;11:15–21.
38. Shirakawa M. Dental treatment for the sick (Yubyoushashikashinryo). Tokyo: Ishiyaku shuppan; 2000. p. 85–8; (in Japanese).
39. Nishida M. Illustrated guidelines for dental treatment of the sick elderly. Tokyo: Quintessence Publishing; 2008. p. 235–7; (in Japanese).
40. Japanese Society of Neurology. Guidelines for the treatment of amyotrophic lateral sclerosis 2013;

https://www.neurology-jp.org/guidelinem/als2013_index.html (in Japanese) https://www.neurology-jp.org/guidelinem/als2013_index.html.

41. Japan ALS Association. Information on treatment research and clinical trials; http://alsjapan.org/2019/06/15/post-2398/. (in Japanese).
42. Ando T. Borderline areas amyotrophic lateral sclerosis misdiagnosed as spinal cord disease neurological diseases that are prone to happen. (Kyoukai ryouiki shitteokitai kinishukusei sokusakukoukashou sekitsu-isekizuishikkan to goshin shiyasui shinkeinaikateki shikkan). Rinseigai. 2018;53(11):1020–2; (in Japanese).
43. Tomomatsu N, et al. A case of amyotrophic lateral sclerosis (ALS)associated with oral symptom (Koukushoujou wo shusoni raiinshita ALS no 1 rei). Nichiguchigaishi. 2014;60(3):142–6; (in Japanese).
44. Umemoto G. How to cooperate with dentistry—to support the lives of the elderly—collaborative care with dentistry for neuromuscular diseases (Shikatono renkeiwo dousuru koureishano seikatsuwo sasaerutameni. Shinkeikinshikkanno shinryou niokeru shikatono renkei). Prog Med. 2017;37(10):1157–61; (in Japanese).
45. Ogino M. Amyotrophic lateral sclerosis. Respiratory care for amyotrophic lateral sclerosis (Kinishukusei sokusakukoukashou. Kinishukuseisokusakukoukashou no kokyukanri). Jpn J Rehabil Med. 2018;55(7):545–50; (in Japanese).
46. Matsuda C, et al. Analysis of resting salivation rate in patients with amyotrophic lateral sclerosis using tracheostomy invasive ventilation (Kikansekkai kayouatsukanki dounyuugo no kinishukusei sokusakukoukashoukanjano anseiji daekibunpitsuryou). Clin Nerve. 2016;56(7):465–71; (in Japanese).
47. Yoshino H. Subjects of regional alliances for amyotrophic lateral sclerosis~from the standpoint of neurology clinic (Kinishukuseisokusakukoukashou no chiikirenkei no kadai. Shinkeinaika clinic no tachibakara). Neurotherapy. 2017;34(3):273–4; (in Japanese).

# Neuropsychiatry Diseases

# 17

Kotaro Otsuka, Seigo Ohba, Asaki Matsuzaki,
Tetsuaki Arai, Tadaharu Kobayashi,
and Norifumi Nakamura

## 1 Schizophrenia

Kotaro Otsuka

### 1.1 Concept, Definition, and Pathophysiology

Schizophrenia is known as a disorder with a high prevalence in adolescents. Schizophrenia is characterized by positive symptoms such as hallucinations, delusions, thought disorder, and disturbance of self-awareness, and negative symptoms such as blunted affect, autism, social withdrawal, and abulia and apathy. In the acute phase, positive symptoms such as hallucinations and delusions appear, and in the chronic phase, negative symptoms such as decreased motivation and blunted affect, and social activities are affected depending on the degree of neurocognitive dysfunction. The diagnosis is made according to the ICD classification or the DSM classification of the American Psychiatric Association. Many patients require long-term, continuous pharmacotherapy. Patients also receive a wide range of care, such as psychiatric rehabilitation and employment support, while leading a social life.

K. Otsuka
Department of Neuropsychiatry, Iwate Medical University School of Medicine, Yahaba, Iwate, Japan

S. Ohba
Department of Regenerative Oral Surgery, Graduate School of Biomedical Sciences, Nagasaki University, Nagasaki, Japan

A. Matsuzaki · T. Arai (✉)
Psychiatric Department, University of Tsukuba, Tsukuba, Ibaraki, Japan
e-mail: 4632tetsu@md.tsukuba.ac.jp

T. Kobayashi
Division of Reconstructive Surgery for Oral and Maxillofacial Region, Department of Tissue Regeneration and Reconstruction, Niigata University Graduate School of Medical and Dental Sciences, Niigata, Japan

N. Nakamura
Kagoshima University, Kagoshima, Japan

Department of Oral and Maxillofacial Surgery, Universitas Indonesia, Jakarta, Japan

### 1.2 Symptoms

#### 1.2.1 Hallucinations

Hallucinations are often observed in schizophrenia, including verbal auditory hallucinations (phantom voices) in which a person's voice can be heard, auditory hallucinations in which a person speaks and responds, and visual hallucinations in which a person's thoughts can be heard as voices. Sensory hallucinations are also often observed, in which abnormalities in bodily sensations are experienced in the form of hallucinations. In addition, tactile hallucination such as "touching the body," olfactory hallucination, gustatory hallucination, visual hallucination are also sometimes observed.


T. Chiba, H. Yamada (eds.), *Internal Medicine for Dental Treatments*,
https://doi.org/10.1007/978-981-99-3296-2_17

#### 1.2.2 Delusion

Delusions are classified into primary delusions, in which we intuitively have false beliefs, and secondary delusions, which are based on other experiences such as emotions and are understandable to some extent. Typical types of delusions include delusion of persecution, delusion of reference, delusion of observation, delusion of pursuit, and delusion of poisoning.

#### 1.2.3 Disturbance of Self-Awareness

Self-consciousness disorder refers to a disturbance in the sense of self-identity, that is, the sense that one's thoughts and actions belong to oneself. For example, in depersonalization, the sense of reality is lost. In addition, the experience of being made (artifice experience) is an experience in which the self is influenced and moved by external forces, deprivation of thought, thought insertion, thought propagation, mind reading are recognized.

#### 1.2.4 Obstacles to Thought Path

Disorders of the thought process are often present, including loosening association, incoherent thinking, blocking of thought.

#### 1.2.5 Abnormalities of Mood

In the acute phase, anxiety, emotional instability, and excitement are also observed, but often there is blunting of emotions and flattening of emotions, which is a state of diminished emotional response to external stimuli. In addition, sometimes the depression may increase when the symptoms are alleviated, and it is necessary to pay attention to the post-schizophrenic depression and the risk of suicide.

#### 1.2.6 Impairment of Motivation

Disorders of motivation may include the following symptoms: stupor, catatonic stupor, abulia, rejection, and stereotypy.

#### 1.2.7 Neurocognitive Dysfunction

In schizophrenia, neurocognitive dysfunction in various domains is observed, including impaired attention, processing speed and fluency, problem-solving ability, memory, and working memory.

### 1.3 Treatment

The goals of care for schizophrenia (WHO) are (1) to identify the illness as soon as possible; (2) to treat the symptoms; (3) to provide the patient and family with skills; (4) to maintain improvement over time; (5) to prevent relapse; and (6) to reintegrate the patient into the community so that he or she can lead a normal life [1]. In order to achieve these goals, the following are important in treatment: (a) pharmacotherapy to control symptoms and prevent recurrence; (b) education and psychosocial interventions to help patients and their families cope with the disease and its complications and to prevent recurrence; and (c) rehabilitation to reintegrate patients into the community and to help them reacquire educational and vocational functions [1].

Psychosocial treatments include psychotherapy, which focuses on the patient's problems while building a trusting relationship with the patient, compliance with medication, and life concerns; psychoeducation, which promotes understanding of the disease; social skill training (SST), which is based on learning social skills; and occupational therapy (OT), which focuses on occupational activities.

Pharmacotherapy is the most important part of treatment. The risk of relapse in first-episode schizophrenic patients with medication interruption is very high, 4.89 times, and 4.57 times for second-episode schizophrenic patients [2], it is important to continue pharmacotherapy. Delay in treatment causes a number of disadvantages, such as delayed recovery, poorer prognosis, reduced psychosocial skills, loss of family and social support, increased suicide risk, and higher health care costs [3].

The mainstay of pharmacotherapy is antipsychotic medication, which includes standard and second-generation (atypical) antipsychotics. Standard antipsychotics, introduced 50 years ago, help to reduce or eliminate symptoms of schizophrenia, such as thought disorder, hallucinations and delusions, and reduce associated symptoms, such as excitement, impulsiveness, and aggression, such as chlorpromazine (1955), levomepromazine (1960) and haloperidol (1964). The side effects of long-term treatment with typical antipsychotics are listed in Table 17.1.

**Table 17.1** Side effects of long-term treatment with standard antipsychotic agents

| | |
|---|---|
| 1. Extrapyramidal symptoms | Parkinsonism, Dyskinesia, Dystonia, Akathisia, Malignant syndrome |
| 2. Anticholinergic action | Constipation, thirst, etc. |
| 3. Antihistamine action | Drowsiness, sedation, weight gain |
| 4. Anti $\alpha_1$ action | Low blood pressure |
| 5. Others | Hyperprolactinemia (amenorrhea), polydipsia (water intoxication), etc. |

Second-generation antipsychotics such as risperidone (1996), olanzapine (2001), quetiapine (2001), perospirone (2001), aripiprazole (2006), blonanserin (2008), clozapine (2009), paliperidone (2011), asenapine maleate (2016), brexpiprazole (2018), and lurasidone (2020) are expected to reduce side effects, reduce neurocognitive impairment, and improve relapse rates and medication adherence as well as positive symptoms. On the other hand, some drugs pose a risk of diabetes mellitus.

## 1.4 Medical Considerations in Dental Interventions

1. **How to proceed with treatment according to the pathophysiology:** In schizophrenia, anxiety, hallucinations, delusions, and the ability to understand the treatment affect the patient's condition. It is necessary to determine whether the patient can fully understand the dental treatment. In schizophrenia, treatment based on the patient's understanding and consent is preferred as much as possible, and therefore, careful and easy-to-understand explanations of treatment are required. On the other hand, when hallucinations or delusions impair the patient's ability to recognize reality, it is desirable to confirm and share information with psychiatrists, family members and other guardians, medical social workers, nurses, and other staff involved in the care of the patient.
2. **Impact on oral hygiene:** Schizophrenia may affect social life and the management of one's own daily life, and oral hygiene activities such as tooth brushing may not be sufficient. Because high goals may prevent the patient from engaging in oral hygiene activities, it is important to set smaller goals and a step-by-step approach to treatment and care, if necessary.
3. **Changes in pain expression due to psychiatric conditions:** Dental-related pain may be modified by anxiety or delusion. In some cases, the patient may not complain of pain due to negative symptoms. Therefore, it is advisable to conduct examinations and checkups, and to make careful and objective evaluations.
4. **Effects of antipsychotic medications:** Dry mouth may be caused by anticholinergic effects, and it is not uncommon for patients to have dry mouth and poor oral hygiene. It is also not uncommon for patients to suffer from lifestyle-related diseases such as diabetes mellitus. On the other hand, it should be noted that gingival hyperplasia may occur in patients taking antiepileptic drugs, for example, due to long-term phenytoin medication.
5. **Medication during dental anesthesia and surgery:** Consideration should be given to the method of administration of psychiatric medications during dental anesthesia, surgery, and fasting. For example, it is desirable to confirm the contents of the medication, to confirm interactions, and to confirm whether it is possible to choose the method of medication or discontinuation of medication, etc. If necessary, it is desirable to consult, inquire about, or confirm information with a psychiatrist who is providing psychiatric treatment. It is also important to keep in mind that discontinuation of antipsychotics may cause serious side effects such as malignant syndrome with high fever, extrapyramidal symptoms, autonomic symptoms, and CK (creatine kinase) elevation.

## 1.5 Notes from Dentistry Perspective

Seigo Ohba

### 1.5.1 Dentist Issues

Schizophrenia is a disease that is observed in approximately 1 in 100 people [4]. It has been suggested that they need oral care because they are unconcerned with oral hygiene, inadequate brushing due to extrapyramidal symptoms, and secretion of saliva is suppressed by the anticholinergic effects of antipsychotic drugs. However, many dentists do not have accurate and sufficient knowledge about this illness [5], thus schizophrenic patients do not have sufficient dental intervention. When patients are well-controlled by their neuropsychiatrists, they usually undergo general dental treatment without troubles. On the other hand, when their condition is unstable, dental intervention may be difficult because of strong beliefs and unpredictable behavior [5]. It is important to manage patients according to their individual condition with correct understanding of the pathophysiology of schizophrenia. Dental treatment of patients with schizophrenia should be performed in collaboration with their attending physician. It is one of the most critical areas requiring collaboration between medical and dental fields. In addition, a good relationship with the key person of the patient is also a necessary process [6].

### 1.5.2 Points to Keep in Mind During Dental Treatment

#### Dental Caries

The manner of pain management is the same as that in normal subjects in dental treatment.

Secondary caries may occur easily in unstable condition because of inadequate self-oral care.

Some antipsychotic drugs have $\alpha_1$-receptor blocking effects. Therefore, when adrenaline-containing lidocaine hydrochloride injection is used for local anesthesia, $\beta_2$ activity may predominate due to the blockade of $\alpha_1$-activity by adrenaline, resulting in decrease in blood pressure [7].

Patients are sometimes unconscious for the esthetics of the anterior teeth region [8].

#### Denture

Patients sometimes do not accept wearing dentures [9].

### 1.5.3 Nagasaki University Hospital

In the Department of Special Care Dentistry, Nagasaki University Hospital, the environment surrounding the patients is changed based on their character and condition. For example, in the case of patients with a possibility of self-injurious behavior, sharp instruments are not placed where they can be seen. In the case of patients with claustrophobia, treatment is performed in open area. In addition, dental treatment is basically performed in a horizontal position, and if necessary, intravenous sedation is performed and body movements are suppressed by using some devices (Fig. 17.1). The number of dental treatments are 26 times in patients, who are under treatment for schizophrenia in the Department of Neuropsychiatry, at the Department of Special Care Dentistry in 2018. The patients were treated mainly for dental caries and new dentures, and the treatments progressed without any problems in all treatments. The patients were able to undergo the same treatment as a healthy person such as imaging exams, local anesthesia, and taking impression. However, some patients did not visit for treatment without contacting, indicating the difficulty of continuous dental intervention for schizophrenic patients.

### 1.5.4 Summary

Dental treatment for schizophrenic patients is usually performed the same as that for normal patients. Each treatment should be performed simple and painless. It is important to understand the pathological condition and respond flexibly because the symptom of schizophrenia shows rise and fall repeatedly. It is also important to create a good relationship with the patient's physician and key persons, and to provide patients with easy-to-understand explanations.

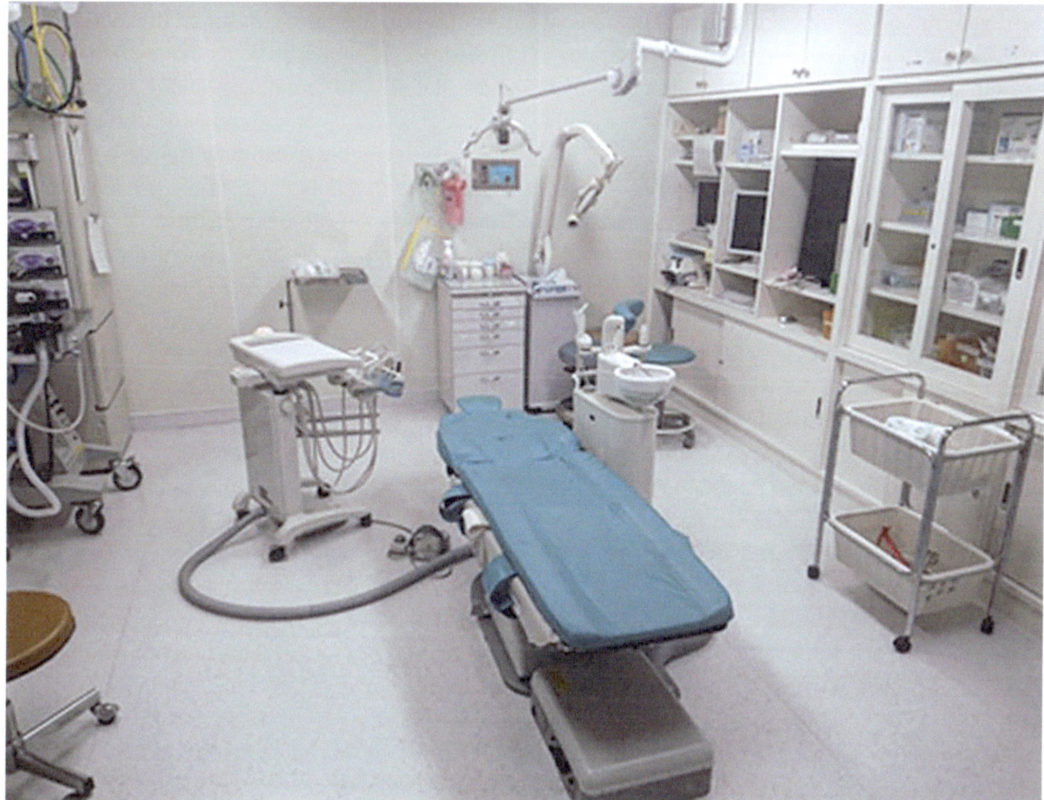

**Fig. 17.1** Clinical scene

## 2 Depression/Bipolar Disorder

Asaki Matsuzaki

### 2.1 Disease Overview

The depressive state is characterized by depressed mood and decreased motivation, while the manic state is characterized by elevated mood and increased activity. Depression (Major depressive disorder) occurs only in the depressed state, and bipolar disorder occurs in both the depressed and manic states. Depression and bipolar disorder are collectively referred to as mood disorders. This article mainly focuses on the diagnostic criteria of DSM-5 (Diagnostic and Statistical Manual of Mental Disorders, Fifth Edition).

### 2.2 Pathophysiology

Everybody experiences a fall and the surge of the feeling, the symptoms of depression and bipolar disorder can be understood as an extension of the mood swings experienced by normal people. However, the medical treatment of depression and bipolar disorder should not be equated with mood swings in normal subjects. Depression is considered to be a dysfunction of the brain caused by several interrelated conditions, including dysfunction of the serotonin, noradrenaline, and dopamine nervous systems, persistently high cortisol levels due to dysfunction of the hypothalamic–pituitary–adrenal system, and hippocampal atrophy. Bipolar disorder is a disorder of biological rhythms. Bipolar disorder is thought to be a dysregulation of biological rhythms. The clinical difficulty lies in the fact that the pathophysiology of both disorders differs greatly, although they are similar in that they both produce mainly depressive states.

### 2.3 Epidemiology

The 12-month prevalence of depression is estimated to be 7%, which is very high. The 12-month prevalence of bipolar disorder, which meets the definition of bipolar disorder, is approximately 1%, but the broader concept of the bipolar spectrum is several times more common. Depression is twice as common in women as in men, and there is almost no difference between men and women in bipolar disorder.

### 2.4 Classifications

Patients may be further classified according to other characteristics after meeting the diagnostic criteria for depression and bipolar disorder. The DSM-5 covers "with melancholic features" is considered to be the core group of depressive states with features such as anorexia, early morning awakening, and morning exacerbation; "with atypical features" such as overeating and hypersomnia; "with anxious distress" with strong anxiety; "with psychotic features" with delusions; "with catatonia" with stupor; "with seasonal pattern" with depression in autumn and winter; "with peripartum onset" with depression during pregnancy and after childbirth. The DSM-5 does not indicate a single condition, but rather the characteristics of symptoms and the timing of onset/exacerbation, which can be both depression and bipolar disorder. Other concepts have been proposed for depression in different situations, such as post-move-out depression, post-promotion depression, empty nest syndrome, and burnout.

There are two types of bipolar disorder: bipolar I disorder, in which patients experience manic (and often depressive) states that require hospitalization or interfere with social life, and bipolar II disorder, in which patients experience depressive states and relatively mild hypomania. Although there is no difference in the treatment itself, it is possible to estimate the strength of the manic state that may occur in the future from the diagnosis. An unstable bipolar disorder that experiences manic or depressive episodes four or more times in 1 year is called "rapid cycling."

### 2.5 Symptoms

In depression, only a depressed state occurs. In bipolar disorder, mania/hypomania and depression can occur, with bipolar I spending an average of more than three times as long in depression as in mania, and bipolar II spending an average of more than 30 times as long in depression as in hypomania. Both depression and bipolar disorder produce approximately the same amount of depression.

Depression in the DSM-5 is defined as 5 or more of following 9 symptoms for 2 weeks or more, depressed mood, decreased interest and pleasure in all things, decreased (or increased) weight and appetite, insomnia (or hypersomnia), psychomotor agitation such as fidgeting and restlessness, and psychomotor inhibition such as slowed speech and movement, fatigue and low energy, feelings of worthlessness and excessive guilt, decreased ability to think and concentrate, difficulty making decisions, and suicidal ideation.

In the DSM-5, the core symptoms of mania are mood changes and increased activity, such as mood elevation and talking to everyone, openness and anger, as well as the diagnostic criteria include the number and duration of the following other seven symptoms: enlarged or exaggerated self-esteem, decreased need for sleep, polyvalence (or the desire to keep talking), and rapid changes in topic (flight of ideas), and the feeling of multiple thoughts rushing in one's mind, distractibility, increased activity and psychomotor agitation, and enthusiasm for shopping, sexual activity, and investing.

## 2.6 Clinical Examination

There are no clinical biochemical or physiological tests to confirm the diagnosis of depression or bipolar disorder. Head imaging and biochemical tests may be used to exclude mood disorders of physical origin.

To screen for depression and assess its severity, self-administered rating scales such as PHQ-9 (Patient Health Questionnaire), QIDS (Quick Inventory of Depressive Symptomatology), BDI (Beck Depression Inventory), and interviewer-administered rating scales such as MADRS (Montgomery Åsberg Depression Rating Scale), HAM-D or HDRS (Hamilton Rating Scale for Depression) may also be used.

## 2.7 Treatment

For everyday depression, general advice and distraction from others may be helpful. However, for those who are medically diagnosed with a mood disorder, medical treatment should be advised rather than general advice and instructions. In other words, we should not lecture or reprimand the patient in an attempt to correct his thinking, and we should not encourage distraction (except voluntarily).

Do not hesitate to ask if the person has suicidal ideation. Frequently, depressed patients have thoughts of dying a rare death. We should then verbalize that we hope they will not commit suicide. When the patient has strong thoughts of dying, they should be hospitalized.

### 2.7.1 Depression

Rest is required. Psychotherapy by a psychiatrist and counseling by a psychologist are useful, and specialized treatment such as cognitive–behavioral therapy may be used. Antidepressants are required for patients with moderate or severe depression. SSRIs (selective serotonin reuptake inhibitors), SNRIs (serotonin–noradrenalin reuptake inhibitors), and NaSSAs (noradrenergic specific serotonergic antidepressants) are mainly used as antidepressants, and sometimes tricyclic and tetracyclic antidepressants with stronger side effects, mainly anticholinergic, are used. Antidepressants are started in small doses and may be associated with nausea in the early stages. The dose is gradually increased to a sufficient level to achieve remission. After satisfactory improvement, continuous treatment for more than 6 months may be required, after which the dose may be tapered and discontinued in some cases, while in other cases, long-term maintenance therapy may be required. Sudden discontinuation of therapy should be avoided, as it may lead to relapse or recurrence. Atypical antipsychotic agents such as aripiprazole may be used in small doses as adjunctive therapy.

### 2.7.2 Bipolar Disorder

Mood stabilizers are drugs used to treat bipolar disorder, including lithium carbonate, valproate, carbamazepine, lamotrigine, and atypical antipsychotic agents (aripiprazole, quetiapine, olanzapine, lurasidone, asenapine, etc). Prolonged use of mood stabilizers is required in depressed, manic, and normal moods, which are neither depressed nor manic. It is also helpful to regulate the rhythm of life, for example, by getting light in the morning and avoiding staying up late.

Mood disorders are often associated with insomnia and anxiety, which are undesirable, but concomitant use of benzodiazepine receptor agonists is not uncommon in actual clinical practice.

## 2.8 Prognosis

### 2.8.1 Depression

The average age of onset is about 30 years, but it can occur at any age, and the onset in old age is not uncommon. The course of the disease varies: some cases are temporary and remission is achieved with treatment and treatment is completed, some cases are remitted with treatment but relapse after treatment is completed and require long-term treatment, and some cases relapse repeatedly or become chronic even with continued treatment. It is not uncommon for a person diagnosed with depression to later be found to have bipolar disorder because of manic symptoms during the course of treatment.

### 2.8.2 Bipolar Disorder

It tends to occur at a younger age than depression, with an age of onset of about 20 years. It is a chronic disease with persistent mood swings if untreated, and remission may be achieved with long-term adherence to effective treatment.

## 2.9 Recent Findings, etc.

Bipolar disorder is more strongly suspected in patients with refractory depression, including recurrent depression, failure of antidepressant medications, recurrent depression despite continued use of seemingly effective antidepressants, and younger onset of depression.

## 2.10 Notes from Dentistry Perspective

Tadaharu Kobayashi

A medical interview is important in the dental care of patients with depression or bipolar disorder to determine the presence or absence of these disorders based on medications and other factors, but patients themselves are often unaware of their condition. Depressed patients often present to medical institutions complaining of physical symptoms rather than psychological symptoms. Patients with depression who visit a dental clinic often complain of unidentified complaints such as xerostomia, tongue pain, taste disorder, denture incompatibility, and temporomandibular joint symptoms. Patients with depression may also present with oral cenesthopathy, which is an incomprehensible oral abnormality localized in the oral cavity. Therefore, it is important to pay attention to the characteristic symptoms of depression during the medical interview and to collaborate with psychiatrists for depressed patients.

When depressive symptoms become severe, psychomotor inhibition decreases interest and motivation to do things, and also decreases motivation to brush, which tends to lead to poor oral hygiene [10]. Sleep disorders such as insomnia also appear frequently, the body's rhythm becomes irregular, and the body and brain remain in a state of fatigue, leading to decreased resistance and an increased susceptibility to dental caries and periodontal disease. In addition, when antidepressants or antipsychotics are prescribed for treatment, their anticholinergic effect suppresses the secretion of saliva, resulting in dry mouth as a side effect and worsening of symptoms such as dental caries and periodontal disease. Dystonia, parkinsonism, and oral dyskinesia may also be observed as extrapyramidal symptoms due to the side effects of antipsychotic drugs.

In the medical examination, listen to the patient's complaints acceptably even if they are verbose and difficult to understand, and proceed with the examination while building a relationship of trust. It is also important not to encourage depressed patients unnecessarily. The patient should be referred to psychiatry or psychosomatic medicine, if deemed necessary. Irreversible treatments such as crown restorations, tooth extractions, extirpation of pulp, occlusal treatment, and new dentures should be avoided when the patient's adaptive capacity is judged to be impaired, and full-scale treatment should be performed after the depressive state improves. Patients with parkinsonism or oral dyskinesia due to the side effects of antipsychotic drugs have unstable jaw position and should be treated with caution.

Because many psychiatric patients receive psychotropic drugs, interactions with dental medications should also be considered. Tricyclic antidepressants and MAO inhibitors inhibit the reuptake of catecholamines at adrenergic nerve endings, increase the concentration of catecholamines at receptors, and potentiate adrenergic neurostimulation. The use of adrenaline-added lidocaine hydrochloride preparations should be minimized, but it is reported that there is no effect on the circulatory system if the number of dental cartridges is up to 2 (3.6 mL) [11].

#### 2.10.1 Epinephrine–Phenothiazine Interaction

Phenothiazine antipsychotics (mainly for the treatment of schizophrenia) have $\alpha_1$ receptor blocking effects, and when used in combination with adrenaline, the $\alpha_1$ effects of adrenaline are blocked and the $\beta_2$ receptor stimulating effects predominate, which may cause a serious decrease in blood pressure. Adrenaline-added lidocaine hydrochloride preparations for medical use are contraindicated in combination with antipsychotic drugs, whereas dental adrenaline-added lidocaine hydrochloride preparations are cautioned against concomitant use with antipsychotic drugs. This may be because the amount of drug routinely used in dentistry is lower than that of medical preparations. In a survey on the use of dental adrenaline-added lidocaine hydrochloride preparations in patients who regularly use antipsychotic drugs in Japan, the frequency of hypotension suspected to be caused by interaction with adrenaline was 0.014%, and no serious cases were reported [12]. Therefore, the risk of hypotension in patients treated with antipsychotic drugs is low if the dose of adrenaline used in routine dental practice is administered, careful observation of hemodynamics is important.

## 3 Alcoholism and Drug Dependency

Kotaro Otsuka

### 3.1 About Dependence Syndrome

There are two types of dependence: mental dependence and physical dependence. Mental dependence is a state of mind in which we cannot help using drugs, and physical dependence is a state in which withdrawal symptoms (tremors, sweating, irritability, insomnia, hallucinations, convulsions, etc.) appear when we stop using drugs. While mental dependence is essential, the characteristics of physical dependence differ depending on the substance.

It is known that the brain reward system (A10 nervous system) from the ventral tegmental area of the midbrain to the nucleus accumbens is involved in the dependence formation and enhances dopamine neurotransmission. In addition, tolerance to the substance emerges, and repeated use of the substance makes it difficult to produce an effect, and the dose increases unintentionally. Furthermore, even if they try to reduce their substance use, they are unable to do so, and they have control problems such as not being able to follow their own prescribed doses. Then, they spend a great deal of money and time to obtain and use substances, and use them even at the expense of their occupation, hobbies, and personal relationships. As a result, they continue to use substances even though they know that they have health, social, and legal problems, because they cannot stop. On the other hand, they often admit to denying the reality of their use, saying that it has nothing to do with the cause of their ill-health.

Alcohol, tobacco, nicotine, and other drugs with age restrictions, stimulants, dangerous drugs, organic solvents, and marijuana are legally regulated. Because dependence can also occur due to prescription medications, therefore it is necessary to check for the formation of dependence when prescribing drugs with dependence potential, and to take pharmacotherapeutic approaches to avoid the formation of dependence.

### 3.2 Diagnosis of Dependence Syndrome and Alcohol Dependence (Table 17.2)

According to ICD-10, a diagnosis should be made only when three or more of the following items are present, usually during the past year [13].

In addition to alcohol dependence, other mental disorders such as depression and dependence on other substance use often overlap.

**Table 17.2** Summary of diagnosis of dependence syndrome (clinical features in parentheses)

| |
|---|
| 1. Strong desire or urgency for substance use (desire to drink alcohol) |
| 2. Apparent impairment of control over the extent to which substance-taking behaviors are initiated, terminated, or used (inability to stop drinking) |
| 3. Physical withdrawal when substance use is reduced or stopped (withdrawal symptoms appear) |
| 4. Evidence of tolerance to the effects of the substance (getting used to it) |
| 5. Being preoccupied with substance use. The pleasures and interests to choose that are important for substance use are completely absent or diminished (you can only see alcohol) |
| 6. Continuing to use a substance despite evidence that it has obvious harmful consequences (knowing it's bad for you, but not being able to stop) |

**Table 17.3** Major physical diseases comorbid with alcohol dependence

| |
|---|
| 1. Acute poisoning |
| 2. Alcoholic hepatitis, fatty liver, liver cirrhosis, liver cancer, liver dysfunction |
| 3. Gastric ulcer, gastritis, gastric cancer, pancreatitis, diabetes mellitus, cancer of the oral cavity and esophagus, esophageal varices, Mallory-Weiss syndrome |
| 4. Hypertension, arrhythmia, cardiomyopathy, bleeding tendency, anemia, dehydration |
| 5. Cerebral atrophy, alcohol withdrawal syndrome, cerebral hemorrhage, vitamin deficiency, Wernicke-Korsakoff syndrome |
| 6. Femur head necrosis, peripheral neuritis, gout |
| 7. Hypothermia, coexistence with other drug intoxication |

## 3.3 Major Physical Diseases Comorbid with Alcohol Dependence (Table 17.3)

Attention should be paid to the possible presence of a variety of physical illnesses that may coexist with alcohol dependence.

## 3.4 Primary Care for Dependency

The change from dependency has the following stages.

1. **Precontemplation phase:** They are not aware of the problem and do not consider the necessity of change.
2. **Contemplation phase:** Thinking about the good and bad points of one's own substance use, but not deciding to change it (insufficient information, unresolved ambivalence).
3. **Preparatory phase: R**eady to take action for change.
4. **Behavioral phase: A**ttempts to change and begins to avoid situations that trigger substance use.
5. **Maintenance phase:** The patient has completely changed and efforts are being made to prevent reversion to use.

We need to "adjust" the information and support we provide to the person based on where they are in the stages, and consider where they are in these stages in their care. For example, if the person is in the precontemplation stage, they may not be ready to change from dependency, so changing the dependency behavior will take time and many steps. It may be necessary to suppress the urge to correct, ask if they want information, and if they express interest, provide them with information about alcohol and drugs and how they may affect them, and discuss how to use them with less harm to their health and how to recognize an overdose. Handing out leaflets on alcoholism in a non-pressured atmosphere is one way of doing this. In the case of a contemplative to preparatory phase, elicit the individual's spontaneity and contemplate the prioritization of values. Understanding the ambivalence of wanting and not wanting to use, and motivational interviewing to elicit language for supportive change of choice are considered effective. On the other hand, overly directive and guilt-tripping approaches, for example, are not always effective because they damage self-esteem.

Another important approach is to discuss options for seeking help from family physicians and specialists, referrals to government health counseling services such as public health centers and mental health welfare centers, referrals to self-help groups such as Alcoholics Anonymous, and referrals to psychiatric and other specialized medical facilities.

In the treatment of addiction, alcohol abstinence and withdrawal is the principle of treatment. However, the concept of harm reduction, which is to reduce harmful use as much as possible, such as reducing the amount of alcohol in the treatment of alcoholism, is spreading.

## 3.5 Medical Considerations in Dental Interventions

### 3.5.1 Alcohol Dependence and Poor Oral Hygiene

In alcohol-dependent patients, dehydration and decreased saliva secretion lead to dryness of the oral cavity and deterioration of the oral environment. The presence of carious teeth and periodontitis is not uncommon. In addition, gingivitis and stomatitis may occur with vitamin deficiency. Plaque and dental calculus may also be present due to insufficient oral hygiene activities.

### 3.5.2 Withdrawal Syndrome Due to Discontinuation of Alcohol Use or Substance Use, and Substance Use

In the inpatient treatment of dentistry, for example, alcohol and substance use may be interrupted due to the need for surgery. After that, withdrawal syndrome may occur, and serious symptoms such as delirium may appear. Therefore, it is necessary to confirm the status of use in advance. In addition, due to the symptoms of dependence, for example, substances may be brought into the hospital ward during hospitalization treatment, leading to use—careful observation is necessary.

### 3.5.3 How to Proceed with Treatment According to the Condition

It is necessary to consider the approach based on the stage of dependence. Naturally, treatment based on the patient's understanding and consent is prioritized as much as possible, and therefore, careful and easy-to-understand explanations are required. On the other hand, there are cases in which legal problems arise, such as drunk driving and dangerous driving in the case of alcohol, and illegal possession and use of drugs in the case of drugs. In difficult cases, cooperation with relevant institutions such as public health centers and the police may be necessary. In addition, if treatment is already underway, it is desirable to confirm and share information with psychiatrists who are treating the mental disorder, family members and other guardians, medical social workers, nurses, and other staff involved in the care.

### 3.5.4 Comorbid Physical Complications

They may present with physical complications due to alcohol or substance use. In addition, they often have lifestyle-related diseases such as diabetes mellitus. The physical condition of the patient should be carefully monitored.

### 3.5.5 Medication During Dental Anesthesia and Surgery

It is necessary to confirm the interaction between alcohol and the drugs used when performing dental anesthesia. In addition, it is necessary to consider selection and dosage of the medicine because cross-resistance to barbiturates and other drugs occurs when tolerance is formed by alcohol dependence.

### 3.5.6 Notes from Dentistry Perspective

Norifumi Nakamura

#### Alcoholism

According to the Ministry of Health, Labour and Welfare (MHLW), Japan, alcohol dependence is "a condition in which the mental and physical functions of the body are continuously or chronically impaired due to dependence on alcohol as a result of repeated and heavy alcohol consumption". Alcoholism is diagnosed when three or more of the following six symptoms (craving to drink, difficulty in controlling drinking behavior, withdrawal symptoms such as headache and irritability, increased tolerance, life centered on drinking, and loss of control over alcohol) have continued for at least 1 month at a time or have appeared repeatedly in the past year [14].

Chronic diseases that may develop in people who drink large amounts of alcohol over a period of years include hypertension, alcoholic hepatitis, and alcoholic gastritis, as well as psychiatric disorders such as alcoholic delirium and hallucinations. The effects of alcoholism on oral health include a higher risk of developing multiple dental caries and gingival disease due to general poor oral hygiene or erosion of the teeth caused by the reflux of gastric juices from frequent vomiting. Salivary glands, especially the parotid gland, may become swollen in long-term drinkers, leading to impaired salivary gland metabolism and excretion, resulting in decreased saliva secretion, which in turn may cause multiple dental caries. In addition, when malnutrition and other factors are added to alcoholism, the immune system is lowered, causing glossitis, angular cheilitis, and gingivitis [15]. Alcohol consumption is considered a potential risk factor for oral cancer, and when consumed with tobacco, it increases the risk of oral cancer.

#### Drug Dependence

Drug dependency is a psychiatric disorder in which continuous use of a drug results in the formation of a drug tolerance that diminishes the effectiveness of the drug, leading to withdrawal symptoms and craving. Major drugs of abuse such as stimulants, sedatives and sleeping pills, and narcotics are regulated by law. Amphetamine-like substances are representative of stimulants, and the severe tooth caries seen in methamphetamine abusers is called "Meth Mouth" (Fig. 17.2) [16]. Methamphetamine tooth caries is caused by a combination of the direct effects of acidic contaminant residues used in the methamphetamine manufacturing process, physiological changes brought about by the inhibition of saliva secretion and xerostomia due to the pharmacological effects of the drug, long-term poor oral hygiene, frequent intake of high-calorie foods and carbonated beverages, and wear caused by teeth clenching.

If alcohol or drug addiction is suspected based on oral symptoms, a dentist should provide oral hygiene guidance and recommend treatment at a specialized medical institution.

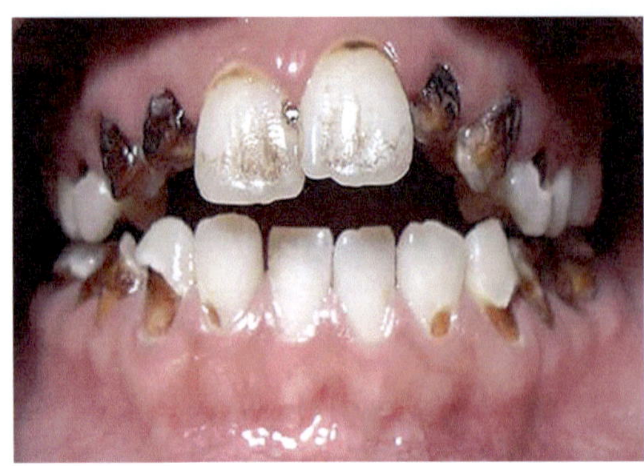

**Fig. 17.2** Oral symptoms that appear to be "Meth Mouth" (reproduced from [16]). Creative Commons Attribution-Share Alike 3.0

## References


1. WHO. The World health report 2001: mental health: new understanding, new hope. Geneva: WHO; 2001. p. 150–5.
2. Binson D, et al. Predictors of relapse following response from a first episode of schizophrenia or schizoaffective disorder. Arch Gen Psychiatry. 1999;56(3):241–7.
3. Mizuno M. Toward the prevention of schizophrenia (Tougoushicchoushou no Yobou ni Mukete). Human Mind. 2005;120:118–23; (in Japanese).
4. Ministry of Health, Labour and Welfare. https://www.mhlw.go.jp/kokoro/know/disease_into.html.
5. Janardhanan T, et al. Dental care and associated factors among older adults with schizorphrenia. JADA. 2011;142:57–65.
6. Nakamura H. A longitudinal study on problems encountered in the long-term dental treatment of a schizophrenic patient (Tougoushicchoushou no Chouki Shikachiryoujyou no Mondaiten nikansuru Jyudanteki Kentou). Japanese J Psychosom Dent. 2008;23:41–5; (In Japanese).
7. Shibutani T. Treatment of patients taking concomitant medication with adrenaline-containing lidocaine hydrochloride products (adrenaline Ganyu lidocaine Ensanenseizai no Heiyouchuuiyaku wo Fukuyousuru Kanjya heno Taisho). Oral Dent Topic. 2017;23:1–6; (in Japanese).
8. Nakamura H, et al. Clinical study on the reaction of schizophrenic patients to damage and treatment of maxillary anterior teeth -comparisons with healthy persons and other patients. (Jyougakuzenshi no Kison oyobi sono Chiryou nitaisuru Tougoushichoushou Kanjya no Hannou nikansuru Rinshouteki Kentou—Kenjyousha oyobi Tashikkan Kanjya tono Hikaku). Japanese J Psychosom Dent. 2003;18:73–9; (In Japanese).
9. Nakamura H, et al. A difficult denture case concerning a patient with schizophrenia due to severe disturbance

of communication (communication no Ichijirushii Shougai notameni Gishichiryou ni Nanjyu shita Seishinbunretsubyou Kanjya no ichirei). Japanese J Psychosom Dent. 2000;15:185–9; (In Japanese).
10. Hashimoto K, Matsuda H, et al. The relation between depressive state in the workplace and subjective symptoms of oral disorders (Shokuba niokeru Yokuutsujyoutai to Koukuu no Jikakushoujyou). J Japanese Soc Disability Oral Health. 2014;35:601–7; (In Japanese).
11. Kaneko Y. Vasoconstrictor (with local anesthetic) and its usage (Kekkan Shushukuyaku (Kyokushomasuiyaku Tenka) to Sono Tsukaikata). J Japan Dent Assoc. 1996;48(12):1282–96; (In Japanese).
12. Ichinohe T, Shimada M. A questionnaire survey regarding the administration of lidocaine hydrochloride solution containing adrenaline for dental use in regular users of antipsychotics. J Japanese Dent Soc Anesthesiol. 2014;42(2):190–5; (In Japanese).
13. Toru M, Nakane Y, Komiyama M (translation supervisor). ICD-10 mental and behavioral disorders: clinical description and diagnostic guidelines. revised ed. Tokyo; Igaku Shoin. 2005; (In Japanese).
14. Japanese Medical Society of Alcohol and Addiction Studies/The Japanese Society of Alcohol-Related Problems eds. Guide to diagnosis and treatment of alcoholism based on the new guidelines for the diagnosis and treatment of alcohol and drug use disorders. 1st ed. Kyoto; Japanese Medical Society of Alcohol and Addiction Studies/Yokosuka; The Japanese Society of Alcohol-Related Problems. 2018. (In Japanese). https://www.jmsaas.or.jp/wp-content/uploads/pdf/Guide-for-diagnosis-and-treatment-of-alcoholism201907.pdf.
15. Khairnar MR, Wadgave U, Khairnar SM. Effect of alcoholism on oral health: a review. J Alcohol Drug Depend. 2017;5(3):266.
16. Wikipedia. Meth mouth. https://en.wikipedia.org/wiki/Meth_mouth.

# 18 Infectious Diseases

Yuki Yamada, Akira Suwabe, Toshihiro Ito, and Satoshi Goto

## 1 Microbial Substitution

Yuki Yamada, Akira Suwabe

### 1.1 Disease Overview and Pathophysiology

Microorganisms (mostly bacteria, but also fungi, viruses, etc.) inhabit on all surfaces of the human body and in contact with the outside world. These microorganisms are called indigenous microbiota, and bacteria in particular are called indigenous bacterial flora or normal bacterial flora. Bacterial flora in humans exists in the skin, eyes, nasopharynx, gastrointestinal tract from the oral cavity to the anus, and urinary and reproductive organs, and the kinds of bacteria present in these areas vary greatly depending on site, age, gender, race, diet, and lifestyle.

Microbial substitution is a phenomenon in which the normal bacterial flora is disturbed by the abnormal growth of bacteria that normally do not exist or exist only in small numbers due to a decrease in the normal flora. When a broad-spectrum antimicrobial agent is administered, not only the target bacteria but also sensitive strain in the normal flora is reduced. As a result, non-sensitive or resistant bacteria multiply abnormally. The causative microorganisms include fungi such as *Candida* spp., *Pseudomonas aeruginosa*, Gram-negative rods such as *Serratia* spp., and anaerobic bacteria. Clinical manifestations of microbial substitution include oral candidiasis in the oral flora and antimicrobial-associated diarrhea and pseudomembranous enteritis caused by *Clostridioides difficile* infection (CDI) in the intestinal flora. In this section, CDI is mainly described.

### 1.2 Epidemiology

*C. difficile* is a spore-forming, obligatory anaerobe, gram-positive bacillus, and is widely present in the environment. Asymptomatic carriers are found in 5–10% of healthy adults and 15–70% of newborns. Risk factors for the development of CDI are disruption of the intestinal microbiota (e.g., administration of antimicrobial agents and antacids), exposure to *C. difficile* (e.g., prolonged hospitalization), and host factors (e.g., advanced age, serious underlying disease, chemotherapy, tube feeding, laparotomy).

Yuki Yamada was deceased at the time of publication.

Y. Yamada · A. Suwabe
Department of Laboratory Medicine, Iwate Medical University School of Medicine, Yahaba, Iwate, Japan

T. Ito (✉)
Department of Infectious Diseases, National Hospital Organization Sendai Medical Center, Sendai, Miyagi, Japan
e-mail: ito.toshihiro.zw@mail.hosp.go.jp

S. Goto
Department of Oral and Maxillofacial Surgery, National Hospital Organization Sendai Medical Center, Sendai, Miyagi, Japan



T. Chiba, H. Yamada (eds.), *Internal Medicine for Dental Treatments*,
https://doi.org/10.1007/978-981-99-3296-2_18

CDI is the most frequently associated with healthcare-associated diarrhea in adults [1].

### 1.3 Symptoms

The main symptoms of CDI are diarrhea, abdominal pain, and fever. Severe cases suffer from pseudomembranous enteritis, toxic megacolon, paralytic ileus, and gastrointestinal perforation. These occur after exposure to incentive drug (antibacterial drug) for a few days to 2 weeks. The pathogenic factors of CDI are toxin A (enterotoxin) and toxin B (cytotoxin), produced by *C. difficile,* which damage the intestinal tract and cause diarrhea and enteritis. Recently, a third toxin, binary toxin, has attracted attention and has been reported to be associated with severe disease as a highly pathogenic strain. PCR ribotype 027 (BI/NAP1/027), a representative strain that produces this toxin, has been spreading in North America and Europe since the 2000s. This strain has not been spreading in Japan, even though a few cases have been reported [2, 3].

### 1.4 Clinical Examination and Diagnosis

CDI is caused by toxins (toxin A and toxin B) produced by *C. difficile* and is diagnosed by confirmation of these toxins. To improve the detection rate, immunochromatographic antigen detection kits that simultaneously detect the glutamate dehydrogenase (GDH) antigen of all *C. difficile* are used. Nucleic acid amplification technique can determine the presence of toxin with high sensitivity. In addition, colonoscopy is performed to check for the presence of pseudomembranes, which are characteristic of the disease.

Because asymptomatic carriers with toxin-producing strains exist in healthy adults, detection of toxin per se in a human without diarrhea is of little clinical significance. The presence of clinical symptoms is important for the diagnosis of CDI. Japanese guidelines state that testing should be performed only when diarrheal symptoms are present [4]. Furthermore, because asymptomatic carrier of *C. difficile* is common in children, testing should not be performed, and the guidelines do not define CDI in children younger than 2 years [4, 5].

### 1.5 Treatment and Infection Control

The treatment of CDI is to discontinue the causative drug as much as possible. Even if the patient is positive for CD toxin test, treatment is not required if the patient does not have diarrhea. Japanese guidelines [4] recommend metronidazole and vancomycin for non-severe cases and fidaxomicin for severe and recurrent cases as antibacterial agents against *C. difficile.* Bezlotoxumab (anti-toxin B antibody) as a relapsing preventer and probiotics as a prophylactic agent are available.

CDI requires contact infection prevention measures. It is known that *C. difficile* spores spread to the hospital environment by adhering to the hands of healthcare workers and caregivers. Because *C. difficile* spores are resistant to heat and desiccation and are very stable in the environment, they can survive for long periods of time. Furthermore, alcohol disinfection is ineffective, so items suspected of being contaminated should be disinfected with sodium hypochlorite. Medical staff should wear gloves and disposable gowns when in contact with patients and wash their hands with running water and soap.

### 1.6 Recent Findings

As many as 100 trillion bacteria are present in the human intestinal tract. Metagenomic analysis of the intestinal microbiota has identified intestinal bacteria associated with various constitutions and diseases by detecting the proportion of the flora and specific bacteria.

## 2 AIDS (Acquired Immunodeficiency Syndrome)

Toshihiro Ito

### 2.1 Introduction

Acquired Immunodeficiency Syndrome (AIDS) was first reported in June 1981 as an outbreak of pneumocystis pneumonia among the gay (male homosexuals) in Los Angeles. Two years later, it was found to be caused by a viral infection. This is human immunodeficiency virus (HIV) infection. Until the discovery of antiretroviral therapy (ART) in the mid-1990s, this infection meant death, and the route of transmission (sexual intercourse, blood transfusion/needlestick, mother-to-child) and the special characteristics of the infected group led the world to panic. Since the start of ART, by the development of drugs and treatment methods, the lifespan has been similar to that of uninfected people. Now, we can consider HIV infection is chronic disease. The most important things for the control of this infection are to know the existence of this virus in the body and to start ART as soon as possible, and to fight against discrimination and prejudice against HIV-infected people based on social customs and systems, and stigma. Unfortunately, discrimination and prejudice against this disease that arose in the early 1980s has not been eradicated even now, and stigma still swirls around.

## 2.2 Disease Overview

HIV infection is defined as the presence of HIV in the body (or more precisely, the presence of HIV in the host DNA as a provirus), and AIDS is defined as the development of some index disease associated with immunodeficiency (23 types in Japan: Table 18.1 [6, 7]).

## 2.3 Pathophysiology

HIV infection is mainly characterized by immunodeficiency caused by HIV-induced decrease in CD4-positive cells, and if not properly diagnosed

**Table 18.1** AIDS indicator diseases (created based on [6])

| | |
|---|---|
| A. Mycosis | 1. Candidiasis (esophagus, trachea, bronchus, lung)<br>2. Cryptococcosis (other than lung)<br>3. Coccidioidomycosis[a]<br>4. Histoplasmosis[a]<br>5. Pneumocystis pneumonia |
| B. Protozoan infection | 6. Toxoplasmic encephalopathy (after 1 month of age)<br>7. Cryptosporidiosis (with diarrhea lasting more than 1 month)<br>8. Isosporiasis (with diarrhea lasting more than 1 month) |
| C. Bacterial infections | 9. Pyogenic bacterial infection[b]<br>10. Salmonella bacteremia (recurrent, excluding those caused by typhoid bacilli)<br>11. Active tuberculosis (pulmonary tuberculosis or extrapulmonary tuberculosis)[a, c]<br>12. Nontuberculous mycobacterial infection[a] |
| D. Viral infections | 13. Cytomegalovirus infection (after 1 month of age, except liver, spleen, and lymph nodes)<br>14. Herpes simplex virus infection[d]<br>15. Progressive multifocal leukoencephalopathy |
| E. Tumor | 16. Kaposi's sarcoma<br>17. Primary cerebral lymphoma<br>18. Non-Hodgkin lymphoma (a) large cell, immunoblastic type; (b) Burkitt type)<br>19. Invasive cervical cancer[c] |
| F. Others | 20. Recurrent pneumonia<br>21. Lymphocytic interstitial pneumonia/pulmonary lymphoid hyperplasia: LIP/PLH complex (<13 years)<br>22. HIV encephalopathy (dementia or subacute encephalitis)<br>23. HIV exhaustion syndrome (general prostration or slim disease) |

[a](a) Disseminated throughout the body; (b) Occurred in a site other than the lung, neck, or hilar lymph nodes
[b]Those under 13 years of age who have had two or more of the following multiple or recurrent events within 2 years due to pyogenic bacteria such as Hemophilus, Streptococcus, etc. (a) septicemia, (b) pneumonia, (c) meningitis, (d) osteoarthritis, (e) abscesses in sites other than the middle ear or cutaneous mucosa, or in deep organs
[c]For pulmonary tuberculosis among C11 active tuberculosis and E19 invasive cervical cancer, only when symptoms or findings suggestive of HIV-induced immunodeficiency are observed
[d](a) Ulceration of the mucous membrane or skin persisting for more than 1 month (b) Bronchitis, pneumonia, and esophagitis after 1 month of age

and treated, AIDS develops and death occurs in about 10 years.

HIV present in the body fluids of an infected person is transmitted through only three routes. They are (1) sexual intercourse (homosexual/heterosexual); (2) blood transfusion/needle stick (medical accident, sharing of injection devices such as stimulants injections, etc.); and (3) mother-to-child (transplacenta, vaginal, lactation). HIV belongs to the retrovirus family of RNA viruses, and its most distinctive feature is its ability to convert RNA to DNA using its own reverse transcriptase enzyme, and to incorporate it into the host cell's DNA using an integrase. CD4 is the receptor of HIV, and CD4-positive cells (CD4-positive lymphocytes and macrophages), which play a central role in the human immune system, are the target of HIV. As long as the infected cells remain alive, HIV is reproduced and the infected cells are eventually destroyed. A fierce battle between CD4-positive cells and HIV is repeated in vivo, resulting in the host's defeat, which leads to immunodeficiency and the development of AIDS. The disease is classified into three phases: acute phase, asymptomatic carrier, and AIDS phase.

## 2.4 Epidemiology

According to the UNAIDS report of 2020 [8], there are about 38 million people living with HIV in the world, two-thirds of whom are in sub-Saharan Africa, and there is little gender difference. It is said that drug users who inject stimulants, gay, commercial sex workers and their partners, transgenders, are a group with a high risk of infection. In Africa, however, more than half of the people living with HIV are infected by male-to-female, mother-to-child transmission than by these high-risk groups. The annual number of new infections is 1.7 million and the number of AIDS-related deaths is 690,000, both of which are on a downward trend due to the spread of ART implementation. In Japan, the total number of new infections was 31,385 at the end of 2019 (excluding victims of blood products), and the annual number of new reports was 1,236 (333 for AIDS), showing a decreasing trend. MSM (men who have sex with men) and heterosexual contact infections accounted for 67.2% and 15.5%, respectively [9].

## 2.5 Symptoms and Diagnosis

There are no specific clinical symptoms of HIV infection. Symptoms appear in the early phase of infection (acute phase) and during the AIDS phase, and the asymptomatic carrier (AC) phase, which accounts for most of the natural course of the disease, follows a course similar to that of uninfected persons. The acute phase is said to resemble infectious mononucleosis, and it is no different from general viral infections, and subclinical infections are also possible. Since the symptoms of AIDS are also due to complications, HIV diagnosis is impossible unless HIV-related blood examination is performed considering the possibility of HIV infection. Screening tests have a certain percentage of false-positives, and definitive diagnosis is made by blood-based HIV antibody confirmation test (WB or immunochromatography:IC method) or detection of HIV-RNA by PCR method [7]. In the acute phase of the disease, the WB or IC method may produce false negatives, so the PCR method should be used in combination with the WB or IC method, and retesting after a period of time is necessary.

## 2.6 Classification

There are two types, HIV-1 and HIV-2, and it is said that in the beginning of the twentieth century (around 1920), Simian immunodeficiency virus (SIV) that had infected primates in Africa mutated and caused human-to-human infection (HIV) [10]. The former (HIV-1) originated in chimpanzees and the latter (HIV-2) in gorillas and orangutans, and HIV-1 is widespread in humans, while HIV-2 is very rare.

## 2.7 Infection Control

Condoms are effective in preventing sexually transmitted infections, including HIV. However, the difficulty of prevention by condoms has been shown by their histories. About HIV, the current prevention method is to suppress HIV in the blood below the detection limit by ART: treatment as prevention (TasP). It has been confirmed that infected people who have been successfully treated are not sexually transmitted (undetectable equals untransmittable: U=U) [11, 12]. Infection can be prevented by taking anti-HIV drugs even for medical contamination accidents (Post-exposure prophylaxis: PEP) [13]. Although not yet common in Japan, pre-exposure prophylaxis (PrEP) [14], in which anti-HIV medication is taken before sexual intercourse, is effective as a preventive measure for non-infected persons during sexual procedure.

## 2.8 Treatment

The therapeutic philosophy is to promote the recovery of CD4 positive cells and restore the immune system by reducing the HIV present in the body to below the detection limit. Once HIV infection is diagnosed, ART should be initiated as soon as possible.

Drugs used in ART are classified by mechanism of action into nucleoside reverse transcriptase inhibitors (NRTIs), non-nucleoside reverse transcriptase inhibitors (NNRTIs), protease inhibitors (PIs), integrase inhibitors (INSTIs), and entry inhibitors, which are categorized as key drugs (more potent in suppressing HIV) and backbone drugs (complementary to key drugs and enhancing viral suppression). In Japan, there are 37 types of drugs as of March 2020 (including different formulations and fixed-dose combinations). Currently, ART is generally performed with a combination of two NRTIs as the backbone and one key drug. Specific drug selection is based on antiviral effects, side effects, and adherence to medications, Since guidelines for HIV managements are frequently updated annually in the field of intense new drug development, the introduction of ART should be asked of a specialist with medical experience. The most recommended combinations for initial treatment are listed in the table (Fig. 18.1) [6].

## 2.9 Prognosis

If ART is successful, the prognosis is good. Life expectancy is similar to that of uninfected persons. However, if treatment fails for any reason, the patient will have a desperate course as in the previous ART era.

## 2.10 Recent Findings

Recent findings are as follows:

1. Aiming for prevention of infection (TasP, PrEP, and PEP), early diagnosis, and early treatment.
2. Continued development of drugs that take into account adherence to medication and reduction of side effects.
3. Control and eradication of the spread of infection have become the main focus.
4. Countermeasures against aging and associated complications (lifestyle-related diseases and malignant tumors) due to improved prognosis are future problems.

## 2.11 Conclusion

Oral lesions are very important in the diagnosis of immunodeficiency diseases, and dentists play an important role in the early diagnosis of HIV infection.

| Combination | Number of medications | Timing of medication | Number of tabletsper day | Tablets to be taken in a day [CH1] |
|---|---|---|---|---|
| BIC/TAF/FTC | 1 | Unlimited | 1 | 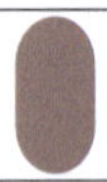 |
| DTG/ABC/3TC | 1 | Unlimited | 1 | |
| DTG + TAF/FTC | 1 | Unlimited | 2 | 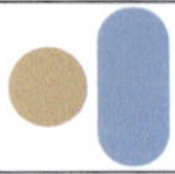 (HT) |
| RAL (600 mg tablet) + TAF/FTC | 1 | Unlimited | 3 | 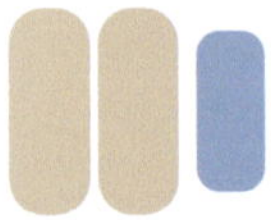 (HT) |
| RAL (400 mg tablet) + TAF/FTC | 2 | Unlimited | 3 | 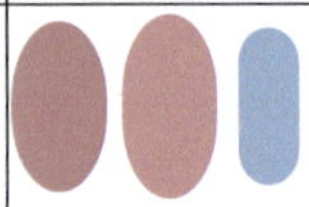 (HT) |
| DRV/cobi/TAF/FTC | 1 | During and immediately after a meal | 1 | 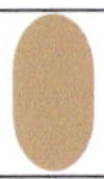 |
| DRV + rtv + TAF/FTC | 1 | During and immediately after a meal | 3 | 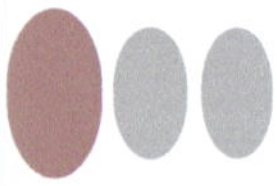 (LT) |
| RPV/TAF/FTC | 1 | During and immediately after a meal | 1 | 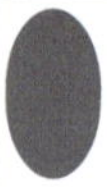 |

BIC: Bictegravir, TAF: Tenofovir alafenamide, FTC: emtricitabine, DTG: Dolutegravir, ABC: Abacavir 3TC: lamivudine, RAL: Raltegravir, DRV: Darunavir, cobi: Cobicistat, rtv: Ritonavir, RPV: Rilpivirine

**Fig. 18.1** Most recommended combinations for initial ART (created based on [6])

## 2.12 Notes from Dentistry Perspective

Satoshi Goto

### 2.12.1 Dental Treatment of Patients with AIDS (HIV Infection)

Since AIDS (acquired immune deficiency syndrome) is a condition in which HIV-infected patients have symptoms caused by immunodeficiency, it is very rare that dental treatment must be performed when patients have AIDS onset. However, because it takes several years from HIV infection to the onset of AIDS, patients may visit a dentist without being aware of their infection. In addition, about 30% of the cases, the infection is known only after the onset of AIDS, and in some cases, oral symptoms lead to the diagnosis of AIDS. Therefore, it is important to understand the main characteristics of oral symptoms caused by the onset of AIDS and to refer patients to specialized medical institutions. Although there are no

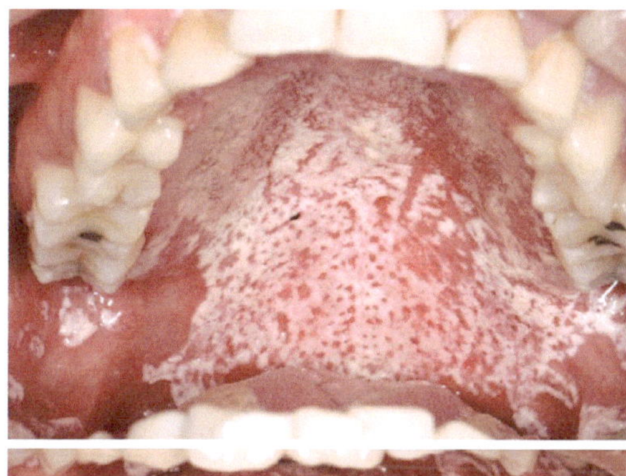

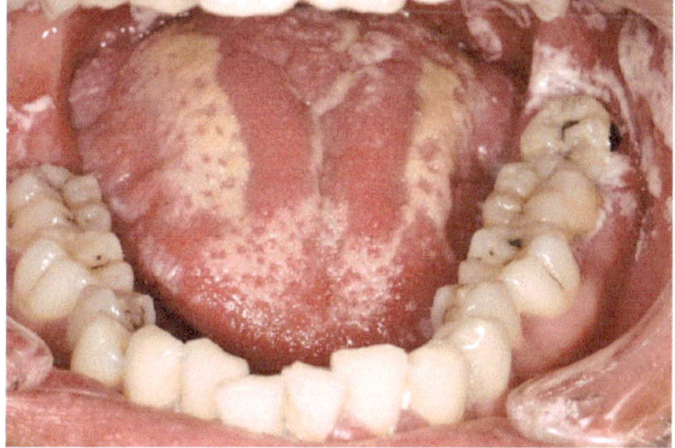

**Fig. 18.2** Oral candidiasis

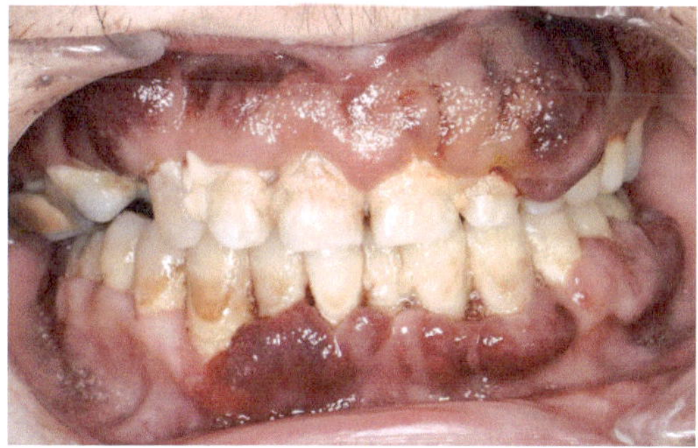

**Fig. 18.3** Gingival Kaposi's sarcoma. (Courtesy of Dr. Yutaka Maruoka, Center Hospital of the National Center for Global Health and Medicine)

diseases specific to the oral cavity in the list of index diseases by the Committee on AIDS Trends of the Ministry of Health, Labour and Welfare, Japan [15], the main oral symptoms include oral candidiasis (Fig. 18.2), Kaposi's sarcoma (Fig. 18.3), lymphoma (Fig. 18.4), and severe marginal periodontitis.

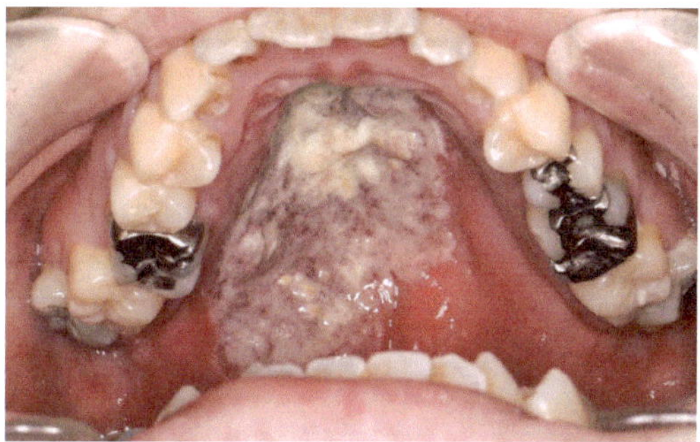

**Fig. 18.4** Malignant lymphoma of the palate. (Courtesy of Dr. Yutaka Maruoka, Center Hospital of the National Center for Global Health and Medicine)

### 2.12.2 Precautions for Dental Treatment

Because of the progress of therapeutic drugs, the viral load of HIV infection can be controlled even after the onset of AIDS, and long-term survival can be expected, the aging of the population and nursing care have become problems. In Japan, the majority of patients are treated at a specialized department. The response rate of therapeutic drugs is high, and the amount of virus in the blood of most patients is said to be below the detection limit if they take the drugs properly. Therefore, dental treatment of patients with controlled disease can be performed in the same manner as that of normal patients, including surgical procedures such as tooth extraction. Dentists should communicate with their primary care physician and receive information on viral load and CD4 levels before undergoing dental treatment. On the other hand, patients with HIV infection may come for dental treatment with a high viral load without being aware of it, so it is important to provide treatment in accordance with standard precautions.

Interactions between HIV medications and other drugs are often a problem in the medical care of HIV-infected patients. The use of antibacterial agents and analgesics frequently used in dentistry does not pose a problem, but the interaction should be checked when sedation is used. In addition, the majority of HIV infections in Japan are sexually transmitted, and it should be kept in mind patients may have a coinfection with other sexually transmitted diseases or viral infections. On the other hand, patients with drug-induced HIV infection have a tendency to bleed because of hemophilia in the background, so it is necessary to communicate with the attending physician if bleeding treatment is necessary.

## References


1. Kachrimanidou M, et al. *Clostridium difficile* infection: a comprehensive review. Crit Rev Microbiol. 2011;37(3):178–87.
2. Rupnik M, et al. *Clostridium difficile* infection: new developments in epidemiology. Nat Rev Microbiol. 2009;7(7):526–36.
3. Knight DR, et al. Diversity and evolution in the genome of *Clostridium difficile*. Clin Microbiol Rev. 2015;28(3):721–41.
4. Kunishima H, et al. The Japanese clinical practice guidelines for management of *Clostridioides (clostridium) difficile* infections. Jpn J Chemother. 2018;66(6):645–90; (in Japanese).
5. McDonald LC, et al. Clinical practice guidelines for *Clostridium difficile* infection in adults and children: 2017 update by the Infectious Diseases Society of America (IDSA) and Society for Healthcare Epidemiology of America (SHEA). Clin Infect Dis. 2018;66(7):987–94.
6. Health and Labor Administration Promotion Research Subsidy for AIDS Control Policy Research Project, HIV Research Group for Overcoming the Challenges of HIV Infections and Their Complications: Guidelines for Anti-HIV Treatment, revised March 2020. (in Japanese). https://hiv-guidelines.jp/pdf/guideline2022.pdf.
7. Committee on AIDS Trends, Ministry of Health, Labour and Welfare. "Ministry of Health, Labour and Welfare, March 8, 2006, Health Inspection Agency No. 0308001, Notification by the Director, Tuberculosis and Infectious Diseases Division, Health Bureau, Ministry of Health, Labour and Welfare. In: HIV infection/AIDS diagnostic criteria for surveillance. Tokyo; Ministry of Health, Labour and Welfare. 2007. (in Japanese). http://www.acc.ncgm.go.jp/information/mhlwinfo/surveillance.html.
8. UNAIDS:FACT SHEET 2020. https://www.unaids.org/sites/default/files/media_asset/UNAIDS_FactSheet_en.pdf.
9. Committee on AIDS Trends, Ministry of Health, Labour and Welfare: 2019 Annual Report on AIDS Outbreaks. 2020. (in Japanese). https://api-net.jfap.or.jp/status/japan/nenpo.html.
10. Faria NR, et al. The early spread and epidemic ignition of HIV-1 in human populations. Science. 2014;346:56–61.
11. Cohen MS, et al. Antiretroviral therapy for the prevention of HIV-1 transmission. NEJM. 2016;375:830–9.
12. Rodger AJ, et al. Risk of HIV transmission through condomless sex in serodifferent HIV transmission through condomless sex in serodifferent gay couples with the HIV-positive PARTNER taking suppressive antiretroviral therapy (PARTNER): final results of a multicenter, prospective, observational study. Lancet. 2019;393:2428–38.
13. Tokyo Metropolitan Collaborating Hospitals for HIV Prevention. Manual for Preventing HIV Infection - Emergency Application in the Event of an Exposure Event - for General Medical Institutions, revised July 2017. (in Japanese). https://www.fukushihoken.metro.tokyo.lg.jp/iryo/koho/kansen.files/manual.pdf.
14. Anderson PL, et al. Emtricitabine-tenofovir concentrations and pre-exposure prophylaxis efficacy in men who have sex with men. Sci Transl Med. 2012;4:151ra125.
15. Aizawa A. General introduction 1. HIV infection/AIDS course. HIV/AIDS manual in the era of long-term care. Tokyo: Manual Japan Medical Journal (Nihon Iji Shinpo Sha); 2014. p. 2–11.

# Pregnancy and Breastfeeding 19

Rie Oyama and Tetsuro Ikebe

## 1 Pregnancy and Lactation

Rie Oyama

### 1.1 Establishment of Pregnancy

#### 1.1.1 Pregnancy

Pregnancy occurs when an egg and a sperm fertilize and that implant into the utrine endometrium lining asn fetrilized egg. Understanding gametogenesis, fertilization, and embryo implantation leads to the understanding of normal and abnormal maternal changes, fetal development, and placentation in pregnancy [1].

### 1.2 Physiology of Pregnancy

Healthy pregnant women have significant physiological changes during pregnancy. Weight gain is approximately 8 to 10 kg during pregnancy due to an increase in the gestational uterus, breasts, and circulating blood volume (or plasma volume), Many changes might almost normalize to their pre-pregnancy state by the end of pregnancy [2].

R. Oyama (✉)
Department of Obstetrics & Gynecology, Iwate Medical University, Yahaba, Iwate, Japan
e-mail: rieoyama@iwate-med.ac.jp

T. Ikebe
Department of Oral and Maxillofacial Surgery, Fukuoka Dental College, Fukuoka, Japan

#### 1.2.1 Material Metabolism

- Maternal insulin resistance begins in the second trimester and peaks in the third trimester.
- There is an increase in total cholesterol and triglyceride levels in pregnancy.
- A pregnant woman requires an increased intake of protein during pregnancy.

#### 1.2.2 Changes in the Cardiovascular System

The resting heart rate increases by about 10 beats per minute. The diaphragm is elevated, the heart is displaced upward to the left, the apex is displaced outward to the left, and shows an enlarged heart on a chest X-ray.

#### 1.2.3 Circulating Blood Volume

At the end of pregnancy, the mean circulating blood volume increases by 40–50% of the non-pregnant level and normalizes to the non-pregnant level within 4–6 weeks after delivery.

#### 1.2.4 Blood Pressure

Peripheral vascular resistance decreases under the influence of progesterone, as the smooth muscle of the blood vessels relaxes and the vessels dilate. As a result, blood pressure remains constant or decreases slightly. In the lower extremities, the gestational uterus compresses the pelvic veins and inferior vena cava, resulting in edema of the lower extremities, varicose veins in the lower extremities and vulva, and


T. Chiba, H. Yamada (eds.), *Internal Medicine for Dental Treatments*,
https://doi.org/10.1007/978-981-99-3296-2_19

hemorrhoids. In the third trimester, the inferior vena cava due to compression of the gestational uterus reduces blood volume in the venous to return into the right ventricular in the supine position, resulting in decreased cardiac output and hypotension.

### 1.2.5 Urinary System

The kidneys enlarge slightly during pregnancy. Glomerular filtration rate (GFR) and renal blood volume increase from early pregnancy, and urine output also increases.

### 1.2.6 Digestive System

The stomach and intestinal tract are compressed by the gestational uterus. Heartburn and constipation are common pregnancy-related digestion symptoms. Constipation and compression of the veins by the gestational uterus predispose to the development of hemorrhoids.

### 1.2.7 Endocrine System

In early pregnancy, maternal free thyroxine (FT4) is mildly elevated and thyroid function is temporarily increased. As pregnancy progresses, Thyroxine binding globulin (TBG) increases, and although total $T_4$ increases with TBG, hyperthyroidism does not occur because TBG causes a loss of thyroid hormone bioactivity.

### 1.2.8 Blood Changes

During pregnancy, the increase in circulating plasma volume exceeds the increase in red blood cells, and hemoglobin, there is a fall in hemoglobin, hematocrit, and red blood cell count. The white blood cell count increases to about 5000–12,000/μL. The platelet count is unchanged or mildly decreased compared with nonpregnant women, averaging 213,000/μL.

## 1.3 Diseases in Early Pregnancy

The most common disorders seen in early pregnancy are hyperemesis gravidarum, miscarriage, ectopic pregnancy, and congenital malformation syndrome related to maternal viral infection.

### 1.3.1 Hyperemesis Gravidarum

Sometimes, the pregnant woman has excessive symptoms such as vomiting almost every day, inability to eat orally, and persistent weight loss with strong positive urine ketone bodies. In addition, it may show liver dysfunction and electrolyte abnormalities due to dehydration and may develop Wernick's encephalopathy due to vitamin $B_1$ deficiency. This is a neurological disorder with various symptoms such as ocular motility disorder, ataxia, and disturbance of consciousness. The prophylactic method is administered 10–50 mg of vitamin B1, B6, B12 with sugar-containing electrolyte solutions [3].

### 1.3.2 Miscarriage

It is defined as an abortion of pregnancy of fewer than 22 weeks in Japan. A spontaneous abortion is defined as an abortion that occurs spontaneously due to fetal or maternal morbidity.

1. Clinical classification.
   (a) Threatened abortion: A condition in which genital bleeding occurs but the uterine cervix is closed and the pregnancy is maintained. In early pregnancy, vaginal spotting is not an entire sign of miscarriage and possible continued pregnancy.
   (b) Inevitable abortion: This is a condition in which the cervix is open and the uterine contents (embryo, villus, a part of gestational sac) are being expelled.
   (c) Missed abortion: A condition in which the fetus remains in the uterus without obvious symptoms, but the fetus has no heartbeat.
   (d) Complete abortion: Complete expulsion of the fetus (or embryo) and fetal tissue.
   (e) Recurrent abortion (miscarriage): Two consecutive miscarriages.
2. Diagnosis

   When a patient with a positive pregnancy test, there is a risk of misdiagnosis of ectopic pregnancy, miscarriage, or hydatidiform mole, if the fetal sac is not obscured due to delayed ovulation. Therefore, a careful interview and ultrasound examination should be performed (Fig. 19.1).

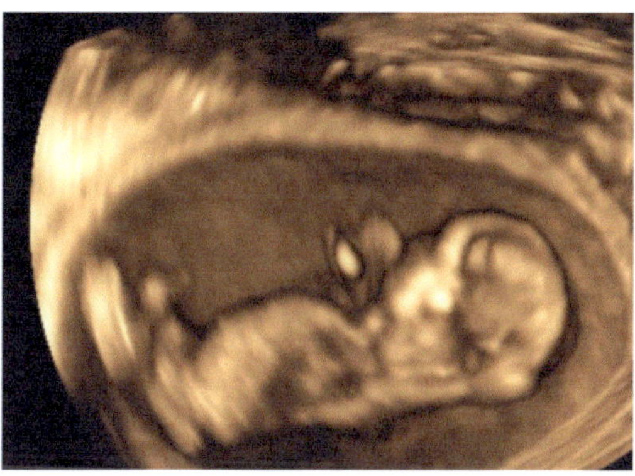

**Fig. 19.1** Three-Dimensional Ultrasound image of a dichorionic diamniotic twins at 10 weeks' gestation

3. Treatment
   (a) Threatened abortion: No effective treatment has been established for threatened abortion at less than 12 weeks' gestation. There is a report that the miscarriage rate was decreased by rest therapy in the case of subchorionic hematoma after the fetal heartbeat was confirmed [4].
   (b) Missed abortion/Inevitable abortion.

   In Japan, the use of drugs such as mifepristone and misoprostol are not approved for the treatment of miscarriages of less than 12 weeks' gestation, so either watchful waiting for a complete abortion or surgical treatment (dilation and curettage or suction evacuation) is selected.

#### 1.3.3 Ectopic Pregnancy

It is a condition in which a fertilized ovum implants in a place other than the uterine cavity and grows to maturity. It can be divided into tubal pregnancy, ovarian pregnancy, and peritoneal pregnancy according to the implantation site of the fertilized ovum [5].

1. Diagnosis
   (a) No evidence of a gestational sac structure in the uterine cavity (after 5–6 weeks gestation).
   (b) A gestational sac-like structure is found outside the uterine cavity.
   (c) Fluid retention in the Douglas pouch is observed.
   (d) A decrease in circulating blood volume (anemia, tachycardia, hypotension) is suspected.
   (e) After probe curettage in the uterine endometrium, no chorionic villi are found in the extracted specimen.
   (f) Indicates acute abdomen.
2. Treatment

   In principle, surgical treatment is performed, but the indications for drug therapy (e.g., methotrexate: MTX) or conservative treatment are determined according to the patient's general condition, implantation site, blood hCG level, presence or absence of fetal heartbeat, mass diameter, and fertility. However, MTX therapy is not covered by insurance in Japan. In case of surgery, either laparotomy or laparoscopy should be chosen.

#### 1.3.4 Maternal Viral Infection

It indicates that a pathogen (virus) infecting the mother infects the child through pregnancy, delivery, and lactation. Currently, rubella is a social problem. In Japan, adult males aged 39 to 56 years who have not been vaccinated against rubella have a great possibility of contracting rubella and transmitting the disease to pregnant women through droplet infection. The Ministry of Health, Labour, and Welfare (MHLW) is recommending rubella vaccination for men aged 39–56 years for 3 years from April 2019 (free of charge in some municipalities). Figure 19.2 shows congenital fetal anomalies caused by maternal infection by pathogens [6].

### 1.4 Pregnancy Complications

Hypertension and diabetes mellitus are the most common complication of pregnancy.

#### 1.4.1 Hypertensive Disorders of Pregnancy

If hypertension develops after 20 weeks of gestation, it is classified as a hypertensive disorder of

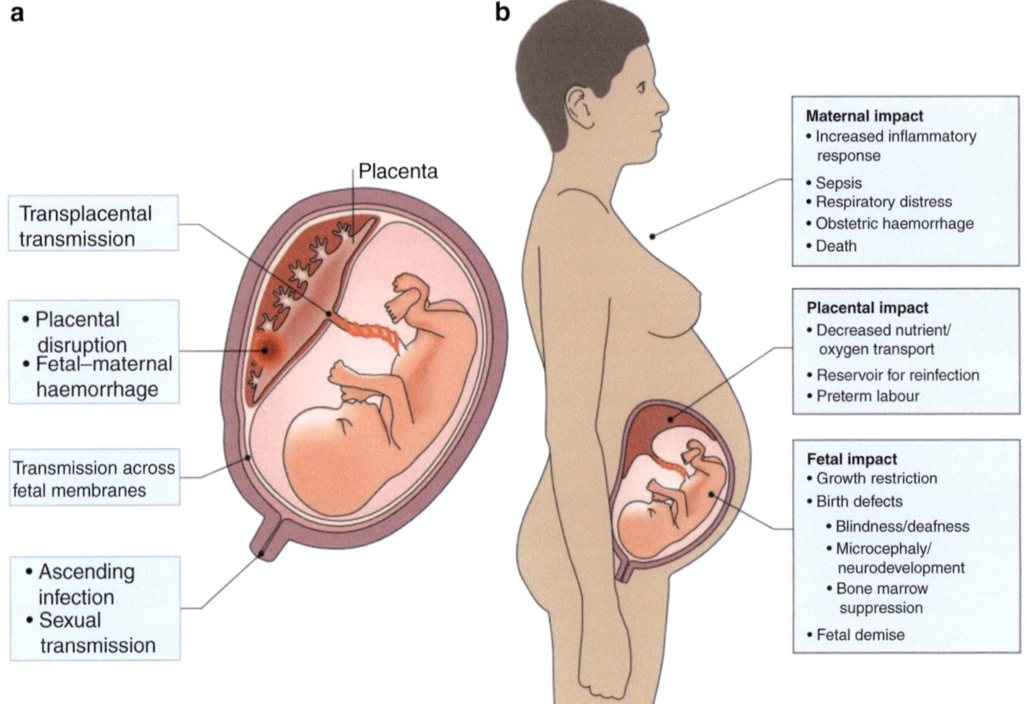


**Fig. 19.2** Routes of transmission across the placenta and consequences of infection (reproduced with permission from [6]). (**a**) TORCH (Toxoplasma gondii, other, rubella virus, cytomegalovirus, herpes simplex virus) pathogens can access the intra-amniotic compartment through multiple mechanisms, including direct transplacental transmission, placental damage or disruption and/or fetal–maternal hemorrhage. In addition, pathogens can be transmitted by ascending the genital tract. (**b**) Infections in pregnancy can affect the maternal host, fetus and/or the placenta itself. The results of infection and the inflammatory response have consequences at each site

pregnancy (HDP), furthermore, if combined with proteinuria,

it may lead to preeclampsia. HDP occurs in approximately 3% to 5% of all pregnancies worldwide. It occurs in 6–8% of first pregnancies, 14–20% of multiple pregnancies, 30% of pregnancies with uterine malformations, and 26% of pregnancies with a family history of hypertension or chronic hypertension [7].

## Pathophysiology and Factors of HDP

In HDP, the failure of trophoblastic cells to invade the spiral arteries of the decidua in the placental bed results in remodeling failure due to narrowing of the diameter of the spiral arteries, leading to fetoplacental circulatory disturbance. This is the first stage of the two-step theory of HDP proposed by Redmann et al. [8]. In the second stage, the production of soluble fms-like tyrosine kinase-1 (sFlt-1), a soluble receptor for a vascular endothelial growth factor (VEGF), and sEng, a soluble receptor for TGF-β1 and β3, increases in chorionic villus cells and enters the fetal placental and maternal circulatory systems due to hypoxia caused by fetoplacental circulatory failure (Fig.19.3).

## Classification by Symptom

1. Mild: Blood pressure: Any of the following cases. Systolic blood pressure of 140 mmHg or more but less than 160 mmHg. Diastolic blood pressure: 90 mmHg or more, less than 110 mmHg. Proteinuria: 0.3 g/day or more.
2. Severe: Blood pressure: Any of the following. Systolic blood pressure of 160 mmHg or higher. Diastolic blood pressure: 110 mmHg or more. Proteinuria: 2 g/day or more.

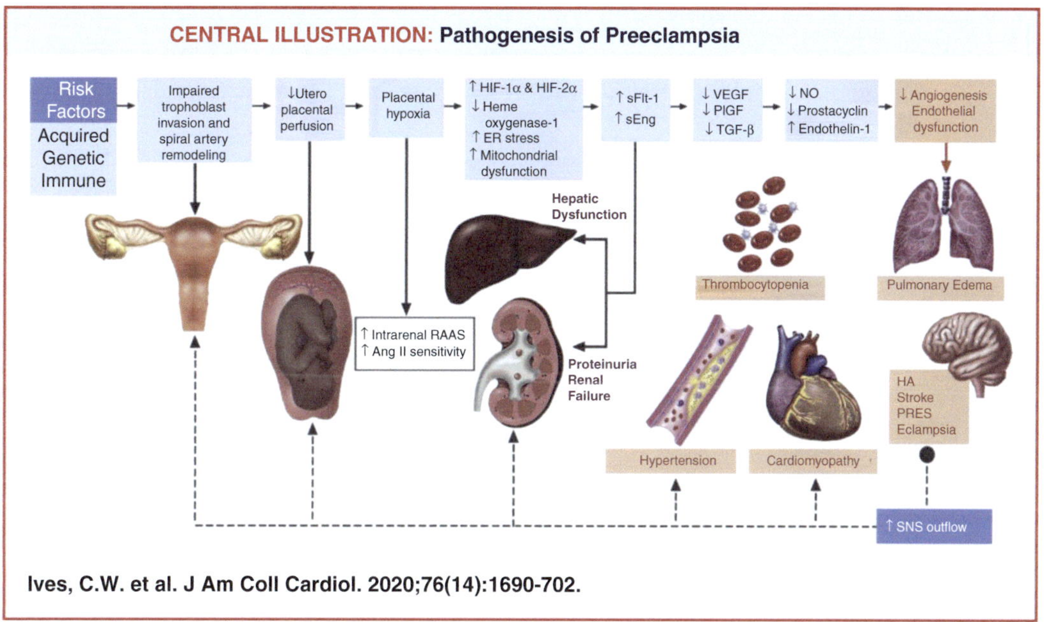


**Fig. 19.3** Pathogenesis of pregnancy-induced hypertension syndrome (reproduced with permission from [9]). Acquired, genetic, and immune risk factors contribute to early placental dysfunction (Stage 1). Placental dysfunction results in release of anti-angiogenic factors, leading to later multiorgan dysfunction (Stage 2). Solid arrows represent progression of disease. Dashed arrows represent SNS effect on respective organs. *Ang II* angiotensin II, *ER* endoplasmic reticulum, *HA* headache, *HIF* hypoxia-inducible transcription factor, *HIF* hypoxia-inducible transcription factor, *NO* nitric oxide, *PlGF* placental growth factor, *PRES* posterior reversible encephalopathy syndrome, *RAAS* renin-angiotensin-aldosterone system, *sEng* soluble endoglin, *sFlt* soluble fms-like tyrosine kinase, *SNS* sympathetic nervous system, *TGF* transforming growth factor, *VEGF* vascular endothelial growth factor. Ivesetal

## Maternal Management and Treatment

Inpatient management is useful because it allows a rapid response to sudden symptom exacerbation.

Caloric intake is calculated according to the individual's age, Body Mass Index (BMI) at non-pregnancy, and physical activity level.

Oral hydralazine or methyldopa is the first-line antihypertensive agent, and if the antihypertensive effect is inadequate, continuous intravenous hydralazine or nicardipine is recommended as the second-line agent. Magnesium sulfate ($MgSO_4$) should be administered to prevent eclampsia associated with hypertension.

## Fetal Management

When fetal growth failure is observed in HDP, fetal well-being should be assessed using the following methods 1 to 4.

1. Non-stress testing (NST).
2. Fetal ultrasound measurement, amniotic fluid volume.
3. Biophysical profiling score (BPS).
4. Blood flow measurement (umbilical artery, middle cerebral artery, uterine artery, etc.)

## Indications for Cesarean Section in HDP

(a) Maternal side factor.
  - When symptoms remain unchanged or worsen in response to hospitalization, bed rest, and medical therapy.
  - Eclampsia, placental abruption, new ocular hemorrhage in the fundus of the eye, increased chest and abdominal fluid, pulmonary edema, intracranial hemorrhage, or HELLP syndrome.
  - If renal dysfunction appears, GFR ≤ 50 mL/min, serum Creatinine≥1.5 mg/dL, serum. Uric

acid≥6 mg/dL, serum BUN≥20 mg/dL, oliguria <300 mL/day or more than 20 mL/day should be decided comprehensively.

- Hemodynamic disorders or abnormalities in blood coagulation, such as hemoconcentration symptoms or DIC (Ht ≥ 40%, platelet count ≤100,000, Fibrinogen≦150 mg/dL) and an increasing DIC score.
- Footnote: The values of 3 and 4 are not absolute, but are indicated when the test is performed over time and an exacerbation trend is observed.

(b) Fetal side factors (in principle, the fetus should be able to live extrauterine).

- Fetal growth restriction: Evaluate the fetal well-being and may need to decide on termination.
- Non-Reassuring Fetal Status (NRFS): fetal heart rate monitoring shows decreased or loss of variability, a sinusoidal pattern, variable deceleration, or prolonged deceleration may be present.

### 1.4.2 Gestational Diabetes and Diabetes Mellitus

Pregnancy is associated with increased insulin resistance due to hormones secreted by the placenta. This tendency increases in the third trimester, and the amount of insulin increases to maintain normal blood sugar levels. There are two types of problems of glucose metabolism in pregnancy: pregnancies complicated by diabetes mellitus, in which diabetes mellitus is present before pregnancy, and the problem of glucose metabolism that is first detected during pregnancy. There are two types of abnormalities of glucose metabolism first detected during pregnancy: GDM, in which blood sugar levels are higher than normal but not high enough to be diagnosed as diabetes mellitus, and diabetes mellitus detected during pregnancy, in which blood sugar levels are high (apparent diabetes mellitus of pregnancy) [10].

#### Diagnosis

Figure 19.4 shows the problems of glucose metabolism and diagnostic criteria in gpregnancy [11].

#### Treatment

(a) Dietary therapy: Non-obese pregnant woman (BMI < 25 at the time of non-pregnancy): Standard weight [height $(m)^2 \times 22$] × 30 + 200 kcal.

(b) Obese pregnant woman (BMI ≥ 25 at non-pregnancy): Standard weight [height $(m)^2 \times$ 22] × 30 kcal.

Pregnancy is characterized by a higher postprandial blood sugar level than that in nonpregnant women. Especially in pregnant women with problem glucose metabolism, the 2-h postprandial blood sugar level increases rapidly. To reduce the fluctuation of blood sugar, it is important to reduce the amount of food per meal and to eat 5 to 6 divided meals to reduce the increase in postprandial blood sugar level.

(c) If the target blood sugar level is exceeded even after diet therapy: Sometimes a woman with gestational diabetes must take insulin [12].

#### Poor Blood Glucose Control

It is known that the risk increases in pregnant women with diabetes who have poor control before and during the first pregnancy trimester. Galindo et al. [13] reported that the incidence of major malformations was 11.7% when the maternal hemoglobin A1c (HbA1c) level was 7–8% and 15.8% when the HbA1c level was 8% or higher.

## 1.5 Postpartum Depression

According to the diagnostic criteria of the American Psychiatric Association, postpartum depression is defined as depressive feelings such as anxiety about baby care, dissatisfaction with

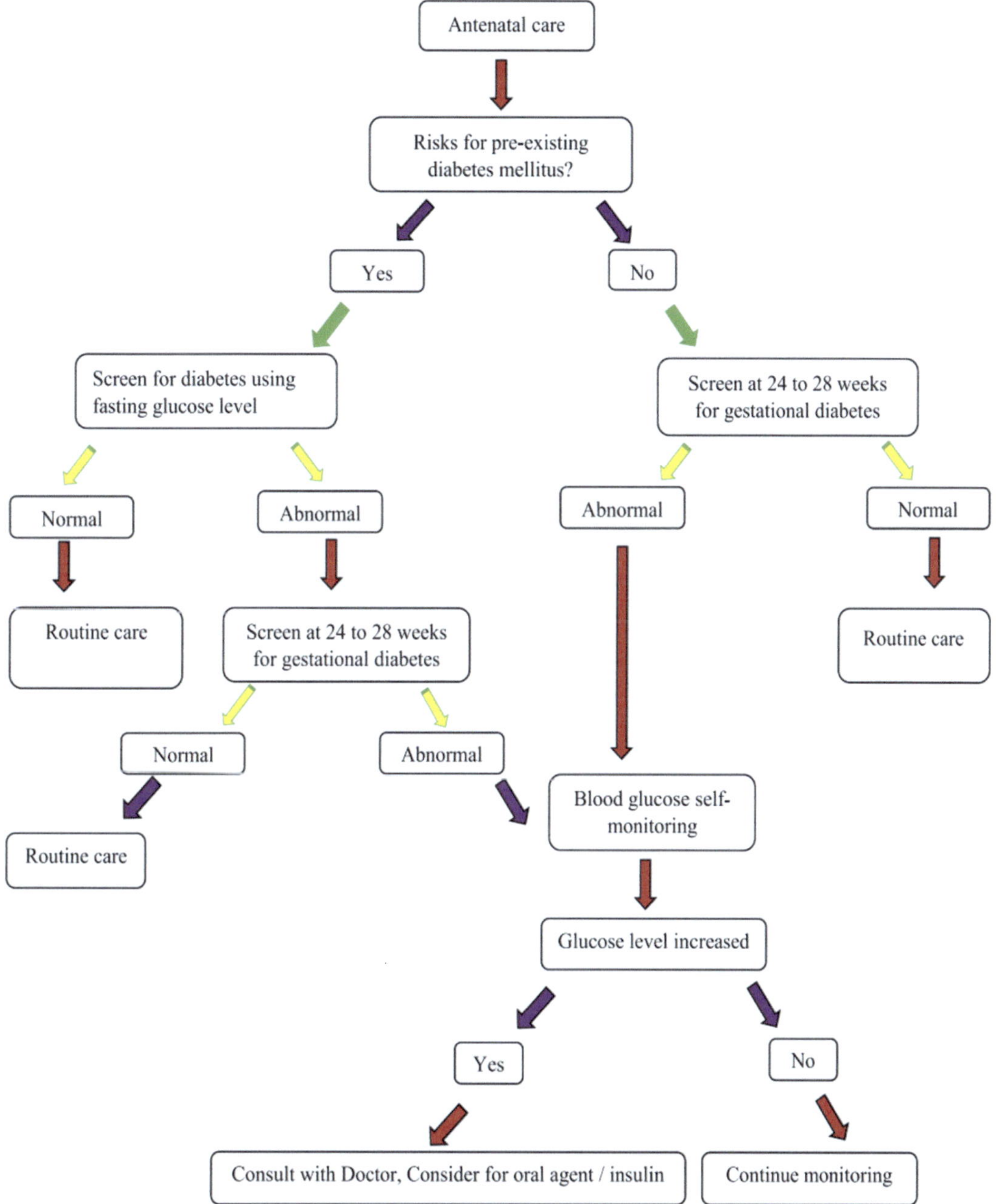


**Fig. 19.4** Screening and Diagnosis of GDM [11]. (Reproduced from Choudhury, V. Gestational diabetes mellitus A metabolic and reproductive disorder. Biomedicine & Pharmacotherapy. 2021; volume 143: 11218. Copyright© 2021. Elsevier Masson SAS. All rights reserved)

housework, excessive worry about the baby's development, and loss of confidence in the mother and new father within 4 weeks after the birth of the baby. The evaluation method is the "Edinburgh Postpartum Depression Scale" [14]. In Japan, if the score is 9 points or more, the possibility of postpartum depression should be considered and an interview with a psychiatrist or psychologist.

## 1.6 Lactation

### 1.6.1 Relationship Between Sex Hormones and Mammary Glands

Once pregnancy is established, the secretion of estrogen and progesterone is stimulated by hCG from the placenta and remains high. This hormonal environment is particularly pronounced after the second trimester, which stimulates lactogenic differentiation, preparing it for milk production and secretion.

### 1.6.2 Hormones Involved in the Structure and Function of the Mammary Gland

Hormones involved in the structure and function of the mammary gland include growth hormone-releasing factor (GRF), corticotropin-releasing factor (CRF), prolactin-inhibitory factor (PIF), luteinizing hormone (LH), follicle-stimulating hormone (FSH), adrenocorticotropic hormone (ACTH), thyroid stimulating hormone (TSH), and estrogen receptor (ER) and others.

### 1.6.3 Maternal Infections and Lactation

1. Human Immunodeficiency Virus (HIV)-infected pregnancies: In Japan, where HIV-infected pregnancies are extremely rare, the proportion of confirmatory test-positive cases (i.e., infected cases) in the pregnant women screening test-positive population (positive predictive value) is extremely low, ranging from 3.8% to 7.7% [15, 16] (6.5% in the *2013* survey). Therefore, confirmatory testing is even more essential for the diagnosis of HIV infection in pregnant women. Perinatal HIV transmission occurs through three routes: placenta, labor, and breastfeeding [17]. Because artificial feeding (milk) prevents mother-to-baby transmission [17–19], therefore milk is recommended immediately after birth [19].
2. Human T-cell Leukemia Virus type 1 (HTLV-1)-infected pregnancy.

   Approximately 95% of mother-to-child transmission (MTCT) of human T-cell leukemia virus type-1 (HTLV-1) is derived from prolonged breastfeeding, which is a major cause of adult T-cell leukemia (ATL) [20]. The routes of infection are MTCT, blood transfer (blood transfusion, organ transplantation), and sexual intercourse (mainly male-to-female). Artificial nutrition, frozen breastfeeding, and short-term (3 months) breastfeeding are presented as options for the prevention of transplacental mother-to-child transmission in HTLV-1 carrier mothers [21].

### 1.6.4 Medication and Breastfeeding

In the drug package inserts, many drugs are described as "transfer to breast milk has been reported and breastfeeding should be avoided." Almost all drugs are secreted into breast milk to varying degrees, and the infant ingests the drug through breast milk [22–24]. It should be noted, however, that drug exposure via breast milk is an order of magnitude less than the level of exposure in the uterine (<10% or even <1%). Drug safety has been investigated based on comparisons with usual doses (theory) and data from previous observational studies [22]. In the drug safety evaluation, "relative infant dose (RID) (%) = total amount of drug ingested via breastfeeding (mg/kg/day)/usual dose of the drug administered to the child (mg/kg/day) × 100" is considered [22]. If the RID is much lower than 10%, depending on the type of drug, the effect on the child is estimated to be small [22]. On the other hand, when the RID is much higher than 10%, considerable caution is required. According to observational studies, many drugs have a little adverse effect on the child when taken by a lactating woman [22]. However, the current situation is insufficient to assess the effects of these drugs. Therefore, we recommend referring to FDA that has introduced the five letter risk categories (A, B, C, D, and X) for the pregnancy and lactation labeling system since 1979, and replaced the former pregnancy risk categories on prescription and biological drugs labeling [25] (Table 19.1). In 2021, the FDA published the new Pregnancy and Lactation Labeling Rule (PLLR or final rule). The PLLR also requires the label to be updated when information becomes outdated. The PLLR removed pregnancy letter categories-A, B, C, D, and X (Fig. 19.5), therefore, physicians should need to notice drug information under the final rule [26].

**Table 19.1** Drug category based on safety during pregnancy (reproduced with permission from 25)

| Category | Drug class | Drugs |
|---|---|---|
| Category A-drugs safe during pregnancy | Over the counter drugs | Folic acid, Vitamin B6, etc. |
| Category B-drugs safe during pregnancy | Antibiotics | Penicillin G, Amoxicillin, Chloramphenicol, Ciprofloxacin, Doxycycline, Levofloxacin, Cephalosporins, Erythromycin, Clindamycin, Metronidazole |
| | Analgesic | Acetaminophen |
| | Synthetic corticosteroid | Prednisone |
| | Hormones | Insulin |
| | NSAID | Ibuprofen |
| | $H_2$-receptor antagonist | Famotidine |
| Category C-drugs likely to cause problems | Antibiotics | Streptomycin, Clindamycin, Gentamicin, Vancomycin, Tobramycin, Ciprofloxacin, etc. |
| | Antidepressant | Tricyclic drugs, monoamine oxidase inhibitors, Serotonergic antidepressant drugs, etc. |
| | Antipsychotic agent | Prochlorperazine |
| | Triazole antifungal drug | Fluconazole |
| Category D-drugs that have clear health risks for the fetus | Anticonvulsant | Phenytoin, Trimethadione, Valproic acid, Carbamazepine, Phenobarbital, etc. |
| | Alcohol | |
| | Antineoplastics (Alkylating agents) | Mechlorethamine, Procarbazine, Cyclophosphamide, Chlorambucil, Melphalan, Lomustine, etc. |
| | Antineoplastics (Taxanes) | Paclitaxel and Docetaxel |
| | Coumarin derivatives | Warfarin |
| | Antidepressant | Lithium |
| Category X-drugs that have been shown to cause birth defects | Sedative | Thalidomide |
| | Retinoids | Vitamin A |
| | Androgenic hormones | Testosterone |
| | Statins | Simvastatin |

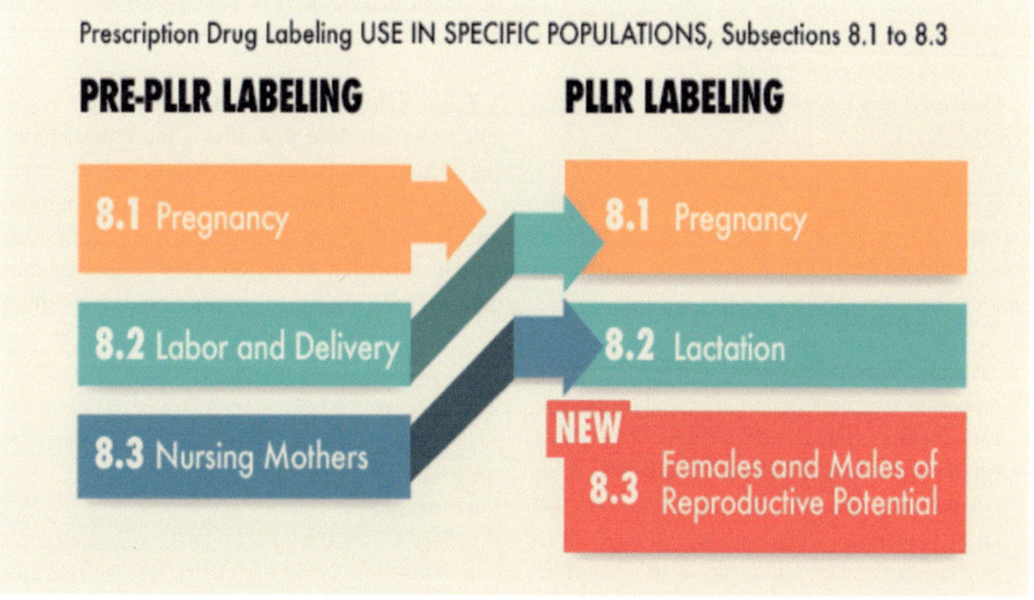


**Fig. 19.5** The new PLLR labeling requirements [26]

## 1.7 Notes from Dentistry Perspective [27–32]

Tetsuro Ikebe

### 1.7.1 Timing Suitable for Dental Treatment (Dental Surgery)

The most important factor in the dental treatment (surgery) of pregnant women is the interview. It is the communication with the patient through the interview. In some cases, the patient voluntarily states that she is pregnant on the questionnaire, but in other cases, she does not describe or declare her pregnancy. The first step is to find out whether or not the patient is pregnant. In addition, since the patient may be undergoing infertility treatment, the interview should be conducted carefully.

In the case of pregnant women, it is essential to know the pregnancy period (weeks or days after conception) to determine the timing for dental treatment (surgery). Therefore, it is necessary for dentists to have a basic knowledge about the pregnancy period. The possibility of teratogenicity, abortion, premature birth, and stillbirth should be considered.

- The gestation period is calculated as 1 week = 28 days, 4 weeks = 1 month.
- The start of the last menstrual period is 0 weeks and 0 days after conception.
- The day of ovulation (fertilization) is 2 weeks (14 days) after conception.
- Delivered at 40 weeks and 0 days (10 months) (280 days).

Based on the above, determine whether the patient's pregnancy is in the first pregnancy trimester, second trimester pregnancy, or third pregnancy trimester of the pregnancy period.

- Two weeks from fertilization to implantation: no connection between mother and fetus.
- First pregnancy trimester: 3 weeks to 12 weeks (up to 4 months of pregnancy): organogenesis period (a period to watch out for teratogenesis).
- Second pregnancy trimester: 5 to 7 months: stable period: appropriate timing for dental treatment (dental surgery) (be careful of fetal toxicity).
- Third pregnancy trimester: 28 weeks of late pregnancy (after 8 months of pregnancy): transfer of drugs to the fetus. The fetus has an immature ability to metabolize drugs.

Particular attention should be paid to the first trimester, from 3 to 12 weeks of pregnancy. This period is the fetal organogenesis period, for example, the period of lip formation is around the first month of pregnancy, and the period of palate formation is around the third month of pregnancy, so if the fetus is affected in any way during this period, it may cause cleft lip or cleft palate. Therefore, the most appropriate time for dental treatment (dental surgery) is between the fifth and seventh months of pregnancy in the second pregnancy trimester. Unnecessary dental treatment (especially surgical treatment, treatment with drugs, and treatment that causes mental or physical stress to the pregnant woman) should wait until this time. The next period when dental treatment is possible is the third pregnancy trimester.

However, even in the first pregnancy trimester, if the patient has severe pain or inflammation and it is decided that treatment is necessary for the health of the pregnant woman, dental treatment should be carried out after being explained about the merit and demerit of dental treatments to the patient.

### 1.7.2 Effects of Dental Radiation

The radiation dose that affects the fetus, including early pregnancy, is 100 mSv or more.

Typical radiation doses during radiography are shown in Table 19.2. There may be no problem in terms of radiation dose when ordinary dental radiography is performed on pregnant

**Table 19.2** Radiation dose during radiography

| | |
|---|---|
| The oral radiograpy | 0.01 ~ 0.03 mSv |
| Panoramic radiography | 0.02 ~ 0.03 mSv |
| Dental CT | 0.1 mSv |
| Medical head CT | 0.5 mSv |
| Chest X-ray | 0.06 ~ 0.15 mSv |

Natural dose of 0.2 mSv when flying between Tokyo and New York and back

women, but its dose should be kept to a minimum and the abdomen where the fetus exists should be protected with a lead apron.

The use of contrast media for CT and MRI should be avoided in pregnant women. If contrast media must be used for lactating women, then, it is better not to breastfeed for 48 h after the use of contrast media.

### 1.7.3 Influence of Dental Medication: Antibiotics and Analgesics (NSAIDs)

When oral or injectable drugs are administered to a pregnant woman, it must be recognized that the drugs are transferred to the fetus through the placenta. Depending on the type and dose of the drug, the fetus may be affected during organogenesis.

Therefore, medication should be avoided, if possible, until 12 weeks (3 months) of pregnancy. The second trimester pregnancy (5 to 7 months) is a safe time for medication and treatment.

In addition, after birth, drugs administered to the mother may be transferred to the infant through breast milk. If the drug is taken immediately after breastfeeding, the concentration of the drug in breast milk can be reduced. Of course, the drug should be administered as little as necessary.

Antibiotics and nonsteroidal anti-inflammatory drugs (NSAIDs) are the most commonly prescribed drugs in dentistry. Attention should be paid to the transplacental passage and breast milk transit of these drugs.

#### Antibiotics

Penicillins or cephem antibiotics (cephalosporin) should be the first choice of antimicrobial agents for pregnant and lactating women. To prevent the emergence of antimicrobial resistance (AMR) bacteria, which has become an international issue, third-generation cephems should be avoided, and penicillins such as amoxicillin are recommended. Amoxicillin is safe throughout pregnancy and is rapidly absorbed and excreted. Its transfer to breast milk is low, and there is little effect on the infant.

If the patient is allergic to penicillins or cephems, macrolide antibiotic should be used. Macrolides are more likely to be transferred to breast milk than penicillins or cephems.

In addition, penicillins, cephems, and macrolides can be used in pediatric patients. However, new quinolones should not be administered to pregnant women or lactating women because their safety for fetuses and infants has not been established.

#### Analgesics

As an analgesic, acetaminophen is safe for pregnant women and nursing mothers. The transfer of acetaminophen (Caronal®) to breast milk is low even when taken during lactation, and there is no problem in administering it in regular doses.

However, NSAIDs should be avoided. NSAIDs are placental transmissible, and when administered to the mother, they are almost always transferred to the fetus and may constrict the fetal ductus arteriosus. This may lead to decreased amniotic fluid and premature birth. It is also transferred to breast milk. Therefore, it should not be used after 28 weeks (7 months) of pregnancy. Diclofenac sodium (Voltaren®), one of NSAIDs, should not be administered to women of childbearing potential.

### 1.7.4 Local Anesthesia

Local anesthetics for dental treatment should be avoided in the first pregnancy trimester and waited until the second pregnancy trimester. However, for emergency treatment such as pulp extirpation or abscess incision, local anesthesia should be administered with the following precautions in mind.

Lidocaine: lidocaine crosses the placenta easily. Fifty percent of the maternal blood concentration becomes the fetal blood concentration.

Adrenaline (vasoconstrictors): easily destroyed and not readily transferred to the fetus.

Propitocaine (Citanest®) and felypressin (Octapressin®): the use of felypressin, a vasoconstrictor, is prohibited because of its delivery (childbirth) accelerating effect.

### 1.7.5 Oral Lesions Due to Pregnancy

#### Pregnancy Gingivitis

Pregnant women are more susceptible to gingivitis because estrogen, a female hormone, affects the growth of periodontal disease bacteria as well as periodontal tissues, which is thought to be associated with progesterone-induced prostaglandin production. The concentration of female hormones are known to be 10 to 30 times higher at the end of pregnancy than during menstruation, and pregnancy gingivitis is more likely to occur during the second and third pregnancy trimesters. Clinically, it is characterized by a rounded swelling of the interdental papillae on the anterior teeth. Pregnant women with periodontal disease are known to be at risk for low birth weight infant and premature birth.

#### Pregnancy Epulis

It is found in about 1% of pregnant women and develops around the third month of pregnancy. After delivery, the lesions spontaneously shrink and fade away. Histopathologically, it often consists of granulomatous or angiomatous tissues. As in usual epulis, it is most frequently seen on the interdental papillae of anterior teeth. The lesions also bleed easily. Since pregnant women are susceptible for periodontitis and dental plaque aggravates the symptoms, plaque control such as brushing instruction is very important for pregnant women. Surgical excision should be waited until after childbirth.

#### Herpes Gestationis (Pemphigoid Gestationis)

Edematous erythema with severe pruritus appears on the abdomen, buttocks, and extremities, and small bullae appear on the erythema, which often occurs in the second and third trimester, or immediately after delivery. Oral mucosal lesions are rare and it is transient and disappears spontaneously. Anti-BP180 autoantibodies cause this lesion.

### 1.7.6 Supine Hypotensive Syndrome

During dental treatment of pregnant women in the third pregnancy trimester, cerebral anemia may occur due to hypotension. When a pregnant woman in this period is placed in the supine position, the uterus presses on the inferior vena cava and the venous return is obstructed, resulting in a decrease in cardiac output and hypotension. It is important to avoid the horizontal position for dental treatment of pregnant women in the third pregnancy trimester. Dental treatment should be performed in the left side down position or in a reclined position.

## References


1. Dey S, et al. How we are born. Citation information. J Clin Invest. 2010;120(4):952–5. https://doi.org/10.1172/JCI42380.
2. Hata J. The wonder of our body that can be understood from the knowledge of junior high school students. http://www.jhata99.org.
3. Baba Y. 068 severe hyperemesis gravidarum (Jyushou Ninshin Oso). In: Essential knowledge of perinatal medicine (Shusanki Igaku Hisshu Chishiki). 8th ed. Tokyo: Editorial Board of Perinatal Medicine; 2016. p. 204–7; (in Japanese).
4. Japan Society of Obstetrics and Gynecology/Japan Association of Obstetricians and Gynecologists, editor. Guidelines for obstetrics and gynecology (Sanfujinka Shinryo Guideline Sankahen). Tokyo: Japan Society of Obstetrics and Gynecology/Japan Association of Obstetricians and Gynecologists; 2020. p. 108–10; (in Japanese).
5. Maeda K. 069 ectopic pregnancy (Ishosei Ninshin). Essential knowledge of perinatal medicine (Shusanki Igaku Hisshu Chishiki). 8th ed. Tokyo: Editorial Board of Perinatal Medicine; 2016. p. 208–10; (in Japanese).
6. Christina J. Infections at the maternal–fetal interface: an overview of pathogenesis and defence. Nat Rev Microbiol. 2022;20:67–82.
7. Kobayashi Y, Yamamoto T. 077 Gestational hypertension (Ninshin Kouketsuatsu Shoukougun). Essential knowledge of perinatal medicine (Shusanki Igaku Hisshu Chishiki). 8th ed. Tokyo: Editorial Board of Perinatal Medicine; 2016. p. 232–5; (in Japanese).
8. Redmman CW, Sargent IL. Latest advances in understanding preeclampsia. Science, 308(5728):1592–1594, 2005.
9. Christopher W. Preeclampsia—pathophysiology and clinical presentations JACC state-of-the-art review. J Am Coll Cardiol. 2020;76(14):2020.
10. The Japanese Society of Diabetes and Pregnancy, editor. Manual of diagnosis and management of abnormalities of glucose metabolism in pregnant women

(Ninshin no Toutaisha Ijyou Shindan Kanri Manual). 3rd ed. Tokyo: Medical View; 2022; (in Japanese).
11. Choudhury V. Gestational diabetes mellitus a metabolic and reproductive disorder. Biomed Pharmacother. 2021;143:11218.
12. Gestational Diabetes and Pregnancy. https://www.cdc.gov/pregnancy/diabetes-gestational.html.
13. Galindo A, et al. Outcome of fetuses in woman with pregestational diabetes mellitus. J Pernat Med. 2006;34(4):323–31.
14. Cox J, et al. Detection of postnatal depression: development of the 10-item edinburgh postnatal depression scale. Br J Psychiatry. 1987;150:782–6.
15. Cathrin B. Hormone action in the mammary gland. Cold Spring Harb Perspect Biol. 2010;2(12):a003178.
16. Preventing Mother-to-Child Transmission of HIV. HIDS info. https://aidsinfo.nih.gov. Accessed 17 Dec 2018.
17. Nduati R, et al. Effect of breastfeeding and formula feeding on transmission of HIV-1. A randomized clinical trial. JAMA. 2000;283:1167–74.
18. Multidisciplinary Study on Measures against HIV Infection in Perinatal, Pediatric, and Reproductive Medicine. Research project on AIDS control. Annual report 2009(II). Tokyo: Ministry of Health, Labour and Welfare; 2009; (in Japanese).
19. Japan Society of Obstetrics and Gynecology/Japan Association of Obstetricians and Gynecologists. Guidelines for obstetrics and gynecology (Sanfujinka Shinryo Guideline Sankahen). Tokyo: Japan Society of Obstetrics and Gynecology/Japan Association of Obstetricians and Gynecologists; 2020. p. 320–2; (in Japanese).
20. Itabashi K, et al. Mother-to-child transmission of human T-cell leukemia virus type 1: mechanisms and nutritional strategies for prevention. Cancers. 2021;13(16):4100. https://doi.org/10.3390/cancers13164100.
21. Japan Society of Obstetrics and Gynecology/Japan Association of Obstetricians and Gynecologists. Guidelines for obstetrics and gynecology (Sanfujinka Shinryo Guideline Sankahen). Tokyo: Japan Society of Obstetrics and Gynecology/Japan Association of Obstetricians and Gynecologists; 2020. p. 326–8; (in Japanese).
22. Ito S. Drug therapy for breast-feeding women. N Engl J Med. 2000;343:118–26; PMID: 10891521.
23. Japan Association of Obstetricians and Gynecologists. Training note no. 81 management of breast disease. Tokyo: Japan Association of Obstetricians and Gynecologists; 2009. p. 1–106; (III) (in Japanese).
24. Kamer MS, et al. Breastfeeding and child cognitive development: new evidence from a large randomized trial. Arch Gen Psychiatry. 2008;65:578–84; PMID: 18458209.
25. Cucullo L. Prenatal development of the human blood-brain barrier; 2009. https://doi.org/10.1007/978-1-60761-287-2_4.
26. U.S Food and Drug Administration. Pregnancy and lactation labeling (drugs) final rule. 2021. https://www.fda.gov.
27. Hirofuji T, et al. Essential handbook for dental residents, 2020 revised medical payment system ed. (Shin Rinsho Kenshui Handbook, 2020-nendo Shinryou Houshu Kaitei Taiouban). Tokyo: Ishiyaku Shuppan; 2020. p. 96–7; (in Japanese).
28. Yamane G, et al. Oral medicine for dental hygienists. Tokyo: Ishiyaku Shuppan; 2019. p. 115–23; (in Japanese).
29. The Japanese Association for Infectious Diseases, Japanese Society of Chemotherapy JAID/JSC infectious disease treatment. Working group on odontogenic infections, Committee for Preparation of treatment guides and guidelines: JAID/JSC treatment guidelines for infectious diseases 2016-dental infections. J Japanese Soc Chemother. 2016;64(4):641–6; (in Japanese).
30. Enomoto S, et al. Oral and maxillofacial surgery (Saihin Kouku Gekagaku). 5th ed. Tokyo: Ishiyaku Shuppan; 2018. p. 221; (in Japanese).
31. Japanese Society of Oral Medicine Committee for terminology and classification. Draft classification of autoimmune bullous disease proposed by the Japanese society of oral medicine. J Jpn Oral Medicine. 2013;19(1):25–8; (in Japanese).
32. Shirasuna K, et al. Oral and maxillofacial surgery (Koukuugekagaku). 4th ed. Tokyo: Ishiyaku Shuppan; 2020. p. 707; (in Japanese).

# Organ Transplantation (Bone Marrow Transplantation, Liver Transplantation)

20

Akira Sasaki, Takeshi Takahara, Tadahide Noguchi, and Yoshiyuki Mori

## 1 Organ Transplantation

Akira Sasaki, Takeshi Takahara

### 1.1 Introduction

Organ transplantation is a medical procedure in which organs are transferred from a donor to a recipient to restore function to a patient whose organ function has been severely impaired by serious illness or accident. Donors are classified into two groups: cadavers and living organisms, and cadavers can be brain dead or in cardiac arrest. Most recipients are experiencing organ failure, and their life expectancies are short or their daily quality of life is significantly impaired. The development and advancement of immunosuppressive drugs have improved the outcome of organ transplantation. After transplantation, if patients take immunosuppressive drugs and are careful about rejection and infections, most of them can lead almost the same daily lives as healthy people.

A. Sasaki
Department of Surgery, Iwate Medical University School of Medicine, Yahaba, Iwate, Japan

T. Takahara (✉)
Department of Surgery, Fujita Health University, Toyoake, Aichi, Japan

T. Noguchi
Department of Dentistry, Oral and Maxillofacial Surgery, School of Medicine, Jichi Medical University, Shimotsuke, Tochigi, Japan

Y. Mori
Department of Dentistry, Oral and Maxillofacial Surgery, Saitama Medical Center, Jichi Medical University, Saitama, Japan

### 1.2 The History of Transplantation Medicine

Liver transplantation and lung transplantation were first performed in the United States in 1963, and heart transplantation was first performed in South Africa in 1967. In Japan, Niigata University performed a temporary kidney transplantation for a patient with acute renal failure in 1956, the University of Tokyo performed a living kidney transplantation for a patient with chronic renal failure in 1964, and Chiba University performed its first liver transplantation in the same year. Organ transplantation in Japan began at about the same time as the rest of the world. In Japan, various problems related to Wada heart transplantation at Sapporo Medical University in 1968 created a sense of distrust toward brain death and organ transplantation, which may have contributed to the slow progress of transplantation in Japan compared to Europe and the United States. Since the Law Concerning Organ Transplantation was enacted in 1997, and the Law Concerning Organ Transplantation was revised in 2009, the number of brain death organ donations has been gradually increasing (Fig. 20.1) [1].


T. Chiba, H. Yamada (eds.), *Internal Medicine for Dental Treatments*,
https://doi.org/10.1007/978-981-99-3296-2_20

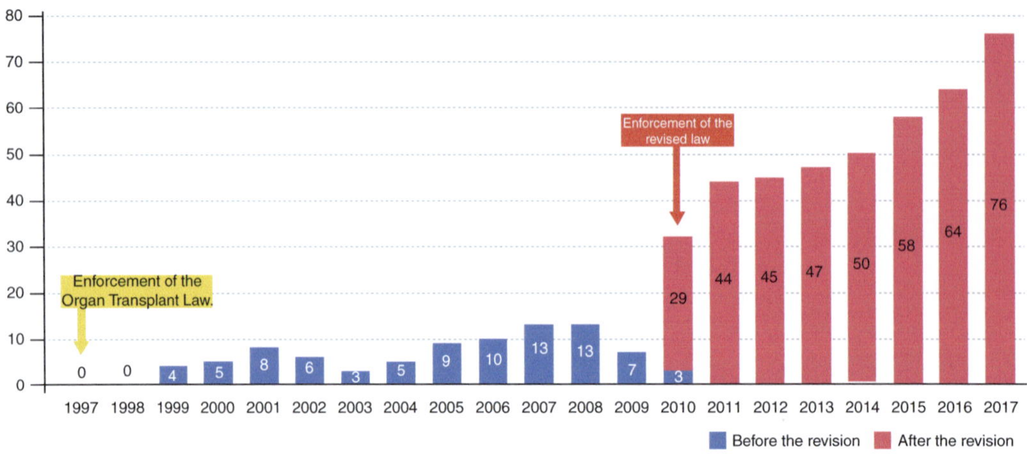


**Fig. 20.1** Number of organ donations (created based on [1])

## 1.3 Organ Donation

Organ donation is possible after brain death or cardiac arrest. In 1997, the Law on Organ Transplantation was enacted to recognize brain death as human death and to allow organ transplantation after brain death as long as the patient expressed in writing the intention to donate organs according to the determination of brain death. The family must also agree to the determination of brain death and organ donation. The International Society for Transplantation (IST) approved Japan's revised Organ Transplant Law in 2008 and the revised Organ Transplant Law in 2010, which allows organ donation with the consent of the family even if the patient's will to donate is unknown. The revised law also includes a lowering of the age limit for organ donation and a ban on organ donation from children suspected of having been abused. The age limit for organ donation is 50 years or younger for the heart, 70 years or younger for the lungs, 70 years or younger for the kidneys, 60 years or younger for the pancreas, and 60 years or younger for the small intestine; there is no age limit for the liver at this time. The following organs can be donated after brain death: heart, lung, liver, kidney, pancreas, small intestine, and eyeball. The organs that can be donated after cardiac arrest are the kidney, pancreas, and eyeball. In the case of organ donation after brain death, the time allowed for the resumption of blood flow after organ's removal from the donor is 4 h for the heart, 8 h for the lungs, 12 h for the liver and small intestine, and 24 h for the pancreas and kidneys.

## 1.4 Rejection

A transplanted organ is non-self to the recipient and is recognized as an antigen by the major histocompatibility complex (MHC). The recipient's immune cells attack the transplanted organ, which results in rejection. Rejection can be divided into three categories: hyperacute rejection, acute rejection, and chronic rejection. Hyperacute rejection is thought to be caused by humoral immunity, and thrombus formation occurs within 24 h after transplantation, resulting in organ ischemia. It is thought to be related to the recipient's existing anti-human-leukocyte-antigen (HLA) antibodies. Acute rejection often occurs between 1 week and 3 months after transplantation, and is mainly related to cellular immunity. Cellular immunity is induced by antigen presentation by MHC class II antigens of donor-derived organs. Chronic rejection often occurs after 3 months of transplantation is thought to be mainly due to the effect of humoral immunity, which has been recently reported to be related to antibody-mediated rejection. It is difficult to control with general immunosuppressive drugs, and retransplantation may be considered.

## 1.5 GVHD

Graft-versus-host disease (GVHD) is a condition in which donor-derived immune competent cells regard the host as an antigen, often due to rejection of hematopoietic stem cells. It can be divided into acute GVHD and chronic GVHD. In acute GVHD, skin symptoms are often the first symptoms, and the main organs affected are the skin, gastrointestinal tract, and liver. Steroids are administered as a treatment. Chronic GVHD refers to GVHD that develops after 100 days of transplantation, and it is believed that more organs are affected by chronic than acute GVHD.

## 1.6 Bone Marrow Transplantation and Peripheral Blood Stem Cell Transplantation

### 1.6.1 Bone Marrow Transplantation

Bone marrow transplantation is the transplantation of normal bone marrow cells from a donor into a patient with leukemia or aplastic anemia by intravenous infusion. When bone marrow transplantation is performed, the donor and recipient must match in terms of HLA, and if incompatible bone marrow cells are transplanted, rejection and GVHD may occur.

### 1.6.2 Peripheral Blood Stem Cell Transplantation

Daily injections of granulocyte colony-stimulating factor (G-CSF), which increases the number of hematopoietic stem cells in the blood, can be administered to donors to obtain enough hematopoietic stem cells from the peripheral blood for transplantation. Depending on the body weight of the recipient, bone marrow transplants require 600 to 1000 cc of infused bone marrow fluid, whereas peripheral blood stem cell transplants often require less than 200 cc. Peripheral blood stem cell transplantation is associated with a higher incidence of GVHD than bone marrow transplantation because of the large number of donor-derived lymphocytes in addition to hematopoietic stem cells. On the other hand, the effect of graft versus leukemia (GVL) is also high, and it is expected to reduce the recurrence rate.

## 1.7 Liver Transplantation

Liver transplantation is a newer medical treatment developed by Starzl et al. in the United States. After overcoming the hardships of its early days, the results of liver transplantation have dramatically progressed through improvements in surgical techniques, organ preservation methods, immunosuppressive drugs, and perioperative management. In the United States, approximately 6000 deceased donor liver transplantation are performed annually. In Japan, the Deceased Donor Liver Transplantation Bill was enacted in October 1997, making deceased donor liver transplantation legally feasible, and the first deceased donor liver transplantation in Japan was performed at Shinshu University in February 1999.

On the other hand, in Japan, living donor liver transplantation, in which a partial liver from a healthy person is transplanted, was first performed at Shimane University in November 1989, followed by Kyoto University and Shinshu University. The cases of living donor liver transplantation have been accumulated solemnly, and the results are better than those of deceased donor liver transplantation. The current indications for liver transplantation are as follows.

### 1.7.1 Indications for Liver Transplantation

**1. Children**

(a) **Post necrotic liver cirrhosis:** congenital liver fibrosis and neonatal hepatitis.
(b) **Cholestatic liver cirrhosis:** biliary atresia, Alagille syndrome, primary biliary cholangitis, secondary biliary cirrhosis, progressive familial bile stasis.
(c) **Fulminant hepatitis:** viral hepatitis, drug-induced liver injury.
(d) **Metabolic diseases:** Wilson's disease, $alpha_1$-antitrypsin deficiency, hemochromatosis, hyperoxaluria, glycogenosis (types I and V), Crigler-Najjar syndrome, Niemann-Pick disease, protoporphyrinemia, hypertyrosinemia.
(e) **Malignant tumor:** hepatoblastoma, hepatocellular carcinoma.

(f) **Benign tumor:** hepatic lymphangioma.
(g) **Others:** hemophilia.

**2. Adults**

(a) **Post necrotic liver cirrhosis:** hepatitis B cirrhosis, hepatitis C cirrhosis, alcoholic cirrhosis, autoimmune cirrhosis, cirrhosis of unknown origin.
(b) **Biliary cholangitis:** primary biliary cholangitis, primary sclerosing cholangitis (PSC).
(c) **Fulminant hepatitis:** viral hepatitis, drug-induced liver injury.
(d) **Metabolic diseases:** Wilson's disease, alpha$_1$-antitrypsin deficiency, hemochromatosis, familial amyloid polyneuropathy, citrullinemia.
(e) **Malignant tumor:** hepatocellular carcinoma.
(f) **Benign tumor:** diffuse cavernous hemangioma, multiple hepatic cysts, cavernous sinusoidal hemangioendothelioma.
(g) **Other:** Budd-Chiari syndrome.

### 1.7.2 Deceased Donor Liver Transplantation

1. **Donor surgery:** In brain death donor surgery, multiple organ harvesting teams proceed in parallel. A midline incision from the upper clavicle to the pubic symphysis is used to remove the abdominal and the thoracic organs (heart, lungs, etc.). A liver biopsy is performed as necessary to confirm that there is no trauma to the liver cirrhosis, or severe fatty liver. The graft is removed by irrigating the abdominal aorta and portal vein with ice-cold preservation fluid (UW solution is commonly used). The graft is then immersed in UW solution and transported ice-cold. The graft can usually be stored for 12 h.
2. **Recipient surgery:** Different transplantation methods, such as whole liver, partial liver, split liver transplantation, and auxiliary partial orthotopic liver transplantation depend on how the grafted liver is transplanted. Depending on the recipient's body size, either whole or partial liver transplantation is selected. To compensate for the recent shortage of donors, a split liver transplantation can save the lives of two recipients by dividing the graft into two parts and using both parts as grafts. In fulminant hepatitis, when the autologous liver is considered regenerable, half of the autologous liver is left, and a partial liver graft is transplanted only during the period when the patient is out of acute liver failure.

   Total hepatectomy of the recipient is performed by the following procedures: hepato-transplantation, hepatic portal dissection (dissection of the hepatic artery, portal vein, and common bile duct), and treatment of the inferior vena cava (taping above and below the liver). The transplantation is completed by removing the recipient's diseased liver and reconstructing the hepatic artery and portal vein as the inflow tracts of the grafted liver and the inferior vena cava and the bile duct as the outflow tracts. If the recipient's inferior vena cava is preserved, the inferior vena cava, portal vein, hepatic artery, and bile duct of the graft should be anastomosed in this order. When the recipient's inferior vena cava is resected, the graft liver is anastomosed in the following order: superior inferior vena cava, portal vein, hepatic artery, inferior vena cava, and bile duct.

### 1.7.3 Living Partial Liver Transplantation

1. **Donor surgery:** The most important factor in donor surgery is safety. The donor is a perfectly healthy person who donates their organs altruistically, and is not a patient. Therefore, postoperative complications that interfere with social life must be prevented.

   In living donor partial liver transplantation, the volume of the liver required by the recipient determines where the graft should be taken from the donor. Based on the recipient's body surface area, a standard liver volume is calculated, and a graft with a volume of at least 40% of the standard liver volume is used. Generally, a lateral zone graft is used in children, and a left or right lobe graft is used in adults.

It is important to note that donor hepatectomy, standard normal hepatectomy, avoids warm ischemia to the graft as much as possible to maintain sufficient graft viability; the hepatic artery and portal vein are separated after the liver dissection. Intraoperative cholangiography is performed to confirm the location of the bile ducts, and the position of the bile ducts is determined. After removal of the graft, the graft is irrigated from the portal vein on a back table with a perfusion fluid, such as UW solution, at a temperature of 4 °C or lower. If necessary, hepatic venoplasty of the graft is performed.

2. **Recipient surgery:** The process of recipient surgery up to total hepatectomy includes hepatotransplantation, hilarization, and dissection of the short hepatic vein. In patients with biliary atresia who have undergone Kasai's operation in the past, there is a high degree of adhesion in the gastrointestinal tract, which must be carefully dissected. After the graft is removed, the hepatic vein and portal vein are anastomosed to restore hepatic blood flow, followed by the hepatic artery and bile duct. The two types of biliary reconstruction are bile duct–jejunal anastomosis and bile duct-bile duct anastomosis (Fig. 20.2).

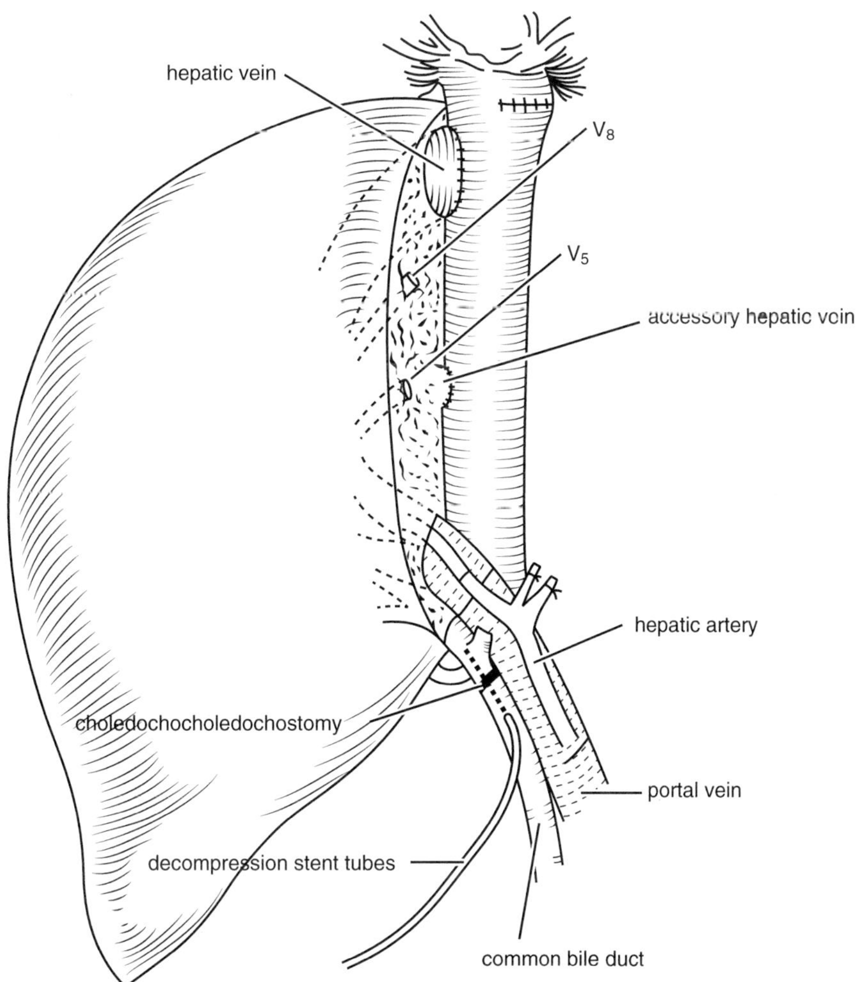


**Fig. 20.2** Right lobe graft (bile duct-bile duct anastomosis)

## 1.8 Notes from Dentistry Perspective

Tadahide Noguchi, Yoshiyuki Mori

### 1.8.1 Pre- and Posttransplant Oral Status and Response

Hematopoietic stem cell transplantation is now used in the treatment of leukemia and malignant lymphoma, but its anticancer drug therapy and systemic radiation therapy can damage the oral mucosa and pose a risk of systemic complications. Therefore, dental treatment and oral care before transplantation should be actively performed.

#### Before Transplantation

**Intraoral examination and dental treatment before transplantation:** Before treatment, check for caries, periodontal disease, and other lesions that may cause problems during treatment. It is desirable to complete dental treatment at least 2 weeks before the pre-transplant procedure, but first-aid should be performed so that the patient can progress without problems until the transplant treatment is completed.

If possible, extract the source of infection (e.g., severely periodontally diseased teeth with deep pockets and pus discharge, periapical pathosis or impacted wisdom teeth with a history of inflammation,) because they may cause dental infection. After extraction, the extraction sockets should be covered with mucosa to prevent exposure of the bone. Prophylactic antibiotics should be administered before proceeding with tooth extraction.

In addition, thorough plaque control should be performed to prevent stomatitis (aiming for a plaque control record [PCR] of 20% or less), and patients should learn self-care to maintain oral cleanliness and prevent xerostomia (moisturizing gel, mouth rinse, aznolene ointment, etc.) during transplant treatment.

#### Treatment of Stomatitis After Pretreatment (Chemotherapy, Total-Body Irradiation) and During Transplantation Therapy

Thorough oral hygiene and symptomatic treatment are essential. Azulene rinses should be used, and if the pain is severe, a rinsing solution containing xylocaine should be used.

#### Oral Care After Transplantation

**Treatment of graft-versus-host disease (GVHD):** There are two types of GVHD: acute GVHD that occurs within 100 days of transplantation and chronic GVHD that occurs later. Acute GVHD presents with redness, erosion, and bleeding of the oral mucosa and resembles radiation stomatitis. In chronic GVHD, oral symptoms are often present at the first sign of disease, and 80% of patients have oral symptoms. Symptoms include lichen planus-like oral mucosal lesions and xerostomia due to salivary gland disorders similar to Sjögren's syndrome (Fig. 20.3). The guidelines of the Japanese Society for Hematopoietic Cell Transplantation state that chronic GVHD should be diagnosed using the

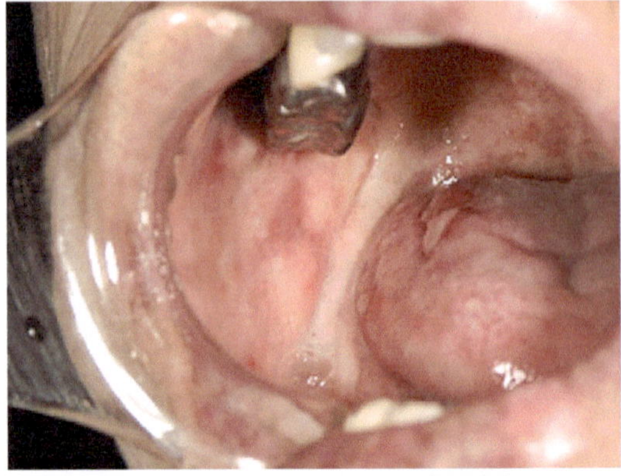

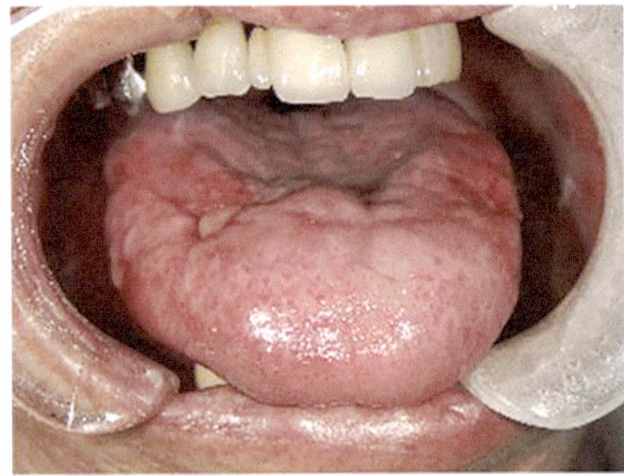

**Fig. 20.3** Chronic GVHD. Upper: a keratotic lesion resembling oral lichen planus is seen on the mucous membrane of the right cheek. Lower: White keratotic lesion on tongue is observed

**Table 20.1** Clinical signs of chronic GVHD

| Clinical signs of chronic GVHD | | | | |
|---|---|---|---|---|
| Organ | Diagnostic signs | Characteristic signs | Other symptoms | Common signs |
| Oral | Lichen planus-like changes | Xerostomia, mucosal atrophy, mucosal cysts, pseudomembranes, ulceration | | Periodontitis, stomatitis, redness, pain |

Created based on [2]

diagnostic criteria proposed by the NIH consensus development project [2] (Table 20.1).

Treatment includes topical steroids or local injections of steroids, and intraoral PUVA (ultraviolet) therapy. At the same time, treatment for xerostomia should be continued.

We have occasionally encountered cases of oral candidiasis caused by the use of steroids or immunosuppressive drugs, and the symptoms have worsened. There are two diagnostic methods for oral candidiasis: (1) isolation and identification of Candida by culture; and (2) observation of mycelium by microscopy. Because Candida is an indigenous bacteria, it is not possible to diagnose oral candidiasis even if it is detected only by culture tests, and it is necessary to detect Candida mycelium in lesions for definitive diagnosis (Fig. 20.4).

If steroid ointment is being applied, it should be temporarily discontinued, and topical application of antifungal agent (miconazole: FLORIDGEL® for oral use) or itraconazole (Itrizole® Oral Solution 1%) should be swallowed after the medication has been distributed throughout the mouth. Alternatively, rinse the mouth with a polyene antifungal agent (amphotericin B: Fungizone®). It is important to use the medication for 1 to 2 weeks because mycelium may remain even after symptoms improve [3].

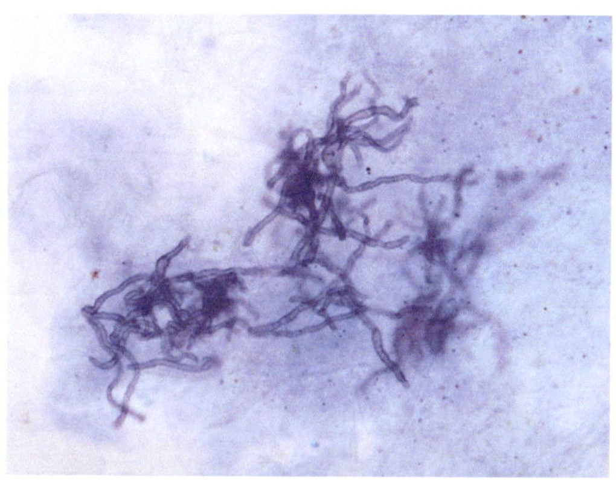

**Fig. 20.4** Microscopic image of Candida mycelium. The presence of mycelium indicates that Candida is pathogenic

## References


1. Yuzawa K. Japanese transplantation registry 2017 annual report. Japanese J Transplant. 2018;53(2/3):79; (in Japanese).
2. The Japan Society for Hematopoietic Cell Transplantation. Guidelines for hematopoietic cell transplantation GVHD. 4th ed. JSHCT monograph, 56: 1–77, 2018; (in Japanese). https://www.jstct.or.jp/uploads/files/guideline/01_02_gvhd_ver04.pdf.
3. Noguchi T. Oral candida not cured (Khoku Candida ga Naoranai). Medicina 8. Tokyo: Igaku Shoin; 2017. p. 1426–31; (in Japanese).

# Correction to: Internal Medicine for Dental Treatments

Toshimi Chiba and Hiroyuki Yamada

**Correction to:**
**Chapters 2 and 8 in: T. Chiba, H. Yamada, *Internal Medicine for Dental Treatments*,**
**https://doi.org/10.1007/978-981-99-3296-2_2**
**https://doi.org/10.1007/978-981-99-3296-2_8**

The book was inadvertently published with an incorrect spelling in Chapter 2, Table 2.1 (Page 19), and additional content has been added on Page 20.

In Chapter 8, additional content has been added on Pages 143 and 144.

Now the correction has been updated in the book.

The updated version of these chapters can be found at
https://doi.org/10.1007/978-981-99-3296-2_2
https://doi.org/10.1007/978-981-99-3296-2_8


T. Chiba, H. Yamada (eds.), *Internal Medicine for Dental Treatments*,
https://doi.org/10.1007/978-981-99-3296-2_21

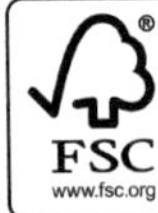
MIX
Papier aus verantwortungsvollen Quellen
Paper from responsible sources
FSC® C105338

If you have any concerns about our products,
you can contact us on
**ProductSafety@springernature.com**

In case Publisher is established outside the EU,
the EU authorized representative is:
**Springer Nature Customer Service Center GmbH**
**Europaplatz 3, 69115 Heidelberg, Germany**

Printed by Libri Plureos GmbH
in Hamburg, Germany